Handbook of
Small Animal
Therapeutics

HANDBOOK of SMALL ANIMAL THERAPEUTICS

Edited by

Lloyd E. Davis, D.V.M., Ph.D.

Fellow, American Academy of Veterinary
  Pharmacology and Therapeutics
Professor of Pharmacology and Veterinary Clinical Medicine
College of Veterinary Medicine
University of Illinois at Urbana-Champaign
Urbana, Illinois

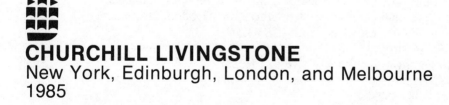

CHURCHILL LIVINGSTONE
New York, Edinburgh, London, and Melbourne
1985

Acquisitions editor: *Gene C. Kearn*
Copy editor: *Michael Kelley*
Production editor: *Michiko Davis*
Production supervisor: *Sharon Tuder*
Compositor: *Maryland Composition Company, Inc.*
Printer/Binder: *The Maple-Vail Book Manufacturing Group*

Distributed in the United Kingdom by Churchill Livingstone,
Robert Stevenson House, 1-3 Baxter's Place, Leith Walk,
Edinburgh EH1 3AF and by associated companies, branches
and representatives throughout the world.

First published 1985

Printed in U.S.A.

ISBN 0-443-08294-4

9 8 7 6 5 4 3 2 1

Library of Congress Cataloging in Publication Data
Main entry under title:

Handbook of small animal therapeutics.

  Includes bibliographies and index.
  1. Dogs—Diseases—Chemotherapy—Handbooks, manuals,
etc. 2. Cats—Diseases—Chemotherapy—Handbooks, manuals,
etc. I. Davis, Lloyd E.   . [DNLM: 1. Cat
Diseases—drug therapy—handbooks. 2. Dog Diseases—
drug therapy—handbooks. SF 985 H236]
SF991.H23 1985   636.7'089   85-4133
ISBN 0-443-08294-4

This book is dedicated to all of the dogs and cats that have been sacrificed in the cause of biomedical science and to the hope that the knowledge gained may be of benefit to our animal patients.

CONTRIBUTORS

Arthur L. Aronson, D.V.M., Ph.D.
Fellow, American Academy of Veterinary Pharmacology and Therapeutics; Professor and Head, Department of Anatomy, Physiological Sciences and Radiology, School of Veterinary Medicine, North Carolina State University, Raleigh, North Carolina

David P. Aucoin, D.V.M.
Clinical Pharmacologist, The Animal Medical Center, New York, New York

Thomas J. Burke, D.V.M., M.S.
Associate Professor of Veterinary Clinical Medicine, College of Veterinary Medicine, University of Illinois at Urbana-Champaign, Urbana, Illinois

Lloyd E. Davis, D.V.M., Ph.D.
Fellow, American Academy of Veterinary Pharmacology and Therapeutics; Professor of Pharmacology and Veterinary Clinical Medicine, College of Veterinary Medicine, University of Illinois at Urbana-Champaign, Urbana, Illinois

Joseph A. DiPietro, D.V.M., M.S.
Associate Professor of Veterinary Clinical Medicine, College of Veterinary Medicine, University of Illinois at Urbana-Champaign, Urbana, Illinois

Bernard F. Feldman, D.V.M., Ph.D.
Associate Professor of Clinical Hematology and Biochemistry, Department of Clinical Pathology, School of Veterinary Medicine, University of California, Davis, California

Richard B. Ford, D.V.M., M.S.
Diplomate, American College of Veterinary Internal Medicine; Associate Professor of Internal Medicine, School of Veterinary Medicine, North Carolina State University, Raleigh, North Carolina

Robert M. Hardy, D.V.M., M.S.
Diplomate, American College of Veterinary Internal Medicine; Associate Professor of Medicine, Department of Small Animal Clinical Sciences, College of Veterinary Medicine, University of Minnesota, St. Paul, Minnesota

Arthur I. Hurvitz, D.V.M., Ph.D.
Diplomate, American College of Veterinary Pathology; Consulting Veterinary Pathologist, The Rockefeller University; Adjunct Assistant Professor, Colum-

bia University; Chairman, Department of Pathology, Director of Research and Vincent Astor Chair of Comparative Medicine, The Animal Medical Center, New York, New York

William L. Jenkins, B.V.Sc., Ph.D.
Fellow, American Academy of Veterinary Pharmacology and Therapeutics; Professor of Veterinary Pharmacology, College of Veterinary Medicine, Texas A & M University, College Station, Texas

Judith S. Johnessee, D.V.M., M.S.
Diplomate, American College of Veterinary Internal Medicine; Eastchester Animal Clinic, Scarsdale, New York

Brent D. Jones, D.V.M.
Assistant Professor of Medicine, Department of Veterinary Medicine and Surgery, College of Veterinary Medicine, University of Missouri, Columbia, Missouri

William J. Kay, D.V.M.
Diplomate, American College of Veterinary Internal Medicine (Internal Medicine and Neurology); Adjunct Professor of Neurology, New York University Medical Center; Chief of Staff, The Animal Medical Center, New York, New York

Mark D. Kittleson, D.V.M., Ph.D.
Assistant Professor, Department of Medicine, School of Veterinary Medicine, University of California, Davis, California

John A. Mulnix, D.V.M., M.S.
Fellow, American Academy of Veterinary Pharmacology and Therapeutics; Carlson Animal Clinic, Fort Collins, Colorado

Carol A. Neff-Davis, B.S., M.S.
Director, Clinical Pharmacology and Endocrinology Laboratory, College of Veterinary Medicine, University of Illinois at Urbana-Champaign, Urbana, Illinois

Carl A. Osborne, D.V.M., Ph.D.
Diplomate, American College of Veterinary Internal Medicine; Fellow, American Academy of Veterinary Pharmacology and Therapeutics; Professor and Chairman, Department of Small Animal Clinical Sciences, College of Veterinary Medicine, University of Minnesota, St. Paul, Minnesota

Allan J. Paul, D.V.M., M.S.
Extension Veterinarian, Small Animal Medicine, College of Veterinary Medicine, University of Illinois at Urbana-Champaign, Urbana, Illinois

David J. Polzin, D.V.M., Ph.D.
Diplomate, American College of Veterinary Internal Medicine; Assistant Pro-

fessor of Medicine, Department of Small Animal Clinical Sciences, College of Veterinary Medicine, University of Minnesota, St. Paul, Minnesota

J. Edmond Riviere, D.V.M., Ph.D.
Fellow, American Academy of Veterinary Pharmacology and Therapeutics; Associate Professor of Pharmacology and Toxicology, Laboratory of Toxicokinetics, School of Veterinary Medicine, North Carolina State University, Raleigh, North Carolina

Robert C. Rosenthal, D.V.M., M.S.
Diplomate, American College of Veterinary Internal Medicine; Assistant Professor, Department of Medical Sciences, School of Veterinary Medicine, University of Wisconsin, Madison, Wisconsin

Philip Roudebush, D.V.M.
Diplomate, American College of Veterinary Internal Medicine; Associate Professor of Medicine, School of Veterinary Medicine, Mississippi State University, Mississippi State, Mississippi

William D. Schall, D.V.M., M.S.
Diplomate, American College of Veterinary Internal Medicine; Professor of Internal Medicine, College of Veterinary Medicine, Michigan State University, East Lansing, Michigan

Danny W. Scott, D.V.M.
Diplomate, American College of Veterinary Dermatology; Associate Professor of Medicine, Department of Clinical Sciences, New York State College of Veterinary Medicine, Cornell University, Ithaca, New York

David C. Seeler, D.V.M., M.S.
Chief of Anesthesiology, Angell Memorial Animal Hospital; Assistant Professor, Department of Surgery, School of Veterinary Medicine, Tufts University, Jamaica Plain, Massachusetts

John C. Thurmon, D.V.M., M.S.
Diplomate, American College of Veterinary Anesthesiology; Chief of Anesthesiology, Professor of Veterinary Clinical Medicine, College of Veterinary Medicine, University of Illinois at Urbana-Champaign, Urbana, Illinois

Kenneth S. Todd, Jr., Ph.D.
Professor of Veterinary Parasitology, Department of Veterinary Pathobiology, College of Veterinary Medicine, University of Illinois at Urbana-Champaign, Urbana, Illinois

William A. Vestre, D.V.M., M.S.
Diplomate, American College of Veterinary Ophthalmologists; Associate Professor of Veterinary Ophthalmology, Department of Small Animal Clinics, School of Veterinary Medicine, Purdue University, West Lafayette, Indiana

Victoria L. Voith, D.V.M., Ph.D.
Director, Animal Behavior Clinic; Assistant Professor of Medicine, School of Veterinary Medicine, University of Pennsylvania, Philadelphia, Pennsylvania

Jeffrey R. Wilcke, D.V.M., M.S.
Assistant Professor of Clinical Pharmacology, Virginia-Maryland Regional College of Veterinary Medicine, Virginia Tech, Blacksburg, Virginia

PREFACE

The *Handbook of Small Animal Therapeutics* will provide the busy practitioner and house officer an up-to-date summary of relevant information necessary to make rational therapeutic decisions.

This handbook was not intended to be a textbook of therapeutics which provides an exhaustive review of the current veterinary medical literature; rather, it is a compilation of therapeutic approaches to various commonly encountered medical disorders of dogs and cats.

Since the clinical problems in dogs and cats usually are related to disorders of one or more bodily systems, this handbook has been organized around these disorders. The authors have made an effort to include in their discussions information concerning the pathophysiology of various disorders, drug dosage, precautions, and potential adverse effects of therapeutic interventions. It is hoped that this information will assist the reader in making risk/benefit assessments and in determining the therapeutic objectives to be attained in the individual patient. Each author has provided a list of suggested readings which may be consulted by the reader who needs more extensive information.

Contributors to the handbook were selected on the basis of their particular clinical specialization and expertise in the management of disorders related to a specific system. All of the authors are recognized experts in their specialties and are actively involved in the problems of patient care. The recommendations for therapy are based on studies reported in the veterinary medical literature and on the personal experience of the authors. The medications described do not necessarily have specific approval by the Food and Drug Administration for treatment of the diseases for which they are recommended. Doses generally should be considered as averages or starting points, and the necessity for individualization should be recognized by the therapist. Because standards of usage change, it is advisable that the veterinarian keep abreast of revised recommendations, particularly those concerning newer drugs.

The editor is indebted to the authors who took time from their busy clinical and academic schedules to share in this undertaking. Thanks are due to Mr. Gene Kearn, Veterinary Editor for Churchill Livingstone, for his patience and assistance in the production of this handbook.

Lloyd E. Davis, D.V.M.

CONTENTS

Handbook of Small Animal Therapeutics

1

General Care of the Patient
Lloyd E. Davis, D.V.M.

The object of therapeutics in the practice of veterinary medicine is to relieve suffering, to restore the patient to a state of health, and to improve the quality of life. In the ensuing chapters, the clinical management of specific diseases or particular modalities of therapy will be discussed. The purpose of this chapter is to outline essential features of the general care of hospitalized patients. This is commonly termed *supportive care*.

ENVIRONMENT

GENERAL COMMENTS

The sick or traumatized dog or cat confined within the unfamiliar surroundings of a veterinary hospital is subjected to stresses and exposed to diseases beyond its primary medical problem. Efforts should be made to minimize environmental sources of discomfort and the potential for nosocomial infections.

TEMPERATURE AND HUMIDITY

The neutral ambient temperature is 75°F. At this temperature there is essentially no expenditure of energy to conserve or to dissipate body heat. It has been shown that the mortality associated with severe trauma increased to 100% with either an increase or decrease of 20°F from this optimum. At a temperature of 75°F the optimal relative humidity is 65%. A greater incidence of mortality, loss of body weight, and digestive disturbances have been noted to occur at low (20–50%) relative humidity rather than at higher values.

CLEANLINESS

Control insects and other arthropods in the environment. Disinfect cages, runs, and other areas of the hospital.

1

I. Surfactants
   Do not mix cationic and anionic detergents as this will result in mutual inactivation.
   A. Anionic surfactants
      Most effective against gram-positive organisms
      1. Soaps
      2. Phisoderm
   B. Cationic surfactants
      Effective against gram-positive and -negative bacteria. Not effective against fungi, viruses, or spores. Inactivated by organic materials such as blood, feces, or exudates.
      1. Benzalkonium (Zephiran, Roccal) 10% solution for disinfection of premises
      2. Benzethonium (Phemerol)
      3. Cetylpyridium (Ceepryn)
II. Halogens
   A. Iodophors
      Effective in presence of organic matter against bacteria, spores, and fungi. Activity is markedly decreased at pH values above 4.0.
   B. Chlorine disinfectants
      Inactivated by organic material. Effective against bacteria and viruses.
      1. Sodium hypochlorite 5% (Clorox). Apply at a rate of 0.5 L/m^2.
      2. Calcium hypochlorite
      3. Chloramine T (Chlorazene). Apply as 1% solution.
III. Coal tar derivatives
   Bactericidal and viracidal. Not effective against spores. If used around cats, these compounds must be thoroughly rinsed from cages and floors so that cats cannot be exposed to them. Phenolics are more toxic to cats than to other species because of slow elimination from the body.
   A. Phenol—too expensive for this use
   B. Cresol
   C. Saponated cresol solution (Lysol)—applied as a 2% solution
   D. Sodium orthophenylphenate—applied as a 1% solution
   E. Orthochlorophenol—3–5% emulsion kills ova and larvae of most nematodes.
IV. Formaldehyde
   Formaldehyde solution contains 40% formaldehyde gas. Effective against bacteria, spores, and viruses and is an excellent deodorizing agent.
   A. For surface application dilute with water to a concentration of 4% formaldehyde gas, i.e., a 1:10 dilution of the solution.
   B. For fumigation of empty quarters. Place 35 ml formaldehyde solution in a vessel for each 35.5 m^3 of room space. Add 17.5 g potassium permanganate to each 35 ml solution. Keep quarters closed for 2 days and follow by thorough airing before returning animals to the facility.

V. Chlorhexidine (Nolvasan)
Effective against bacteria, viruses, and fungi. Active in presence of organic matter.

VENTILATION

Provisions should be made for adequate exchange of room air.

FLUIDS

I. Provisions must be made for assuring adequate fluid intake by all patients. Quantities and mode of presentation will be dictated by the clinical situation and should be specified on the orders for the patient. Fluid, electrolyte, and acid-base disorders are discussed in Chapter 2.

II. Maintenance Requirements
   A. Normal water intake will vary with diet, activity, and environment but averages about 60 ml/kg/day.
   B. Approximately 2.5 ml water are consumed for each gram of dry food (90% dry matter).
   C. Less drinking water is consumed if a canned food is provided.

III. Requirements will be increased by fever, polyuria, vomiting, diarrhea, or high environmental temperature.

IV. If there is no need for fluid restriction or extra fluids, leave an order for fluids ad libitum. Cages should be checked periodically to confirm that a source of clean, fresh water is available.

V. Fluids must be administered IV or SQ if the patient cannot consume them orally. The rate of IV infusion should be slow when providing maintenance requirements. In patients with expanded extracellular fluid volumes the central venous pressure should be monitored.

VI. If sodium intake is restricted and water is available ad libitum, dilutional hyponatremia may occur (see chapter 2). Water restriction rather than administration of hypertonic solutions is the preferred treatment for this condition.

NUTRITION

Adequate nutritional support of the patient is an important consideration which is often neglected. Sick animals are often anorectic as a result of their disease and change of environment. Dietary manuals (such as *Nutrition and Management of Dogs and Cats* published by Ralston Purina Co.) should be consulted for specific nutritional information. Malnutrition can increase severity of infectious disease, prolong convalescence, and impair healing following surgery of trauma.

NUTRIENT REQUIREMENTS OF ADULT DOGS
AND CATS

I. Daily metabolizable energy requirements
   A. Dogs— 88 kcal/kg
   B. Cats—85 kcal/kg
   C. These requirements are increased during growth, gestation, and lacta-
      tion. They are decreased during senescence.
II. Requirements for individual nutrients are listed in Table 1-1.
    A. The daily requirement per kilogram of body weight for individual nu-
       trients can be obtained from Table 1-1 by multiplying by a factor of

TABLE 1-1. NUTRIENT REQUIREMENTS OF DOGS AND CATS (PERCENTAGE OR
AMOUNT PER KILOGRAM OF FOOD, DRY BASIS)[a]

Nutrient	Unit	Requirement Dogs[b]	Requirement Cats[c]
Protein	%	22.0	28.0
Fat	%	5.0	9.0
Linoleic acid	%	1.0	1.0
Arachidonic acid	%	—	0.1
Minerals			
Calcium	%	1.1	1.0
Phosphorus	%	0.9	0.8
Potassium	%	0.6	0.3
Sodium chloride	%	1.1	0.5
Magnesium	%	0.04	0.05
Iodine	mg	1.54	1.0
Iron	mg	60.0	100.0
Copper	mg	7.3	5.0
Manganese	mg	5.0	10.0
Zinc	mg	50.0	30.0
Selenium	mg	0.11	0.1
Vitamins			
Vitamin A	IU	5,000	10,000
Vitamin D	IU	500	1,000
Vitamin E	IU	50	80
Thiamine	mg	1.0	5.0
Riboflavin	mg	2.2	5.0
Pantothenic acid	mg	10.0	10.0
Niacin	mg	11.4	45.0
Pyridoxine	mg	1.0	4.0
Folic acid	mg	0.18	1.0
Biotin	mg	0.10	0.05
Vitamin B_{12}	mg	0.02	0.02
Choline	mg	1,200	2,000

[a] Based on a diet with an energy concentration of 4 kcal/g dry matter.
[b] Nutrient requirements of dogs—revised 1974, National Academy of Science, National Research Council, Washington, DC.
[c] Nutrient requirements of cats—revised 1978, National Academy of Science, National Research Council,
Washington, DC.

0.022. For example, the daily requirement for thiamine in dogs would be 1.0 mg/kg food × 0.022 kg food/kg body weight/day = 0.022 mg/kg body weight. Similarly, in the cat 5.0 mg × 0.022 = 0.11 mg/kg
B. The cat differs from the dog in nutritional requirements for
   1. Arachidonic acid
   2. Taurine
   3. Vitamin A
   4. Thiamine and other B vitamins

DIETS

I. Liquid diets
   A. Indicated for patients following gastrointestinal surgery, acutely ill patients that cannot eat, initial feedings following NPO (nothing per os) orders for acute gastroenteritis. Clear broth is a readily available clear liquid food.
   B. Liquid diets generally consist of broths, sugar, electrolytes, water, milk, eggs. Such diets are deficient in protein, B vitamins, iron, and some minerals. Vitamin and mineral supplements should be given.
   C. Recipe for tube feeding

   1 pt whole milk
   1 pt cream
   4 oz raw liver
   4 raw eggs
   2 tsp brewer's yeast
   7.5 oz sugar or corn syrup
   4 tsp whole milk powder
   4 tsp casein
   4 tsp applesauce, pectin, or apple powder
   1 tsp iodized salt

   Mix and liquify in a blender.
   D. Care should be taken not to introduce volumes of air into the stomach through pharyngostomy tubes. Avoid distending the stomach; smaller, more frequent feedings are desirable.
   E. Dehydration, azotemia, and hypernatremia may be produced by excessive solute loads with inadequate water during tube feeding. Attention must be given to provide adequate amounts of water to the animal.
II. Soft bland diets
   A. Soft bland diets contain foods having a low residue and providing easily assimilated protein and carbohydrates. They may be fed during the transition from a liquid diet to a regular diet and during convalescence from severe gastrointestinal (GI) disorders. Vitamins and minerals should be supplemented.

B. Recipe

> $\frac{1}{2}$ cup farina cooked to make two cups
> $1\frac{1}{2}$ cup creamed cottage cheese
>   1 egg, hard-cooked
>   2 tbsp brewer's yeast
>   3 tbsp sugar
>   1 tbsp corn oil
>   1 tbsp potassium chloride
>   2 tbsp dicalcium phosphate
>   Yields 2 lb containing 440 kcal/lb

(From *Nutrition and Management of Dogs and Cats*. Ralston Purina Co., St. Louis, MO, 1979).

REGULAR DIETS

Animals that have an appetite and are able to eat should be fed maintenance quantities of a good-quality balanced dog or cat food.

IV FEEDING

I. Parenteral alimentation may be required for patients with protracted vomiting. Strict aseptic techniques must be followed and continuous slow infusions are required.
II. Solution
Equal quantities of 50% dextrose solution and 10% protein hydrolysate solution are mixed aseptically in a 1-L infusion bottle. A volume containing the appropriate number of calories is infused slowly over a period of 16 hours. This solution contains approximately 1,200 kcal/L. B vitamins are administered IM or SQ.
III. The patient's electrolyte and acid-base balance should be carefully monitored.

BOWEL FUNCTION

GENERAL COMMENTS

I. Physiologic bowel action should be encouraged in hospitalized dogs and cats. Animals may become constipated if not provided with clean litter boxes or access to runs. House-trained pets are strongly conditioned and may not defecate unless they are walked or have access to papers.
II. If the patient has been anorectic or fed a low-residue diet the colon may be nearly empty so as not to provide an adequate stimulus for the defecatory reflex.

III. Animals may develop diarrhea during hospitalization as a result of dietary change, tube feedings with diets having a high water content, or psychogenic stimuli.

TREATMENT OF CONSTIPATION

I. Cathartics exert their action on the bowel by stimulating motility, adding water to intestinal contents, providing lubrication, or increasing bulk of the contents.
II. Treatment with cathartics may be useful for
  A. Hospitalized patients that cannot or will not defecate of their own volition
  B. Animals with painful lesions of the anus or perineal area
  C. Patients in which straining at stool may have undesirable consequences (severe heart failure, prolapses, hernias)
  D. Drug-induced constipation (following barium studies, anticholinergic or opiate drugs)
III. Contraindications include abdominal pain, intestinal obstruction, and gastric dilatation
IV. Preparations
  A. Mineral oil (liquid petrolatum, USP)
       An inert oil which lubricates the fecal mass and facilitates passage. Useful to assist in removal of hair balls from cats. Excessive use (rare in veterinary practice) interferes with absorption of fat-soluble vitamins. Care must be taken that mineral oil not be introduced into the trachea as it produces fatal lipid pneumonia. Dose: dogs 5–30 ml; cats 2–6 ml.
  B. Anthraquinone cathartics
       Stimulate the colon only, as the glycoside is inactive and requires the action of colonic bacteria to release emodin which acts locally. Action results in passage of a formed stool 6–8 hours following administration. Most nearly mimics normal defecatory reflex.
       1. Cascara sagrada extract. Dose: dogs 1–4 ml; cats 0.5–1.5 ml.
       2. Senna. Dose: dogs 1–8 g; cats 0.1–0.3 g.
       3. Danthron. Dose: dogs 25–45 mg/kg; cats 15–20 mg/kg.
  C. Castor oil
       Hydrolyzed in small intestine to ricinoleic acid which stimulates secretion and motility. Prompt action (1–2 hours) with watery feces. Used for cleansing bowel prior to diagnostic studies or surgery. Dose: dogs 5–25 ml; cats 3–10 ml.
  D. Saline cathartics
       They act to increase water volume in small and large intestine through osmotic effect. Rapid onset of action (1–2 hours), fluid feces, and moderate colic. Used to prepare bowel for special examinations or to empty

alimentary canal following intoxications. Magnesium salts are not to be administered to animals with renal insufficiency.

1. Magnesium sulfate (Epsom salt). Dose: dogs 5–25 g; cats 2–5 g.
2. Sodium sulfate (Glauber's salt). Dose: dogs 5–25 g; cats 2–5 g.
3. Magnesium hydroxide (milk of magnesia). Dose: dogs 5–10 ml; cats 2–6 ml.

E. Hydrophilic colloids

   Increase the indigestible residue in feces which stimulates peristalsis. Most physiologic means for regularizing activity of the bowel.

1. Psyllium (Metamucil) may be added to the food. Dose: dogs 3–10 g; cats 3 g.
2. Methylcellulose. Dose: dogs 0.5–5 g; cats 0.5–1 g.
3. Bran may be mixed with the food ration. Dose: dogs 1–4 g; cats 0.5–2 g.

F. Surfactants

   Increase the wetting effectiveness of water by lowering surface tension. This has the effect of softening inspissated fecal material. Should not be given simultaneously with mineral oil as it may promote absorption of the oil which acts as a foreign body to produce granulomas in lymph nodes and liver.

   Dioctyl sodium sulfosuccinate (DSS, Colace, Doxinate). Dose: dogs and cats 2 mg/kg.

V. Enemas

   May be used to evacuate the colon for diagnostic procedures or prior to rectal or anal surgery. Useful to relieve obstipation of the colon.

A. Tap water or saline
B. Soap suds
C. Glycerin suppositories will stimulate defecation.
D. Dioctyl sodium sulfosuccinate, 1% solution. One part may be added to nine parts of tap water for removal of desiccated stool.
E. Fleets disposable enemas are convenient for inducing rapid emptying of the colon.

TREATMENT OF DIARRHEA

I. General comments

A. Episodes of diarrhea are frequently self-limiting in nature and may not require treatment. In cases of severe or protracted diarrhea, attempts should be made to determine etiology so that specific therapy can be instituted. Possibilities to be considered include parasitic, bacterial, or viral diseases, malabsorption syndromes, endocrine disorders, toxicoses, and allergic or neoplastic diseases. Diarrhea may result from primary GI disorders or may be secondary to systemic diseases.
B. The GI tract should be placed at rest by initiating NPO orders or limiting food to a clear liquid diet (see Nutrition, Diets, I, B, above).

C. Primary attention should be given to providing replacement of fluids and electrolytes and maintenance of normal acid-base balance. This is generally accomplished by parenteral therapy (see Chapter 2) but glucose-electrolyte solutions are available for oral replacement (Pedialyte, Gatorade, Lectade).

II. Antidiarrheal drugs that alter GI motility and secretion

A. Opiates are spasmogenic and hence increase segmental tone while decreasing propulsive movement. They also have been shown to decrease water and electrolyte secretion by the intestinal muscosa. By contrast, anticholinergic drugs decrease both segmental tone and peristaltic activity, which provides an open conduit for the passage of diarrheal fluids from the body.

1. Diphenoxylate (Lomotil). Dose: dogs and cats 0.5–1 mg/kg. (The dose of atropine included in Lomotil is subtherapeutic. It is added to discourage drug abuse.)
2. Camphorated tincture of opium (Paregoric). Dose: dog 2–15 ml.
3. Morphine may be administered parenterally for intractable diarrhea. Dose: dogs 0.2 mg/kg, cats 0.1 mg/kg.

B. Protectants coat the surface of inflamed GI mucosa and exert a demulcent/adsorbent effect. Efficacy is unproven but probably little risk is associated with their use. These drugs are common interactants limiting absorption of some drugs.

1. Kaolin-pectin (Kaopectate). Dosage: dogs and cats 1–2 ml/kg every 4–6 hours.
2. Activated charcoal. Dosage: dogs and cats 0.3–5 g every 8 hours (messy to administer).
3. Barium sulfate
4. Bismuth subsalicylate (Pepto-Bismol) 1.75% suspension. Dose: dog 10–30 ml every 4–6 hours; cat not established. Probably is best choice as it exerts protectant, anti-inflammatory, antitoxin, and antiprostaglandin effects on the bowel.

FEVER

GENERAL COMMENTS

I. An increase in body temperature may be caused by bacterial or viral infections; immune-mediated, neoplastic, or granulomatous diseases; drugs; dehydration; high environmental temperature; and toxicoses.

II. Fevers less than 105°F seldom are of danger to the patient and may serve the useful purpose of inhibiting proliferation of pathogens (particularly viruses). The mode of onset and severity of fever may be a useful clue to diagnosis and guide in assessing efficacy of specific drug therapy, i.e., in the case of bacterial infections.

III. Body temperatures in excess of 106°F may lead to brain damage, cardiac dysrhythmias, dehydration, increased tissue catabolism, and disseminated intravascular coagulation. This constitutes a medical emergency and measures must be taken to quickly reduce body temperature to safe levels. Cool baths or cool water enemas are used and shivering may be a problem. A phenothiazine derivative such as promazine or acepromazine may facilitate defervescence but temperature must be monitored closely as hypothermia may result from external cooling of a patient which has received a phenothiazine.

ANTIPYRETIC DRUGS

Antipyretic drugs act to reduce the set point of the hypothalamic temperature regulating center with subsequent increase in heat loss.

I. Salicylates are the first choice of antipyretics for use in dogs and cats. They are equal in efficacy to other antipyretics but have a superior risk/benefit ratio.
   A. Aspirin
      Insoluble in water, must be administered orally. Dosage: dog 10 mg/kg every 12 hours; cat 10 mg/kg every 48 hours.
   B. Sodium salicylate
      May be added to water for injection or saline for IV administration. Dosage: same as for aspirin.
II. Acetaminophen
      Is as effective as aspirin as an antipyretic but may produce more serious toxicity, particularly in cats. Acetaminophen has caused considerable morbidity in cats which was characterized by Heinz body anemia and hepatic necrosis. Dosage: dogs 10 mg/kg every 12 hours; cats—should not be used.
III. Pyrazolon derivatives
      Pyrazolon derivatives are employed primarily as anti-inflammatory drugs (see Chapter 5), but they exert antipyretic effects comparable to aspirin. Again, the risk/benefit ratio is less favorable for this group than for aspirin as they may produce blood dyscrasias, gastrointestinal disturbances, hepatitis, and nephropathy in dogs and cats.
   A. Phenylbutazone
      Dosage: dogs 22 mg/kg every 8 hours.
   B. Dipyrone
      Dosage: dogs 25 mg/kg every 8 hours. Dipyrone should not be given to dogs that have been treated with phenothiazine compounds as hypothermia may result.

RELIEF OF PAIN

GENERAL COMMENTS

I. This is an important therapeutic objective to pursue in the overall management of animal patients as it fulfills our ethical obligation to relieve

suffering, facilitates the conduct of a thorough physical examination, encourages rest, and forestalls the possible development of neurogenic shock.
II. As pain is a subjective perception experienced by the patient it is difficult for the veterinarian to objectively evaluate the intensity, degree of suffering, and extent of the painful experience in creatures with which we are unable to communicate.
III. Reactions to pain may be manifested by vocalization, adoption of unusual postures, defensive reactions to palpation, autonomic responses, and muscular splinting of the affected body region.
IV. Response to painful stimuli will vary with temperament of the individual animal, severity, chronicity, etiology, and setting. Because of the many variables it frequently is difficult to be certain that a patient hurts. If, the nature of the disorder or injury and its location suggest that it may be painful it is my policy to provide analgesia. This is one of the very few areas of therapeutics in which I would advise that if in doubt—treat.
V. The nature of pain and groups of drugs expected to be effective in providing relief vary with location of the receptors and the nature of the stimulus. Superficial or deep somatic pain of mild to moderate intensity is obtunded by the nonsteroidal anti-inflammatory analgesics, whereas relief of severe somatic or visceral pain requires administration of central-acting, narcotic analgesics.

NON NARCOTIC ANALGESICS

I. Exert their actions peripherally and centrally at the thalamus. Particularly effective in moderating or obtunding pain resulting from inflammatory reactions.
II. These drugs are discussed in detail in Chapter 5.
III. Administration or prescription of these drugs is warranted to relieve pain and discomfort from
A. Incisions of body wall (except for thorax)
B. Arthritis, tendonitis, muscular injuries
C. Cystitis.
D. Cutaneous or mucosal lesions
E. Dental injuries
F. Mild gastroenteritis
IV. Aspirin will generally provide adequate relief of discomfort. It is inexpensive, generally well tolerated by most dogs and cats and, importantly, the pharmacokinetics are known in these species.
A. Dosage
1. Dogs
The usual dose is 10 mg/kg, repeated at 12-hour intervals. The dose may be increased to 25 mg/kg in patients with rheumatoid arthritis or mild lupus erythematosus.
2. Cats
The dose is 10 mg/kg repeated every 48 hours. For chronic ther-

apy of arthritis in an average-sized cat, I recommend one 1.25 gr (infant aspirin) tablet every Monday, Wednesday, and Friday with no medication on the weekend. This is a convenient schedule for the client to follow and the omission of treatment during the weekend prevents accumulation of the drug in the patient.

B. Toxicity
  1. Toxic effects of aspirin are generally dose-related. Few problems are associated with the lower dosage or with intermittent use. Occasionally, individual dogs or cats will not tolerate aspirin and will exhibit signs of gastritis, vomiting, and GI bleeding. There is little evidence that buffered aspirin alleviates this problem. Allergic reactions to aspirin are rare but have been observed in dogs.
  2. Severe toxicity may occur with acute overdosage, particularly in cats. It is characterized by vomiting, hyperpnea, pyrexia, coma, severe metabolic acidosis, and GI ulceration and bleeding.

C. Contraindications
  1. Gastric or intestinal ulcers
  2. Renal insufficiency
  3. Asthma
       Inhibition of synthesis of prostaglandin E_1 may be deleterious because this mediator causes compensatory bronchodilation in this condition.
  4. Lymphomas produce an unusual sensitivity to salicylates characterized by hypothermia. This has been reported in human patients but has not been documented in dogs or cats.

V. Other drugs
  A. Acetaminophen
       No advantage, except in dogs that are intolerant to aspirin. Should not be used in cats.
  B. Phenacetin
       A component of APC tablets (Anacin, Empirin). Metabolized to acetaminophen and should be avoided in cats. No advantage over aspirin.
  C. Propoxyphene (Darvon)
       Related in structure to methadone but is not a narcotic. When combined with aspirin the analgesic effect is potentiated. Has been abused by drug users. Offers little advantage in veterinary therapeutics.

Narcotic Analgesics

I. Opiates are the primary drugs which are effective for providing relief of severe, agonizing, somatic, or visceral pain. Also useful for control of severe cough and diarrhea and in the management of acute pulmonary edema. There are a number of drugs available but morphine remains the drug of choice in the dog and cat.

A. Pharmacologic effects

Produce analgesia with a moderate degree of sedation and alteration of behavioral response to pain. The opiates and opioids (in equianalgesic doses) are spasmogenic, causing bronchoconstriction, increased sphincter tone, contraction of biliary ducts and ureters, increased segmental tone, and decreased peristalsis of intestine. They depress the respiratory and cough centers in the medulla, initially stimulate and then depress the emetic center, and stimulate release of antidiuretic hormone (ADH) which causes an antidiuretic response. Tachyphylaxis occurs with repeated administration. Induces relaxation of splanchnic capacitance vessels which may cause hypotension. Pupils of the eye are dilated in cats and constricted in dogs. Morphine increases cerebrospinal fluid (CSF) pressure and stimulates the spinal cord.

B. Preparations

1. Morphine sulfate or hydrochloride is generally administered IM or SQ with onset of action in 15 minutes and a duration of action of 6 hours. May be administered IV but stimulates release of histamine and causes transient excitement. Dose: dog 0.25 mg/kg; cat 0.1 mg/kg. May be repeated every 6 hours if necessary. Overdosage produces maniacal excitement in the cat and progressive depression in the dog.

2. Codeine phosphate

Analgesic potency is about $\frac{1}{10}$ that of morphine. Commonly employed with aspirin for relief of moderate pain. Used alone as an antitussive. Dosage: dog 2 mg/kg every 6 hours; cat—not established.

II. Opioids

A. Semisynthetic derivatives of morphine or codeine or synthetic drugs. At equianalgesic doses the effects are similar to morphine.

B. Preparations

1. Methadone (Dolophine)

Similar to morphine in potency and duration of action. More expensive.

2. Dihydromorphinone (Dilaudid)

More potent than morphine with shorter duration of action

3. Meperidine (Demerol)

Satisfactory as a preanesthetic agent but duration of analgesia is too short (45 minutes) for relieving severe pain in the dog and cat. Approximately 90% of the dose is metabolized within 1 hour following administration to dogs or cats. Overdosage produces convulsions. Dose: dog 10 mg/kg IM; cat 5 mg/kg IM. Meperidine should not be injected SQ as it is quite irritating.

4. Oxymorphone (Numorphan)

More potent than morphine. Does not produce as much sedation and has little effect on the cough center. Drug of choice for relief of pain in patients which need to be able to cough, e.g., postthoracotomy. Dose: dogs 0.03–0.05 mg/kg, IM; cats—not established.

III. Narcotic antagonists

A. Act to block the opiate receptors in the central nervous system (CNS) and GI tract. Administration will reverse the pharmacologic effects of the opiate and opioid drugs. Some of the drugs in this group act as both agonists and antagonists at the receptor. If administered alone, these drugs will produce analgesic and antitussive effects. When given to an animal that has received a narcotic they will antagonize its effects.

B. Preparations

1. Naloxone (Narcan)

A pure antagonist which will reverse the action of narcotics. Has no effect in animals which have not received a narcotic, e.g., it neither increases nor decreases depression from barbiturates. Dose: dogs and cats 40 µg/kg IV.

2. Nalorphine (Nalline)

An agonist-antagonist drug. Produces narcosis in animals which have not received other narcotics. Naloxone is preferred for reversal of narcotic depression. Dose: dog and cat 1 mg/kg IV.

3. Pentazocine (Talwin)

An agonist-antagonist. Used as an analgesic but duration of action is very short in dogs and it appears to produce dysphoria in cats. Dose: dogs 2 mg/kg.

4. Butorphanol (Stadol, Torbutrol)

Potent analgesic and antitussive in the dog. Newer drug. Dose: dog 0.05–0.1 mg/kg, every 6–8 hours.

IV. Precautions in use of narcotic drugs

A. These drugs should be used only under the direct supervision of the veterinarian. They should very rarely be dispensed or prescribed unless the client is well known to the doctor. The majority of these drugs are controlled substances which have been subjected to a great deal of abuse by some members of society. We must not contribute to their problem.

B. Most conditions in which narcotics are indicated are acute in nature. Seldom should a veterinary patient require therapy for more than 24–48 hours. We don't have the problem which the physician faces of having to provide long-term analgesia during the terminal stages of malignant disease as we have available the more merciful option of euthanasia.

C. Animals with head injuries should not receive narcotics as the increase in CSF pressure may contribute to brain damage.

D. Side effects such as vomition and hypotension are less frequent in recumbent patients than when they are ambulatory.

E. Do not use narcotics in animals with signs of spinal convulsions (strychnine, tetanus).

F. Phenothiazine derivatives potentiate the effects of narcotics. Decrease the dose of narcotic to half if you have given a tranquilizer.

G. In animals with narcotic-induced depression of respiration the principal effect is abolition of the response to CO_2. Accordingly, one must be cautious in providing oxygen therapy as the primary drive to the respiratory centers is hypoxia.

H. Caution should be taken in the use of narcotics in patients with respiratory insufficiency or asthma.

I. Good clinical judgment should attend the use of these drugs as the analgesia and euphoria produced may mask important clinical signs which may be needed for making a diagnosis.

SEDATION AND RESTRAINT

I. Patients that are frightened, anxious, hyperactive, or vicious may require drugs to render them manageable for proper examination and treatment, to prevent self-inflicted injury, and to provide rest during their hospitalization.

II. The objective is to produce a reduction in response to aversive stimuli without impairment of the animal's ability to eat, drink, defecate, urinate, and change posture.

III. Whenever it is practical, sedatives should be given orally. Extra care must be given to choice of drug in patients with cardiac, renal, or hepatic disorders; hypotension; high fever; pulmonary disease; electrolyte and acid-base disturbances. In animals with renal insufficiency or hepatic disease select a drug that is not eliminated by the affected organ, i.e., pentobarbital may be given to an animal with renal failure while phenobarbital may be administered to a patient with hepatic disease.

IV. Make certain that the source of restlessness or anxiety is not the result of a condition which can be more rationally corrected by other means. The patient could be experiencing pain (analgesics), inadequate cerebral perfusion from hypovolemia (intensify fluid therapy), or need to defecate or urinate (remove from cage).

BARBITURATES

I. May be selected on the basis of duration of action. Long-acting drugs (barbital, phenobarbital) produce sedation in 69–90 minutes and the effect lasts 6–8 hours. They are excreted primarily by the kidneys. Pentobarbital is short-acting with an onset of action of 30–45 minutes and duration of 4–5 hours. It is entirely eliminated by biotransformation in the liver.

II. Barbiturates, in sedative doses, have a high margin of safety with few side effects. With chronic use they induce microsomal enzymes in the liver and may cause drug interactions.

III. Dosage
    A. Phenobarbital. Dogs and cats: 2 mg/kg, orally, every 8–12 hours
    B. Pentobarbital. Dogs and cats: 2–4 mg/kg, orally, every 6 hours

PHENOTHIAZINE DERIVATIVES

  I. Exert more of an effect on behavioral responses to external stimuli than true sedation. This is manifested as a taming effect in vicious animals and a lack of concern for what would normally be threatening stimuli. This group produces little impairment in the animal's ability to eat, drink, eliminate, or ambulate.
 II. They may be administered either orally or parenterally but are most commonly injected.
III. The phenothiazines have a number of actions in the body. They block cholinergic, α-adrenergic, serotonin, histamine, and dopaminergic receptors and stimulate the extrapyramidal system. They are effective in inhibiting the chemoreceptor trigger zone and thereby exert an antiemetic effect. They impair thermoregulation and an animal may develop hypothermia or pyrexia, depending on the ambient temperature.
IV. Preparations
    A. Acepromazine. Dose: dog and cat 0.1–0.5 mg/kg
    B. Chlorpromazine (Thorazine). Dose: dog and cat 3 mg/kg, orally 0.5 mg/kg IM or IV
    C. Promazine (Sparine). Dose: dog and cat 2–4 mg/kg IM or IV
 V. Clinical uses
    A. Behavioral modification (see chapter 17)
    B. Control intractable hiccups
    C. Relieve pruritis [particularly trimeprazine (Temaril) and methdilazine (Tacaryl) which block effects of both histamine and serotonin in inflamed skin].
    D. Facilitate lowering of body temperature in heat stroke
    E. Antiemetic—not effective in motion sickness
    F. Potentiate analgesic effect of narcotics
VI. Adverse effects
    A. Xerostomia
    B. Constipation
    C. Inhibition of ejaculation in male
    D. Paradoxical behavioral reactions have been reported in which a docile animal becomes vicious following treatment.
    E. Due to effect on extrapyramidal system phenothiazines should not be given to patients with tetanus or strychnine intoxication.
    F. An occasional animal will develop severe hypotension and collapse following treatment with a phenothiazine derivative. This is due to peripheral adrenergic blockade and may be fatal if untreated. *Epinephrine*

should not be given as it may worsen the situation by epinephrine reversal. Phenylephrine or levarterenol should be given IV to restore blood pressure.
- G. Rarely, allergy to phenothiazines has been observed.
- H. Cats eliminate phenothiazines slowly in comparison to dogs. Care should be taken to prevent drug accumulation.

OTHER SEDATIVES

Diazepam (Valium)

I. Decreases anxiety, increases seizure threshold in brain, supresses polysynaptic activity in spinal cord, and decreases activity in reticular system. Following single doses, the effects of diazepam subside rapidly due to distribution into nonneural tissues. The drug is metabolized rather slowly and active metabolites are formed. Thus, repeated administration may lead to drug accumulation. The principal adverse effects are dose-related ataxia and paradoxical aggression. Dosage: 0.25 mg/kg, every 8 hours, orally
II. Antihistamics such as diphenhydramine (Benadryl) and promethazine (Phenergan) exert prominent sedative effects and may be used when use of barbiturates or phenothiazines may be inadvisable. Dosage: diphenhydramine 4 mg/kg, orally, every 8 hours in dogs or cats.

CARE OF SKIN, COAT, AND EYES

I. Dogs and cats in the hospital are generally confined to less space than may be optimal and when ill they are unlikely to groom themselves.
II. Provisions should be made for them to keep dry and their coats should be groomed to prevent matting of hair and to maintain cleanliness.
III. If there are draining exudates or if the animal is incontinent the exposed areas of skin should be coated with petrolatum to prevent scalding.
IV. The eyes should be kept clean and if lachrymal secretion is inadequate, orders should be given for periodic instillation of methylcellulose drops.

ORDERS FOR PATIENTS

HOSPITAL ORDERS

I. Orders should be written in the chart and revised as often as necessary. They should be complete, clear, and explicit to avoid misinterpretation. They are to be signed and dated by the attending veterinarian.
II. Previous orders are canceled before new orders are written.

III. A system should be followed routinely to avoid omissions and should include:
  A. General observations to be made and frequency, e.g., temperature, pulse, respiration, (TPR), central venous pressure, attitude, and so forth
  B. General care: exercise, fluids, diet, bowel care
  C. Symptomatic treatment: pain, fever, cough, and the like
  D. Specific therapy: antimicrobials, cardiac drugs, parasiticides, diuretics, oxygen, and the like.
  E. Prevention of complications: skin and eye care, cage pads, frequent turning, external heat

HOME ORDERS

Orders for drugs to be dispensed for home use should be written in terms that are understandable to the client. Avoid use of medical jargon and technical terms.

PRESCRIPTIONS

  I. Should include the name, breed and sex of the animal, the name and address of the client, the date, name of drug, dose, amounts to be dispensed, the number of refills allowed, explicit instructions on how the medication is to be administered, the signature of the veterinarian and his or her Drug Enforcement Administration (DEA) number if the prescription is for a controlled substance.
  II. Use metric system for expressing dosage.
  III. Specify generic rather than proprietary names in most cases.
  IV. Write in ink.
  V. The name of the drug and the number and size of tablets or capsules should be included on the label. This permits rapid identification in case of accidental ingestion by a human being.
  VI. Do not use abbreviations or chemical formulae for ingredients on a prescription.
  VII. Keep a duplicate copy of the prescription in the patient's record.

SUGGESTED READINGS

Carter JM, Freedman AB: Total intravenous feeding in the dog. J Am Vet Med Assoc 171:71, 1977

Catcott EJ (ed): Canine Medicine. 4th Ed. American Veterinary Publications, Santa Barbara, CA, 1979

Davis LE: Clinical pharmacology of the gastrointestinal tract. p. 277. In Anderson NV (ed): Veterinary Gastroenterology. Lea and Febiger, Philadelphia, 1980

Davis LE: Drug presentation and prescribing. p. 13. In Booth NH, McDonald LE (ed): Veterinary Pharmacology and Therapeutics. 5th Ed. Iowa State University Press, Ames, 1982

Davis LE: Emergency drugs. p. 287. In Zaslow IM (ed): Veterinary Trauma and Critical Care. Lea and Febiger, Philadelphia, 1983

Ettinger SJ (ed): Textbook of Veterinary Internal Medicine. Diseases of the Dog and Cat. 2nd Ed. WB Saunders, Philadelphia, 1983

Kirk RW (ed): Current Veterinary Therapy. Vol. 7. WB Saunders, Philadelphia, 1983

Kronfeld DS: Feeding cats and feline nutrition. Compend Contin Ed 5:419, 1983

Nutrition and Management of Dogs and Cats. Ralston Purina Co., St. Louis, Mo, 1979

2

Fluid and Electrolyte Disorders

David C. Seeler, D.V.M.
John C. Thurmon, D.V.M.

Fluid and electrolyte therapy is an integral part of the management of various diseases. Proper management requires a knowledge of the pathogenesis of the fluid and/or electrolyte disturbance, clinical evaluation of the patient, and a knowledge of the composition of commercially available fluids. Specific therapeutic regimens should be based on the fluid and/or electrolyte alteration. Factors to be considered include: (1) existing volume of body fluids; (2) serum osmolality; (3) alteration of acid-base status, and (4) electrolyte composition of body fluids. In addition, renal and cardiovascular function should be assessed prior to therapy.

Life-threatening alterations must be attended to first. Preexisting deficits are determined and corrected. Continuing abnormal losses and basal or maintenance needs should be evaluated and then met. It is prudent to evaluate the response to therapy during administration of the calculated corrective dose.

GENERAL PRINCIPLES

BODY FLUID AND ELECTROLYTE COMPOSITION

I. Volume and distribution of body fluids in healthy animals remain relatively constant despite wide variations in water intake. Total body water accounts for up to 80% of the body weight at birth, decreasing to approximately 60% of total body weight at maturity. Obese animals have a proportionately lower body water content (40–50% total body weight) than lean animals.

II. Compartmentalization of body water occurs into intracellular, extracellular, and transcellular fluids.

   A. Intracellular fluid (ICF) makes up approximately 40% of the total lean body weight.

B. Extracellular fluid (ECF) consists of 20% of total lean body weight and is divided into the interstitial and plasma fluid compartments.
1. The interstitial fluid is contained within a gelatinous ground substance transversed with collagen fibers. The normal pressure of the interstitial fluid space ranges from -8 to -4 mmHg. While the interstitial fluid comprises only 15% of total lean body weight, its volume may expand rapidly under disease conditions. As fluid accumulates, the interstitial pressure increases toward zero, at which point there is a precipitous increase in compliance of the interstitial space, favoring further fluid accumulation and edema formation.
2. The plasma volume (intravascular fluid) makes up 5% of the total lean body weight. Due to its protein content, plasma volume is maintained at the expense of the interstitial fluid volume.
III. Approximately 1–3% of the body fluids are in specialized compartments (transcellular fluid) such as that in the cerebrospinal fluid or the gastrointestinal tract.
IV. Electrolyte composition of the various body fluids is presented in Table 2-1 and the constituents of plasma for the dog and cat are presented in Table 2-2.

COMMERCIAL FLUIDS

I. The composition of various commercial fluids is listed in Table 2-3.
II. Points to consider
A. Potassium-free fluids should be given in acute renal failure.
B. Calcium-containing fluids should not be administered through the same intravenous administration set as used for whole blood.

TABLE 2-1. APPROXIMATE ELECTROLYTE COMPOSITION OF BODY FLUIDS (mEq/L)

Ion	ICF	ISF	Plasma
Cations			
Na^+	13	145[a]	142[a]
K^+	155[a]	4	5
Ca^{2+}	2	3	5
Mg^{2+}	35	2	2
Anions			
Cl^-	2	115[a]	106[a]
HCO_3^-	10	30	24
Phosphates	113[a]	2	2
Sulfates	20	1	1
Organic acids	0	5	5
Protein	60	1	16

Abbreviations: ISF, interstitial fluid; other abbreviations as in text.
[a] Major ionic component of the respective compartments.

TABLE 2-2. REFERENCE VALUES OF IMPORTANT CONSTITUENTS OF
CANINE-FELINE PLASMA

Constituent	Units	Canine	Feline	Conversion Factor to SI Units (mmol/L)
Na$^+$	mEq/L	140–154	147–156	1.00
K$^+$	mEq/L	3.7–5.2	4.0–5.0	1.00
Ca^{2+} [a]	mg/dl	9.0–11.0	7.0–10.0	0.2495
Mg^{2+} [b]	mg/dl	1.5–2.5	1.5–2.5	0.4114
Cl	mEq/L	108–120	110–123	1.00
HCO$_3^-$	mEq/L	17–24	17–24	
PCV	%	37–55	24–45	0.01 (L/L)
TP	g/dl	6.0–7.5	6.0–8.0	10 (g/L)
A/G ratio		0.8–1.1	0.9–1.1	
BUN	mg/dl	10–20	20–30	0.3570
Creatinine	mg/dl	0.5–1.5	0.5–2.0	88.40 (μmol/L)
Glucose	mg/dl	65–110	60–100	0.05551
Serum osmolality	mOsm/kg	282–292	282–292	1.00 (mmol/kg)

Abbreviations: A/G = albumin/globulin ratio; BUN, blood urea nitrogen; PCV, packed cell volume; TP, total protein.
[a] To convert to mEq/L of calcium: mg/dl × 0.5 = mEq/L.
[b] To convert to mEq/L of magnesium: mg/dl × 0.82 = mEq/L.

C. Use intravenous solutions containing the preservative benzyl alcohol with caution.

D. Use of solutions with an excess of chloride ions (i.e., isotonic saline) induces metabolic acidosis and is contraindicated in acidotic patients.

E. Potassium should be added to maintenance fluids to prevent hypokalemia (see section on Potassium, II, C, 2, below).

F. Solutions should be warmed to body temperature before administration to prevent hypothermia in small patients.

G. Drugs added to intravenous fluids may be inactivated or form precipitates due to pH difference or interaction with substances contained in the solution. Some incompatibilities are listed in Table 2-4.

CLINICAL ASSESSMENT

I. A thorough history and physical examination in most instances will reveal the patient's state of hydration (Tables 2-5 and 2-6) and identify the probable underlying disease process.

II. Laboratory procedures should include determination of packed cell vol-

TABLE 2-3. COMPOSITION OF SOME COMMERCIALLY AVAILABLE FLUIDS (mEq/L)

Solution	Na$^+$	K$^+$	Ca^{2+}	Mg^{2+}	Cl$^-$	HCO$_3^-$ Acetate	Gluconate	Lactate	Dextrose (g/L)	Calories per Liter	Tonicity Salt	Total	mOsm per Liter	Approx. pH
5% dextrose (D5W)	—	—	—	—	—	—	—	—	50	171	Hypo	Hypo	252	5.0
10% dextrose (D10W)	—	—	—	—	—	—	—	—	100	342	Hypo	Hyper	505	5.0
0.9% saline	154	—	—	—	154	—	—	—	0	0	Iso	Iso	308	5.7
0.45% saline	77	—	—	—	77	—	—	—	0	0	Hypo	Hypo	154	4.5–7.0
Ringer's	147	4	4.5	—	156	—	—	—	0	0	Iso	Iso	310	5.0–7.0
Lactated Ringer's (LRS)	130	4	3	—	109	—	—	28	0	9	Iso	Iso	272	6.7
Normosol R	140	5	—	3	98	27	23	—	0	18	Iso	Iso	295	6.4
Normosol M in D5W	40	13	—	3	40	16	—	—	50	175	Hypo	Hyper	368	5.5
Plasma Lyte 148 in H$_2$O	140	5	—	3	98	27	23	—	0	21	Iso	Iso	294	4.0–6.5
D5W in LRS	130	4	3	—	109	—	—	28	50	179	Iso	Hyper	525	5.1

TABLE 2-4. INCOMPATIBILITIES OF DRUGS ADDED TO INTRAVENOUS
SOLUTIONS

Solution	Incompatible Drugs
Albumin, canine	Protein hydrolysate
Blood, whole	Dextrose solutions, levarterenol, metaraminol, phytonadione. In general, no drug should be added to blood transfusion
Calcium chloride or gluconate	Cephalothin, chlorpheniramine, nitrofurantoin, sodium bicarbonate, tetracyclines, magnesium sulfate, streptomycin, prochlorperazine
Dextrose	Kanamycin, phenytoin, warfarin, vitamin B_{12}, novobiocin, whole blood, digoxin, digitoxin, morphine, meperidine[a]
Lactated Ringer's	Amphotericin B, calcium EDTA, cortisone acetate, ethanol, metaraminol, phenytoin, sodium bicarbonate, sulfadiazine, tetracyclines, thiopental, warfarin, digoxin, digitoxin, morphine, meperidine[a]
Magnesium sulfate	Calcium gluconate, procaine, sodium bicarbonate, protein hydrolysate
Potassium chloride	Protein hydrolysate
Preservatives in water for injection	Amphotericin B, nitrofurantoin
Protein hydrolysate	ACTH, albumin, aminophyllin, digoxin, digitoxin, hydralazine, meperidine, metaraminol, nitrofurantoin, pentobarbital, potassium chloride, magnesium sulfate, thiopental
Ringer's	Amphotericin B, ethanol, calcium EDTA, cortisone acetate, sodium bicarbonate, thiopental
Sodium bicarbonate	ACTH, ethanol, calcium salts, insulin, levarterenol, magnesium sulfate, meperidine, methadone, morphine, pentobarbital, procaine, promazine, phenytoin, protein hydrolysate, lactated Ringer's, Ringer's, sodium lactate, streptomycin, tetracyclines, thiopental, vitamin B complex
Sodium chloride	Amphotericin B, levarterenol, phenytoin, digoxin, digitoxin
Sodium lactate	Sodium bicarbonate, sulfadiazine, succinylcholine

Abbreviations: ACTH, adrenocorticotropic hormone; other abbreviations as in text.
[a] Digitalis glycosides and opiates should not be dissolved in infusion fluids. They may be injected slowly into the Y-tube of administration sets.

ume, total serum protein, blood urea nitrogen (BUN), glucose, serum electrolytes, and urinalysis.

III. If precise concentrations of serum electrolytes are unknown, then treatment may be based on the consideration of the pathophysiology of the disease process (Table 2-5).

IV. Serum osmolality may either be measured or estimated with reasonable accuracy using one of the following formulas:

A. $mOsm = 1.86 (Na^+ + K^+) + \dfrac{Glucose}{18} + \dfrac{BUN}{2.8} + 9$

B. $mOsm = 2 \times Na^+ + \dfrac{Glucose}{20} + \dfrac{BUN}{3}$

TABLE 2-5. DISEASE PROCESSES AND TYPICAL FLUID AND ELECTROLYTE LOSSES

Clinical Disorder	Changes in Plasma								Changes in Total Body Content				Recommended Fluids
	Na	K	Cl	PCV	TSP	Osmolality	pH	HCO	H₂O	Na	K	Cl	
Loss of whole blood	N[a]	N	N	N/↓	N/↓	N/↓	↓/↓	↓	↓	↓	↓	↓	a–d
Loss of plasma	N	N	N	↑	↓	N/↓	V[b]	V	↓	↓	↓	↓	b–d
Dehydration													
6–8%	N	N	N	↑	↑	↑	N	N	↓	↓	↓	↓	H, I
10–12%	↑	↑	↑	↑	↑	↑↑↑	V	V	↓↓	↓↓	↓↓	↓↓	H, I
Vomition	N/↓	N/↓	↓↓↓	↑	↑	N	↑↑	↑↑	↓	↓	↓	↓	e, f
Diarrhea	N/↓	V	N/↓	↑	↑	N	↓	↓	↓	↓	↓	↓	d, g
Gastric torsion/dilation	V	V	V	V/↑	V/↑	V/↑	V	V	↓↓↓	N	↓	↓	d

Abbreviations: a, whole blood; b, plasma; c, plasma expanders; d, balanced electrolyte solution; e, isotonic saline; f, acidifying solutions; g, alkalinizing solution; H, hypotonic solutions; I, D5W, PCV, packed cell volume; TSP, Total serum protein.
↓, slight decrease; ↓↓, moderate decrease; ↓↓↓, extreme decrease; ↑, slight increase; ↑↑, moderate increase; ↑↑↑, extreme increase.
[a] No change.
[b] Variable.

TABLE 2-6.   CLINICAL SIGNS ASSOCIATED WITH DEGREE OF DEHYDRATION

Observation	Minimal[a] (4%)	Moderate (6–8%)	Severe (10–12%)
Skin resiliency	Pliable	Leathery	No pliability
Skin tenting[b]	Twist disappears immediately and tent persists for up to 2 seconds	Twist disappears immediately and tent persists 3 seconds or more	Twist and tent persists indefinitely
Eye	Bright Slightly sunken	Dull Sunken	Cornea Dry Markedly sunken
Capillary refill	Normal	Slightly increased	Greater than 3 seconds
Mouth	Moist, warm	Sticky to dry Warm	Dry, cyanotic Warm to cold
Bicarbonate deficit	2 mEq/kg	4 mEq/kg	8 mEq/kg

[a] Based on history of fluid loss.
[b] Mid-lumbar area.

C. The second formula will tend to underestimate serum osmolality during uremia or hyperglycemia.

V. Acid-base status may be measured directly or bicarbonate deficits may be estimated based on clinical examination and knowledge of the pathophysiology of the disease process (Tables 2-5 and 2-6).

VI. The anion gap represents the difference between the normally measured serum cation and anion concentrations. It is customarily calculated as $(Na^+ + K^+) - (Cl^- + HCO_3^-)$ with normal values ranging from 12 to 16 mEq/L. It may be used in the differentiation of the various causes of metabolic acidosis (Table 2-7).

TABLE 2-7.   DIFFERENTIATION OF VARIOUS CAUSES OF METABOLIC ACIDOSIS USING THE ANION GAP (AG)

Normal AG[a]	Increased AG
Diarrhea[b]	Ketoacidosis
Renal tubular acidosis[b]	Uremia
Early renal failure acidosis	Exogenous poisoning
Drugs	Salicylates
Acetazolamide[b]	Methanol
Acidifying agents (NH_4Cl)[b]	Paraldehyde
Hyperalimentation	Starvation
	Lactic acidosis

[a] Generally referred to as a hyperchloremic acidosis although a normal AG may occur without hyperchloremia in dilutional acidosis or dilutional hypernatremia.
[b] Associated with hypokalemia.

PRINCIPLES OF FLUID THERAPY

  I. Fluid therapy is divided into three phases:
      A. Replacement of deficits
      B. Replacement of continuing losses
      C. Providing maintenance requirements
 II. The type and degree of fluid and/or electrolyte disturbance is determined
     by history, physical examination, and laboratory tests.
III. Continuing or ongoing losses should be measured or accurately estimated
     and replaced during the course of therapy.
 IV. Fluids may be administered orally, intravenously or subcutaneously.
      A. In general, oral administration of fluids is recommended unless the
         animal is severely dehydrated, in shock, or has gastrointestinal dis-
         ease. Force feeding may be required when food and water are refused
         by animals not having gastrointestinal disturbances.
      B. Only nonirritating, isotonic solutions may be administered subcuta-
         neously. These solutions may safely contain more potassium than
         those administered intravenously. If dehydration is severe, rate of
         absorption from the subcutaneous tissues may be inadequate due to
         decreased peripheral circulation.
      C. The intravenous route will result in rapid and accurate correction of
         volume and electrolyte deficits. It is the method of choice for severe
         dehydration. Strict aseptic technique must be utilized in placement
         of intravenous catheters and the patient should be monitored for signs
         of sepsis or phlebitis. Catheters should be replaced every 48–72 hours.
  V. Replacement therapy corrects preexisting fluid volume, electrolyte def-
     icits, and acid-base disturbances.
      A. Volume deficits may be determined by changes in body weight if the
         animal's previous weight is known or by multiplying the clinically
         determined percent dehydration by the body weight in kilograms. As
         1 L of water weighs 1 kg, the fluid deficit in liters is easily determined.
      B. The appropriate fluid should be chosen based on the pathophysiologic
         alterations associated with the disease (Table 2-6).
      C. Acid-base abnormalities may be treated empirically (Table 2-7) or the
         acid-base status may be measured and sodium bicarbonate adminis-
         tered based on base excess according to the following formula:

      1. mEq HCO_3^- req. = Base excess $\times$ f $\times$ weight (kg)

      2. Base excess may be determined by using standard nomograms such
         as the Siggard-Andersen alignment nomogram.
      3. The diffusion constant (f) ranges from 0.3 to 0.6. The value used
         depends on patient age and duration of the disease process.
      4. The factor 0.3 is generally utilized and one half to two thirds of
         the bicarbonate deficit may be administered over a period of 30–

90 minutes with the remainder administered over the duration of replacement therapy.

   D. The rate of fluid administration for volume and electrolyte replacement depends on the severity of the condition.

      1. Rates up to 90 ml/kg/hr are acceptable in the initial treatment of shock. Length of time over which rapid rates are administered is generally determined by clinical signs of improvement.

      2. Where the degree of dehydration is not severe, fluid deficit may be corrected over a 24-hour period in addition to replacement of continuing losses and maintenance requirements. This generally results in a fluid administration rate of less than 10 ml/kg/hr when maintenance levels are included.

      3. Alternatively, two-thirds to three quarters of the deficit may be replaced over a 6-hour period at which time the patient is reevaluated. The remaining deficit should be adjusted accordingly and then replaced over the next 18 hours.

  VI. Continuing losses should be estimated and included in the daily maintenance requirement.

 VII. Maintenance fluid requirement is 40 ml/kg/24 hr and should be administered concurrently with replacement fluids. In some instances the subcutaneous route is satisfactory, particularly when the fluid deficit has been corrected and ongoing losses have stopped.

   A. Parenteral caloric supplementation is generally not required if the duration of therapy is less than 5 days.

   B. When the animal is able to maintain its own fluid and electrolyte balance orally, parenteral therapy is discontinued.

VIII. Monitoring of the cardiopulmonary and urinary system to evaluate response to therapy and to prevent complications associated with fluid and electrolyte therapy should be conducted on an ongoing basis.

   A. Serial laboratory tests should also be included in the monitoring regimen.

   B. Potential problems include circulatory overload, iatrogenic fluid and electrolyte imbalances, thrombophlebitis, pyrogenic reactions, and endocarditis.

  IX. Intraoperative fluid therapy should include replacement of maintenance fluid deficits incurred during the preoperative fasting period. This also includes replacement of fluid losses due to the primary disease process and the operative procedure.

   A. The severity of translocation of body fluid during surgery is determined by the type of surgery and the degree of surgical trauma.

   B. The greatest rate of translocation will occur during the first 2 or 3 hours of the procedure.

   C. While it is generally agreed that edema fluid accumulates at the operative site, there is no consensus as to the benefit of increasing the ECF volume in compensation.

   D. Intraoperatively, hypotonic solutions may be utilized to replace water deficits which occurred during the fasting period.
1. The amount given is equal to the number of hours without fluids times hourly maintenance requirements (1.7 ml/kg).
2. Isotonic solutions may be utilized for maintenance fluids at a rate of 2.0–10.0 ml/kg/hr depending upon the degree of trauma associated with the surgery.
3. Intraoperative blood losses should be accurately estimated and replaced with an isotonic solution at a volume of two to three times that of the blood loss.
4. If whole blood loss exceeds 20% of the blood volume, whole blood should be administered.

PRIMARY ELECTROLYTE IMBALANCES

Sodium

I. Sodium: Na^+; 1 mEq = 23 mg; normal plasma concentration = 140–156 mEq/L.
   A. Sodium is the primary extracellular cation and is the primary crystalloid involved in the maintenance of osmotic pressure. Sodium constitutes about 90% of the crystalloid osmotic pressure of the ECF. Electrolytes provide approximately 98% of ECF fluid osmolality.
   B. Sodium is involved in regulating ECF volume, the maintenance of cell membrane potential, and regulating transmission of nerve impulses, and is important in cell depolarization.
   C. Sodium and water requirements are generally met by dietary intake. While sodium may fluctuate on a daily basis, total body sodium content fluctuates very little over long periods.
   D. Sodium excretion is primarily accomplished by the kidney. Ninety percent of the sodium filtered at the glomeruli is passively reabsorbed.
1. Antidiuretic hormone (ADH) plays an important role in maintaining water balance and ultimately determines ECF osmolality. Osmolality of the ECF is increased by water loss or the gain of a solute. Increased tonicity is sensed by osmoreceptors and results in the release of ADH. The osmoreceptors respond to a change in tonicity of 1–2%. The primary effects of ADH are an increase in thirst and increased permeability to water in the renal distal convoluted tubules and collecting ducts to water. Release of ADH may also occur secondarily to baroreceptor stimulation. Hypotonic ECF results in a loss of water through the kidneys and reabsorption of sodium chloride. In addition, regulation of ECF tonicity is related to the ECF volume.

2. The primary determinant of the ECF volume is body sodium content which is regulated by the kidney through the effects of aldosterone. A decrease in blood volume and ultimately ECF volume is sensed by both the baroreceptors and the juxtaglomerular apparatus, resulting in the release of ADH and stimulation of the renin-angiotensin system. The subsequent release of aldosterone due to activation of the renin-angiotensin system increases reabsorption of sodium chloride and water in order to keep ECF isotonic.

E. Physiologic disturbances in fluid balance may occur from: (1) ECF volume depletion (isotonic loss), (2) ECF volume excess (isotonic gain), (3) hyponatremia (hypotonic gain or hypertonic loss), and (4) hypernatremia (hypertonic gain or hypotonic loss).

II. Hyponatremia (hypo-osmolality)

A. In general, hyponatremia will result in a decrease in tonicity of the ECF.

1. In diabetes mellitus, hyperlipidemia, and hyperproteinemia the ECF tonicity will either be normal or increased.

2. Vomiting or diarrhea, salt-wasting renal disease, and Addison's disease will result in hypovolemia and hyponatremia.

3. Hypervolemia and hyponatremia may be caused by acute renal failure, advanced congestive heart failure, or the nephrotic syndrome.

4. Appropriate or inappropriate ADH release, acute congestive heart failure, and glomerular nephritis may result in normovolemia and hyponatremia.

5. Hyperlipidemia will result in normovolemia and hyponatremia while diabetes mellitus and hyperproteinemia may result in either hypovolemia or normovolemia in conjunction with hyponatremia.

B. Hyponatremia exists when the serum sodium concentration is less than 135 mEq/L.

1. Clinical signs appear when the serum sodium concentration is 120 mEq/L or less and may include weakness, stupor or coma, vomiting, tachycardia, hypotension, decreased skin turgor, and cold extremities.

2. Seizures may occur when serum sodium is less than 102 mEq/L.

3. The electrocardiogram (EKG) may reveal a widened QRS complex with an elevated S-T segment. Ventricular tachycardia or fibrillation may occur when the serum sodium concentration is less than 100 mEq/L.

4. In addition to a thorough history and physical examination, a urinalysis and measurement of serum electrolyte concentrations and osmolality should be performed.

5. The patient's state of hydration should be determined in order to establish a rational therapeutic approach.

C. Identify and treat the underlying cause of hyponatremia first. If serum osmolality is normal, this may be all that is required.

    1. When the tonicity of the ECF is increased, the underlying cause must be corrected and isotonic fluids administered to expand the ECF volume.

    2. When the tonicity of the ECF is decreased, treatment depends on the degree of correction of patient hydration and the underlying cause.

    3. When hypovolemia exists, isotonic fluids should be given to expand the ECF volume. In addition to replacement fluids, maintenance fluids may also be required.

    4. When the ECF volume is normal or slightly increased, dilutional hyponatremia should be ruled out prior to treatment.

    5. Hypertonic saline solutions such as 3% sodium chloride may be utilized to replace sodium and chloride with a minimum of water when clinical signs of hyponatremia are severe. Three percent sodium chloride contains 520 mEq/L sodium and has a tonicity of 1,040 mOsm/L.

    6. The sodium deficit in mEq/L is equal to normal serum sodium concentration minus the actual serum sodium concentration times body weight in kilograms times 20%. Half of the sodium deficit may be corrected during the first 24 hours. Serum concentrations of sodium should be monitored during this time.

    7. If the clinical signs are not severe, restriction of water intake and treatment of the underlying cause may be sufficient. With marked increases in ECF volume, primary treatment of the sodium imbalance is unwarranted unless the hyponatremia is acute in onset and is severe.

III. Hypernatremia (hyperosmolality, dehydration)

    A. Hypernatremia is caused by a gain of sodium ions or, more commonly, the loss of water.

        1. Salt gain is uncommon but when it occurs it is generally iatrogenic in origin and is associated with the excessive administration of saline or hypertonic sodium bicarbonate solutions.

        2. With hypernatremia an increase in the ECF volume occurs due to a shift of water from the ICF space.

        3. Loss of water in excess of sodium loss from the body will result in a decrease in both the ECF and ICF volumes.

        4. Hypernatremia may be associated with diabetes insipidus, decreased water intake, increased insensible water loss (heat prostration, hyperventilation), chronic diabetes mellitus, or primary aldosteronism.

    B. Clinically, serum sodium concentrations above 160 mEq/L constitute hypernatremia.

        1. Clinical signs include lethargy, confusion, seizures, coma, muscle weakness, and myoclonus.

        2. The severity of clinical signs depends on the rate of onset and degree of hypernatremia. In severe hypernatremia, death may result from

neuronal dehydration. The underlying cause should be determined prior to treatment.

C. When the serum sodium concentration is less than 160 mEq/L, solute-free fluids may be administered orally. In more severe cases, fluids should be administered intravenously. While D5W alone may be effective, too rapid an administration may result in cerebral edema and convulsions.

   1. If dextrose solutions are used, they should be administered slowly over a period of 2–3 days, with frequent evaluations of the serum sodium concentration.

   2. Alternatively, one third of the water deficit may be replaced with a hypotonic saline solution (0.225 or 0.45%) over a 4-hour period. The remaining water deficit may be corrected over 2–3 days with D5W and normal maintenance fluids.

   3. Potassium should be added to these fluids to prevent hypokalemia.

   4. The volume of water necessary to return the serum sodium concentration to normal is as follows:

    a) Normal body water (L) = 0.6 × body weight (kg)

    b) Current volume body water

$$= \frac{\text{Normal serum } [Na^+] \times \text{normal body water}}{\text{Measured serum } [Na^+]}$$

    c) Body deficit = normal volume − current volume

POTASSIUM

I. Potassium: K^+; normal plasma concentration = 3.7–5.2 mEq/L

A. The primary intracellular cation, potassium is essential for transmission of nerve impulses, muscular function, maintenance of normal renal function, acid-base regulation, and the maintenance of intracellular tonicity.

B. While serum potassium represents only 1.5–2.5% of the total body potassium, a normal concentration is critical for normal neuromuscular and cardiac function.

C. Daily potassium intake is required as there is little body storage. Most commercial diets contain enough potassium to meet daily requirements. Daily requirement of potassium in the dog ranges from 1 to 2 mEq/kg.

   1. Precise regulation of the serum potassium concentration is accomplished by the kidney which eliminates up to 92% of the potassium excreted. The remaining 8% is lost through gastrointestinal excretion. Aldosterone promotes passive potassium secretion in exchange for active sodium reabsorption in the distal renal tubule. Increased tubular flow will also promote renal excretion of potassium.

   2. The serum potassium concentration is also influenced by the pa-

tient's acid-base status. This occurs as potassium is the predominant cation which moves in exchange for hydrogen across cell membranes. Acidosis increases the serum potassium concentration 0.6 mEq/L for each 0.1 unit decrease in pH while alkalosis has the opposite effect. Other factors which increase potassium movement intracellularly include increased circulating growth hormone, insulin, androgens, or catecholamines.

II. Hypokalemia

  A. Hypokalemia generally results from either an increased gastrointestinal loss or an increased urinary loss. In addition, hypokalemia will be present to some degree in both acute and chronic illnesses. Decreased serum potassium levels may occur in starvation as there is an obligatory renal loss of potassium or it may occur due to the excessive use of potassium-free intravenous fluids.

  1. Vomiting and diarrhea may cause major losses of potassium.
  2. Renal losses occur in renal tubular disorders such as the salt-wasting nephropathies or during recovery from acute renal necrosis. Diuresis through volume overload or the use of various diuretics such as the osmotic diuretics, the Henle loop blockers (furosemide, ethacrynic acid), the mecurials, or the thiazides will result in hypokalemia.
  3. Stress, including major surgery or the use of corticosteroids, increases urinary potassium excretion. Increased mineralocorticoid levels or hyperaldosteronism will result in retention of sodium and increased urinary losses of potassium.
  4. Hypokalemia, due to a shift of potassium intracellularly, will occur during alkalosis, alkali administration, or with hyperinsulinemia.

  B. Clinically, hypokalemia exists when the serum potassium concentration is less than 3.5 mEq/L. Clinical manifestations are not apparent until the serum concentration decreases below 3.0 mEq/L.

  1. Clinical signs are related mostly to neuromuscular dysfunction and include severe muscular weakness, muscular tenderness, and lethargy. Anorexia, vomiting, and decreased motility of the bowel may occur.
  2. As hypokalemia renders the tubular epithelium unresponsive to ADH, polydipsia/polyuria may occur.
  3. Cardiac dysrhythmias with increased myocardial sensitivity to digitalis will also be present. The EKG abnormalities appear when the serum potassium concentration decreases below 3.0 mEq/L. They include flattened or inverted T waves, depressed ST segments, prolonged PR intervals, tall P waves, and prolonged QRS intervals. Severe cardiac manifestations of hypokalemia include: sinus bradycardia, heart block, and A-V dissociation (Fig. 2-1).

  C. Prior to therapy renal and cardiac function should be assessed. As the true body deficit is unknown, and aggressive therapy may result in cardiotoxic levels of serum potassium, the serum potassium level

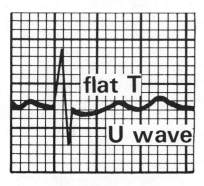
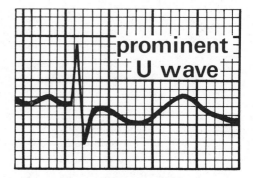

Moderate   Extreme

Fig. 2-1 Appearance of electrocardiogram in hypokalemia. Moderate hypokalemia, 3.5 mEq/L, will cause the T wave to flatten and a U wave will appear. With extreme hypokalemia, 2.5 mEq/L, the U wave becomes more prominent and the T wave disappears (Modified from Dubin D: Rapid Interpretation of EKG's. Cover Publishing, Tampa, FL, 1972.)

should be closely monitored. This is especially important if there is a concurrent volume deficit.

1. Generally, potassium supplementation should occur over 3–5 days to allow equilibration between the intracellular and extracellular pools.
2. Patients receiving parenteral maintenance fluids for prolonged periods should receive supplemental potassium. Potassium at a level of 35 mEq/L of fluid may be used for maintenance purposes.
3. Patients receiving diuretics, corticosteroids, or amphotericin B therapy should receive dietary potassium supplementation.
4. Potassium concentrations should be monitored in digitalized patients. It is generally agreed that the minimal acceptable serum potassium in digitalized patients for elective surgery is 3.5 mEq/L. In chronic hypokalemic patients 3.0 mEq/L is acceptable.
5. If acidosis is present with hypokalemia, then potassium acetate, potassium citrate, or potassium bicarbonate should be administered. Potassium chloride should be administered to alkalotic, hypokalemic patients.
6. Oral administration of potassium salts is recommended when hypokalemia is not life threatening.
   a) Therapy should extend over a minimum of 3 days to ensure replacement of the total body potassium deficit without inducing clinical signs of potassium toxicity.
   b) Gavage with commercial diets has been recommended as their potassium content is adequate for this purpose. Alternatively, oral potassium elixirs (Kay Ciel, potassium gluconate) containing 10% potassium chloride or gluconate may be utilized. These prepa-

rations contain 20 mEq potassium/15 ml fluid. In dogs, the daily
dose would be 5–15 mEq while in cats the dose is one half that
for dogs. To ensure palatability, these preparations should be diluted with three to four parts water.

   c) The serum potassium concentration should be monitored daily
and the dose adjusted by 4–8 mEq/day as required. Generally,
the dose will need to be increased. Potassium chloride enteric-
coated tablets should be avoided as they can result in small intestinal irritation or ulceration.

  7. Parenteral administration of potassium should be considered when
oral supplementation is not feasible or severe hypokalemia exists.
If vomiting or diarrhea prevents oral therapy, potassium may be
administered subcutaneously. Maintenance fluids containing up to
35 mEq/L potassium may be given subcutaneously without signs of
local irritation or systemic toxicity.

   a) Moderate hypokalemia with minimal EKG changes may be
treated using the following formula: patient's weight (kg) $\times$ 3 =
maximum dose (mEq) in a 24-hour period. One half of this calculated dose is administered intravenously in D5W over 12 hours.
The serum potassium concentration is then evaluated to assess
response and the remainder is given over the next 12 hours. The
serum potassium concentration is again measured with further
therapy depending on the current potassium deficit. If the serum
potassium concentration is normal, then all maintenance fluids
utilized should contain 35 mEq/L potassium.

   b) Severe hypokalemia (less than 2.0 mEq/L) is life-threatening. Potassium may be administered in D5W at a rate of 0.5 mEq/kg/hr
up to a maximum dose of 3 mEq/kg over 24 hours.

   c) In critical situations the potassium may be administered in isotonic saline due to the fact that D5W may actually decrease serum
potassium levels initially.

   d) The EKG should be used to monitor electrical activity of the heart
during potassium administration (Figs. 2-1 and 2-2). If the T wave
becomes isoelectric or slightly peaked, serum potassium should
be evaluated.

III. Hyperkalemia

  A. Hyperkalemia is not generally associated with an increase in total body
potassium even though the serum potassium concentration is increased.
Increased potassium intake rarely causes hyperkalemia if there is adequate renal function. Hyperkalemia does occur with acute renal failure
or oliguria. It is uncommon for hyperkalemia to occur in chronic renal
failure.

   1. Rapid cellular release of potassium may occur postoperatively, with
systemic acidosis, or catabolic states due to muscle trauma or extensive infections.

    2. Hyperkalemia also occurs in Addisonian crisis as a decreased aldosterone concentration results in the excretion of sodium and retention of potassium.

    3. Iatrogenic hyperkalemia may occur by overdosage with potassium salts or by the rapid administration of potassium penicillin G which contains 1.7 mEq K^+/1,000,000 U.

B. Hyperkalemia exists when the serum potassium concentration exceeds 5.5 mEq/L. Serum concentrations above 7.5 mEq/L are life-threatening and require immediate therapy.

    1. Clinical signs are primarily neuromuscular and cardiac in origin. As the serum potassium concentration reaches 6.5 mEq/L, myocardial contractility decreases, and there is a marked decrease in conduction velocity and a resultant bradycardia. At 7.0–8.0 mEq/L the EKG will reveal peaked T waves and a decrease in the size of the P waves. Over 8.0 mEq/L the P-R interval increases and the P wave disappears. The QRS complex gradually widens until it assumes a sine-wave appearance and A-V dissociation occurs (Fig. 2-2). Eventually asystole or ventricular fibrillation ensues.

    2. When serum potassium concentration reaches 8.0 mEq/L, skeletal muscle weakness results because of inability to repolarize. Hyporeflexia and paralysis are commonly associated with hyperkalemia although hyperreflexia has also been reported.

C. Hyperkalemia may be treated by increasing potassium loss from the body or by increasing the movement of potassium from serum into cells. Agents (such as calcium salts) that antagonize the cardiotoxic effects may be utilized in severe toxicity so as to allow time for more conventional treatment. The degree of hyperkalemia will dictate which therapeutic measure is chosen.

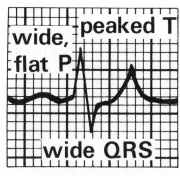
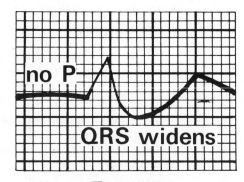

Moderate   Extreme

Fig. 2-2 Electrocardiographic changes observed in hyperkalemia. Increasing serum potassium concentration (6.0 mEq/L) will cause the P wave to become wide and flat and the T wave to become peaked. In extreme hyperkalemia (8.0 mEq/L) the P wave disappears and the QRS complex widens. (Modified from Dubin D: Rapid Interpretation of EKG's. Cover Publishing, Tampa, FL, 1972.)

1. A serum concentration greater than 7.5 mEq/L requires immediate therapy in addition to correction of the underlying cause.
2. If the hyperkalemia is not life threatening, correction of the underlying disease and diuresis may be sufficient.
3. If hyperkalemia accompanies severe acidosis, correction of the initiating cause and the acid-base status may result in hypokalemia. This is particularly true in diabetic ketoacidosis where the total body potassium is depleted despite the hyperkalemia. The serum potassium concentration should be monitored so that aggressive therapy does not result in hypokalemia.
4. Fluids: if the hyperkalemia is renal in origin, the cause should be determined and treated. If acidosis is not a problem, D5W or isotonic saline may be administered to correct the dehydration and to initiate and promote diuresis. Hypertonic saline may help to restore the rate of membrane polarization, in addition to having a dilutional effect.
5. Diuretics such as mannitol or furosemide may be administered to promote diuresis. Mannitol (25%) may be diluted with an equal volume of isotonic saline and 0.5–2.0 g/kg administered slowly intravenously. The maximum dose is 2.0 g/kg in 24 hours. If there is no effect in 1 hour, furosemide, 2 mg/kg, may be administered intravenously.
6. Correction of the bicarbonate deficit will result in an intracellular shift of potassium in exchange for hydrogen ions. The degree of acidosis correlates with the degree of dehydration with 2 mEq/kg, 4 mEq/kg, and 8 mEq/kg being used to correct the base deficit in minimal (4%), moderate (6–8%), or severe (10–12%) dehydration, respectively. Even if acidosis is not present, alkalinization of the blood may be used to treat hyperkalemia although it is not as effective as in acidotic states. Excessive or rapid administration of bicarbonate solutions may result in hyperosmolar states (40 mEq HCO_3^- equals 90 mOsm) or in paradoxical CSF acidosis.
7. Calcium antagonizes the myocardial toxic effects of potassium and allows time for other therapeutic measures. Calcium helps restore membrane potential. While its onset of action is rapid, its action is short-lived (0.5–1.5 hours). Calcium gluconate (10%) may be administered intravenously at a rate of 0.5–1.0 ml/kg over 5–10 minutes. The EKG should be monitored and calcium administration discontinued when the dysrhythmias disappear. If the dysrhythmias are still present after treatment, the dosage may be repeated after 5 minutes. Further use of calcium beyond this point is unlikely to be of benefit.
8. As potassium is a cofactor in the action of enzymes effecting the movement of glucose into cells, both the use of insulin and/or dextrose will result in a shift of potassium intracellularly. Dextrose 10% (D10W) alone may be infused slowly at a dose of 1.0 ml/kg body

weight, to prevent a hyperosmolar state occurring with rapid volume expansion. The osmolality of 10% dextrose (D10W) is 505 mOsm/L.

   a) One-half to 1.0 U regular insulin/kg may be administered in conjunction with 2.0–3.0 g dextrose/U insulin.

   b) Insulin and dextrose may be added to 1 L of potassium-free solution which is then administered to effect or to the point that 50% of the calculated dehydration is corrected within 3 hours. The remainder should be given over the next 24 hours. A response should be noticeable within 1 hour. It is unlikely that insulin-dextrose mixtures are more efficacious than the use of dextrose alone.

   c) To prevent hypoglycemia, dextrose should be infused for 8 hours after the administration of regular insulin.

9. Sulfonic acid exchange resins such as disodium polystyrene sulfonate may be administered orally or rectally to decrease the serum potassium concentration. If vomiting is not a problem 20–50 g/day may be administered orally in divided doses. If vomiting is a problem, 50 g may be diluted in 100 ml water and given as a high enema for a period of 30–45 minutes every 3–4 hours until serum potassium is less than 5.5 mEq/L. Theoretically, each gram of polystyrene sulfonate will bind 3 mEq of potassium, but practically it should be assumed that only 1 mEq is bound per gram of resin by exchanging sodium for potassium.

CALCIUM

I. Calcium: Ca^{2+}; normal plasma concentration = 7.0–11.0 mg/dl.

   A. Calcium is the fifth most abundant element in the body with over 90% contained in the bony structure. Calcium in bone is in a steady state of exchange with the calcium of the interstitial fluids.

   B. Calcium ensures the functional integrity of both the nervous and muscular tissues by regulating cell membrane permeability to sodium and potassium. It is also necessary for muscle contraction, blood coagulation, and capillary permeability.

   C. Fifty to 60% of serum calcium is bound to protein, primarily albumin. The physiologically active portion is nonprotein-bound and ionized. The serum ionized calcium is pH-dependent with alkalosis decreasing serum-ionized calcium levels. Total serum calcium content is serum protein-dependent as well. A change in total serum calcium concentration of approximately 0.8 mg/dl occurs for each 1.09 g/dl change in serum albumin levels.

   D. If vitamin D and parathormone levels are normal, daily calcium requirements are met by dietary intake. Glucocorticoids inhibit calcium uptake by the gut.

E. Calcium is excreted in the gastrointestinal tract, saliva, and through the kidney. Parathormone stimulates the reuptake of calcium by the kidney while calcitonin inhibits proximal tubular reabsorption.

II. Hypocalcemia may be caused by hypoparathyroidism, pseudohypoparathyroidism, acute pancreatitis, acute renal failure due to hyperphosphatemia, or during the transfusion of large volumes of citrated blood.

  A. It is, however, most commonly encountered clinically in eclampsia or puerperal tetany. Hypocalcemia will not occur during prolonged therapy with calcium-free fluids as bone acts as a reservoir or serum calcium.

  B. Signs of hypocalcemia occur when the serum concentration of calcium is less than 8.0 mg/dl in the dog and 7.0 mg/dl in the cat.

    1. With hypoalbuminemia, total serum calcium may be decreased but the ionized fraction may be normal, resulting in the absence of clinical signs of hypocalcemia. When albumin concentrations are abnormal, the corrected calcium value is equal to the calcium concentration minus the albumin concentration plus 3.5.

    2. Clinical signs of hypocalcemia are a direct result of a decreased threshold of excitability resulting in neuromuscular irritability leading to spontaneous discharge of nerve impulses causing tetany or convulsions. Paresthesia and muscle cramps may also occur.

    3. Hypocalcemia causes a prolonged action potential with an increase in the QT and ST segments of the EKG (Fig. 2-3).

    4. Hyperkalemia potentiates the cardiac and neuromuscular irritability associated with hypocalcemia and vice versa.

  C. Acute hypocalcemia requires immediate therapy. The use of calcium salts is indicated when hypocalcemic tetany is present. Calcium glu-

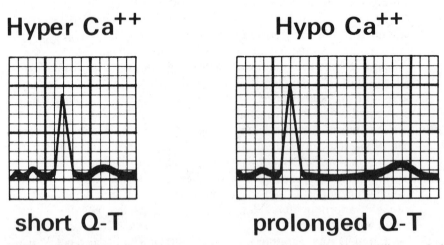

Hyper Ca^{++} # Hypo Ca^{++}

short Q-T   ## prolonged Q-T

Fig. 2-3. Effects of deviation of serum calcium concentration on the electrocardiogram. In hypercalcemia the QT interval is shortened while it is lengthened in hypocalcemia. (Modified from Dubin D: Rapid Interpretation of EKG's. Cover Publishing, Tampa, FL, 1972.)

conate (10%) or calcium chloride (10%) are the most commonly used agents.

1. Calcium chloride preparation is a more irritating and acidifying salt and in some instances may cause hypotension.
2. Calcium gluconate may be administered intravenously, after being warmed to body temperature, at a rate of 0.5–1.5 ml/kg (50–150 mg/kg) over 20–30 minutes. The infusion should be stopped if bradycardia develops.
3. Prolonged therapy following treatment of an acute crisis involves infusion of 10.0–15.0 ml/kg over a 24-hour period.
4. Renal function should be assured and the serum calcium concentration should be monitored in order to prevent a rebound hypercalcemia.
5. Calcium salts should not be added to fluid containing bicarbonate, phosphate, or citrated blood because of incompatibility (Table 2-4).
6. As calcium potentiates the effects of digitalis, it should be administered with caution in digitalized patients.
7. Long-term therapy of asymptomatic hypocalcemia includes correction of the initiating factor and increasing gastrointestinal absorption of calcium by increasing dietary calcium and vitamin D. Calcium lactate may be added to the diet at a rate of 0.5–2.0 g/day for the dog and 0.2–0.5 g/day for the cat. Vitamin D may be supplemented orally in dogs at a rate of 70–175 IU daily for 1 week and then twice weekly thereafter.

III. Hypercalcemia is unlikely to occur due to increased intake as long as renal function is normal.

A. It rarely occurs in cats but is diagnosed in the dog, especially in hyperparathyroidism or secondary to renal failure.
   1. Pseudohyperparathyroidism secondary to lymphosarcoma will also induce hypercalcemia as will osteolytic metastasis of malignant neoplasms.
   2. Disuse atrophy may occasionally result in hypercalcemia, especially after trauma to large body surface areas.
   3. Eventually, renal failure will occur if hypercalcemia is not corrected.

B. Clinical signs of hypercalcemia occur when the serum concentration is above 12.0 mg/dl. An increased serum calcium concentration results in an increased threshold for excitability of contractile tissue.
   1. Signs may include anorexia, vomiting, constipation, polyuria/polydipsia, dehydration, and muscular weakness.
   2. Rapid increases of serum calcium above 15.0 mg/dl may cause vagal stimulation leading to extreme bradycardia and/or cardiac arrest.
   3. Electrocardiographic signs of hypercalcemia include bradycardia and variable effects on the ST segment (Fig. 2-3).
   4. As hypercalcemia is associated with neoplastic disorders, an extensive workup ruling out such disorders is required.

C. Of paramount importance in the treatment of hypercalcemia is rehydration of the patient. Then one may increase renal excretion of calcium or increase deposition in bone or soft tissues in order to reduce serum calcium concentration.
   1. Isotonic saline or 0.45% saline may be used for rehydration and to enhance renal calcium excretion. Saline will promote diuresis and reduce tubular reabsorption of calcium through competitive inhibition by sodium reabsorption. Saline is infused at a rate of 80–120 ml/kg/day as long as there is adequate cardiovascular and renal function.
      a) Monitoring will prevent fluid overload.
      b) Once volume replacement is complete, a diuretic agent (furosemide 3–5 mg/kg, BID) may be used to further enhance diuresis. Electrolyte concentrations should be monitored and if hypokalemia occurs, potassium should be added to the fluids.
      c) If hypernatremia occurs, the saline infusion should be stopped.
   2. Isotonic sodium sulfate contains 38.9 g sodium sulfate decahydrate per liter and may be infused IV to further enhance calcium diuresis. The sulfate anion further inhibits tubular reabsorption of calcium. As the infusion of sodium sulfate will result in hypokalemia, potassium should be added to the IV fluids. Sodium sulfate may be infused at similar rates to which saline is infused as long as cardiac and renal function are normal. As isotonic sodium sulfate is hypertonic with respect to sodium, serum sodium levels should be monitored in order to prevent iatrogenic hypernatremia. Sodium sulfate is not now presently available in injectable form and solutions must be prepared from the dry salt.
   3. Prednisolone has been used at a dose of 2–3 mg/kg BID to decrease the serum calcium concentration in patients with pseudohyperparathyroidism associated with lymphoma.
   4. As ethylenediaminetetraacetic acid (EDTA) may result in serious renal toxicity, it should only be used in acute, life-threatening situations when the serum calcium concentration reaches 20mg/dl. Ethylenediaminetetraacetic acid combines with ionized calcium to form a soluble complex which is excreted by the kidney. Sodium EDTA is infused at a rate of 25–75 mg/hr. Serum calcium concentration should be closely monitored.

MAGNESIUM

I. Magnesium: Mg^{2+}; normal plasma concentration = 1.5–2.5 mg/dl
   A. One third is bound to protein and the remainder exists as free ions. Magnesium is a cofactor for adenosine triphosphate (ATP) enzyme reactions involved in phosphate transfer. It is associated with calcium ion movement and cellular distribution.

B. Clinically, magnesium deficiency appears similar to and is often associated with hypocalcemia. Hypomagnesemia may accompany hypokalemia and thus contribute to digitalis toxicity. The incidence of hypomagnesemia in dogs and cats is not extremely high but it does occur.
   1. Clinical signs of magnesium deficiency include neuromuscular excitation, convulsions, and cardiac dysrhythmias.
   2. Electrocardiogram alterations are similar to those associated with hypercalcemia (Fig. 2-3).
   3. Ventricular tachycardia, resistant to therapy with potassium, lidocaine, procainamide, and phenytoin has been treated successfully with intravenous magnesium sulfate.
C. Treatment is with magnesium sulfate solution intravenously or intramuscularly. Dosage will depend on magnitude of deficiency but generally ranges from 5 to 15 ml of 25% magnesium sulfate given over a period of 1–2 hours. Calcium gluconate should be readily available to counteract magnesium intoxication should overdosage occur.
D. Hypermagnesemia is most commonly encountered in association with advanced renal disease or as a complication of magnesium sulfate therapy.
   1. Clinical signs include drowsiness, muscular weakness, hypotension bradycardia, and increased electrocardiographic Q-T interval as with hypocalcemia.
   2. Cardiac arrest is likely when serum concentration reaches 7–8 mmol/L. Preceding cardiac arrest, neuromuscular activity is affected because of impaired acetylcholine release.
   3. Even with paralysis of the extremities, the diaphragm continues to support limited breathing.
E. Treatment consists of respiratory support (i.e., positive pressure ventilation) and administration of calcium gluconate, or as an alternative, glucose-potassium-insulin to promote intracellular shift of magnesium.

SUGGESTED READINGS

Brobst D: Pathophysiologic and adaptive changes in acid-base disorders. J Am Vet Med Assoc 183:773, 1983

Clark DR, Adams HR: Symposium on circulatory shock. J Am Vet Med Assoc 175:77, 1979

Muir WW, DiBartola SP: Fluid therapy. p. 28. In Kirk RW (ed): Current Veterinary Therapy, VIII. WB Saunders, Philadelphia, 1983

Polzin DJ, Stevens JB, Osborne CA: Clinical application of the anion gap in evaluation of acid-base disorders in dogs and cats. Compend Contin Ed 12:1021, 1982

3

Antimicrobial Drugs and Infectious Diseases

Richard B. Ford, D.V.M.
Arthur L. Aronson, D.V.M.

GENERAL PRINCIPLES

HOST-AGENT-ENVIRONMENT INTERACTION

An animal, as host to a known disease-producing agent, will respond with some degree of predictability to that infection. However, other factors capable of altering a patient's response to infection must be taken into consideration during the course of therapy.

I. Host factors

  A. Age

    Morbidity and mortality rates of infectious diseases are highest among the very young and the very old.

  B. Immunologic responsiveness

    Although immunologic responsiveness is difficult to measure quantitatively, it can easily be attenuated pharmacologically, e.g., cancer chemotherapy, long-term corticosteroid therapy.

  C. Genetics

    Although difficult to document, it is possible that a genetic predisposition to become infected and to develop clinical signs of disease exists among certain breeds.

  D. Concurrent disease

    Primary or secondary disease, either occult of overt, must be considered in the clinical management of any patient. The ability of one infection to predispose the host to a second infection is well recognized as a determinant factor in the outcome of any disease.

II. Agent factors

  The ability of an organism to produce signs of disease will depend, at least in part, on the virulence of that organism, the route of exposure and the amount (concentration of agent in the host's environment) of exposure.

III. Environmental factors

   The environment in which the host was housed at the time of exposure, the time that signs developed, and the environment in which the host is treated significantly affect the outcome of an infectious disease. Population density, frequency of animal interchange, sanitation, temperature, humidity, and air exchange are significant environmental factors to be considered in the management of any infected patient.

TREATMENT CONSIDERATIONS

   Successful therapeutic management of an infection cannot be determined by antimicrobial therapy alone. Several factors must be considered first.

   I. Lesion management

   Routine wound cleaning, delayed surgical closure, foreign body removal, drainage of abscesses, relief of obstruction are among the primary concerns of managing infection. Attempts to manage advanced local or regional infections with antimicrobial drug therapy alone is inappropriate and associated with a higher incidence of treatment failure.

   II. Supportive care measures

   Monitoring caloric, water and electrolyte needs, urination, defecaton, exercise, development of decubitus, and sanitation, are essential and treatment should be vigorously applied as appropriate.

   III. Predisposing factors

   Hyperadrenocorticism, severe periodontal disease and cancer, must be seriously considered in the overall management in order to prevent a relatively mild infection from becoming a fatal infection.

ANTIMICROBIAL DRUG THERAPY

   Should be considered as supplemental to the host's natural defence mechanisms. Hence, procedures described above, i.e., supportive care and lesion management are of primary concern. These procedures also will facilitate distribution of an antimicrobial drug to the site of infection and create an optimal environment for the drug to exert its antimicrobial effect. Consider that three fundamental conditions must be met for an antimicrobial drug to be clinically effective:

   I. Bacterial sensitivity

   The infecting organism must be sensitive to the drug. Sensitivity tests are especially important for organisms showing considerable variation in sensitivity, e.g., *Staphylococcus*, coliforms, enterococci, *Proteus*, *Pseudomonas*, and *Salmonella*. The Kirby-Bauer test currently is most commonly employed, but quantitative measurements of minimum inhibitory concentration (MIC) and minimum bactericidal concentration (MBC) are being employed with increasing frequency in veterinary hospitals.

II. Drug distribution.

    Distribution to the site of infection in adequate concentration following drug administration is the pharmacokinetic phase. An infectious process can enhance, but usually impedes, drug distribution.

    A. Enhanced distribution

        Penicillin G will cross inflamed meninges more readily than normal meninges.

    B. Decreased distribution

        Can occur because of edema or fibrinous and purulent material associated with an infectious process.

III. Environmental conditions

    Environmental conditions must be favorable at the site of infection for drug action (pharmacodynamic phase). Drug action can be adversely affected by:

    A. Slowing bacterial growth

        Conditions in purulent material may not support rapid bacterial growth which is necessary for the action of penicillins and cephalosporins.

    B. Binding the drug

        Aminoglycosides and polymyxins bind markedly to intracellular constituents present in purulent material.

    C. Degrading the drug

        Penicillin G has been shown to be rapidly degraded in samples of intracranial pus.

    D. Interaction with metals

        Calcium can antagonize the action of aminoglycosides and polymyxins against *Pseudomonas aeruginosa*. This is the basis for incorporating complexing agents in certain topical preparations.

    E. pH

        The action of drugs that must cross the cell membrane to exert their effect intracellularly (inhibitors of intermediary metabolism and protein and nucleic acid synthesis) can be markedly affected by changes in pH. Weak acids, including nitrofurantoin, novobiocin and tetracyclines (acidic isoelectic point), are increasingly effective as pH decreases. Weak bases, including aminoglycosides and macrolides, are increasingly effective as pH increases.

IV. Clearly, procedures described under lesion management and supportive care will not only maximize drug distribution to the site of infection, but also will improve the environment in which the drug exerts its antimicrobial effect.

SELECTION OF AN ANTIMICROBIAL DRUG

    The following points should be kept in mind when considering the pharmacology of antimicrobial drugs.

I. The organism must be sensitive to the drug

Unless complicated by bacterial infection, viral infections (e.g., feline leukemia virus) are not treated with antibacterial drugs. The only possible exception to this is the treatment of infectious tracheobronchitis in dogs; there is some evidence that certain viruses associated with ITB are susceptible to tetracyclines.

II. Rapidity in instituting therapy

Culture and sensitivity tests generally require 2 to 3 days. However, newer technology is reducing this time to slightly over one day. Is the risk of withholding therapy (until culture and sensitivity is known) greater than the risk of starting therapy with an inappropriate drug? If not life-threatening, it may be better to wait.

III. Route of administration

Consider the iv route in hypotension or serious infections. Oral, im, or sc routes are safer and thus preferable in less demanding circumstances.

IV. Bactericidal drugs are generally superior, especially if immunologic deficiency exists or if steroids are being used concurrently.

V. Duration of therapy

The treatment of acute, uncomplicated infections (e.g., bacterial cystitis) should be discontinued only if the patient has been afebrile and free of clinical signs for 72 hours. Chronic bacterial infections (e.g., bacterial endocarditis) may require several weeks of therapy for adequate control.

PHARMACOLOGY OF ANTIMICROBIAL DRUGS

CLASSIFICATION

I. General comments
   A. Classification is according to site and/or mechanism of action. This classification:
      1. Facilitates grouping of bactericidal and bacteriostatic drugs, and
      2. Facilitates rational selection of combinations of antimicrobial drugs in those instances where they are indicated. Combinations which include an inhibitor of cell wall synthesis (e.g., carbenicillin or ticarcillin) with a bactericidal inhibitor of protein synthesis (e.g., gentamicin or amikacin) have proven effective in difficult infections due to gram-negative organisms (e.g., *Pseudomonas* infections).
II. Inhibitors of cell wall synthesis (includes penicillins, cephalosporins, bacitracin and vancomycin)
III. Labilizers of cell membranes (includes polymyxins, amphotericin B, ketoconazole)
IV. Bactericidal inhibitors of protein synthesis (includes aminoglycosides)
V. Bacteriostatic inhibitors of protein synthesis (includes chloramphenicol, tetracyclines, macrolides and lincosamides)

VI. Inhibitors of nucleic acid synthesis (includes nalidixic acid, griseofulvin, ketoconazole and metronidazole)
VII. Inhibitors of intermediary metabolism (antimetabolites and inhibitors of electron transport) (includes nitrofurans, sulfonamides, and hydroxyquinolines)
VIII. Dosage information and pharmacokinetic data for antimicrobials in the dog and cat, compiled by the Clinical Pharmacology Studies Unit, University of Illinois, constitutes Table 3-1.

INHIBITORS OF CELL WALL SYNTHESIS

Penicillins

I. General comments
   A. The penicillins as a group remain among the most effective and least toxic (except for hypersensitivity reactions) of antimicrobial drugs.
   B. Penicillin G still is indicated more commonly than any other antimicrobial agent and it is the least expensive.
II. Chemistry
   A. The penicillins are weak acids, pKAs around 2.7 and they are moderately lipid soluble.
   B. Units of penicillin G
      1. 1 unit = 0.6 μg Na penicillin G; 0.627 μg K penicillin G
      2. 1 mg Na penicillin G = 1667 units; 1 mg K penicillin G = 1595 units; 1 mg procaine penicillin G = 1009 units
      3. 1 million units of Na penicillin G weighs 0.6 grams. This dose will provide 1.7 mEq. or 38.7 mg Na. May be an important consideration if patient suffers from Na retention.
      4. 1 million units of K penicillin G weighs 0.627 grams. This dose will provide 1.7 mEq. K or 65.8 mg K. May be an important consideration if patient suffers cardiac dysfunction.
   C. Isolation of the 6-aminopenicillanic acid (6-APA) nucleus provided for the synthesis of semisynthetics that, relative to penicillin G, can enhance:
      1. Resistance to destruction by gastric acidity
      2. Resistance to β-lactamase
      3. Antibacterial spectrum against gram-negative organisms
III. Mechanism of action and spectrum of activity
   A. Penicillins and cephalosporins act as structural analogues of D-alanyl-D alanine, an essential metabolite for cell wall synthesis.
   B. In growing and dividing bacteria, a defective cell wall results as a consequence of failure of transpeptidation reactions.
   C. The defective cell wall renders the bacteria susceptible to osmotic lysis.

TABLE 3-1. DOSAGE INFORMATION AND PHARMACOKINETIC DATA FOR ANTIMICROBIALS IN THE DOG AND CAT (CLINICAL PHARMACOLOGY STUDIES UNIT, UNIVERSITY OF ILLINOIS)

	Route	Percent Absorbed Orally	Suggested Dosage Range (mg/kg)	Dosage Interval	$T_{\frac{1}{2}}$	V'd (L/kg)	CL_T ml/kg/min	Plasma Concentration Needed for MIC of Susceptible Organisms (μg/ml)	Cost[d] of 1 Days Therapy	Urine Concentrations Achieved (μg/ml)
K+ and Na+ Penicillin G.	IM, IV		20,000–40,000 u/kg	q 6 h	30.0 min (dog)	0.156	3.6	≤0.12		294
Procaine Penicillin G.	IM, SQ		22,000 u/kg[a]	q 12 h	30.0 min	0.156	3.6	≤0.12		
Ampicillin Trihydrate	IM, SQ		10–50 (dog)	q 6–8 h (dog)	30–60 min (dog)	.270–.400 (dog)	3.87–7.74 (dog)	≤1.0	2.00–4.00	
Na+ Ampicillin	IM, IV		10–20 (cat)	q 8–12 h (cat)	73 min (cat)	0.166 (cat)	1.57 (cat)		13.20–26.40	
Ampicillin (oral)	Oral	50 (dog) 18–42 (cat)							0.45–0.80	309.0
Amoxicillin (Amoxi drops)	Oral	80	11–22	q 8 h–q 12 h	60–90 min	0.20	1.54–231	≤1.0	0.50–1.05	201
(Amoxi tabs)	Oral	80	11–22	q 8 h–q 12 h						
Carbenicillin (Geocillin)	Oral		15–50[b]	q 6 h–q 8 h	60–90 min	0.18–0.20	1.46–2.21	≤32.0	2.25–4.50	
(Pyopen)	Inject								5.00–10.00	
Hetacillin (Hetacin-K)	Oral		as for Ampicillin						2.25–4.00	300
Methicillin	IV, IM		20–40	q 4 h–q 6 h	30 min	0.20	4.62	0.12–2.0	5.60–11.00	
Oxacillin (Prostaphlin)	IM		7	q 8 h	30 min	0.30	6.93			
	Oral	50	8–15							
Cloxicillin	IM		10	q 6 h	30 min	0.20	4.62			
Dicloxicillin	Oral	50–85	10–25	q 8 h	40 min	0.20[f]	3.465		1.20–1.95	
Dicloxin			11–55							
Cephalothin (Keflin)	IM, IV SQ		15–35	q 6–8 h	42–51 min	.435	5.9–7.18	≤8.0	10.90–14.40	
Cefoxitin (Mefoxin)	IM, IV		6–40	q 4–6 h	40 min	0.20[f]	3.46	≤8.0		
Cephradine (Velosef)	Oral IM, IV	70–90	12 6–25	q 6 h	84 min	.334	2.7		2.80	
Cefamandole (Mandol)	IM, IV	60–70	15	q 4–6 h	30–54 min	0.30	3.3	≤8.0		
Cephalexin (Keflex)	Oral	94–98	8–30	q 6–8 h	80–165 min	.274	1.15–2.4		2.40–6.93	805

Drug	Route	(%)	Dose (mg/kg)	Interval	Half-life			MIC (≤)		Cost[d]
Cephapirin (Cefadyl)	IM, IV		30	q 4–6 h	25 min	0.32	8.87			
Cephaloridine (Loridine)	IM, SQ		10–15	q 8 h	72–106	0.20	1.13–1.93			
Cefazolin (Ancef) (Kefzol)	IM	80	15–25	q 6–8 h	48–90 min	0.70	10.1–5.39			
Gentamicin	IM, IV SQ		2–4	q 6–8 h	52–76 min	.30–.35	3.00–4.39	≤4.0	3.84–7.68	107
Kanamycin (Kantrim)	IV, IM, SQ		5–15	q 6, 8, 12 h	42–58.9 min	0.225–0.280	2.96–4.17		1.30–3.90	530
Streptomycin	IM, SQ		11	q 6, 8, 12 h	2.5 hr	0.20	0.924			
Sulfisoxazole	Oral		50	q 8 h	4.5 hr	0.300	0.770			1466
Sulfadiazine	Oral		110	q 12 h	3.9 hr					
Tobramycin	IM, SQ			q 8 h	1.5–2.2 hr	0.26	1.36–2.00	≤4.0		66
Amikacin	IV, IM, SQ		5	q 8 h	51 min	0.23[f]	3.125	≤16.0	21.51	342
Trimethoprim-Sulfadiazene (Tribrissen)	Oral SQ		5 TMP[e] 25 SDZ	q 12 h	TMP = 2.51 hr SDZ = 9.84 hr	TMP = 1.49 SDZ = 1.02	TMP = 6.86 SDZ = 1.20		0.80	26 (TMP) 79 (SDZ)
Chloramphenicol	Oral IM, IV	70–75	40–50	q 6–8 h (dog) q 8–12 h (cat)	4.2 hr (dog) 5.1 (cat)	1.77 (dog) 2.36 (cat)	4.87 (dog) 5.34 (cat)	≤8.0		123.0
Tetracycline	Oral, IM IV	77	Oral = 25 4.4–11	q 6–8 h q 8–12 h	5–6 hr	1.20–1.30	2.41–2.89	≤1.0	0.20	138
Oxytetracycline	IV		10 (Prime) 7.5 (Maint.)	q 12 h	6.02 hr	2.096	4.23			
Doxycycline	Oral	90–100		q 12 h	10 hr	0.9–1.8	1.04–2.08			
Erythromycin	Oral	60	5–20	q 8 h	60–90 min	2.0	15.4–23.1	≤0.5	.30–.45	
Tylosin (Tylocine)	IM		6.6–11.0	q 12 h–q 24 h	54 min	1.7	22.0		0.40–0.60	
Lincomycin (Lincocin)	Oral IM		15–25 (Oral) 10 (IM)	q 12 h q 12 h	5 hr[f]	0.49[f]	1.13		0.50–1.00	
Clindamycin	Oral, IM		10	q 12 h	14.5 hr	5.78	4.60	≤0.5		

[a] Penicillin G, dose may go as high as 80,000 u/kg daily. Higher doses required for *Actinomyces* infections. (100,000–200,000 u/kg IM daily.

[b] Carbenicillin, 15–50 mg/kg is the dose recommended for urinary infection. Severe systemic infections require much higher dose, 100–150 mg/kg for systemic infection. Use with gentamicin when treating *Pseudomonas*.

[c] 25–100 mg/ml needed for *Pseudomonas*.

[d] Cost based on 1 day of therapy for a 15 kg dog. Prices are based on the prices charged to client at University of Illinois pharmacy as of July 1, 1983.

[e] TMP/SDZ dose should be doubled for *Nocardia* infection.

[f] These values are only estimates. Dog and cat pharmacokinetic data are not available.

IV. Physiologic disposition of penicillins
   A. The absorption varies with the penicillin and the salt. See individual drugs.
   B. Distribution generally is limited to extracellular fluids, and these include joint and wound fluids. Distribution into ocular and cerebrospinal fluids is poor, except when the meninges are inflamed.
   C. Binding to plasma proteins is generally moderate, but it is high (95%) for oxacillin, cloxacillin and dicloxacillin.
   D. Serum half-lives range from 30 to 60 minutes.
   E. Biotransformation is minimal; less than 10% of a dose is degraded to penicilloic acid.
   F. Excretion is mainly renal and tubular secretion is prominent. Serum half-lives may increase to several hours if renal insufficiency exists. Concentrations in bile are greater than in serum; this route increases in importance in renal insufficiency.
 V. Potential adverse drug reactions
   A. Hypersensitivity reactions may range from urticaria, pruritis, wheals to acute anaphylaxis characterized by salivation, dyspnea and collapse (treat with epinephrine).
   B. Guinea pigs and hamsters develop fatal diarrhea at doses which are therapeutic in other species.
   C. Concentrations of penicillin G in excess of 10 μg/ml in CSF can produce convulsions, but these are reversible.
   D. Methicillin is occasionally nephrotoxic in human patients.
   E. Care must be exercised that procain penicillin G is not injected intravenously; pulmonary embolism can result.
VI. Examples of beta-lactamase (penicillinase)-sensitive penicillins.
   A. Penicillin G
      1. Is effective against most gram-positive organisms (except penicillinase-producing staphylococci) and many gram-negative organisms at high concentrations (as obtained in urine at conventional doses).
      2. The procaine ester can be given either im or sc
      3. The benzathine ester will produce serum concentrations for one to two weeks, but high enough only for the most sensitive organisms.
      4. Although considerable degradation occurs at gastric pH (about 50%), the Na or K salt may be given orally for urinary tract infections.
   B. Phenoxymethyl penicillin (penicillin V)
      1. Same spectrum as penicillin G, but more reliable absorption following oral administration because of resistance to destruction by gastric acid
      2. Is generally used after another penicillin has been given parenterally
   C. Ampicillin
      1. An extended-spectrum penicillin active against several gram-neg-

ative organisms including (non-penicillinase producing) *E. coli, Shigella* spp. and *Proteus mirabilis*

    2. Available as the Na or trihydrate salt. Although prolonged concentrations result from giving the trihydrate, they are sufficient only for the most sensitive organisms.

D. Hetacillin

    A formulation of ampicillin designed to enhance its bioavailability following oral administration. Hetacillin is hydrolyzed to ampicillin and acetone in body fluids.

E. Amoxicillin

    Antimicrobial spectrum is similar to ampicillin, but it is more readily absorbed and it persists for a longer time period in the body. Food decreases absorption less prominently than in the case of ampicillin.

F. Carbenicillin and ticarcillin

    1. These extended-spectrum penicillins are active against *Pseudomonas* spp. and *Proteus vulgaris*, especially when given concurrently with an aminoglycoside.

    2. Ticarcillin can be given at about one-half the dose of carbenicillin in pseudomonas infections because it is more active against this organism. This can be a marked advantage if excess Na load could compromise the patient.

VII. Examples of beta-lactamase (penicillinase)—resistant penicillins

A. These include methicillin and the isoxazolyl group (oxacillin, cloxacillin and dicloxacillin).

B. Use only for infections due to penicillinase-producing staphylococci.

VIII. New developments with the penicillin group of drugs.

A. The ureidopenicillins, including piperacillin, mezlocillin and azlocillin, have greater activity against gram-negative organisms, especially Pseudomonas.

B. Efforts are being made to incorporate clavulanic acid, a potent inhibitor of beta-lactamases, into preparations of ampicillin and amoxicillin. If successful, the efficacy of these drugs against beta-lactamase producing bacteria would be markedly enhanced.

Cephalosporins and Cephamycins

I. General comments

A. Are beta-lactam antibiotics, closely related to penicillins with respect to chemistry, mechanism of action, physiologic disposition and toxicity.

    1. An important difference in distribution may be penetration of cephalosporins into the CSF is undependable, even with inflamed meninges.

    2. Biotransformation of cephalothin and cephapirin occurs; the metabolites have about one-half the activity of the parent compound.

    B. Positive features relative to the penicillins include:
       1. Greater resistance to inactivation by beta-lactamases produced by staphylococcus and many gram-negative organisms.
       2. Sometimes can be given to patients allergic to penicillins.
       3. Often more effective against *Klebsilla.*
    C. Generally more expensive than penicillins. Except for the above three reasons, cephalosporins usually not used as first-line drugs.
    D. Usually classified as first-, second-, and third generation cephalosporins, cephamycins and 1-oxacephalosporins.
       1. Generation is determined by activity against microorganisms, especially gram-negative organisms.
       2. All clinically useful cephalosporins are semisynthetic being derived from 7-aminocephalosporanic acid (7-ACA).
       3. A total of four sites for chemical modification on the 7-ACA nucleus are possible; consequently, the opportunity for development of new drugs is greater than is the case for penicillins (only one site for chemical modification).
  II. First-generation cephalosporins
    A. Antibacterial spectrum includes gram-positive cocci including many beta-lactamase-producing staphylococci, *E. coli, Salmonella, Shigella, Proteus* and *Klebsiella.*
    B. Because of cost, first-generation cephalosporins will likely have more use in veterinary medicine than second- and third generation cephalosporins.
    C. Examples suitable for oral administration include cephalexin, cephadroxil, cephradine and cefaclor.
    D. Examples suitable for parenteral administration include cephalothin, cephazolin, cephradine and cephapirin.
 III. Second-generation cephalosporins
    A. Antibacterial spectrum includes gram-negative rods resistant to first-generation drugs.
    B. Examples suitable for parenteral administration include cefamandole, cefotiam, cefuroxime, ceforanide and cefoxitin (a cephamycin).
 IV. Third-generation cephalosporins
    A. Enhanced antibacterial activity, increased resistance to beta-lactamases and increased effectiveness against *Pseudomonas aeruginosa* and *Haemophilus influenzae*
    B. Examples suitable for parenteral administration include cefotaxime, cefoperazone, cefmenoxime, cefsulodin and moxalactam (the latter is actually a 1-oxacephalosporin).
       1. Moxalactam has the widest antibacterial spectrum of all current beta-lactam antibiotics;
       2. Excellent activity reported for moxalactam against *Pseudomonas aeruginosa.* Wide spectrum of activity may decimate the intestinal

flora, including vitamin K-producing microorganisms. Supplemental vitamin K should be considered to minimize a reported side effect of bleeding.

Vancomycin

  I. Principal use is for staphylococcal infections that respond to nothing else.
 II. Chemistry
     A. Obtained from *Streptomyces orientalis*, structure unknown
     B. Highly water soluble
III. Mechanism of action—prevents formation of the linear peptidoglycan in cell wall synthesis.
 IV. Physiologic disposition
     A. Absorption
        1. Not absorbed following oral administration; give orally for staphylococcal enterocolitis
        2. Preparations are available for parenteral administration
     B. Distribution
        1. Limited to extracellular fluid following iv administration
        2. Binding to serum proteins about 10%
     C. Excretion—mainly renal
  V. Potential adverse reactions—ototoxic and nephrotoxic potential is high

LABILIZERS OF CELL MEMBRANES

Polymyxins

  I. General comments
     A. Used to be major drugs against pseudomonas infections. The advent of newer aminoglycosides, penicillins and cephalosporins has diminished this indication markedly.
     B. Must be used with great care if renal dysfunction.
     C. Potential for nephrotoxicity and respiratory paralysis is high.
     D. Polymyxin B reported to bind endotoxin, but the clinical significance is not established.
     E. Useful for "bowel sterilization", and peritoneal lavage (care must be exercised with dose since polymyxins are absorbed well from the peritoneal cavity).
 II. Chemistry
     A. Several polymyxins (named A, B, C, D, E and M) have been isolated from *Bacillus polymyxa*.
     B. Two have been used clinically
        1. Polymyxin B
        2. Polymyxin E (colistin)

III. Mechanism of action and antibacterial spectrum
  A. Act as surface-active agents
  B. Associate with phospholipid on membranes by ionic attraction
  C. Bactericidal effect on susceptible organisms is rapid (1 to 10 minutes); thus useful for emergency "bowel sterilization"
  D. Bactericidal to either growing or resting bacteria
  E. Antibacterial spectrum is limited to gram-negative organisms. Especially effective against *Pseudomonas* spp.; *Proteus* spp. are uniformly resistant.
  F. Antibacterial activity of polymyxins is markedly affected by:
    1. Pus: binding to constituents is considerable; one ml pus has been shown capable of binding 1500 μg polymyxin B. This emphasizes the importance of establishing drainage of infected areas.
    2. Acidic phospholipids in cell membranes bind polymyxins. This results in a high degree of binding to tissues in vivo as described below under distribution.
IV. Physiologic disposition
  A. Absorption
    1. Activity limited to within the gastrointestinal tract when given orally
    2. Rapidly absorbed following parenteral routes
    3. Commonly incorporated in topical preparations
  B. Distribution
    1. Marked differences between the sulfate and methane sulfonate salts following parenteral administration
    2. Binding to plasma proteins approximately 70 to 90% for polymyxin B; approximately 10% for colistimethate
    3. Binding to tissues occurs with both salts, but especially the sulfate. This is an important disadvantage with both drugs.
  C. Excretion—primarily glomerular filtration
V. Potential adverse effects
  A. Nephrotoxicity
    1. Early signs include cellular casts, albuminuria, azotemia, and depression of GFR.
    2. Colistimethate is less likely than polymyxin B sulfate to produce nephrotoxicity.
  B. Respiratory paralysis
    1. Curare-like effect
    2. Can occur when:
      a) Preexisting renal dysfunction and dosage not modified
      b) Rapid IV administration
      c) Use of too much drug in peritoneal lavage—these drugs are absorbed well from the peritoneal cavity
  C. CNS effects including depression, hyperpyrexia and anorexia may occur with polymyxin B sulfate after a few days of therapy.

Amphotericin B

I. Chemistry—polyene antibiotic from *Streptomyces nodosus*

II. Mechanism of action and antifungal spectrum

    A. Combines with sterols (ergosterol) in cell membranes of susceptible fungi. Pores are created through which molecules can leak.

    B. Broad spectum of activity against pathogenic fungi. Shown to be effective against fungi causing histoplasmosis, blastomycosis, coccidioidomycosis, cryptococcosis, candidiasis, mucormycosis, phycomycosis, aspergillosis and sporotrichosis.

    C. Selective toxicity. Bacterial membranes do not contain sterols. Cholesterol of mammalian membranes is a less suitable ligand than ergosterol, but enough to cause toxicity problems.

III. Physiologic disposition

    A. Absorption

        1. Oral absorption poor

            Given orally only for fungal infections in the gastrointestinal tract

        2. Preparations are available for intravenous and intrathecal administration

    B. Distribution

        Concentrations can be produced in the body that are effective in clinical infections.

    C. Excretion

        Slow excretion in the urine.

IV. Potential adverse reactions

    A. Nephrotoxicity of primary concern; do not exceed a dose of 2 mg/kg in the dog.

    B. Other life-threatening adverse reactions include cardiac arrhythmias, acute hepatic failure and anaphylaxis.

    C. Other problems include nausea, emesis, fever, phlebitis and hemolytic anemia.

Nystatin

I. Same mechanism of action as amphotericin B

II. Use only for local therapy because of systemic toxicity. Preparations are available for oral and topical administration.

Miconazole

I. Synthetic imidazole compound

II. Spectrum of activity essentially limited to fungi causing coccidioidomycosis, candidiasis and cryptococcosis

III. Is given IV for systemic fungal infections

IV. Ketoconazole probably will largely replace the use of miconazole because it can be given orally, has a broader spectrum of activity against pathogenic fungi and it has considerably less potential to produce toxicity.

Ketoconazole

I. Chemistry
   Synthetic imidazole compound
II. Mechanism of action and spectrum of antifungal activity
   A. Probably exerts antifungal activity at two sites:
      1. Alters membrane permeability by interfering with biosynthesis of ergosterol.
      2. Enhanced permeability may facilitate penetration of drug into cell resulting in inhibition of precursors of nucleic acid synthesis.
   B. Antifungal spectrum almost as broad as for amphotericin B. Shown to be effective against fungi causing candidiasis, coccidioidomycosis, blastomycosis and sporotrichosis (not useful for aspergillus or phycomycetes).
III. Physiologic disposition
   A. Absorption
      Well-absorbed following oral dose. Recommend giving with food since gastric acidity is required to dissolve tablets.
   B. Distribution
      Well-distributed throughout the body, but not to the CSF.
   C. Biotransformation
      Extensively degraded by o-dealkylation and aromatic hydroxylation
   D. Excretion. Mainly biliary
IV. Potential adverse reactions
   Inhibits steroidogenesis in adrenal gland. This effect is reversible but will cause abnormal ACTH challenge test results.

BACTERICIDAL INHIBITORS OF PROTEIN SYNTHESIS

Aminoglycosides

I. General comments
   A. Streptomycin and neomycin were discovered in the 1940s.
   B. Kanamycin, discovered in the 1950s, provided for an antibiotic bactericidal against several gram negative organisms that had become resistant to streptomycin.
   C. Gentamicin, discovered in the 1960s, was a very important addition to the armamentarium of drugs effective against infections due to gram-negative organisms.

D. Newer aminoglycosides include tobramycin, amikacin, sisomycin and netilmicin.

II. Chemistry

    A. Are called aminoglycosides because these compounds are composed of amino sugars connected by glycosidic linkages

    B. Are organic bases, pKA's approximately 7.8, and are highly water soluble

    C. Except for streptomycin and dihydrostreptomycin, aminoglycosides are inactivated by penicillins in solution; avoid in vitro mixing

III. Mechanism of action and antibacterial spectrum

    A. Taken up by sensitive bacteria by active transport. Anaerobic conditions are inhibitory to this process.

    B. All aminoglycosides bind to the 30S ribosomal subunit of bacteria; P10 protein-binding is common to all. Various aminoglycosides have additional binding sites on the 30S subunit.

    C. All inhibit protein synthesis and alter the genetic code, but the mechanism of bactericidal effect is not known.

    D. Spectrum of activity includes aerobic gram-negative bacilli. Considerable differences exist in the activity of the various aminoglycosides against these organisms.

    E. Bacterial resistance to aminoglycosides is accomplished by enzymatic alteration of the drug through acetylation of amino groups and/or phosphorylation or adenylation of hydroxyl groups.

        1. Several of these enzymes have been identified; by 1983 ten were identified that inactivate kanamycin, seven that inactivate gentamicin, and three that inactivate amikacin.

        2. Thus an organism resistant to one aminoglycoside may still retain sensitivity to another.

    F. Antibacterial activity of aminoglycosides is markedly affected by:

        1. pH

            The antibacterial activity of aminoglycosides increases with increasing pH. Minimum inhibitory concentrations (MIC) may change several-fold within the pH range 6 to 8.

        2. Pus

            One ml pus has been shown capable of binding 700 μg gentamicin. Broken cells release acidic proteins and nucleic acids that are known to bind aminoglycosides. This emphasizes the importance of establishing drainage of infected areas.

IV. Physiologic disposition

    A. Absorption.

        1. Given orally for "bowel sterilization" or infections localized within the gastrointestinal tract. Inappropriate route for systemic therapy.

        2. Well absorbed following im or sc administration; peak concentrations achieved within one hour.

B. Distribution
   1. Binding to plasma proteins less than 20%.
   2. Limited essentially to extracellular fluid.
   3. Accumulates in cells of renal cortex; important in nephrotoxic potential of this group of drugs.
C. Biotransformation is nil
D. Excretion
   1. Kidney by glomerular filtration.
   2. If renal dysfunction the serum half-life of aminoglycosides can increase from 1–2 hours to days. The dose and dosage schedule must be modified if renal dysfunction is present.
V. Potential adverse effects
   A. Nephrotoxicity
      1. All aminoglycosides have the potential; related to the number of amino groups per molecule. Thus streptomycin the least and neomycin the greatest potential for nephrotoxicity; the others are intermediate.
      2. Monitor BUN, serum creatinine, creatinine clearance, urine osmolality or specific gravity and appearance of albumin, cylinduria and increased urine output.
   B. Ototoxicity
      1. Both auditory and vestibular branches can be affected.
      2. Predisposing factors
         a) Failure to adjust dose if preexisting renal dysfunction.
         b) Concurrent administration of furosemide.
   C. Respiratory/cardiac failure
      1. Predisposing factors.
         a) Excessive dosage when using aminoglycosides in peritoneal lavage in an anesthetized patient (aminoglycosides are absorbed well from the peritoneal cavity).
         b) Endotoxin shock
            Cardiotoxic effects of gentamicin have been demonstrated when given during endotoxin shock. It is likely that the occurrence of this adverse effect can be minimized by restoring fluid balance in the patient before administering the drug.
VI. Examples of individual aminoglycosides
   A. Streptomycin and dihydrostreptomycin
      1. Antibacterial spectrum of both drugs is virtually identical.
      2. Dihydrostreptomycin not used in human because of the risk of irreversible deafness.
      3. Many organisms once sensitive are now resistant.
      4. Bacterial resistance can rapidly develop during treatment.
   B. Neomycin
      1. Most toxic of all aminoglycosides in current use
      2. Preparations are available for parenteral use, but main use is for

oral, topical (often combined with polymyxin B), ophthalmic and irrigating preparations.
3. Prolonged oral use may cause diarrhea, malabsorption (reversible), suprainfections.
C. Kanamycin
    Effective against more organisms than dihydrostreptomycin, but fewer than gentamicin.
D. Gentamicin
    1. Currently the most widely used aminoglycoside in veterinary and human medicine.
    2. Effective against most gram-negative organisms and some gram-positive organisms.
        a) Restrict use to infections caused by gram-negative organisms.
        b) Use other drugs for infections due to gram-positive organisms, e.g., staphylococcal infections.
        c) Bacterial resistance to this valuable drug is increasing.
E. Tobramycin
    1. Antibacterial spectrum similar to gentamicin
    2. More effective against *Pseudomonas aeruginosa*
F. Amikacin
    1. Effective against many gram-negative organisms that have developed resistance to other aminoglycosides, especially *Pseudomonas* and *Klebsiella*.
    2. Should not be used as a first-line drug. Preserve its use for those situations where other aminoglycosides do not work. This will help delay the emergence of bacteria resistant to amikacin.

BACTERIOSTATIC INHIBITORS OF PROTEIN SYNTHESIS

Tetracyclines

I. General comments
    A. Chlortetracycline was isolated from *Streptomyces aureofaciens* in 1944; the first "broad-spectrum" antibiotic.
    B. Several other tetracyclines have been isolated from fungi or have resulted from the chemical manipulation of the basic tetracycline molecule. Objectives of chemical manipulation: improve gastrointestinal absorption, enhance tissue distribution, prolong retention in the body, and enhance antimicrobial activity.
    C. Seven tetracyclines currently are available for clinical use in the U.S. (chlortetracycline, oxytetracycline, tetracycline, demeclocycline, methacycline, doxycycline and minocycline).
        1. Tetracycline is the most useful member of the group in small animal medicine.

    2. Doxycycline and minocycline are newer tetracyclines that have not been used much, but may have potential, for use in veterinary medicine.

II. Chemistry

  A. All tetracyclines have a common hydronaphthacene nucleus and are amphoteric.

    1. The isoelectric point of most tetracyclines occurs about pH 5.6; with minocycline it occurs about 6.6.

    2. With minocycline, the point of maximal lipid solubility is closer to physiologic pH than is the case of other tetracyclines. This may explain the greater ability of this tetracycline to distribute throughout the body.

  B. Doxycycline and minocycline are the most lipophilic tetracyclines.

III. Mechanism of action and antimicrobial spectrum

  A. Enter susceptible bacteria by active transport

    1. Active transport process appears to be favored by lipid solubility of the tetracycline.

      a) Greatest antimicrobial activity when pH close to the isoelectric point

      b) Minocycline and doxycycline show greater in vitro activity against organisms than other tetracyclines.

      c) Minocycline shown to be active against staphylococci that are resistant to other tetracyclines

    2. Resistance to tetracyclines. Bacteria carry an R factor that induces synthesis of an inhibitor of active transport.

  B. Mechanism of bacteriostatic effect due to reversibly binding to the 30S ribosomal subunit and blocking the binding of aminoacyl-tRNA to the mRNA-ribosome complex.

  C. Selective toxicity

    1. Tetracyclines, especially chlortetracycline, can inhibit protein synthesis in cell-free preparations of mammalian as well as bacterial cells.

    2. Active transport provides for intracellular penetration in susceptible bacteria.

    3. Intracellular penetration in mammals does not occur appreciably except if high serum concentrations due to:

      a) Overdosage

      b) Conventional doses if preexisting renal dysfunction.

  D. Spectrum of antimicrobial activity

    1. Probably the broadest antimicrobial spectrum of any drug; however, many organisms, once sensitive are now resistant.

    2. Includes many gram-positive and gram-negative bacteria, chlamydia, rickettsia, protozoa, mycoplasma and leptospira.

IV. Physiologic disposition
  A. Absorption
    1. Oral route
      a) Absorption of most tetracyclines is not complete, but is satisfactory for treating systemic infections.
      b) Absorption of doxycycline and minocycline is virtually complete, even in the presence of food.
      c) Ca, Mg, and Al-containing materials (dairy products, antacids) chelate with tetracycline (much less with doxycycline and minocycline) and prevent absorption. Must separate the administration of tetracycline and these materials by 2 hours.
      c) Fe-containing preparations reduce absorption and effectiveness of all tetracyclines.
    2. Parenteral preparations are available for IV and IM routes. Irritating by IM, however.
  B. Distribution
    1. Much variation in binding to plasma proteins reported (25 to 65% for tetracycline and 70 to 90% for doxycycline and minocycline).
    2. Tetracyclines with greater lipophilicity concentrate to a greater extent in tissues and body fluids. Thus, doxycycline and minocycline distribute to a greater extent than tetracycline to the CSF, brain, ocular and vitreous humor, saliva, tears, lungs, bronchial secretions and prostate gland.
    3. Incorporated as a tetracycline-Ca orthophosphate complex into newly-formed bone or teeth
  C. Biotransformation
    1. Reported to be negligible in dogs
    2. Doxycycline and minocycline reported to be biotransformed in man
  D. Excretion
    1. Kidney—major route for most tetracyclines
    2. Intestinal mucosa—major route for doxycycline in the dog and probably other species
      a) Active drug passes through intestinal mucosa and then becomes bound as a stable complex (antibacterially inactive) in intestinal content.
      b) Doxycycline disturbs normal intestinal flora to a lesser extent than other tetracyclines.
      c) Doxycycline can be given to patients with renal dysfunction without dosage modification.
    3. Bile. Actively transported into bile.
V. Potential adverse effects
  A. Gastrointestinal upsets most common
    1. May cause nausea, emesis and diarrhea in dogs.

    2. Cats do not tolerate tetracyclines well. Common are diarrhea, colic, emesis, depression, fever and anorexia.

B. Suprainfection

    1. Broad spectrum of activity may decimate the normal bacterial flora, providing for an ecologic niche in which a resistant pathogen may flourish.

    2. Keep in mind, that in the experimental production of a fungal infection, it is common to administer a tetracycline and corticosteroid concurrent with the fungal agent.

C. Tooth discoloration

    1. Due to the affinity and chelation of tetracyclines and Ca; the drug concentrates where Ca utilization is occurring—bones and teeth.

    2. Avoid tetracyclines in the last 2 to 3 weeks of pregnancy and the first month of life.

D. Hepatotoxicity

    1. Associated with excessive doses or even conventional doses to patients with impaired kidney function

    2. Tetracyclines can produce an antianabolic effect; decreased utilization of amino acids leading to a rise in BUN (azotemia).

E. Minocycline has been reported to produce severe vestibular effects in human patients. However, very high doses of minocycline have been given to dogs with brucellosis (i.e., 27.5 mg/kg q12 hr for 14 days) with minimal side effects.

Chloramphenicol

I. Chemistry

  A. Isolated from *Streptomyces venezuela.*

  B. Neutral compound with high lipid solubility.

  C. Solubilized with propylene glycol for delivery in an aqueous medium.

  D. Two esters are useful.

    1. Palmitate ester masks bitter taste for oral use.

    2. Succinate ester is highly water soluble and facilitates parenteral use.

II. Mechanism of action and antimicrobial spectrum.

  A. Mechanism of bacteriostasis is reversible binding to the 50S ribosomal subunit of bacteria (similar binding site for macrolides and lincosamides) with subsequent inhibition of peptide bond formation and protein synthesis.

  B. Resistance to chloramphenicol

    Bacteria acquire an R factor by conjugation that induces an acetyl transferase enzyme which acetylates chloramphenicol to an inactive compound.

  C. Selective toxicity

    1. Chloramphenicol does not bind to the 80S cytoplasmic ribosomes of

mammalian cells, but it does bind to mammalian mitochondrial ribosomes (many similarities to bacterial ribosomes).

2. Basis for bone marrow depression (not aplastic anemia).

D. Spectrum

Broad spectrum of activity against gram-positive and gram-negative aerobic bacteria, most all anaerobic bacteria, chlamydia, rickettsiae, and some protozoa

III. Physiologic disposition

A. Well-absorbed following oral administration

B. Distribution

1. Probably more extensively distributed throughout the body than any other antimicrobial drug.

2. Binding to plasma protein ranges 30 to 60%.

C. Biotransformation

1. Extensive biotransformation by endoplasmic reticulum; nitro reduction and conjugation to the glucuronide via glucuronyl transferase.

2. Cats lack the ability to form glucuronides with exogenous compounds. Thus the frequency of dosage is less in cats than in other species.

3. Several weeks of age are required for the biotransforming mechanism to become fully functional. Thus the frequency of dosage in neonates is less than in adults.

D. Excretion

1. Kidney the major route

a) Excreted primarily as the glucuronide

b) Between 5 to 10% of a dose is excreted in active form; generally this is sufficient for urinary tract infections caused by susceptible organisms.

2. Bile

Concentrations in bile exceed those in serum.

IV. Potential adverse reactions

A. Aplastic anemia in humans

1. Idiosyncratic reaction; not dose-related; usually fatal

2. Occurrence in humans is rare (about 1 in 40,000).

3. Exercise care in handling preparations of this drug for administration to animals.

B. Bone marrow depression

1. Reported in all species.

2. Dose-related and reversible (if diagnosed in time).

3. Due to ability of chloramphenicol to inhibit mammalian mitochondrial protein synthesis.

C. Inhibition of drug biotransformation

1. Chloramphenicol, given concurrently with other drugs, can inhibit their biotransformation resulting in a prolongation of the duration of effect.

2. A therapeutic dose of chloramphenicol has been shown to
    a) Prolong the duration of pentobarbital anesthesia 120% in dogs and
       260% in cats.
    b) Precipitate signs of phenytoin toxicity in dogs receiving that drug.
  D. Inhibition of the immune response. Animals should not be immunized
     while receiving chloramphenicol.

Macrolides

 I. General comments
    A. Erythromycin discovered in 1952 from *Streptomyces erythresus*.
    B. Members of this group include erythromycin, tylosin, carbomycin,
       oleandomycin, troleandomycin and spiramycin.
    C. Erythromycin and tylosin are available for oral or parenteral use in
       treating individual animals. The others are used mainly as feed addi-
       tives.
    D. Often classified as "penicillin substitutes". Can be given to patients
       allergic to penicillins and there may be activity against beta-lactamase-
       producing staphylocci.
 II. Chemistry
    A. Called macrolides because they contain a large lactone ring with one
       or more deoxy sugars attached.
    B. Organic bases, pKAs range 6 to 9 (erythromycin 8.6, tylosin 7.1).
    C. Erythromycin is acid labile. Various forms of erythromycin designed
       to improve oral absorption and facilitate im and iv injection include the
       stearate, ethylsuccinate, estolate, glucoheptonate and lactobionate.   •
III. Mechanism of action and antimicrobial spectrum
    A. Very similar to that described for chloramphenicol.
       1. Erythromycin shown capable of preventing the binding of chlor-
          amphenicol to the 50S ribosomal subunit
       2. May antagonize the action of chloramphenicol
    B. Antimicrobial effect markedly pH-dependent.
       1. Antimicrobial activity increases with increasing pH.
       2. Even though erythromycin distributes well to the prostate gland, the
          low pH of prostatic fluid precludes effective antimicrobial activity.
    C. Antimicrobial spectrum.
       1. Primarily gram-positive organisms, including many beta-lactamase-
          producing staphylococci.
       2. Some activity against mycoplasma, rickettsia and chlamydia.
       3. Gram-negative organisms are resistant.
IV. Physiologic disposition.
    A. Absorption
       1. Generally given orally; absorbed well.
       2. Can also be given iv or im (often painful).

B. Distribution
   1. High tissue concentrations relative to serum.
   2. High concentrations in prostatic fluid, but the drug loses antimicrobial effectiveness at low pH.
C. Biotransformation
   Some of the drug may be inactivated by demethylation.
D. Excretion
   1. Between 2 to 5% of the dose excreted in the urine in active form. High urine pH favors antimicrobial effectiveness.
   2. High concentrations are found in bile.
V. Potential adverse effects
   A. Adverse effects seldom reported in dogs and cats.
   B. In human patients, the use of erythromycin estolate has been associated with cholestatic hepatitis. Probably should avoid the estolate if liver function is impaired.
   C. Whereas macrolides are tolerated well by dogs and cats, this group of drugs induces severe diarrhea in horses.

Lincosamides

I. General comments
   A. Members of this group include lincomycin and clindamycin.
   B. Often classified as "penicillin substitutes" for the same reasons as are the macrolides.
II. Chemistry
   A. Lincomycin produced by *Streptomyces lincolnensis*
   B. Clindamycin is 7-chlorolincomycin
   C. Organic bases, pKas about 7.6, moderately lipophilic
III. Mechanism of action and antimicrobial spectrum.
   A. Very similar to that described for chloramphenicol
      1. Binding site overlaps the chloramphenicol and erythromycin binding site.
      2. Erythromycin can prevent binding of lincomycin.
      3. These drugs probably should not be given in combination.
   B. Spectrum of activity
      1. Essentially gram-positive cocci, except enterococci. Effective against some beta-lactamase-producing staphylococci. Especially useful in patients sensitive to penicillins.
      2. Clindamycin generally is more potent than lincomycin. Especially useful for anaerobes such as *Bacteroides fragilis*.
IV. Physiologic disposition. Several important differences between lincomycin and clindamycin.
   A. Absorption
      1. Lincomycin incompletely absorbed following oral administration, but well enough to produce effective systemic concentrations.

2. Clindamycin is completely absorbed following oral administration. Must use capsules or the palmitate ester to mask its bitter taste.
3. Preparations of both drugs are available for im and iv administration.
B. Distribution
   1. Significant concentrations of both drugs achieved in most tissues of the body
   2. Poor penetration of cerebrospinal fluid
   3. Both drugs distribute to bone in appreciable concentrations. Useful in staphylococcal osteomyelitis.
C. Biotransformation
   1. No reports on lincomycin
   2. Appreciable biotransformation of clindamycin in dogs. About 36% of a dose is excreted as unchanged clindamycin. Antimicrobial activity of metabolites ranges from no activity for the glucuronide (28%), one-fourth activity of the parent compound for the sulfoxide (28%), and 4 times activity of the parent compound for N-demethyl clindamycin (9%).
D. Excretion
   1. Bile a major route of excretion for both drugs; quantitatively more than in the urine.
   2. Exercise care in dosing if hepatic dysfunction exists.
V. Potential adverse effects.
   A. Loose stools and emesis may occur on oral dosing.
   B. Hemorrhagic diarrhea reported in dogs
   C. Severe diarrhea reported for horses, rabbits, guinea pigs and hamsters; avoid use in these species.
   D. Fatal pseudomembraneous colitis can occur in people.

INHIBITORS OF NUCLEIC ACID SYNTHESIS

Nalidixic Acid

I. This drug has produced toxicities in dogs and cats characterized by neurologic reactions, epileptiform seizures and often death.
II. An example of where a human dose (12 mg/kg q 6 h) is too large for dogs and cats.
   A. Has been reported that 3 mg/kg q 6h can be given safely to dogs and cats
   B. Useful in urinary tract infections caused by gram-negative organisms, especially those caused by *Pseudomonas sp*

Griseofulvin

I. Chemistry
   A. Antibiotic from *Penicillium griseofulvin dierckx*
   B. Virtually insoluble in water

C. Particle seize is important for absorption (microsize and ultramicrosize).
II. Mechanism of action and antimicrobial activity
  A. Enter susceptible fungi by active transport
  B. Antifungal effect due to disruption of the mitotic spindle, thus arresting the metaphase of cell division
  C. Spectrum of activity limited to dermatophytes causing ringworm
III. Physiologic disposition
  A. The drug is given orally.
    1. Between 25 to 70% absorbed for microsized form
    2. Virtually 100% absorbed for ultramicrosized form
    3. High dietary fat facilitates absorption
  B. Distribution
    1. Deposited in keratin of skin, hair and nails
    2. Can be detected in stratum corneum within a few hours of dosing
  C. Biotransformation
    Degraded by o-dealkylation to 6-dimethylgriseofulvin in the endoplasmic reticulum
  D. Excretion
    1. Less than 1% excreted in the urine unchanged
    2. Unabsorbed griseofulvin excreted in the feces
IV. Potential adverse effects
  A. Include gastrointestinal upsets, photosensitization, depressed spermatogenesis
  B. Shown to be teratogenic to cats
  C. Drug interactions; phenobarbital shown to depress absorption of griseofulvin

Ketoconazole

I. Systemic antifungal drug discussed under Labilizers of Cell Membranes.
II. Enhanced permeability may facilitate penetration of ketoconazole into the cell where the drug inhibits precursors of nucleic acid synthesis.

Metronidazole

I. Chemistry
    A nitroimidazole synthetic compound
II. Mechanism of action and antimicrobial spectrum
  A. The nitro group is reduced in susceptible organisms. The reduced form inhibits DNA synthesis and/or degrades existing DNA.
  B. Spectrum of activity
    1. Probably the broadest spectrum of activity against pathogenic protozoa of any drug. Includes organisms causing trichomoniasis, giardiasis, amebiasis, balantidiasis and trypanosomiasis.
    2. Bactericidal to many anaerobic bacteria including *Bacteroides* sp

III. Physiologic disposition
   A. Well-absorbed following oral administration
   B. Distribution
      1. Low degree of binding to plasma protein
      2. Widely distributed in the body
      3. Distributes well into the CSF
   C. Biotransformation is extensive
   D. Excretion is primarily renal
IV. Potential adverse effects
   A. No major concerns reported, but gastrointestinal upsets may occur.
   B. Shown to be carcinogenic to rats and mutagenic to bacteria

INHIBITORS OF INTERMEDIARY METABOLISM

Nitrofurans

I. General comments
   A. Several members of this group are used in veterinary medicine.
   B. Nitrofurazone (topical use) and nitrofurantoin (urinary tract infections) probably have received widest use in small animal medicine.
II. Chemistry
   A. Synthetic compounds derived from 5-nitrofuran.
   B. Nitrofurantoin a weak acid, pKa 7.2 and it is moderately lipophilic.
III. Mechanism of action and antimicrobial spectrum.
   A. Bacteriostatic effect may be due to blocking oxidative decarboxylation of pyruvate to acetyl CoA.
   B. Antimicrobial effect markedly pH-dependent; acidify urine when used in urinary tract infections.
   C. Spectrum of activity includes gram-positive and gram-negative bacteria, some protozoa.
IV. Physiologic disposition
   A. Absorption
      1. Oral absorption is enhanced when taken with food.
      2. Delayed gastric emptying allows for more complete dissolution of the drug.
   B. Distribution
      1. Widely-distributed in the body, but concentrations are very low.
      2. Concentrations high enough for systemic antimicrobial activity would be toxic.
   C. Biotransformation occurs, but poorly defined.
   D. Excretion is renal.
      1. About 50% excreted in active form
      2. Involves glomerular filtration, tubular secretion and tubular reabsorption

3. Urinary acidification promotes tubular reabsorption, thereby decreasing urine concentrations. However, concentrations in urine still are sufficiently high. Urine must be acidic to enable the drug to diffuse across the bacterial cell membrane.
V. Potential adverse reaction
   A. Includes emesis, diarrhea, gastrointestinal bleeding and sensitivity reactions
   B. Nitrofurantoin contraindicated if preexisting renal dysfunction. Peripheral neuritis, pulmonary complications and hepatitis reported in people.

Sulfonamides

I. General comments
   A. First antimicrobial drugs that could safely be given systemically.
   B. Inexpensive drugs, but considerable bacterial resistance has developed.
II. Chemistry
   A. Weak acids, pKas' range 4.8 to 10.4 (about 6.5 for those most active) and moderately lipophilic.
   B. Sodium salts are most common. Some sulfonamide solutions have a pH of 9 to 10. These solutions can cause tissue sloughs if injected perivascularly.
   C. The presence of one sulfonamide does not appreciably affect the solubility, hence the "law of independent solubility". Basis for the use of "triple sulfas".
   D. Acetylated sulfonamides are less soluble than the parent compound, except for the sulfapyrimidines (e.g., sulfadiazine, sulfamerazine and sulfamethazine).
III. Mechanism of action and antimicrobial spectrum.
   A. Bacteriostatic effect is due to interference with the incorporation of p-aminobenzoic acid (PABA) into folic acid.
      1. Onset of bacteriostasis is slow (approximately 3 to 4 hours) while endogenously-formed folic acid is being used up by the bacteria.
      2. Organisms that utilize preformed folic acid are insensitive to this effect. Basis of selective toxicity since mammals use preformed folic acid.
   B. Spectrum of activity is considered broad and may include gram-negative and gram-positive bacteria, some chlamydia and protozoa (coccidia).
      1. Unfortunately, many organisms now are resistant.
      2. Combination of a sulfonamide with a diaminopyridine (e.g., trimethoprim or pyrimethamine) may markedly enhance antimicrobial activity.

IV. Physiologic disposition
  A. Absorption
    1. "Enteric" and "systemic" forms are available for oral administration.
      a) "Enteric" sulfonamides are used for infections confined within the intestinal tract, for example sulfathalidine (phthalylsulfathiazole).
      b) "Systemic" sulfonamides are well-absorbed.
  B. Distribution
    Most are distributed well throughout the body, including the cerebrospinal fluid.
  C. Biotransformation
    1. Acetylation to an inactive metabolite occurs in all species except dogs (net acetylation of primary amines does not occur in dogs).
    2. Some oxidation of the benzene ring and subsequent conjugation with glucuronic acid and sulfate occurs.
  D. Excretion
    1. Renal excretion is the major route.
    2. In addition to glomerular filtration, tubular secretion and/or reabsorption occurs depending on the drug
      a) Low urinary pH favors tubular reabsorption.
      b) Differences in urinary pH partially explain differing rates of elimination of sulfonamides in different species.
    3. "Long-acting" sulfonamides
      a) Are extensively reabsorbed by the renal tubules
      b) May undergo enterohepatic recycling
V. Potential adverse reactions
  A. Crystalluria resulting from precipitation of sulfonamide in the kidney is the major concern. It is caused by
    1. Excessive dosage
    2. Dehydration and low urine volume
    3. Acidosis and low urinary pH is a contributing factor since the solubility of sulfonamides decreases with decreasing pH in the physiologic range
  B. Allergic reactions, e.g., pruritis and photosensitization have been reported.
  C. Alopecia may occur on long-term therapy.
VI. Sulfonamides for systemic use may be classified according to the duration of effective concentration in the body following a therapeutic dose.
  A. "Short-acting" (less than 12 hour duration).
    1. Examples include sulfathiazole, sulfisoxazole, sulfamethizole and sulfacetamide.
  B. "Intermediate-acting" (12 to 24 hour duration)
    Examples include sulfadiazine, sulfamerazine, sulfamethazine, sulfamethoxypyridazine and sulfachlorpyridazine.

    C. "Long-acting" (about 24 hours)
        Examples include sulfadimethoxine and sulfamethylphenazole.

Diaminopyridines

  I. General comments
    A. Synthetic compounds developed on the basis that dihydrofolate reductases from various species (e.g., bacteria, protozoa and mammals) differed in sensitivity to these drugs.
    B. Trimethoprim—effective against bacteria
    C. Pyrimethamine—effective against protozoa
    D. Major use of these drugs is in combination with sulfonamides.
 II. Mechanism of action of the combination of sulfonamide (sulfadiazine) and diaminopyridine (trimethoprim):
    A. Sequential blockade in the formation of tetrahydrofolate
      1. Sulfadiazine blocks the incorporation of PABA into dihydrofolate.
      2. Trimethoprim inhibits dihydrofolate reductase.
    B. Explanation of the synergistic effect
        Sulfadiazine may enhance the activity of trimethoprim by decreasing the formation of substrate (dihydrofolate).
III. Physiologic disposition
    A. Given orally; absorbed well
    B. Distribution
      1. Both drugs widely distributed in the body
      2. A fixed-dose ratio of 1:5 provides approximately the optimal ratio in tissues of 1:20.
IV. Potential adverse effects
    A. See sulfonamides
    B. Possibility of inducing folate deficiency
    C. Has been given to pregnant dogs with no apparent ill effects.

UPPER RESPIRATORY TRACT INFECTION

  Secondary bacterial infections of the upper respiratory tract are considered more common in small animal practice than are primary bacterial infections. In dogs, nasal foreign bodies, dental disease, trauma and neoplasia are the most common factors predisposing to bacterial infection. In cats, acute and chronic viral upper respiratory infections are the most common causes of secondary bacterial infection.

Diagnosis

  I. Clinical signs and history
      Paroxysms of sneezing, accompanied by a serous to serosanguinous or mucopurulent nasal discharge, are typically described by the client. Epi-

sodes of heavy discharge may be followed by several days of normal behavior and no nasal discharge. Bilateral epistaxis, particularly when there is no history of trauma, is more likely to be caused by coagulopathy than by infection. Occasionally, coughing is a prominent complaint in animals with chronic pharyngeal and laryngeal disease.

II. Laboratory

Severe infections of the upper respiratory tract can be associated with mild leukocytosis in both dogs and cats. Routine laboratory tests are of minimal diagnostic value in patients with upper respiratory tract infections.

III. Radiology

A careful radiographic study of the upper airways is indicated. Views should include at least a lateral skull, ventrodorsal view of the nasal cavity, and an anterior-posterior view of the frontal sinuses. Radiographs should be examined for evidence of asymmetry and bone destruction.

IV. Physical exam

Nasal biopsy may be obtained through the nostrils. Additionally, it may be possible to obtain nasal flushings through a polyethylene catheter inserted into the affected nostril. Alternate flushing and aspiration may yield material suitable for diagnostic cytology and culture.

V. Cytology

Cytologic exam is of diagnostic value when performed on tissue biopsied from the nasal cavity. Bacterial cultures are routinely positive. However, normal nasal flora and opportunistic bacteria are typically recovered. It is unlikely that bacteria recovered from nasal discharges are primary offenders.

GENERAL THERAPEUTIC CONSIDERATIONS

I. Fluid therapy

In dehydrated patients, intravenous rehydration will decrease the viscosity of nasal secretions and enhance the animal's ability to clear obstructing secretions from the nasal cavity.

II. Topical decongestants

Phenylephrine HCl 0.5% (q4h) or oxymetazoline HCl 0.05% (q24h) effectively decrease swelling of congested nasal mucous membranes. The obvious relief provided by these drugs will be transient; they should not be used in long-term treatment regimens.

ANTIBIOTIC THERAPY

I. Bacterial infections of the upper respiratory tract are predominately secondary to some underlying condition, e.g., viral rhinitis, traumatic sinusitis, neoplasia. In dogs and cats a mixed population of Staphylococcus spp. and Streptococcus spp. is most likely to be involved. Oral ampicillin (10–20 mg/kg, q6h) in dogs and cats, trimethoprim-sulfadiazine (15 mg [combined]/kg, q12h) in dogs or tetracycline (20 mg/kg, q8h) in dogs and cats will effectively manage bacterial infections and control the associated clinical signs. However, exacerbation following withdrawal of the antibacterial therapy can be expected until the primary disorder is identified and treated.

II. *Bordetella bronchiseptica* and mycoplasma may also be identified in cultures from the upper respiratory tract of dogs with chronic rhinitis. Tetracycline is the preferred antibiotic to use against these organisms. However, the role of *Bordetella* and mycoplasma as primary pathogens of the upper respiratory tract is not yet established.

COMPLICATIONS

Bacterial pneumonia is the most serious complication of upper respiratory tract infection, particularly in kittens with viral upper respiratory disease. Longstanding bacterial infections of the upper respiratory tract, whether primary or secondary, may cause permanent, anatomic injury to the supporting tissues of the upper respiratory tract.

BACTERIAL EAR INFECTIONS

Bacterial otitis externa is among the most common and potentially most serious bacterial infections that occur in dogs. Bacterial ear infections in cats do occur but with a lower frequency than in dogs. Table 3-2 lists the most commonly encountered primary causes of bacterial ear infections in dogs and cats.

DIAGNOSIS

I. Physical exam

Diagnosis of bacterial otitis is based on otoscopic examination of the external ear canal. Characteristically, pain or pruritus is manifested during manipulation of the affected ear. Additional evidence of self-induced trauma, e.g., laceration of the pinna or hematoma, may be seen. Additional diagnostic studies are indecated if the etiology cannot be established during the visual exam.

II. Bacterial culture and sensitivity

These are important if bacterial otitis is to be successfully managed. Table 3-3 lists the most common pathogens recovered from dogs with chronic otitis externa.

III. Additional diagnostic studies that may be useful in cases of chronic otitis nonresponsive to antibiotic therapy include: cytology, skin scrapes, fungal cultures, thyroid function tests, intradermal skin test, and biopsy.

TABLE 3-2.   COMMON CAUSES OF BACTERIAL EAR INFECTION

Foreign bodies	Plant material; water; dried medication
Parasites	Mites (*Otoclectes cynotis, Demodex canis, Sarcoptes scabei, Notoedres cati*); ticks
Mycoses	*Microsporium* spp.; *Trichophyton* spp.; *Aspergillus* spp. *Candida* spp, and *Malassezia pachydermitis* (*Pityrosporum*)
Endocrinopathies	Hypothyroidism, male feminizing syndrome, Sertoli cell tumors.
Allergies	Atopy, food and contact allergies.
Trauma	Oftentimes self-inflicted
Seborrhea	Seborrhea sicca; seborrhea oleosa (ceruminous otitis).
Immune mediated diseases	Pemphigus foliaceus; lupus erythematosis.
Neoplasia	Adenomas are more common than adenocarcinoma.
Miscellaneous	Confirmation of ear canal; position of pinae; hair growth in the external canal.

GENERAL THERAPEUTIC CONSIDERATIONS

Prior to prescribing therapy, it is important that both ear canals be thoroughly cleaned and examined. The proximal (horizontal) ear canal should be cleaned by flushing rather than with cotton-tipped swabs. Examination of the external ear canal should include visual evaluation of the tympanic membrane, since chronic infections may lead to degeneration of the membrane, rupture and secondary otitis media.

TABLE 3-3.   PATHOGENIC BACTERIA RECOVERED FROM EARS OF DOGS WITH OTITIS EXTERNA

Staphylococcus aureus	Common isolate; occasionally recovered from dogs with normal ears.
Other *Staphylococcus* spp.	Common.
β-*Streptococcus* spp.	Common isolate; occasionally recovered from dogs with normal ears.
Pseudomonas spp.	Most commonly recovered from dogs with chronic infections; painful otitis
Proteus spp.	Rarely recovered from normal ears; common in chronic infections; painful otitis.

Coliforms
  E. coli
  Kelbsiella spp.
  Enterobacter spp.
	Are relatively common in chronic infections; have occasionally been recovered from normal ears.

ANTIBIOTIC THERAPY

Topical preparations of chloramphenicol, aminoglycoside antibiotics (neomycin, polymixin, gentamicin) are most commonly prescribed in the treatment of bacterial infections associated with otitis externa. Successful treatment depends on the ability of medication to contact the skin of the ear canal. Attempts to treat an ear filled with cerumen, blood or other debris wastes medication, can inactivate the antibiotic and is unnecessarily expensive.

Commercial ear preparations available are oftentimes combined with corticosteroids. The objective is to decrease tissue inflammation and pruritus associated with the infection. There is no evidence to suggest that the use of topical corticosteroids impairs the antimicrobial efficacy of the antibiotic preparation with which it is combined.

DURATION OF THERAPY

Topical antibiotic preparations may be used 4–6 times daily for as long as needed to control the bacterial infection. Chronic administration of aminoglycoside antibiotics, however, has been associated with ototoxicity in animals having a ruptured tympanic membrane.

COMPLICATIONS

Otitis media may develop secondary to chronic otitis externa if the tympanic membrane is ruptured. Peripheral neuropathy associated with cranial nerves V & VII may become evident clinically.

Occasionally, bacterial otitis interna will develop in dogs and cats with ruptured tympanic membranes. Bacterial meningitis can develop subsequently, but the occurrence appears to be more likely among cats than dogs. In these cases, systemic antibiotic therapy with chloramphenicol should be pursued.

BACTERIAL INFECTIONS OF THE CENTRAL NERVOUS SYSTEM

Compared to human cases, bacterial and fungal infections of the CNS in animals are rare. When they do occur, the meninges are the most likely to be colonized. Bacteria can enter the CNS by at least four routes: 1) ascending bacterial neuritis from a bite wound abscess, 2) hematogenous, 3) bacterial otitis interna and 4) penetrating injury to the cranium or spinal cord. The most common organisms recovered from animals with bacterial meningitis are *Pasturella multocida, Staphylococcus aureus, Staphylococcus epidermidis* and *Staphylococcus albus. Cryptococcus neoformans* is the most common cause of fungal meningitis in dogs and cats.

DIAGNOSIS

I. Clinical signs of bacterial or fungal meningitis include seizures, disorientation, cranial nerve deficits, generalized hyperesthesia and rigidity. Evidence of disease in other body systems may not be evident.

II. Laboratory
Neutrophilic leukocytosis and monocytosis may be seen on routine hematology. CSF examination may reveal excess numbers of neutrophils, large quantities of protein and elevated intracranial pressures. Occasionally, bacteria may be seen on gram-stained cytologic exam of the CSF. If bacterial infection is confirmed, treatment should begin immediately rather than waiting for culture and sensitivity results. Cryptococcus neoformans is usually identified on direct examination of CSF in animals with fungal meningitis. This is particularly so when the CSF is examined with an India ink preparation (organisms won't stain) or Gram's stain (large gram-positive organisms).

GENERAL TREATMENT CONSIDERATIONS

I. Sepsis must be ruled out in any patient with evidence of bacterial meningitis.

II. Overhydration with I.V. fluids can contribute to brain swelling and increased CSF pressure.

III. Fever. Salicylates, acetaminophen, and tepid water baths should be used to keep the temperature below 106°F. (See chapter 1)
ANTIBIOTIC THERAPY
Positive identification of bacteria in the CSF (Gram's stain) is diagnostic; treatment should not be delayed for laboratory confirmation since bacterial meningitis is life-threatening. Therefore, the type of antibiotic used is likely

TABLE 3-4. ANTIBIOTIC THERAPY OF BACTERIAL MENINGITIS

Organism	Drug of Choice	Alternatives

A. Gram Positive
   Staphylococcus spp.
   Streptococcus spp.
	Cephalothin, I.V.
	20–30 mg/kg, q6h
		a) Na or K Penicillin G,
		I.V. @ 50,000 units/kg
		q6h
		b) Chloramphenicol
		succinate, I.V.
		50 mg/kg q8 (dog)
		50 mg/kg q12h (cat)

B. Gram Negative
   Pasteurella multocida
   Enteric gram-negative
	a. Na or K Penicillin G,
	I.V. @ 50,000 units/kg
	q6h
	b. Gentamicin sulfate IM or
	I.V. 2–3 mg/kg q8h[a]
		a. Ampicillin, I.V. 10 mg/kg
		q6h
		b. Chloramphenical
		succinate I.V.
		50 mg/kg q8H (dog)
		50 mg/kg q12h (cat)

[a] Total daily dosage should not exceed 7–9 mg/kg.

to depend on whether the organism is gram-positive or gram-negative. Table 3-4 summarizes the antimicrobial regimens for bacterial meningitis.

SEPSIS/BACTERIAL ENDOCARDITIS

Uncontrolled colonization and proliferation of bacteria in one or more body regions or compartments represents sepsis. The pathophysiologic consequences of sepsis are directly attributable to bacterial organisms and/or the production of endotoxin produced by gram-negative bacteria. The clinical picture is one of deterioration of multiple organ system functions, particularly cardiovascular, renal, pulmonary, gastrointestinal, hepatic, hematopoietic/coagulation and reticuloendothelial and culminates in the syndrome known as septic shock.

DIAGNOSIS

I. Patients at risk

In many respects, sepsis is an occult disease with either short- or long-term duration. The time required to confirm sepsis in a patient may exceed the time that a septic animal can survive. Therefore, it is important to identify those animals at risk of becoming septic and institute appropriate therapy in an attempt to prevent the occurrence of sepsis.

II. Clinical signs

Signs associated with sepsis are highly variable depending on the organism and the organ system(s) involved at the time of presentation. Clinical signs are not diagnostic. Clinical features include: prolonged febrile illness characterized by lethargy and cachexia, heart murmur, arthralgia, petechiation associated with thrombocytopenia, anemia, regional cellulitis, acute onset congestive heart failure (a poor prognostic sign), jaundice, hepatic failure (particularly in dogs), acute renal failure, gastrointestinal hemorrhage, and, in the terminal stages, DIC.

III. Laboratory findings

A. Hematology

Leukocytosis with a left shift (degenerative shift in advanced cases), normocytic, normochromic anemia without evidence of regeneration; progressive thrombocytopenia is a common finding.

B. Biochemistry profiles

Results are highly variable depending on which organ(s) are involved and the extent of disease. Sequential profiles are most valuable in assessing the patient's response, or failure to respond, to therapy.

C. Coagulation profiles

Bleeding diathesis seen in septic patients has been associated with thrombocytopenia in the early phase of disease, decreased production

of clotting factors (hepatic failure or consumptive coagulopathy such as DIC) in the terminal phase. (See Chapter 8)
D. Blood cultures
Three blood cultures are collected within 24 hours, or are collected within a 2–3 hour period in the febrile patient.

SUPPORTIVE THERAPY

While antibacterial therapy is the principal modality in treating septic shock, supportive care must supplement therapy in clinical cases. (See Chapter 9)
I. Fluid therapy
Sustained I.V. infusions of lactated Ringer's solution, 10–12 ml/kg/hr or 10% Dextran-40, 0.5 to 1.5 ml/kg/hr (maximum total daily dose = 15 ml/kg/24 hrs) are necessary in the early stages of disease. If available, enough plasma should be given intravenously to maintain plasma oncotic pressure. (See Chapter 2)
II. Corticosteroids
Long-term use of corticosteroids in septic patients is not indicated. Short-term use of aqueous corticosteroid preparations are used early in septic shock but treatment duration is limited to one day only.
III. Nonsteroidal anti-inflammatory drugs have been shown to increase survival time in both endotoxic and septic shock. (See Chapter 5)
IV. Cardiovascular drugs shown to have efficacy in septic shock are Dopamine (5–10 mcg/kg/min, I.V.) and Dobutamine (5–20 mcg/kg/min, I.V.). Both drugs have positive inotropic and chronotropic effects. These drugs should be used only after fluid volume replacement has been achieved.

ANTIBIOTIC THERAPY

The treatment of septic patients is limited to bactericidal antibiotics.
I. Table 3-5 summarizes the guidelines for antibiotic administration to septic patients.
II. The duration of therapy is determined by individual patient response to treatment. Parenteral therapy (I.V.) should be continued for a minimum of 10–14 days followed by oral administration of the appropriate antibiotic for an additional four to eight weeks.

PROGNOSIS

The prognosis of any patient in septic or endotoxin shock is poor. Generally those patients with gram-negative sepsis have a poorer prognosis than those with gram-positive sepsis.

TABLE 3-5. ANTIBIOTIC THERAPY IN SEPSIS

Organism	Primary Drug	Alternate
A. *Gram-positive:* *Staphylococcus aureus* *Streptococcus* spp. Anerobic bacteria (excluding *Bacillus fragilis*) *Corynenbacterium* spp.	NA or K Penicillin G, I.V. 25,000 u/kg, q6h	Cephalothin,[a] I.V. 20–30 mg/kg q6h
B. *Gram-negative:* *E. coli* *Klebsiella* spp. *Pseudomonas aeruginosa* *Proteus* spp. *Enterobacter* spp.	Gentamicin sulfate,[c] I.V. 1–3 mg/kg, q8h	Gentamicin sulfate, I.V. 1–3 mg/kg, q8h, *coadministered with:*[b] Carbenicillin I.V. 15 mg/kg, q8h or Cephalothin,[a] I.V. 20–30 mg/kg, q6h

[a] May be given IM but injections are painful.
[b] Aminoglycoside antibiotics are often synergistic with beta-lactam antibiotics.
[c] Gentamicin nephrotoxicity is potentiated by dehydration and metabolic acidosis, both of which are common clinical findings in septic patients.

COMPLICATIONS

Complications reported in animals recovering from sepsis/bacteremia include congestive heart failure, renal failure subsequent to infarction or immune complex glomerulonephropathy, sustained (up to two weeks) anorexia, gastrointestinal bleeding, and reversible nephrogenic diabetes insipidus.

ENTERIC INFECTIONS

Among the known causes of acute onset diarrhea in dogs and cats, bacterial enteritis is uncommon and is probably limited only to a few species of bacteria that are not normally part of the bowel flora.

Several local factors have a role in preventing colonization of the bowel by transient bacteria: 1) the normal bacterial flora, 2) production of bacteriocidal compounds by the normal flora, 3) propulsive movements of the bowel and, 4) secretory immunoglobulins. Disruption of any of these factors, e.g., viral enteritis, oral antibiotics, bowel obstruction, etc., will predispose an animal to bacterial enteritis.

DIAGNOSIS

I. Inoculation of appropriate media should be made from scrapings of the rectal mucosa rather than from feces or rectoanal swabs.

II. Two organisms most likely to cause bacterial enteritis in dogs and cats are *Salmonella* spp. (especially, *S. typhimurium*) and *Campylobacter jejuni*.

A. *Salmonella* spp: Levine eosin-methylene blue agar and MacConkey agar—clear, uncolored colonies without setters; nonlactose fermenting. Brilliant green agar, pink to red colonies surrounded by intense red zone.
B. *Campylobacter* spp.: Campy agar, a selective medium, inhibits most enteric bacteria (42°C incubation temperature). Pinpoint colonies develop in 24 hours; 2–3 mm grey colonies by 48 hours.
C. *Salmonella* spp. have been isolated from stools of normal dogs.

III. Treatment

Guidelines are not established. Antibiotic therapy in animals with Salmonella enteritis may lead to chronic shedding and the development of resistant strains. If antibiotics are used, chloramphenicol and gentamicin are reported to be effective, Erythromycin is effective against Campylobacter; however, the relationship of a positive stool culture and enteritis is difficult to establish.

IV. Complications

A. Salmonella readily develop resistance to many antibiotics and are capable of transferring this resistance to other bacteria.
B. Antibiotic therapy in human patients with salmonellosis is known to be associated with patients becoming chronically infected.

PERIODONTAL DISEASE

The colonization of bacteria in the gingiva initiates the insidious, destructive processes leading to gingival ulceration and erosion, recession of alveolar bone, and loose teeth that characterize severe periodontal disease. Bacterial peridontitis is the most common primary regional bacterial infection seen in small animal practice. Periodontitis is estimated to exist in 85% of all dogs in the U.S. that are six years of age or older. Routine dental prophylaxis in animals with moderate to severe periodontal disease will result in transient bacteremia. Age and the presence of underlying systemic disease appear to be important factors in determining those patients at risk of becoming septic following routine dental procedures.

ANTIBIOTIC THERAPY

I. General considerations. The numbers and types of bacteria present in the oral cavity justifies the prophylactic use of oral antibiotics at least 24 hours prior to routine cleaning or scheduled oral surgery and for at least three to five days post-cleaning/surgery. The prophylactic use of antibiotics prior to dental surgery may be of particular importance in elderly animals. Routine prophylactic procedures in young animals are unlikely to necessitate prophylactic antibiotic therapy. Several antibiotics will effectively reduce the concentration of bacteria in the oral cavity; oftentimes the halitosis associated with periodontal disease can be eliminated with antibiotics alone.

II. A variety of broad-spectrum antibiotics may be used in the pre-and post-dental prophylaxis therapy of dogs:
  A. Tetracycline at 20 mg/kg, q8h, orally.
  B. Ampicillin/hetacillin at 20 mg/kg, q8h, orally.
  C. Chloramphenicol at 50 mg/kg, q8h, orally.

COMPLICATIONS

The majority of problems associated with bacterial periodontitis can be eliminated through early diagnosis and treatment. Neglected cases, patients with severe periodontal disease and other systemic diseases, and those patients with moderate to severe periodontitis that undergo operative dental procedures without receiving antibiotics are at greatest risk of developing complications
  I. Recession of alveolar bone and tooth loss. The loss of teeth, either through infection or extraction does affect the integrity of adjacent teeth and periodontium. Following the loss of a tooth, it has been shown that the periodontium of the antagonist tooth atrophies resulting in potentially severe malocclusion.
  II. Periapical abscess is likely to result in pulpitis and pressure necrosis of the pulp and death of the affected tooth. Bone necrosis and the development of oronasal fistulae are possible sequellae.
  III. Chronic necrotizing stomatitis and gingival ulceration.
  IV. Bacterial osteomyelitis of the mandible and/or maxilla.
  V. Septicemia and bacterial endocarditis are the most severe potential complications arising from untreated bacterial periodontitis.

PEDIATRIC BACTERIAL INFECTIONS

GENERAL CONSIDERATIONS

  I. Neonatal metabolism and dosage considerations
    Serveral physiologic factors unique to neonates and young animals affect drug uptake, distribution and excretion. Increased intestinal absorption, immaturity of the blood brain barrier, hypoproteinemia, decreased renal excretion of drug, and particularly, the deficiency of hepatic microsomal enzymes contribute to the increased sensitivity of young animals, particularly neonates (birth to four weeks) to drugs. Objective criteria by which drug efficacy and toxicity can be predicted in neonatal and juvenile animals have not been established. However, general acceptance of the increased likelihood of inducing drug toxicity in neonates is followed with the general recommendation that dose or dosage interval be reduced neonates. The amount by which dose should be reduced is arbitrary.

It is not possible to predict which drugs or class of drug is more likely to cause toxicity in neonates. Each drug must, as must each individual patient, be evaluated individually in light of the condition being treated.

II. Antibiotics

Although antibiotics are generally well absorbed from the neonatal gastrointestinal tract, ingestion of food at the time of drug administration may reduce the absorption of some antibiotics: e.g., ampicillin, penicillin-G, many of the penicillinase-resistant penicillin derivatives, and the cephalosporins. Milk or calcium containing milk replacers may combine with orally administered tetracycline thereby reducing the overall bioavailability of the antibiotic.

TREATMENT OF SPECIFIC CONDITIONS

I. Neonatal septicemia
   A. Typically associated with death at 1–4 days of age, neonatal septicemia is a leading cause of death among puppies 1 to 4 days old. The condition frequently results from hemolytic streptococcal infection of the navel at birth or shortly thereafter. Other bacteria thought to cause this condition include *E. coli, Brucella canis*, toxoplasma spp. and staphylococcus spp.
   B. Diagnostic confirmation is generally made during postmortem exam. Death is rapid following the onset of signs, therefore, treatment is seldom initiated. When suspected, administration of antibiotics to the bitch may be the most effective means of treating the nursing neonate. Ampicillin at 10–20 mg/kg/q6h, given S.C. or P.O. is indicated. The administration of ampicillin at 5 mg/kg P.O. q6h or amoxicillin, 5 mg/kg P.O. q12h may be administered to pups with suspected infections.

II. Puppy septicemia
   A. This severe bacterial infection occurs between one and 40 days of life. Infections by staphylococcal spp., streptococcal spp., *E. coli, Proteus* and *Pseudomonas* are reported. In contrast to neonatal septicemia, the navel is not necessarily the route through which infection occurs. Septicemia has been associated with mastitis and/or metritis in the bitch.
   B. Attempts to prevent puppy septicemia in a high risk bitch, entail administering a 5-day course of antibiotics at the time of breeding followed by a second 5-day course of antibiotics beginning 48 hours prior to the anticipated whelping date.
   C. Infected pups may be treated with chloramphenicol palmitate given orally at 10–20 mg/kg q8h. In addition, pups suspected of having puppy septicemia should not be permitted to nurse. Furthermore, it is recommended that the environmental temperature be maintained at 85°F.

III. Juvenile (pyoderma) cellulitis
   Also called "puppy strangles," juvenile cellulitis is a condition of young dogs that is characterized by severe cervical and mandibular lymphade-

nopathy and cellulitis of the ears and face. The condition is not contagious. Secondary bacterial infection can develop in affected dogs. Ampicillin, 10–20 mg/kg q8h, P.O., should be given for five to seven days. It is recommended that treatment be supplemented with corticosteroids to reduce the complications associated with severe cellulitis.

IV. Neonatal conjunctivitis (ophthalmia neonatorum)

A localized infection that occurs beneath the unopened eyelids of neonatal dogs and cats. Pyogenic bacteria such as staphylococcal spp. are typically recovered from affected animals. In cats, bacterial infection may be secondary to viral conjunctivitis caused by feline herpesvirus or calicivirus.

Treatment includes gently separating the eyelids and flushing pus and debris from the conjunctiva and cornea with an irrigating solution. An ophthalmic preparation of broad-spectrum antibiotics should be administered topically (e.g., neomycin, bacitracin, polymixin B or chloramphenicol). Ideally, drops should be administered every half hour during the day; an ointment may be administered once in the evening.

OSTEOMYELITIS

Although radiation therapy, corrosion from implants and trauma are capable of causing osteomyelitis, the most common cause of bone inflammation in companion animals is bacterial infection. Bacterial osteomyelitis is clearly one of the most difficult infections to manage; it is most commonly caused by gram-positive organisms. Staphylococcal spp. are recovered in 45–50% of the cases in small animals. β-hemolytic *Streptococcus* and *Brucella canis* are also reported to cause osteomyelitis in dogs, particularly discospondylitis.

DIAGNOSTIC METHODS

The diagnosis of osteomyelitis is confirmed by radiography and positive culture results on specimens collected by fine needle aspirates or bone culture. A tube agglutination test for *B. canis* should be performed on all cases of discospondylitis. Cultures taken at the skin surface of a draining sinus tract are an unreliable means of confirming bone infection.

The clinical signs of osteomyelitis include heat, swelling over the affected bone, draining tracts, and lameness. Leukocytosis is not a consistent finding.

GENERAL THERAPEUTIC CONSIDERATIONS

Antibiotic therapy must be considered as an adjunct in the management of osteomyelitis. Treatment usually involves surgical intervention with decompression and drainage at the affected site. Surgical management of osteomyelitis is discussed elsewhere in the veterinary literature (Claywood DD: Osteomyelitis. Vet Clin N Am 13:43–53, 1983).

Antibiotic Therapy

The following treatment regimens are recommended in the management of osteomyelitis:
  I. Staphylococcus spp:
    A. Cephradine—20 mg/kg q8h, orally, or
    B. Cephalexin—30 mg/kg q12h, orally, or
    C. Cloxacillin—10 mg/kg q6h, orally.
  II. β-hemolytic streptococcus:
    A. Ampicillin—20 mg/kg q6h, orally, or
    B. Sodium penicillin G—20,000 u/kg q4h, I.V.
  III. *Brucella canis:*
    A. Tetracycline HCL—20 mg/kg q8h, orally for three weeks, combined with
    B. Streptomycin—20 mg/kg q12h I.M. for five days. Rest three weeks; repeat for five additional days.
    C. Minocycline—50 mg/kg, q12h, orally for 20 days (expensive). Best when combined with streptomycin.

Duration of Therapy

Animals with bacterial osteomyelitis caused by staphylococcal spp. or streptococcal spp. should be treated for a minimum for four to six weeks.

Complications

Any bone may become infected; the severity of complications are clearly related to the location (e.g., vertebrae vs. the digits), the surgical accessibility to the lesion, the cause of the infection, and the duration/extent of the infection.

SYSTEMIC MYCOSES

General Considerations

The systemic mycoses of importance in small animal medicine include histoplasmosis, blastomycosis, coccidioidomycosis and cryptococcosis. Clinical signs referrable to lymph nodes, skin, the gastrointestinal tract (including liver, small bowel and colon) the CNS and bone do occur in addition to the respiratory tract. Infections are usually chronic and are typically associated with progressive debilitation and weight loss.

I. Drug toxicity

Amphotericin B and ketoconazole are the two most commonly used drugs in the management of systemic mycoses. Amphotericin B is a polyene antibiotic that has both fungicidal and fungistatic activity. The most serious side effect is a dose-related nephrotoxicity. Renal damage evident on routine laboratory tests (BUN, creatinine, urinalysis) warrants immediate dosage reduction or total discontinuation of drug.

At therapeutic doses, ketoconazole is considered to be nearly devoid of significant toxicity in dogs even when administered over long periods of time.

II. Patient condition

Thorough evaluation of the patient's status before and during therapy is important since these fungi can disseminate systemically. Response to therapy is not rapid; several weeks may be required before physical signs of remission are evident. Generally, the greater the delay between infection and onset of treatment, the greater the likelihood of dissemination and the poorer the prognosis.

The systemic mycoses in dogs and cats are not contagious diseases, nor are they considered zoonotic infections.

DIAGNOSTIC METHODS

I. Serology

Antibody titers are of some diagnostic value. Test results must be interpreted in light of clinical signs and other laboratory findings.

II. Identification of organism

Direct visualization of the organism during cytologic examination of tissue or fluid collected from the patient is diagnostic.

A. Direct smears/cytology

Exudates, scrapings from superficial lesions (skin, rectum), lymph node aspirate, bone marrow and body fluids (CSF) should be stained and examined microscopically for the presence of fungi.

B. Culture

Sabarouds media should be heavily streaked with representative specimens and held a minimum of six weeks. This is the least efficient means of diagnosing mycoses.

C. Histopathology

Biopsy of affected tissues should be placed in 10% buffered formalin. The use of specific fungal stains, such as periodic acid-Schiff, should be used for identification of spores in tissue specimens.

Treatment Protocols

I. Amphotericin B

A stock solution of drug is prepared by adding 10 ml of sterile water (without preservatives) or 5% dextrose in water to a single 50 mg vial of crystalline amphotericin B (Note: use of electrolyte solutions such as saline or lactated Ringer's solution to reconstitute the drug will cause *in vitro* precipitation) yielding a final concentration of 5 mg/ml. The entire stock solution may be added to 240 ml of 5% dextrose and water yielding a more dilute concentration of 0.2 mg amphotericin B per ml of solution.

Amphotericin B is administered intravenously over 20–30 minutes at doses ranging from 0.15 to 0.5 mg/kg per treatment and is given at alternate day intervals. In practice, the lower dose is used initially; drug is gradually increased during the second and third treatment week as long as complications, such as significant azotemia (BUN > than 50 mg/dl) does not occur. In cats, a maximum dose of 0.25 mg/kg per treatment day is recommended.

Treatment may be given on an outpatient basis for six to eight weeks; this usually entails 20–22 injections.

II. Ketoconazole

This is a water soluble antifungal drug which is available for oral administration. In veterinary medicine, the drug is recommended for treating blastomycosis and coccidioidomycosis. Ketoconazole is given at a dose of 10–30 mg/kg orally q8h for two to six months.

III. Flucytosine (5-flurocytosine, 5FC)

An oral drug used in the treatment of certain systemic mycoses has received little attention in the veterinary literature. The drug can be combined with amphotericin B therapy. However, development of drug resistance by Candida and Cryptococcal isolates is reported in the human literature.

Flucytosine is not licensed for use in dogs and cats.

SUGGESTED READINGS

Aronson RL, Kirk RW: Antibiotic therapy. p 15–22. In Kirk RW (ed): Current Veterinary Therapy V. WB Saunders, Philadelphia, 1974.

Chester DK: Bacterial and rickettsial diseases. In Catcott EJ (ed): Canine Medicine. 4th Ed. American Veterinary Publications, Santa Barbara, 1979.

Davis LE: Antimicrobial therapy. pp 2–16. In Kirk RW (ed) Current Veterinary Therapy VII. WB Saunders, Philadelphia, 1980.

Ling GV, Hirsh DC: Principles of antimicrobial therapy. In Kirk RW (ed): Current Veterinary Therapy VIII. WB Saunders, Philadelphia 1983

Macy DW, Small E: Deep Mycotic Diseases. pp 237–269. In Ettinger SJ (ed): Textbook of Veterinary Internal Medicine. 2nd Ed. WB Saunders Co. Philadelphia, 1983.

Mandell GL, Douglas RG Jr, Bennett JE (eds): Principles and Practice of Infectious Diseases. John Wiley and Sons, New York. Vols 1 & 2, 1979

Pratt WB: Chemotherapy of Infection. Oxford University Press, New York. 1977

Youmans GP, Paterson PY, Sommers HM: The Biologic and Clinical Basis of Infectious Diseases. 2nd ED. WB Saunders, Philadelphia, 1980

4

Parasitic Diseases

Kenneth S. Todd, Jr., Ph.D
Allan J. Paul, D.V.M.
Joseph A. DiPietro, D.V.M.

This chapter has been prepared to provide veterinarians and veterinary students with a convenient means for finding information on treatment of small animal parasites. No recommendations are given for a drug of choice. The best treatment is usually left to the veterinarian who is familiar with the individual animal and its environment. Although treating an animal to rid it of parasites is often a means of control, it should be stressed that good sanitation and hygiene are the best means of control. Good management and nutrition and the immune state of the host are among the factors that also influence parasite control. The key to the entire problem is often the veterinarian's knowledge of the parasite's life cycle, evaluation of the host-parasite relationship, and how these factors apply to each individual animal.

Ideally, antiparasitic drugs are administered to rid an animal of infection or infestation. They can be used to keep parasites at a manageable level. Although some compounds are nearly 100% efficacious in ridding an animal of parasites, the environment is often a source of reinfection and periodic treatment must be done. Prophylactic use of drugs to maintain an animal free of parasites can be successfully done with only a few—ascarids, hookworms, and heartworms.

Some of the drugs listed do not have Food and Drug Administration (FDA) approval and are named for informational purposes only. They are used at the veterinarian's risk and each veterinarian should be aware of the ethical and legal aspects of using such compounds. Even though a drug has label approval, the veterinarian should use it prudently and properly. Contraindications are not available for some compounds, especially those that have not been properly evaluated. Good judgment, such as not treating any severely debilitated or sick animal with an antiparasitic drug, is needed.

NEMATODE INFECTIONS

ASCARIDS–*Toxocara* spp., *Toxascaris leonina*

Clinical Features

I. Dogs
   A. Migratory larvae
      1. Peritonitis
      2. Septicemia
      3. Liver damage
      4. Verminous pneumonia
   B. Aberrant migration—adults
      Depends on organ involved
   C. Intestinal
      1. More common in young animals
      2. Gastrointestinal disturbances
      3. Unthriftiness
      4. Dull hair coat
      5. Vomiting
      6. Diarrhea
      7. Alternating diarrhea and constipation
      8. Anemia
      9. Nervous signs ("worm fits")
      10. Distended abdomen
      11. Aspiration pneumonia
      12. Rupture of bowel (rare)
II. Cats
   A. Migratory—larvae
      1. Usually not as severe as in dogs
      2. *T. leonina*—no tracheal migration
   B. Aberrant migration—adults, same as dogs
   C. Intestinal—same as dogs

Diagnosis

   I. Clinical signs
  II. Kennel or cattery history
 III. Worms in feces or vomitus
 IV. Fecal flotation

Treatment

   I. n-Butyl chloride (l-chlorobutane), Nemantic, BuChlorin, (available in many over-the-counter preparations)
      A. Dosage
         Dog—under 2.3 kg—1 ml; 2.3–4.5 kg—2 ml; 4.5–9.0 kg—3 ml; 9.0–18.2 kg—4 ml; over 18.2 kg—5 ml
      B. Comments
         Overnight fasting and the use of a cathartic increases efficacy.

C. Contraindications
None known
II. Dichlorvos, Task
A. Dosage
Dog—26–33 mg/kg
B. Comments
Dichlorvos is a cholinesterase inhibitor. Do not use simultaneously or within a few days after treatment with or exposure to cholinesterase-inhibiting drugs, pesticides, or chemicals. Antidote—atropine
C. Contraindications
Do not administer in conjunction with any other anthelmintic (except diethylcarbamazine), muscle relaxants, or tranquilizers. Do not administer to dogs with constipation, intestinal blockage, impaired liver function, circulatory failure, or dogs recently exposed to or showing signs of infectious disease. Do not use in dogs infected with *D. immitis*. Do not use in animals other than dogs or dogs weighing less than 2 pounds.
III. Dichlorvos, Task Tabs
A. Dosage
Dog and cat—11 mg/kg
B. Comments
Do not use in animals under 10 days of age or under 1 lb body weight. See Task, above.
C. Contraindications
See Task, above.
IV. Diethylcarbamazine (available under a number of trade names)
A. Dosage
Dog and cat—55–110 mg/kg
B. Comments
May be used as a preventative medication for ascariasis when given at 6.6 mg/kg daily to dogs
C. Contraindications
Do not use in dogs infected with *D. immitis*.
V. Dithiazanine iodide, Dizan
A. Dog: 22 mg/kg for 3–5 days
B. Comments
Vomiting, diarrhea, and anorexia may occur. The compound is a cyanine dye that stains fabrics, skin, and hair. The compound in feces or vomitus will also cause stains.
C. Contraindications
Do not administer to dogs sensitive to dithiazanine iodide or to dogs with reduced renal function.
VI. Fenbendazole, Panacur
A. Dosage
50 mg/kg daily for 3 days

   B. Comments
      Vomiting is a rare side effect
   C. Contraindications
      None known
VII. Mebendazole, Telmintic
   A. Dosage
      Dog—22 mg/kg for 3 days
   B. Comments
      Hepatic dysfunction (sometimes fatal) has been reported occasion-
      ally in dogs. Vomiting and diarrhea or soft stools are the most fre-
      quently reported side effects.
   C. Contraindications
      None known
VIII. Piperazine salts (available under a number of trade names, including Ver-
   mizine, Piperate, Pipertab, Piperson, Pipzine, Piperate tablets, Pipcide,
   Thenatol (also contains thenium closylate)
   A. Dosage
      In calculating the dose the percent of base needs to be considered.
      Cats and dogs 45–65 mg base/kg.
   B. Comments
      Avoid vapors and skin or eye contact. May exaggerate the extra-
      pyramidal effects of phenothiazine derivatives.
   C. Contraindications
      Do not use in animals with long-standing renal or hepatic disease.
IX. Pyrantel pamoate, Nemex
   A. Dosage
      Dog—5.0 mg base/kg
   B. Contraindications
      None known
X. Toluene, Methacide, Wurm Caps, Vermiplex, Difolin, Anaplex, Paracide
   (all also contain Dichlorophen), Nemantic (also contains n-butyl chlo-
   ride), Anthol (also contains arecoline)
   A. Dosage
      Dog and cat—see label for individual product
   B. Comments
      Best results are obtained if food is withheld 12 hours prior to treat-
      ment and 1 or 2 hours after. Toluene irritates the mucous membranes.
      Overdosage may result in transistory incoordination, vomiting, and
      possible central nervous system (CNS) depression. Gastric instillation
      of mineral oil delays drug absorption. Use oxygen therapy for severely
      depressed animals. Avoid epinephrine, digestible fats, oils, and al-
      cohol.
   C. Contraindications
      Do not use in severely debilitated animals.

Prevention

  I. Sanitation
 II. Periodic treatment
III. Treat puppies as early as possible after birth.
IV. Prevent cats from eating transport hosts.

Public Health Implications

Visceral larva migrans

Hookworms—*Ancylostoma* spp., *Uncinaria* spp.

Clinical Features

 I. Dogs
   A. Larval skin penetration
     1. Pruritis
     2. Dermatitis
     3. Secondary bacterial infections
     4. Usually a problem in interdigital area
   B. Migratory stage
     1. Usually not a problem
     2. Massive larval penetration—pneumonia
   C. Intestinal stages
     1. Peracute (death before prepatent period)
     2. Massive blood loss and anemia
     3. Enteritis
       a) Microcytic hypochromic anemia
       b) Diarrhea
       c) Malabsorption
       d) Leukocytosis
       e) Eosinophilia
       f) Most common in young nonimmune animals
       g) Occurs in older immune animals that are immunosuppressed
       h) Exacerbated by malnutrition
     4. Chronic
        Items a–e, above
II. Cats—same features as dogs

Diagnosis

 I. Anemia
II. Black tarry feces

III. Enteritis
IV. History of hypoproteinemia
 V. Fecal flotation
VI. Baermann technique for soil and grass samples from animal's habitat

Treatment

    I. Butamisole hydrochloride, Styquin
       A. Dosage
          Dog—0.22 ml/kg SQ
       B. Comments
          Animal should be weighed accurately and the dose measured care-
          fully. Do not inject more than 3 ml at one site.
       C. Contraindications
          Do not use concurrently with bunamidine hydrochloride. Do not
          administer to dogs infected with *D. immitis*. Do not use in breeding
          females prior to the third week of pregnancy. Do not use in puppies
          less than 8 weeks of age.
   II. Dichlorvos—see Ascarids, above.
  III. Disophenol, DNP
       A. Dosage
          Dog—0.22 ml/kg SQ
       B. Comments
          Animal should be weighed accurately and the dosage measured
          carefully before administration. Do not repeat treatment in less than
          14 days, do not give IM. In large dogs, the dose may be divided and
          given in two sites. In case of overdosage, use oxygen therapy and
          keep the animal in a cool environment.
  IV. Dithiazanine iodide, Dizan—22 mg/kg for 7 days.
   V. Styrylpyridium-diethylcarbamazine, Styrid Caricide
       A. Dosage
          Dog—5.5 mg/kg
       B. Comments
          For control of ascarid and hookworm infections and prevention of
          heartworm.
       C. Contraindications
          Do not use in dogs infected with *D.immitis*.
  VI. Tetrachlorethylene, Nema, Tetracap
       A. Dosage
          Dog and cat—0.22 ml/kg
       B. Comments
          Animal must be on a fat-free diet 48 hours prior to treatment, no
          food or water should be given 12 hours prior to and 4 hours after
          treatment.

C. Contraindications

Do not use in tapeworm-infected dogs. Do not use in animals weighing less than 2 lb. Do not use in nursing animals or in sick animals.

VII. Thenium closylate, Canopar, Thenatol (also contains piperazine phosphate)

A. Dosage

Dog—2.3–4.5 kg—$\frac{1}{2}$ of a 500-mg tablet twice daily; 4.5 kg and over—one 500-mg tablet as a single dose

B. Comments

Do not feed milk or other fatty foods during treatment. Rare reactions of a toxic or anaphylactic nature, sometimes fatal, have been reported following use; this occurs more commonly in Airedales than in other breeds

C. Contraindications

Do not use in suckling puppies and those weighing less than 2.3 kg.

VIII. Fenbendazole, Panacur—see Ascarids, above.

IX. Mebendazole, Telmintic—see Ascarids, above.

X. Pyrantel pamoate, Nemex—see Ascarids, above.

XI. Toluene—see Ascarids above.

Prevention

I. Prompt removal of feces

II. Strict sanitation

III. Larvae are killed by direct sunlight, drying, or heat.

IV. Treat dirt runs with sodium borate.

V. Use flame or steam to kill larvae in runs.

VI. Protect pregnant or lactating bitches from larvae.

VII. Periodic treatment

Public Health Implications

I. Cutaneous larva migrans (creeping eruption)

II. Loeffler's syndrome

WHIPWORMS—*Trichuris vulpis*

Clinical Features

I. Dogs

A. Light infections—usually asymptomatic

B. Severe infections

1. Enteritis

2. Secondary bacterial infections

    3. Anemia

    4. Weight loss

    5. Diarrhea

    6. Unthriftiness

    7. Blood in feces

II. Cats

    Infections are rare or probably nonexistent in North America.

Diagnosis

 I. Clinical signs

II. Fecal flotation

Treatment

  I. Butamisole hydrochloride, Styquin—see Hookworms above.

 II. Dichlorvos, Task, Task Tabs—see Ascarids, above.

III. Dithiazanine iodide, Dizan—see Ascarids, above.

IV. Fenbendazole, Panacur—see Ascarids, above.

 V. Mebendazole, Telmintic—see Ascarids, above.

Prevention

 I. Sanitation

II. Periodic treatment

HEARTWORMS—*Dirofilaria immitis*

Clinical Features

 I. Dogs

    A. Depends on health of dog, length and severity of infection.

    B. Right ventricular hypertrophy

    C. Right ventricular failure—pulmonary, hepatic, and renal involvement

    D. Left heart compensation

    E. Endocarditis

    F. Pulmonary endarteritis

    G. Pulmonary thrombosis and embolism

    H. Emphysema

    I. Passive pulmonary and hepatic congestion

    J. Perivascular hemorrhage

    K. Ascites

    L. Hydrothorax

    M. Edema

N. Chronic cough
O. Lack of stamina
P. Collapse after exercise
Q. Vena caval syndrome
II. Cats
    Same as dog
III. See chapter 9.

Diagnosis

I. Clinical signs
II. Identification of microfilariae in blood
III. Serologic tests

Treatment

I. Adults
    A. Thiacetarsamide sodium, Caparsolate Sodium, Filaramide
        1. Dosage
            Dog—0.22 ml/kg IV twice daily for 2 days
        2. Comments
            Perivascular leakage must be avoided. Dogs with severe heart-
            worm disease are poor risks for treatment. The compound is po-
            tentially hepatotoxic and nephrotoxic. If impaired kidney, liver, car-
            diovascular, or pulmonary function is not amenable to improvement,
            the drug should not be used. Any signs of nephrotoxicity or hepa-
            totoxicity should cause treatment to be halted. If treatment is inter-
            rupted, the full treatment regime must be started again 2–3 weeks
            later. Persistent vomiting is reason for discontinuing therapy. The
            animal should be kept quiet 4–6 weeks following treatment to min-
            imize the effect of pulmonary emboli caused by dead worms.
        3. Contraindications
            If signs of pulmonary embolism occur, supportive therapy should
            be implemented. Dogs with the vena caval syndrome of heartworm
            disease should not be re-treated until recovery from surgery to re-
            move the parasites.
II. Microfilariae
    A. Dithiazanine iodide, Dizan
        1. Dosage
            Dogs—6.6–11.0 mg/kg daily (8.8 mg/kg daily for 7 days).If mi-
            crofilaremia persists, increase dosage to 13.2–15.4 mg/kg daily until
            negative for microfilariae.
        2. Comments
            See Ascarids, above. Vomiting and diarrhea are side effects. These
            can be minimized by avoiding higher dosages unless low dosages fail

to clear microfilariae. If microfilaremia persists after 20 days of treatment, another microfilaricide might be used. If microfilaremia persists after treatment with other drugs, consideration should be given to a second treatment to remove adults.

    3. Contraindications

        See Ascarids, above.

  B. Levamisole

    1. Dosage

        Dog—11.0 mg/kg orally for 6–12 days

    2. Comments: Does not have FDA approval. Examine blood on the sixth day of treatment. Discontinue treatment when negative for microfilariae. Vomiting, neurologic signs, severe behavioral changes, and death have been reported following use. Treatment beyond 15 days increases the risk of toxicity.

    3. Contraindications

        Do not use concurrently with organophosphates or carbamates, or in animals with chronic renal or hepatic disease.

III. Preventative

  A. Diethylcarbamazine (available under a variety of trade names)

    1. Dosage

        Dog—6.6 mg/kg daily from the beginning of the mosquito season and for 2 months thereafter. Give all year where mosquitoes are active year around.

    2. Comments

        See Ascarids, above. Dogs on the preventative program should be examined 3 months after its beginning and at 6-month intervals thereafter for microfilariae.

    3. Contraindications

        See Ascarids, above. Do not use in dogs with *D. immitis* microfilariae.

  B. Styrylpyridium-diethylcarbamazine

    1. Dosage

        Dog—6.6 mg/kg

    2. Comments

        See Hookworms, above.

    3. Contraindications

        See Hookworms above. Do not administer to dogs with *D. immitis* microfilariae.

  C. Thiacetarsamide sodium, Caparsolate Sodium, Filaramide

    1. Dosage

        Dog 0.22 ml/kg twice daily for 2 days at 6-month intervals.

    2. Comments

        See thiacetarsamide sodium adult treatment for *D. immitis* above. If dogs cannot tolerate diethylcarbamazine, they should be given a therapeutic regimen of thiacetarsamide sodium twice yearly. This

may cause elimination of parasites in the heart before clinical signs develop.
3. Contraindications

See thiacetarsamide sodium adult treatment for *D. immitis*.

Prevention

Use preventative medication.

Public Health Implications

Human cases have been reported but risk is minimal.

Lungworms—Cats—*Aelurostrongylus abstrusus* (also see section on *Capillaria aerophila* in dogs, below)

Clinical Features

I. Usually asymptomatic
II. Moderate infections
    A. Coughing and sneezing
    B. Anorexia
    C. Respiratory distress
III. Severe infections (rare)
    A. Severe cough
    B. Dyspnea
    C. Anorexia
    D. Emaciation
    E. Hydrothorax
    F. Polypnea

Diagnosis

I. Clinical signs
II. Fecal examination by Baermann technique

Treatment

I. Levamisole, Tramisol
    A. Dosage
        Cat—100 mg daily PO every other day for five treatments
    B. Comments
        Does not have FDA approval. This compound may be toxic in cats.
Adverse reactions include salivation and vomiting. There are reports

of cats being killed by the compound. Fifteen minutes before treatment, 0.5 mg atropine sulfate should be given SQ.

   C. Contraindications

      Do not use concurrently with organophosphates or carbamates or in animals with chronic renal or hepatic disease.

II. Levamisole, Tetramisole

   A. Dosage

      Cat—15 mg/kg per os every other day for three treatments, 3 days later 30 mg/kg followed 2 days later by 60 mg/kg

   B. Comments

      See above. Experimentally, cats salivated profusely, but no other side effects were seen.

   C. Contraindications

      See above.

III. Fenbendazole, Panacur

   A. Dosage

      Cat—20 mg/kg once daily for 5 days, repeat after 5 days.

   B. Comments

      Does not have FDA approval for use in cats.

   C. Contraindications

      Experimental—none known.

Prevention

  I. Avoid contact with intermediate hosts—snails and slugs

 II. Avoid contact with transport hosts—lower vertebrates, mice, and birds.

Public health implications

  None known

LUNGWORMS—DOGS AND CATS—*Capillaria aerophila*

Clinical signs

  I. Chronic cough

 II. Bronchitis (rare)

III. Rhinitis (rare)

Diagnosis

  I. Clinical signs

 II. Fecal flotation

Treatment

I. Levamisole
   A. Dosage
      Cat—4.4 mg/kg SQ for 2 days then 8.8 mg/kg for 1 day 2 weeks later OR 5 mg/kg daily PO for 5 days, followed by 9 days of no treatment; repeat two times
   B. Comments
      See *A. abstrusus*, above.
   C. Contraindications
      See *A. abstrusus*, above.
II. Mebendazole, Telmintic
   A. Dosage
      Dog—6 mg/kg twice daily for 5 days
   B. Does not have label approval in dogs for this parasite—see Ascarids above.
   C. Contraindications—None known

LUNGWORMS—DOGS—*Filaroides osleri*

Clinical Signs

   I. Dyspnea
  II. Coughing
 III. Emaciation
 IV. Chronic tracheobronchitis
  V. Respiratory distress after exercise
 VI. May be asymptomatic

Diagnosis

   I. Bronchoscopy
  II. Tracheal washing
 III. Fecal examination with Baermann technique

Treatment

Albendazole
   I. 9.5 mg/kg for 55 days OR 25 mg/kg twice daily for 5 days. Repeat treatment in 2 weeks.
  II. Does not have FDA approval
 III. Experimental—none known

Prevention

  I. Sanitation
 II. Treat infected animals prior to breeding.

LUNGWORMS—DOGS—*Filaroides hirthi*
and *Filaroides milksi*

Clinical Signs

  Usually asymptomatic

Diagnosis

  Fecal examination with Baermann technique

Treatment

  I. None known for *F. milksi*
 II. Albendazole
    A. Dosage
       25–50mg/kg twice daily for 5 days
    B. Comments
       Does not have FDA approval. A severe tissue reaction to dead parasites has been reported.
    C. Contraindications
       Experimental, none known

Prevention

  I. Treat infected bitches prior to breeding.
 II. Sanitation

LUNGWORMS—DOGS—*Crenosoma vulpis*

Clinical Signs

   I. Bronchopneumonia
  II. Tracheitis
 III. Coughing and sneezing
 IV. Nasal discharge
  V. Emaciation
 VI. Anemia

Diagnosis

I. Clinical signs
II. Fecal examination with the Baermann technique

Treatment

I. Levamisole
  A. Dosage: 8 mg/kg as a single dose
  B. Does not have FDA approval—see *D. immitis*, above.
  C. Experimental—see *D. immitis*, above.
II. Diethylcarbamazine
  A. Dosage
    80 mg/kg every 12 hours for 3 days
  B. Comments
    Experimental. No signs of toxicity were noted—see *D. immitis*, above.
  C. Contraindications
    See *D. immitis*, above.

Capillaria plica AND *Capillaria feliscati*

Clinical Features—Cat and Dog

I. Usually asymptomatic
II. Cystitis
III. Difficulty in urination

Diagnosis

Finding eggs in urinary sediment

Treatment

I. *C. plica*—Fenbendazole, Panacur
  A. Dosage
    Dog—50 mg/kg once daily for 3 days; single 50 mg/kg dose 3 weeks later
  B. Comments
    Does not have label approval
  C. Contraindications—None known
II. *C. feliscati*—no treatment known

Prevention

I. *C. plica*—earthworms are intermediate hosts
II. *C. feliscati*—life cycle unknown

Dioctophyma renale

Clinical Features—Dogs

I. May be asymptomatic
II. Dysuria
III. Hematuria

Diagnosis

I. Finding eggs in urinary sediment
II. Radiologic examination

Treatment

I. No compounds have been evaluated.
II. Surgical removal

Prevention

Do not feed raw fish.

Dipetalonema reconditum

Clinical Features—Dogs

None

Diagnosis

I. Examination of blood for microfilariae
II. Microfilariae may be confused with those of *D. immitis*.

Treatment

I. None known or needed.
II. Parasites are not considered to be pathogens.

Prevention

Avoid contact with intermediate hosts.

Dracunculus insignis

Clinical Features

I. Lesion in skin
II. Worm protrudes after wetting skin.

Diagnosis

Observation of protruding worm

Treatment

Surgical excision

Prevention

Prevent animals from drinking water containing *Cyclops*.

Ollulanus tricuspis

Clinical Features

I. Usually none
II. Gastritis
III. Chronic vomiting

Diagnosis

I. Examination of stomach washings with a microscope
II. Use 0.44 mg/kg xylazine to induce vomiting. Examine vomitus with a microscope.

Treatment

Levamisole
I. Dosage
    Cat—5 mg/kg SQ
II. Comments
    See *A. abstrusus* and *D. immitis*, above.

III. Contraindications
> See *A. abstrusus* and *D.immitis*, above.

Prevention

Prevent cats from eating vomitus of infected animals

Pelodera strongyloides (syn. *Rhabditis strongyloides*)

Clinical Features

Dermatitis

Diagnosis

Finding nematodes in skin scraping

Treatment—Dog

I. Infections usually clear spontaneously if the animal is provided clean dry bedding.
II. Lindane
> A. Dosage
>> Bathe in 0.5% solution and again 1 week later.
> B. Comments
>> Does not have FDA approval. May be hepatotoxic.

Prevention

Avoid wet bedding, especially straw.

Physaloptera spp.

Clinical Features—Dog and Cat

I. Gastritis
II. Vomiting
III. Black tarry feces
IV. Anemia
V. Hematemesis

Diagnosis

I. Clinical signs
II. Fecal flotation

Treatment

I. Pyrantel pamoate, Nemex
   A. Dosage
      Dog—5 mg pyrantel base/kg
   B. Comments
      Does not have label approval but is highly efficacious. See Hookworms, above.
   C. Contraindications—None known
II. Dichlorvos, Task
   A. 22–33 mg/kg
   B. See hookworms, above.
   C. See hookworms, above.

Prevention

Avoid contact with intermediate hosts, e.g., cockroaches, crickets, or beetles.

Spirocerca lupi—Dogs

Clinical Features

    I. May be asymptomatic
   II. Dysphagia
  III. Vomiting
   IV. Esophageal neoplasia
    V. Aortic aneurysm
   VI. Hypertrophic pulmonary osteoarthropathy
  VII. Anemia
VIII. Spondylitis
   IX. Hematemesis
    X. Pleuritis
   XI. Peritonitis
  XII. Respiratory distress
XIII. Anorexia
XIV. Coughing
 XV. Hypersalivation

Diagnosis

  I. Clinical signs
  II. Eggs may be found in feces. Periodic discharge of eggs often requires repeated fecal flotation.
  III. Radiologic evidence of spondylitis in thoracic vertebrae

Treatment

  Disophenol, DNP
  I. Dosage
    7.7 mg/kg SQ followed by the same dosage 1 week later
  II. Comments
    Does not have FDA approval. See Hookworms, above.
  III. Contraindications
    See Hookworms, above.

Prevention

  I. Avoid contact with intermediate and especially transport hosts.
  II. Keep outside dogs on wire floors above ground in highly endemic areas.

Strongyloides stercoralis

Clinical Features

  I. Penetration—secondary bacterial infections, pruritus
  II. Intestinal
    A. Diarrhea
    B. Dehydration
    C. Anemia
    D. Enteritis
    E. Necrosis and sloughing of intestinal mucosa
    F. Anorexia
    G. Rapid weight loss
    H. Usually a problem in young animals

Diagnosis

  I. Clinical signs during hot humid weather
  II. Usually a problem only in kennels
  III. Finding larvae in feces

Treatment

  I. Dithiazanine iodate, Dizan

    A. Dosage
        22 mg/kg for 10–12 days
    B. Comments
        See Hookworms, above.
    C. Contraindications
        See Hookworms, above.
II. Thiabendazole, TBZ, Omnizole
    A. Dosage
        50–60 mg/kg
    B. Comments
        Does not have FDA approval. Vomition is a possible side effect.
    C. Contraindications
        Experimental. Dachshunds may be especially sensitive to the compound.
    D. Public health implications—may be transmitted to man.

Thelazia spp.

Clinical Features

    I. Usually none
  II. Lacrimation
 III. Conjunctivitis
 IV. Photophobia

Diagnosis

    I. Clinical signs
  II. Observation of worms in the conjunctival sac
 III. Eggs in tears

Treatment

Manual removal under local anesthesia

Prevention

Avoid contact with flies.

CESTODE INFECTIONS

Taenia spp., *Dipylidium caninum,*
Mesocestoides spp., *Echinococcus*
granulosus, Dibothriocephalus latus,
Spirometra spp.

Clinical Features

Dog and cat
  I. Often nonpathogenic
  II. Depends on numbers present
  III. Vague clinical signs
  IV. Chronic diarrhea and enteritis
  V. Abdominal discomfort
  VI. Vomition
  VII. Weight loss
VIII. Poor growth rate
  IX. Possible nervous signs
  X. Alternating constipation and diarrhea
  XI. Anal pruritis

Diagnosis

  I. Clinical signs
  II. Presence of perianal proglottids
  III. Proglottids in feces
  IV. Proglottids in animal's environment
  V. Fecal flotation—least reliable except for *D. latus* and *Spirometra* spp.
  VI. History of contact with intermediate host
  VII. *E. granulosus*—purgation and examination of ingesta and feces

Treatment

  I. *Dipylidium caninum* and *Taenia* spp.
    A. Arecoline acetarsol, drocarbil, Nemural
       1. Dosage
          Dog and cat—5 mg/kg
       2. Comments
          Give in milk 3 hours after principal meal; vomiting, salivation,
          restlessness, ataxia, and labored breathing are possible side effects.
          May cause excessive salivation in cats. Antidote—atropine
       3. Contraindications
          Do not give to puppies 3 months of age or cats under 1 year. Do
          not use in febrile animals, those with catarrhal enteritis, or animals
          with severe cardiac or circulatory disturbances. Do not use with
          organophosphates.
    B. Arecoline hydrobromide, Areco Canine
       1. Dosage
          Dogs and cats—0.4–1.0 mg/kg
       2. Twice the recommended dosage may cause side effects including

vomition, ataxia, unconsciousness, and sudden collapse. Use after a preliminary fast. Excessive salivation has been reported in cats. Antidote—atropine

3. Contraindications

See Arecoline acetarsol.

C. Arecoline carboxyphenylstilbonate, Anthelin

1. Dosage

Dogs—10.3 mg/kg to a maximum dose of 211.5 mg for dogs 20.5 kg and over.

2. Comments

Withhold food except milk for 24 hours prior to treatment. If catharsis does not occur within 3 hours, give an enema. Toxic signs are depression, vomiting, and abdominal pain. If toxic signs appear, feed the dog 1 hour after treatment. If no toxic signs, feed 4–8 hours after treatment.

3. Contraindications: do not use in sick or undernourished animals. See Arecoline hydrobromide, above.

D. Bunamidine hydrochloride, Scolaban

1. Dosage

Dog and cat—25–50 mg/kg

2. Comments

Give on an empty stomach after a 3- to 4-hour fast. The drug is irritating to the conjunctiva—use care in handling. If the tablet is crushed, it is irritating to the oral mucosa. Side effects include vomition and mild diarrhea. Sudden collapse and death have been reported following use.

3. Contraindications

Do not use in animals with cardiac disease. Do not use male dogs for breeding within 28 days of treatment. Do not use concurrently with butamisole or in animals with impaired liver function. Do not use in severely debilitated animals. Do not retreat within 14 days.

E. Dichlorophen, Diphenthane-70, Vermiplex, Wurm Caps, Difolin, Anaplex (all also contain toluene; Nemantic (also contains n-butyl chloride)

1. Dosage

Dog—0.3 g/kg; cat— 0.1–0.2 g/kg

2. Comments

See Hookworms, above.

3. Contraindications

See Hookworms, above.

F. Fenbendazole, Panacur

1. Dosage

Dog—50 mg/kg daily for 3 days

2. Comments

For *Taenia* spp. only. See Hookworms, above.

    3. Contraindications

        None known

  H. Praziquantel, Droncit

    1. Dosage

        Dog and cat—refer to the label. Smaller animals require higher dosages per kilogram.

    2. Comments

        Fasting is not recommended.

    3. Contraindications

        Do not use in puppies less than 4 weeks of age or in kittens less than 6 weeks of age.

  I. Mebendazole, Telmintic

    1. Dosage

        Dog—22 mg/kg daily for 3 days.

    2. Comments

        For *Taenia* spp. only. See Hookworms, above.

    3. Contraindications

        See Hookworms, above.

  J. Niclosamide, Yomesan

    1. Dosage

        Dog and cat—71.4 mg/kg

    2. Comments

        Fast overnight. The drug is well tolerated at therapeutic dosages.

    3. Contraindications

        None known.

II. *Echinococcus granulosus*

  A. Arecoline compounds

    1. Dosage

        See *Taenia*, above

    2. Comments

        Label claims are not made, but all are evidently effective—see *Taenia*, above.

    3. Contraindications

        See *Taenia*, above.

  B. Bunamidine hydrochloride, Scolaban

    1. Dosage

        See *Taenia*, above.

    2. Comments

        See *Taenia*, above.

    3. Contraindications

        See *Taenia*, above.

  C. Praziquantel, Droncit

    1. Dosage

        See *Taenia*, above.

2. Comments
   See *Taenia*, above.
3. Contraindications
   See *Taenia*, above.

III. *Mesocestoides* spp.
   A. Arecoline compounds
      1. Dosage
         See *Taenia*, above.
      2. Comments
         Gives variable results in individual dogs. See *Taenia*, above.
      3. Contraindications
         See *Taenia*, above.
   B. Bunamidine hydrochloride, Scolaban
      1. Dosage
         See *Taenia*, above.
      2. Comments
         Drug of choice. see *Taenia*, above.
      3. Contraindications
         See *Taenia*, above.

IV. *Dibothriocephalus latus* and *Spirometra* spp.
   A. Arecoline compounds
      1. Dosage
         See *Taenia*, above
      2. Comments
         Label claims are not made, but the compounds are reported to be effective. See *Taenia* above.
      3. Contraindications
         See *Taenia* above.
   B. Other compounds have not been evaluated for these parasites; however, bunamadine hydrochloride, niclosamide, and praziquantel may be effective.

Prevention

I. Avoid contact with intermediate hosts.
II. Do not feed raw viscera to dogs or cats—*Taenia* spp., *E.granulosus*.
III. Eliminate fleas—*D. caninum*.
IV. Do not feed raw or undercooked fish—*D. latus* and *Spirometra* spp.
V. Do not allow animals to roam and hunt.
VI. Periodic treatment of infected animals

Public Health Importance

I. *D.caninum*
   A. Human infection occurs when infected fleas are ingested.

B. Kissing animals that have chewed fleas may result in ingestion of larval stages from fur or skin.
C. Eliminate fleas.
II. *E. granulosus*
A. May be a severe human pathogen
B. If in endemic areas, use care in handling canine feces.
C. Avoid feeding raw viscera.
D. Do not allow dogs to run free.
E. Periodic treatment of dogs in endemic areas is recommended.

TREMATODE INFECTIONS

Paragonimus kellicotti

Clinical Features

I. Bronchopneumonia
II. Productive cough
III. Hemoptysis
IV. Dyspnea

Diagnosis

I. Finding eggs in feces or sputum
II. Radiographic examination

Treatment

I. Albendazole
A. Dosage
Cat—30 mg/kg once daily for 6 days; dog—30 mg/kg daily for 12 days
B. Comments
Does not have FDA approval
C. Contraindications
Not known, experimental
II. Fenbendazole
A. Dosage
Dog—50–100 mg/kg daily in two divided doses for 10–14 days.
B. Comments
Does not have label approval
C. Contraindications
Not known, experimental

Prevention

Avoid contact with intermediate host.

Platynosomum fastosum

Clinical Features—Cat

  I. Vomiting
 II. Diarrhea
III. Icterus

Diagnosis

 I. Finding eggs in feces
II. History of eating lizards.

Treatment

Praziquantel, Droncit
  I. Dosage
     Cat—20 mg/kg as a single dose
 II. Comments
     Does not have label approval
III. Contraindications
     Not known, experimental. May be toxic.

PROTOZOAN INFECTIONS

Giardia spp.

Clinical Features—Dogs and Cats

   I. Many infections are asymptomatic.
  II. Chronic diarrhea
 III. Mucoid diarrhea
 IV. Flatulence
  V. Abdominal pain
 VI. Poor appetite
VII. Weight loss

Diagnosis

  I. Clinical signs
 II. Trophozoites in diarrheal smears
III. Cysts in fecal flotation with zinc sulfate solution

Treatment

I. Metronidazole, Flagyl
   A. Dosage
      Dog—initial loading dose of 44 mg/kg followed by 22 mg/kg every 8 hours for 5 days
   B. Comments
      Does not have FDA approval. Side effects include neurologic disorders, hepatotoxicity, hematuria, and vomition.
   C. Contraindications
      Do not use in pregnant or lactating animals or in severely debilitated animals.
II. Quinacrine, Atabrine
   A. Dosage
      Dogs—50–100 mg/dog every 12 hours for 3 days, repeat in 3 days. Another recommended dosage is: large breeds—200 mg/dog three times on the first day and twice daily on 6 subsequent days. Small breeds—100 mg/dog twice on the first day and once daily for 6 subsequent days. Puppies—50 mg/dog twice on the first day and once on 6 subsequent days.
   B. Comments
      Does not have FDA approval. Side effects include yellowness of the skin, anorexia, nausea, diarrheic, pruritis, blurred vision, and behavioral changes. Use sodium bicarbonate concurrently to reduce vomition. The drug crosses the placental barrier. Hepatic toxicity, toxic psychoses, aplastic anemia, fatal agranulocytosis, and hypersensitivity have been reported in human patients following use.
   C. Contraindications
      Do not use in pregnant animals.

Prevention

  I. Strict sanitation
 II. Treat carrier animals.
III. Public Health Implications—may be transmitted to man

Isospora spp.

Clinical Features

  I. Diarrhea
 II. Enteritis
III. Weight loss
IV. Decreased food and water intake
 V. Dehydration

Diagnosis

I. Clinical signs
II. Finding oocysts by fecal flotation

Treatment

I. Treat symptomatically for secondary bacterial infections.
II. Amprolium, Amprol
A. Dosage
Dog—110–220 mg/kg of powder in food for 7–12 days; preventive—1–2 tbsp of 9.6% solution in 1 gallon water. Give to bitch 10 days prior to whelping as the only water source.
B. Comment
Does not have FDA approval. Amprolium is a thiamine inhibitor. Side effects after prolonged usage include vomiting, anorexia, diarrhea, and nervous symptoms. Treatment should be stopped and animals treated with thiamine, calcium gluconate solution, and fluids.
C. Contraindications
Experimental; none known
III. Sulfadimethoxine, Albon
A. Dosage
Dog—day 1–55 mg/kg; days 2–4 or until asymptomatic—27.5 mg/kg
B. Comments
Does not have FDA approval. Supportive treatment is recommended.
C. Contraindications
Not known, experimental

Toxoplasma gondii

Clinical Features—Cat

I. Usually asymptomatic
II. Fever
III. Hepatitis
IV. Bilirubinemia
V. Pneumonia
VI. Dyspnea
VII. Anemia
VIII. Leukopenia
IX. Encephalitis
X. Myositis
XI. Myocarditis
XII. Enteritis
XIII. Lymphadenitis

Diagnosis

  I. Clinical signs
  II. Intestinal stages—finding oocysts in feces
  III. Systemic infections—serology—paired sera indicating a rising titer

Treatment

  I. Systemic infections
    A. Sulfadiazine and pyrimethamine
      1. Dosage
          Cats—sulfadiazine—60 mg/kg/day divided into four to six daily doses plus pyrimethamine at 0.5–1.0 mg/kg/day
      2. Comments
          Does not have FDA approval. Sulfamerazine, sulfamethazine, or sulfadoxine or combinations may be substituted for sulfadiazine. If treatment exceeds 2 weeks, platelet and leukocyte counts are advised. When platelets or leukocyte counts drop to $\frac{1}{2}$ or $\frac{1}{4}$ of normal, antagonists should be used with the treatment or prophylactically. Antagonists are: folic acid 1 mg/kg/day and baker's yeast—100 mg/kg/day. Kidney and urinary tract disturbances may follow use. Side effects are anorexia, depression, hematuria, crystallinuria, and elevated blood urea nitrogen (BUN).
      3. Contraindications
          Experimental
  II. Oocyst shedding phase
    A. Sulfadiazine and pyrimethamine
      1. Dosage
          Cat—sulfadiazine at 120 mg/100 g in the diet or 60 mg/100 g plus 0.5 mg/100 g pyrimethamine in the diet
      2. Comments
          See above
      3. Contraindications—See above

Prevention

  I. Do not feed raw or undercooked meat.
  II. Do not allow cats to roam freely and hunt.
  III. Empty litter boxes daily and clean thoroughly.

Public Health Implications

  I. Human infections usually result from ingesting sporulated oocysts of *T. gondii*, eating raw or undercooked meat, and by transplacental transmission.
  II. Ingestion of oocysts from cat feces may result in human infection.

*Balantidium coli, Entamoeba
histolytica,* and *Trichmonas* spp.

These protozoa have been considered to be pathogens in rare cases. Little is known about clinical features or treatment.

EXTERNAL PARASITES

FLEAS—*Ctenocephalides canis, C. felis*

Clinical Features

Dogs and cats
I. Skin irritation
II. Pruritus
III. Self-mutilation
IV. Anemia
V. Flea allergy dermatitis
   A. Severe pruritis
   B. Alopecia
   C. Crusted miliary lesions on lower back and spinal regions

Diagnosis

I. Clinical signs
II. Presence of fleas
III. Presence of flea excreta
IV. Presence of *Dipylidium caninum* proglottids
V. Intradermal skin testing with flea antigen

Treatment

I. General comments
   A. Numerous insecticides are available to kill fleas on pets.
   B. Insecticides can be toxic and should be used with care.
   C. Cats are more sensitive to insecticides than dogs.
   D. Never use a product on a cat unless specifically recommended for that species.
   E. Use of flea medications may render both dogs and cats more susceptible to toxicoses due to accidental exposure to insecticides.
   F. Concurrent use of flea medications and certain anthelmintic compounds may result in poisoning.
II. Commonly used compounds
   A. Organophosphates
      1. Generally considered to contain some of the most potent insecticidal compounds

    2. Should be used only with extreme caution in cats

    3. Should not be used on kittens

    4. Some resistant flea populations have developed.

  B. Carbamates

    1. Less toxic than organophosphates

    2. Can be used on cats but not kittens

    3. Should be used with care on puppies

  C. Pyrethrins

    1. Least toxic

    2. Contact poisons with rapid, strong action

    3. Can be used on kittens

III. Methods of use

  A. Flea collars, medallions

    1. May be useful in reducing the flea population, but are not adequate for management of the allergic patient

    2. May be irritating to skin

    3. Usually contain organophosphates and/or carbamates

  B. Shampoos

    1. Good knockdown but no residual effect

    2. Completely useless as sole method of flea control

  C. Sprays

    1. Good knockdown but poor residual activity

    2. May be messy, alarming to animal, and difficult to apply correctly

  D. Powders

    1. Fair residual activity usually for 3–7 days

    2. Must be worked well into coat when applied

  E. Dips

    Most effective and best residual activity—usually 7 days

  F. Systemic insecticides

    Proban—an organophosphate which is administered orally. Fleas are killed by ingesting the drug from the body fluid.

Prevention

  I. Treat all animals in the household.

 II. Treat the environment.

  A. Vacuum carpets and animal's bedding.

  B. Sprays

  C. Foggers

  D. Commercial exterminators

Public Health Implications

Dipylidium caninum—see section on Cestodes, above

TICKS—*Rhipicephalus sanguineus, Dermacentor variabilis, D. andersoni, D. occidentalis, Ixodes scapularis, Otobius megnini, Amblyomma americanum, Amblyomma maculatum*

Clinical features

Dogs and cats
I. Most ticks tend to be found on the head, ears, and toes.
II. Site of attachment may become irritated or infected.
III. Anemia may occur in young animals with heavy infestations.
IV. Tick paralysis.
V. Ticks can serve as vectors of bacterial, rickettsial, viral, and protozoan diseases.

Diagnosis

I. Close visual inspection of animal
II. Examination of bedding

Treatment

I. If numbers are small, manual removal
II. If large numbers of ticks are present, dipping with an insecticide that is effective against ticks is recommended.
III. Powders or shampoos may also be used.

Prevention

I. Household infestations with ticks may require foggers or professional exterminators.
II. Destroy tick habitat by cutting and burning brush and grass.
III. Tick collars may provide some relief.

Public Health Implications

Some of these ticks will also feed on people, and some are vectors of human pathogens.

MITES—*Sarcoptes* spp., *Notoedres cati*

Clinical Features

I. Dogs—*Sarcoptes* spp.
A. Intense pruritus

    B. Highly contagious

    C. External ears are sites of predilection. The extremities, especially the elbows and hocks, are also involved frequently

    D. Affected areas show partial alopecia, erythema, excoriations, thickening, and crusting.

    E. Self-inflicted trauma

    F. Secondary bacterial infections

II. Cats—*Notoedres cati*

    A. Lesions similar to those in dogs

    B. Found primarily on ears, face, eyelids, and neck

Diagnosis

  I. History

  II. Clinical signs

  III. Skin scrapings

  IV. Potassium hydroxide—sugar-centrifuged sedimentation

  V. Skin biopsy

Treatment

  I. Isolation

  II. All animals on premises should be treated

  III. Gentle clipping and cleansing of affected areas to remove hair and crusts

  IV. Antiseborrheal shampoos to remove scales and debris

  V. Corticosteroids to relieve pruritus

  VI. Acaricidal dips to eradicate mites. For cats, 2% lime sulfur solution is the agent of choice.

Prevention

  I. Isolation of infected animals

  II. Mites do not persist long off the host so eradication procedures are not necessary for the environment.

Public Health Implications

  I. Mites may infest people temporarily, causing a pruritic, papulocrustous dermatitis.

  II. Mites do not multiply on people and infections are self-limiting.

MITES—*Demodex canis, D. cati*

Clinical features

I. Dogs
  A. Localized form—one to five small, well-circumscribed, scaly, erythematous, nonpruritic areas of alopecia around eyes, ears, lips, and forelegs
  B. Generalized form
    1. Severe disease which can be fatal
    2. Large areas of the body may be affected with alopecia, edema, erythema, seborrhea, pyoderma, and pruritus.
    3. Peripheral lymphadenopathy is a consistent finding.
II. Cats—same as dogs

Diagnosis

  I. History
 II. Physical examination
III. Skin scrapings

Treatment

 I. Localized form
    Daily treatment with topical acaricidal preparations such as rotenone, benzyl benzoate, or benzoyl peroxide gel until hair growth is evident
II. Generalized form
  A. Antibiotics when deep pyoderma is present
  B. Gently clip all hair on the affected areas and remove matted crusts.
  C. Antiseptic baths and gentle shampoos
  D. Numerous compounds have been tried with variable results for treating demodectic mange. The current drugs of choice are:
    1. Dogs—Amitraz, Mitaban
      a) Dosage
        See label for complete instructions.
      b) Comments
        Animals should not be stressed for a period of at least 24 hours posttreatment. The most frequently observed adverse reaction is transient sedation.
      c) Contraindications
        Fertility, reproductive, and safety studies have not been conducted in dogs less than 4 months of age.
    2. Cats—2% lime-sulfur dips—safe and economical

Prevention

  Dogs with generalized demodicosis should not be used for breeding.

Mites—*Cheyletiella* spp.

Clinical Features

Dogs and cats
I. Mild pruritus
II. "Walking dandruff"—yellow-gray scales along the dorsum and on the rump, top of the head, and nose
III. Asymptomatic carriers ·

Diagnosis

I. History
II. Physical examination
III. Skin scrapings

Treatment

I. Antiseborrheal shampoos to remove scales
II. Corticosteroids for pruritus
III. Most insecticides are effective

Prevention

I. Treat all animals on premises.
II. Destroy bedding and treat environment.

Public Health Implications

Cheyletiella spp. can infest people.

Mites—*Otodectes cynotis*

Clinical Features

I. Dogs
  A. Highly contagious
  B. Pruritus
  C. Self-trauma
  D. Head-shaking
  E. Aural hematomas
  F. Inflammation and probably a hypersensitivity reaction
  G. Thick, crusty, brown-black exudate in external ear canal
II. Cats—same as dogs

Diagnosis

I. History
II. Physical examination
III. Presence of mites in ear canal

Treatment

I. Thorough cleansing of ear canal
II. Instillation of acaricidal otic preparation such as Mitox or Canex
III. Antibiotic—glucocorticoid preparation
IV. Total body pyrethrin-carbamate powders may be necessary to kill mites outside of ear.

Prevention

Treat all animals on premises.

Public Health Implications

People may be transiently affected with a papular eruption.

LICE—*Trichodectes canis, Felicola subrostatus*

Clinical Features

I. Dogs
  A. Contagious disease
  B. Usually associated with neglect, debilitation, and poor sanitary conditions
  C. Found primarily on neck and shoulders
  D. Restlessness
  E. Pruritus
  F. Skin inflammation
  G. Alopecia
II. Cats—same as dogs

Diagnosis

I. Clinical signs
II. Demonstration of the parasite and its egg

Treatment

I. Isolation
II. Lice are susceptible to all insecticidal agents.
III. Apply weekly for 4 weeks.

Prevention

I. Treat all animals on premises.
II. Correct any predisposing causes.

Public Health Implications

None

SUGGESTED READINGS

Dunn AM: Veterinary Helminthology. 2nd Ed. William Heinemann, London, 1978

Georgi JR: Parasitology for Veterinarians. 3rd Ed. WB Saunders, Philadelphia, 1980

Roberson EL: Chemotherapy of Parasitic Diseases. In Booth NH, McDonald LE (eds): Veterinary Pharmacology and Therapeutics. 5th Ed. Iowa State University Press, Ames, 1982

Soulsby EJL: Helminths, Arthropods, and Protozoa of Domesticated Animals. 7th Ed. Lea and Febiger, Philadelphia, 1982

5

Pharmacologic Control of Inflammation

William L. Jenkins, B.V.Sc.

A host of injurious agents may be responsible for an inflammatory reaction in any tissue of the body. The physiopathologic responses are essentially protective against the noxious insult. The resultant lesions may be localized or generalized and the clinical course may vary from peracute to chronic. Although defensive in nature, inflammation associated with a number of disease conditions may of itself be harmful or incapacitating. Thus, the pharmacologic modulation of the processes involved often becomes a critical feature of a successful therapeutic regimen. The object of this chapter is to outline the salient components of inflammatory reactions that can be modified pharmacologically and to review the characteristics of the antiinflammatory drugs that may be employed for this purpose.

PHYSIOPATHOLOGY OF INFLAMMATORY REACTIONS

CAUSES OF TISSUE INJURY

Nonimmunological

I. Physical
   Trauma, temperature extremes, electromagnetic radiation
II. Chemical
   Inorganic or organic compounds
III. Biochemical
   Harmful metabolites, destructive enzymes, active peptides
IV. Biological
   Infectious agents, ectoparasites, endoparasites, toxins

Immunologic

I. Type I hypersensitivity reactions
   Several inflammatory mediators
II. Type III hypersensitivity reactions
   Immune complexes and complement, inflammatory mediators
III. Type IV or delayed hypersensitivity reactions
   Cell mediated (lymphokines, monokines), inflammatory mediators
IV. See Chapter 6

CLINICAL SIGNS OF INFLAMMATION

Acute Inflammation

I. Active hyperemia
   Due to increased blood supply
II. Heat
   Due to increased metabolism and blood supply
III. Swelling
   Due to engorgement and enhanced capillary permeability
IV. Pain
   Due to stimulation of nociceptors by inflammatory mediators
V. Loss of function
   Due to tissue damage or destruction
VI. Systemic manifestations
   Malaise, inappetence, fever, leukocytosis, elevated erythrocyte sedimentation rate (ESR) and plasma fibrinopeptide levels, hypoferremia, others

Chronic Inflammation

I. Granulation tissue (granulomas)
   Due to fibroblasts and high vascularity
II. Fibrous tissue (scars)
   Due to collagen deposition and reduced vascularity
III. Suppuration
   Due to extensive cellular (leukocyte) destruction
IV. Some signs of acute inflammation
   May persist in chronic processes
V. Systemic manifestations
   As for acute inflammation with hypoalbuminemia, hypergammaglobulinemia, others

GENERAL INFLAMMATORY-REPARATIVE RESPONSES

Depending upon the nature of the noxious insult and subsequent tissue reactions, several reparative responses are possible (Fig. 5-1).

PATHOGENESIS OF THE ACUTE INFLAMMATORY REACTION

General Sequence of Events

This sequence is often independent of the noxious agent's nature; several variations are possible.

I. Damage to vascular walls

Leakage of protein-rich fluid and blood cellular elements

II. Platelet aggregation, fibrin formation, and local edema

Platelets release vasoactive substances, clotting and related sequences initiated

III. Margination and subsequent emigration of leukocytes

Facilitated by chemotactic factors and increased capillary permeability, neutrophils, eosinophils or monocytes (macrophages) involved, many mediators produced by these leukocytes

IV. Injured and dying cells release provocative substances

Lysosomal and other enzymes, oxygen-derived radicals, prostaglandins, leukotrienes, histamine, platelet activating factors, and other mediators

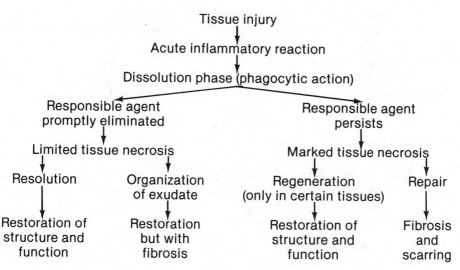

Fig. 5-1. Reparative responses to noxious insult and subsequent tissue reactions

V. Clotting and kinin cascades proceed with concurrent activation of the fibrinolysin system

Fibrinopeptides and kinins actively contribute to inflammatory response

VI. Dissolution commences

Noxious agent destroyed or neutralized, tissue debris and fibrin products removed by leukocytes (neutrophils and macrophages)

VII. Subsequent course of inflammatory process determined by degree and rapidity of injury and tissue necrosis, persistence of causative agent, organ system involved, and other considerations

Immunologically-Mediated Sequence of Events (Dependent on Types of Hypersensitivity Reactions Involved)

Many reactions as for general sequence, plus:

I. T-derived lymphocytes

Cytotoxic cellular destruction and release of lymphokines

II. B lymphocytes and plasma cells

Produce immunoglobulins

III. Complement system

Activated by immune complexes, cytolytic and chemotactic actions, interplay with fibrinogenesis, fibrinolysis, and kinin generation

IV. Immediate hypersensitivity (allergic) reactions

Humorally mediated [immunoglobulin E (IgE)], onset 5–15 minutes, duration up to 1 hour, basophils and eosinophils infiltrate, histamine and leukotrienes major mediators

V. Immune complex reactions

Humorally mediated [immunoglobulin G (IgG)], onset up to 6 hours, duration 24 hours or longer, neutrophils and eosinophils infiltrate, complement major mediator

VI. Delayed hypersensitivity

Cell mediated, onset up to 24 hours, duration 72 hours or longer, basophils and mononuclear cells infiltrate, lymphokines and monokines major mediators

INFLAMMATORY MEDIATORS

Successful pharmacologic intervention is based on the capability of drugs to modify both cellular and humoral components of the inflammatory process.

Cell-Derived Mediators

I. Granular constituents

A. Histamine

Released from mast cells and basophils, produces vasodilation and increased capillary permeability, stimulates nociceptors to cause pain,

initial effects mediated by H_1 receptors, during subsequent events histamine effects result mainly from H_2 actions and are modulatory
  B. Serotonin (5-hydroxytryptamine)
       Released from platelets, produces vasodilation or vasoconstriction, may increase vascular permeability, stimulates pain receptors, two groups of receptors involved (5-HT$_1$ and 5-HT$_2$) role in inflammation not clearly understood
II. Lysosomal constituents
    Released from phagocytic and other cells, many potential inflammatory mediators
  A. Cationic proteins
       Chemotactic factors and increase vascular permeability
  B. Acid proteinases
       Degrade membranes and other structural components of cells
  C. Neutral proteinases
       Chemotactic factors and degrade collagen, elastin, cartilage and fibrin, release kinins from kininogens
III. Oxygen-derived radicals—released from damaged tissues or from leukocytes attracted to the site, highly destructive agents
  A. Superoxide anion (O_2^-)
       Converted to H_2O_2 by intracellular superoxide dismutase (SOD)
  B. Hydrogen peroxide (H_2O_2)
       Inactivated by catalase and by glutathione peroxidase, which also catalyzes the destruction of membrane lipid hydroperoxides
  C. Hydroxalradical (OH·)
       Extremely harmful, scavenged by mannitol and dimethylsulfoxide (DMSO)
IV. Arachidonic acid metabolites
    Many important mediators are derived from arachidonic acid and other essential polyunsaturated acids found in membrane phospholipids. The prostaglandins are produced by the cyclo-oxygenase enzyme system. The hydroperoxy derivatives and leukotrienes are produced by the lipoxygenase system.
  A. Prostaglandins (PGs)
       Responsible for several manifestations of inflammatory reactions, act as both mediators and modulators, synthesis and degradation rapid; see Figure 5-2.
       Thromboxane produced in platelets. Prostacyclin synthesized by vascular endothelial cells and lungs. Prostaglandins [prostaglandin E_2 (PGE_2), prostaglandin D_2 (PGD_2), prostaglandin F_2 (PGF_2), and several others] are generated in all tissues except mature erythrocytes.
  B. Leukotrienes (LTs) and hydroperoxy-derivatives (5-hydroperoxyeicosa tetraenoic acid or HPETE and 5-hydroxyeicosatetraenoic acid or HETE).
       Very potent mediators and modulators, active from 30 minutes to

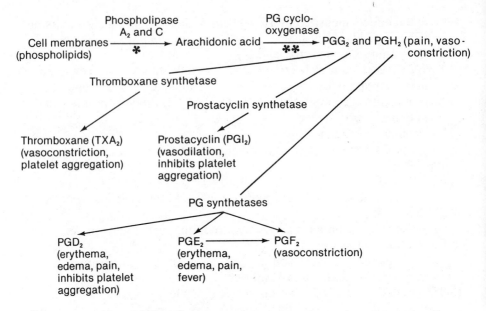

Fig. 5-2. Key elements of prostaglandin synthesis

several hours following initial insult, induce contraction of smooth mus-
cle (e.g., SRS-A and bronchoconstriction); see Figure 5-3.
  C. Lipoxygenases in platelets, leukocytes and lungs, LTC$_4$, LTD$_4$ and
     LTE$_4$—vasoconstriction, increased vascular permeability, bronchocon-
     striction, LTB$_4$—neutrophil stimulator.
  V. Acetylated alkyl phosphoglycerides
     Very potent lipid autacoids produced by a variety of inflammatory cells,

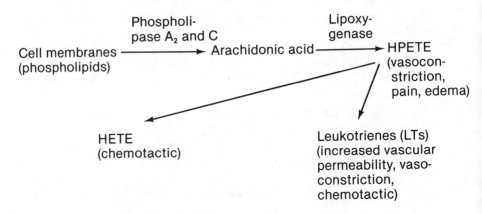

Fig. 5-3. Key elements of leukotriene synthesis

recruit platelets and evoke all the cardinal signs of acute inflammation, inactivated by phospholipases

A. Acetyl glyceryl ether phosphorylcholine (AGEPC) or platelet activating factor (PAF)—stimulates release reaction of platelets and neutrophil aggregation, chemotaxis, secretion of granule enzymes, production of superoxide anion and, if injected IV, produces anaphylactic shock reaction

B. Others?

Plasma-Derived Mediators

I. Kinin system

Kinins (bradykinin and kallidin) are derived from plasma precursors (kininogens) by the action of an enzyme kallikrein. Kallikrein activity is promoted by the Hageman factor (factor XII), a change in pH, and by contact with foreign substances. The kinins are potent vasodilators, producing an increase in capillary permeability and local edema. They also stimulate peripheral pain receptors. An interrelationship exists between the generation of kinins, the clotting sequence, fibrinolytic system, and the complement cascade (see Figure 5-4).

II. Fibrinopeptides

Fibrinopeptides, released from fibrinogen by the action of thrombin during clotting and by plasmin during proteolysis of fibrin, are inflammatory mediators. They enhance the effects of bradykinin, induce vascular leakage, and act as chemotactic factors. Plasmin promotes fibrinolysis, and activates Hageman factor and several complement subcomponents (see Figure 5-4).

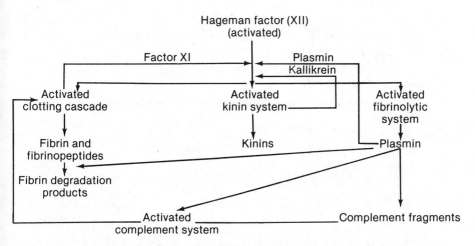

Fig. 5-4. Interactions that occur between complement and the other plasma-derived mediators.

III. Complement

The complement pathways may be activated immunologically or non-immunologically. Complement is capable of mediating the lytic destruction of many cells. Several complement system by-products possess major inflammatory effects. C3a and C5a fragments (anaphylatoxins) produce histamine release and vascular leakage. C3 and C5 fragments and the C567 complex are chemotactic for neutrophils. A C5 fragment acts as a lysosomal enzyme releasing factor.

The interactions that occur between complement and the other plasma-derived mediators—clotting, fibrinolysis, and kinin production—are illustrated in Figure 5-4.

CLASSIFICATION OF ANTI-INFLAMMATORY AGENTS

HORMONAL AGENTS—MEMBRANE AND METABOLIC EFFECTS

Corticosteroids

NONSTEROIDAL ANTI-INFLAMMATORY DRUGS (NSAIDS)

The following inhibit prostaglandin cyclo-oxygenase and other enzyme systems in some cases.
  I. Salicylates and related drugs
     Acetylsalicylic acid (aspirin), sodium salicylate, salicylamide, diflunisal (Dolabid)
  II. Fenamates
     Mefenamic acid (Ponstel), meclofenamic acid (Meclomen, Arquel)
  III. Nicotinic acid derivative
     Flunixin meglumine (Banamine)
  IV. Phenylacetates
     Fenoprofen (Malfon), ibuprofen (Motrin, Rufen), aclophenac, and diclofenac
  V. Indole—Acetates
     Indomethacin (Indocin), sulindac (Clinoril)
  VI. Pyrrole—Acetates
     Tolmetin (Tolectin)
  VII. Naphthalene—Acetates
     Naproxen (Naprosyn)
  VIII. Pyrazolidinediones
     Phenylbutazone (Butazolidin), oxyphenbutazone (Oxalid, Tandearil), dipyrone (Novin)

IX. Benzothiazines
    Piroxicam (Feldene)
X. Others
    Many other acidic and nonacidic agents possess antiinflammatory activity. A number are currently being developed for clinical use. Several have been withdrawn, e.g., benoxaprofen (Oraflex).

ENZYME-RELATED PREPARATIONS

The following inhibit or enhance enzyme-mediated reactions associated with inflammation.
I. Proteolytic enzymes
    Reduce fibrin deposition or inactivate fibrinopeptides
    A. Trypsin/chymotrypsin (Orenzyme)
    B. Fibrinolysin activators—streptokinase (Streptase, Kabikinase), urokinase (Abbokinase, Breokinase)
    C. Plant-derived proteolytic enzymes—bromelains (Ananase), papains (Papase)
II. Superoxide dismutase (SOD)
    Superoxide radical scavenger—orgotein (zinc copper SOD) (Palosein)
III. Selenium and vitamin E
    Prevent peroxidative damage to cellular elements—sodium selenite and vitamin E (Seletoc)
IV. Trypsin/chymotrypsin inhibitor
    Prevents proteolytic destruction in acute pancreatitis—aprotinin (Trasylol—not available at present)

ANTIHISTAMINIC AGENTS (H$_1$-blockers)

These agents inhibit effects of histamine released *early* in inflammatory reactions. The role of H$_2$-blockers is still uncertain.

AGENTS USED TO CONTROL IMMUNE-MEDIATED INFLAMMATORY REACTIONS (see chapter 6)

I. Immunosuppressants
    A. Alkylating agents
        Cyclophosphamide, busulphan, chlorambucil
    B. Antimetabolites
        Azathioprine, 6-mercaptopurine, 6-thioguanine, cytosine arabinoside, methotrexate
    C. Antibiotics
        Actinomycin D

D. Natural products
   Vincristine, vinblastine, L-asparaginase
E. Others
II. Immunomodulators
    Levamisole, thiabendazole, D-penicillamine, 5-mercaptopyridoxine, dapsone, others
III. Organic gold compounds
    Gold sodium thiomalate (Myochrysine), aurothioglucose (Solganal)

MISCELLANEOUS AGENTS

I. Dimethylsulfoxide/DMSO (Domoso, Rimso)
   Hydroxal radical scavenger and membrane effects
II. Hyaluronic acid (Healon)
    Intraarticular and intraocular administration
III. Mucopolysaccharide polysulfuric acid esters (Arteparon)—intraarticular administration

STEROIDAL ANTI-INFLAMMATORY AGENTS

Adrenocortical steroids and synthetic analogs commonly used for their antiinflammatory actions include the following:
   I. Betamethasone
  II. Cortisone
 III. Dexamethasone
  IV. Flumethasone
   V. Fluocinolone
  VI. Fluprednisolone
 VII. Flurandrenolone
VIII. Hydrocortisone/cortisol
  IX. Methylprednisolone
   X. Paramethasone
  XI. Prednisolone
 XII. Prednisone
XIII. Triamcinolone
 XIV. Others

ROUTE OF ADMINISTRATION AND FORM

I. Intravenous
   Sodium salts of succinate and phosphate esters
II. Intramuscular
    Acetates, dipropionates, hexacetonides, and water-soluble salts noted above

III. Intraarticular
   Water-soluble suspensions and acetates
IV. Oral
   Nonesterified forms or esters
 V. Topical
   Valerates, acetonides, pivalates, and nonesterified forms

MECHANISMS OF ANTIINFLAMMATORY ACTION

Corticosteroids inhibit early and late stages of inflammatory process. Mechanisms are not entirely understood. Only tissue responses and clinical signs are suppressed. There is *no* antagonism to noxious agent.

Select Features

   I. Suppress T-lymphocyte functions
   II. Inhibit monocyte-macrophage activities
   III. Decrease lysosomal release from neutrophils, neutrophil chemotaxis inhibited by large doses
   IV. Inhibit endogenous pyrogen release
   V. Decrease release of arachidonic acid from membrane phospholipids and thereby depress prostaglandin and leukotriene synthesis.
   VI. Suppress antibody production
   VII. May alter complement metabolism in some species
VIII. Inhibit kinin cascade and plasminogen activation
   IX. Suppress fibroblast functions and collagen deposition
   X. Induce vasoconstriction due to permissive action at adrenergic sites

Net Effects

Inhibit edema formation, fibrin deposition, capillary dilatation, leukocyte migration, and phagocytic activity as early manifestations of inflammation. Later depress capillary and fibroblast proliferation and collagen deposition.

PHARMACOLOGIC EFFECTS

See chapter 19 for review of general glucocorticoid and mineralocorticoid actions.

KINETIC FATE

  I. Absorption
    A. Oral—readily absorbed
    B. IM or SQ—rapid absorption unless depo-form

C. Intraarticular—significant absorption can take place

D. Topical—absorption may occur, especially from inflamed areas

II. Distribution

A. Widely distributed in tissues—penetrate readily

B. Plasma protein bound—corticosteroid-binding globulin and albumin (up to 90%)

III. Biotransformation

A. Hepatic

Reduction reactions and conjugation (glucuronides and sulfates)

B. Cortisone and prednisone are pro-drugs

Converted to active hydrocortisone and prednisolone, respectively

IV. Excretion

A. Renal and biliary—conjugated and unconjugated.

B. Enterohepatic cycles common.

V. Elimination kinetics

A. Plasma half-lives short—60 minutes for prednisolone, 300 minutes for betamethasone and dexamethasone

B. Biological half-lives long [correlate with metabolic, antiinflammatory, and hypothalamic-hypophyseal-adrenal axis (HHAA) suppression]

1. Short-acting (<12 hours), e.g., hydrocortisone

2. Medium-acting (12–36 hours), e.g., prednisolone

3. Long-acting (>36 hours), e.g., betamethasone, dexamethasone

THERAPEUTIC INDICATIONS

I. Immune-mediated syndromes

A. Affecting skin and mucous membranes

1. Food allergies (not continuous therapy)

2. Atopy or allergic inhalation dermatitis

3. Drug allergy, drug reaction, drug eruption

4. Insect bite allergy

5. Allergic contact dermatitis

6. Urticaria and angioneurotic edema

B. Autoimmune disorders

1. Pemphigus vulgaris

2. Pemphigus foliaceus

3. Pemphigus vegetans

4. Systemic lupus erythematosus

5. Cutaneous lupus erythematosus

C. Affecting other organ systems

1. Multiple myeloma

2. Polymyositis and eosinophilic myositis

3. Allergic rhinitis and bronchitis, bronchial asthma

4. Eosinophilic enteritis and intestinal granulomas

      5. Glomerulonephritis
      6. Chronic active hepatitis
      7. Polyarteritis nodosa
    D. Immune-mediated arthritides
      1. Rheumatoid arthritis
      2. Idiopathic polyarthritis
      3. Plasmacytic-lymphocytic synovitis
      4. Other forms of erosive and nonerosive arthritis
  II. Musculoskeletal conditions
    A. Musculoskeletal trauma
    B. Myositis
    C. Tendonitis
    D. Tenosynovitis
    E. Osteoarthritis
    F. Osteitis and periostitis
    G. Others
 III. Endotoxemic shock
 IV. Cerebral and spinal edema—efficacy is questionable
  V. Snake bite
 VI. Ulcerative colitis
 VII. Lick granuloma
VIII. Otitis externa
 IX. Ocular disease
    A. Conjunctivitis
    B. Keratitis–*not* corneal ulcers
    C. Chemosis
    D. Pannus
    E. Uveitis

PRINCIPLES OF CORTICOSTEROID THERAPY

Guidelines which should be followed when corticosteroids are administered include the following:

   I. Use at correct dosage rate and frequency for a defined and appropriate indication.
  II. Single large dose of a glucocorticoid unlikely to be harmful.
 III. Prolonged therapy, at doses above substitution level, may produce harmful effects.
 IV. Depression of the HHAA may occur and several months are required for recovery to take place.
  V. For long-term therapy, early morning alternate-day administration minimizes detrimental effects on the HHAA (use short- or medium-acting corticosteroids).
 VI. Taper off doses gradually in chronic cases and administer adrenocorti-

cotropic hormone (ACTH) to promote function of depressed adrenal cortex (see Chapter 19).
VII. Recognize disadvantages of long-acting corticosteroids and depo-preparations—especially with regard to HHAA supression.
VIII. Long-term therapy should be accompanied by dietary supplementation with high-quality protein, potassium, vitamin A, and vitamin D.
IX. The risk/benefit ratio of the concurrent use of corticosteroids and antimicrobial agents should be appraised in each case. Bactericidal antibiotics are preferred.
X. Where acute inflammatory reactions may produce lifelong impairment of an organ's function, early effective doses of corticosteroids are vital.
XI. Always recognize that corticosteroids may obscure clinical signs because of the euphoric effects produced, together with improved appetite, reduced fever, pain alleviation, and diminished inflammatory reaction.
XII. Intrasynovial use of corticosteroids should always be followed by a prolonged period of rest to allow complete healing.

POTENTIAL SIDE-EFFECTS AND PRECAUTIONS ASSOCIATED WITH THE STEROIDS

I. Acute adrenal insufficiency from too rapid withdrawal
II. Large repetitive doses or prolonged therapy with corticosteroids will result in iatrogenic hypercorticism.
   A. Fluid and electrolyte disturbances with sodium and water retention, potassium loss, and hypokalemic alkalosis
   B. Hyperglycemia and glycosuria ("steroid diabetes"). Incipient diabetes mellitus may be precipitated.
   C. The catabolic effect of the corticosteroids results in a negative nitrogen balance and an increased urea synthesis
   D. Abnormal fat deposition may occur
   E. Polydipsia with polyuria, and polyphagia
   F. Osteoporosis as a result of calcium loss and an increased proneness to fractures
   G. Decreased linear growth in growing animals
   H. Myopathy, characterized by muscular weakness
   I. Acute pancreatitis (rare)
   J. Susceptibility to infection may be increased and encapsulated lesions may break down. Normal wound healing may also be impaired.
   K. Suppression of normal immune mechanisms
   L. Hypercoagulability of blood has been reported.
   M. Lymphocytopenia, eosinopenia, and neutrophilia
   N. Temperament changes. An apparent increased feeling of well-being may mask a deterioration in the clinical condition.
   O. The corticosteroids have been incriminated in the exacerbation of seizures in epileptic patients.
   P. Peptic ulceration

Q. Reversible hepatopathy has been described in dogs.
R. Induction and inhibition of drug-metabolizing microsomal enzymes may alter the duration of an animal's response to other drugs.
III. Possible harmful effects following local use of corticosteroids include the following
   A. Contact dermatitis
   B. Crystal-induced synovitis following intraarticular administration
   C. Prolonged use in the eye may lead to an increase in intraocular pressure and ultimately glaucoma. Posterior subcapsular cataracts have been reported.
IV. Major contraindications to corticosteroid therapy include the following:
   A. Early pregnancy
      Teratogenicity has been recognized, particularly cleft palate.
   B. Late pregnancy
      Abortion or premature birth may occur, especially if the drug is given
      IV. Ruminants are particularly prone.
   C. Simultaneous vaccination
      A poor immunologic response may occur.
   D. Corneal ulceration
      Danger of bulbar rupture.
V. Effects on laboratory findings may include
   A. Blood
     1. Neutrophilia, moncytosis, lymphopenia, eosinopenia
     2. Mild polycythemia (?)
     3. Hyperglycemia
     4. Blood urea nitrogen (BUN) and creatinine—normal or low
     5. Serum alkaline phosphatase (SAP) increased
     6. Alanine aminotransferase (AAT) and γ-glutamyl transpeptidase (GGT) increased
     7. Lipemia and hypercholesterolemia
     8. Increased sulfobromophthalein (BSP) retention
     9. Elevated sodium, depressed potassium, elevated calcium (?)
   B. Urine
     1. Dilute urine (S.G. < 1.007)
     2. Glycosuria
     3. Calciuria

PREPARATIONS AND DOSAGE (see Table 5-1)

NONSTEROIDAL ANTI-INFLAMMATORY DRUGS (NSAIDs)

A variety of NSAIDs have been useful for the treatment of acute and chronic inflammatory conditions affecting the musculoskeletal and other organ systems in small animals. The most frequently employed include salicylates and phen-

TABLE 5-1. ADRENOCORTICOSTEROID—PREPARATIONS AND DOSAGE

Drug	Preparations	Dose	Route	Frequency	Comments
Cortisone acetate	Cortone	6 mg/kg	IM	24 hr	Requires conversion to hydrocortisone in liver. Ineffective topically.
Hydrocortisone	Cortef	5 mg/kg	IM, IV	24 hr	Very high doses are used for shock
	Hydrocortone	5 mg/kg	PO	12 hr	
Prednisolone	Deltra Deltasone Meticortin	0.5–1.25 mg/kg	IM	12 hr	For allergy
		2.0–3.0 mg/kg	IM	12 hr	Immune suppression
Prednisolone Sodium succinate	Solu-Delta-Cortef Meticortelone Soluble	5.5–11.0 mg/kg	IV	1, 3, 6, or 10 hr	Endotoxemic or septic shock
Methylprednisolone	Medrol	1.0 mg/kg	PO	8 hr	—
Methylprednisolone acetate	Depo-Medrol	1.0 mg/kg	IM	14 days	—
Dexamethasone	Decadron Azium	0.15 mg/kg	IV, IM PO	24 hr 24 hr	Lack electrolyte-retaining effects Cat dosage half canine dosage
Dexamethasone Sodium phosphate	Decadron phosphate Hexadrol phosphate	5 mg/kg	IV		Endotoxemic or septic shock
Betamethasone	Betasone	0.17–0.35 mg/kg	IM	3–6 wk	Depo-form
Triamcinolone	Vetalog Aristocort Kenacort	0.11–0.22 mg/kg	PO	24 hr	0.5 mg maximum for cat
		0.11–0.22 mg/kg	IM, SQ	24 hr	
Flumethasone	Flucort Methagon	0.06–0.25 mg/kg	PO IV, IM	24 hr	—
Fludrocortisone	Florinef	0.05–0.3 mg	PO	24 hr	Cat—0.1–0.2 mg

ylbutazone. Other NSAIDs, listed in the section on Classification of Antiinflammatory Agents, above, are either not used or little information is available
about their clinical pharmacology in small animals.

MECHANISMS OF ANTI-INFLAMMATORY ACTION

  I. Inhibition of prostaglandin cyclo-oxygenase—common to all NSAIDs
 II. Some NSAIDs actually depress PG actions (salicylates, fenamates)
III. Inhibit formation of kinins (salicylates)
IV. Uncouple oxidative phosphorylation (several)
 V. Depress biosynthesis of mucopolysaccharides (indomethacin)

GENERAL PHARMACOLOGIC PROPERTIES

  I. Weak acids, only penetrate damaged and inflamed tissue (acidic environ-
     ment)
 II. Highly bound to plasma proteins—prolonged effects
III. Extracellular distribution
IV. Excreted by glomerular filtration and tubular secretion
 V. Often latent period prior to onset of action due to high tissue concentrations
    of PGs

KINETIC FATE

  I. Absorption
     A. Oral—readily absorbed
     B. IV—solutions often irritant because of alkalinity
 II. Distribution
     A. Extracellular
     B. Highly plasma protein bound (often >90%)
III. Biotransformation
     A. Hepatic—microsomal
     B. Conjugation reactions common
IV. Excretion
     A. Mainly renal—glomerular filtration and tubular secretion
     B. Often pH dependent
 V. Elimination kinetics
     A. Notable species differences
           e.g., plasma $T_{\frac{1}{2}}$ of salicylate
        1. Dog—8 hours
        2. Cat—38 hours
        3. Horse—1 hour
     B. Prolonged elimination for most NSAIDs in dog and cat. Great caution
        necessary. Dosage frequency often 24–72 hours.

THERAPEUTIC INDICATIONS
  I. Soft tissue trauma and inflammation
  II. Osteoarthritis and other musculoskeletal disorders
  III. Immune-mediated disease syndromes
  IV. Postsurgical swelling
  V. Endotoxemic shock (Banamine)

POTENTIAL SIDE EFFECTS AND PRECAUTIONS

  I. Potential toxic effects include:
     A. Gastrointestinal ulceration and bleeding (administer with food to avoid gastrointestinal irritation)
     B. Nephrotoxicity, papillary necrosis, sodium and water retention
     C. Impaired platelet adhesion and bleeding disorders
     D. Delayed parturition
     E. Altered pattern of ductus arteriosus closure
     F. Hypersensitivity reactions
     G. Bone marrow-related disorders are not common in animals but may occur in rare instances—e.g., aplastic anemia, agranulocytosis, pancytopenia
  II. Major contraindications include:
     A. Gastroenteritis
     B. Gastric ulceration
     C. Bleeding tendency
     D. Nephritis and other nephropathies
  III. Pharmacokinetic interactions include:
     A. Delayed absorption from gastrointestinal tract when administered with antacids
     B. Displacement of other agents from plasma protein binding sites
          Coumarins, oral hypoglycemics, sulfonamides, ethacrynic acid, other NSAIDs
     C. Microsomal enzyme induction (phenylbutazone)
     D. Urinary acidifiers—delay excretion
     E. Urinary alkalinizers—enhance renal elimination
     F. Delayed excretion due to competition for tubular secretory mechanisms
          Penicillins, cephalosporins, NSAIDs, probenecid, furosemide, glucuronides
  IV. Effects on laboratory findings may include:
     A. Blood
          1. Interfere with thyroid function tests
          2. Interfere with platelet function tests
          3. Blood glucose (salicylate effect variable)
          4. Elevated bilirubin levels possible
     B. Urine
          1. False-negative tests for urine glucose by glucose oxidase methods (salicylates)

TABLE 5-2.   NSAID—PREPARATIONS AND DOSAGE

Drug	Preparations	Dose	Route	Frequency	Comments
Aspirin	Many	10–20 mg/kg	PO	12 hr	Dog
		10 mg/kg	PO	48 hr	Cat
Flunixin meglumine	Banamine	0.5–1 mg/kg	IM/IV	—	Single dose only do not repeat
Ibuprofen	Motrin Rufen	10 mg/kg	PO	24–48 hr	Slow elimination— caution
Naproxen	Naprosyn	5 mg/kg	PO	Initial	Slow elimination— caution
		1.2–2.8 mg/ kg	PO	24 hr	
Phenylbutazone	Butazolidine	10–15 mg/kg	IV	12 hr	—
		10 mg/kg	PO	12 hr	Reduce dose progressively

2. Ketone test (Gerhardt test) impaired by salicylates
3. Exacerbate proteinuria

PREPARATIONS AND DOSAGE (see Table 5-2)

MISCELLANEOUS ANTI-INFLAMMATORY AGENTS

ORGANIC GOLD COMPOUNDS

I. Used for treating rheumatoid arthritis (chrysotherapy)
II. Mechanisms of action unclear but
    A. Depress macrophage phagocytosis
    B. Inhibit lysosomal enzyme release
    C. Decrease levels of rheumatoid factor and immunoglobulins
    D. Suppress cellular immunity
III. Few reports of serious side effects in dogs but experience is limited.
IV. Preparations and dosage schedules
    A. Auriothioglucose (Solganal)—test doses of 5 mg or 10 mg IM, then 1 mg/kg IM, weekly
    B. Gold sodium thiomalate (Myochrysine)—1 mg/kg IM weekly

PROTEOLYTIC ENZYMES

I. Most useful for treating soft tissue trauma (accidental or surgical)
II. Mechanism of action probably based on depolymerization of fibrin and inactivation of fibrinopeptides

III. Efficacy of proteolytic enzymes as antiinflammatory agents is equivocal
IV. Few side effects
    A. Septicemia or bacteremia due to release of encapsulated microorganisms.
    B. Disrupted hemostatic mechanisms
    C. Hypersensitivity reactions
  V. Preparations and dosage schedules (see table 5-3)

ORGOTEIN (Cu-Zn superoxide dismutase)

  I. Indicated for acute and chronic inflammatory conditions
 II. Mechanism of action based on the ability of SOD to inactivate destructive superoxide radicals released during the inflammatory reaction. May also prevent disruption of lysosomal membranes.
III. Evidence for efficacy equivocal—SOD is large enzyme which may not reach inflamed areas. Superoxide dismutase does not penetrate normal membranes.
IV. Side effects uncommon. Superoxide dismutase is a weak immunogen.
  V. Preparation and dosage schedule—dog:
    Orgotein—"Palosein"—5 mg SQ every day for 6 days, then 5 mg SQ every 48 hours for 8 days

SELENIUM AND VITAMIN E (Tocopherol)

  I. Indicated for inflammation and pain, associated with various arthropathies
 II. Mechanism of action based on the ability of tocopherol to block lipid peroxidation of polyunsaturated fatty acids which leads to the formation of free radicals and hydroperoxides. Selenium is a component of glutathione peroxidase which catalyzes the destruction of H_2O_2 and lipid hydroperoxides. Tocopherol appears to potentiate immune mechanisms at pharmacologic doses.
III. Selenium and tocopherol preparations often used to supplement action of other antiinflammatory agents.

TABLE 5-3.   PROTEOLYTIC ENZYMES—PREPARATIONS AND DOSAGE

Drug	Preparations	Dose	Route	Frequency	Comments
Bromelains	Ananase	100,000 U	PO	6 hr	Human
Papains	Papase	20,000 U	PO	6 hr	Human
Trypsin (tryp)/	Orenzyme	100,000 U (tryp)	PO	6 hr	Human
chymotrypsin (chym)		8,000 U (chym)			

IV. Side effects uncommon if dosage schedule followed carefully (selenium may be toxic).
   A. Nausea and vomiting
   B. Gastroenteritis
 V. Preparation and dosage schedule—selenium/vitamin E (see table 5-4)

DIMETHYLSULFOXIDE (DMSO)

   I. Has been used both topically and parenterally as an antiinflammatory agent
  II. Mechanism of action as an antiinflammatory agent appears to be multi-faceted and complex.
   A. Hydroxal radical scavenger, reduction metabolite dimethylsulfide (DMS) is a free oxygen radical scavenger.
   B. Membrane stabilization—substantially enhances corticosteroids' effects on lysosomal membranes
   C. Blocks conduction in pain fibers
   D. Possesses a thermal effect in tissues—enhances blood flow
   E. Blocks polymerization of hyaluronic acid initiated by hydroxal radical. Softens collagen.
   F. May modulate local immune responses
 III. Clinical uses of DMSO
   A. Topical
      1. Localized ophthalmic conditions
      2. Otitis externa
      3. Dermal hypersensitivity reactions and dermatitis
      4. Acute and chronic musculoskeletal conditions—traumatic injuries, myositis, rheumatoid arthritis, osteoarthritis, bursitis, tendonitis, and so forth
      5. Tissue trauma and burn wounds
      6. Postsurgical edema.
   B. Parenteral (IV)
      Brain and spinal cord trauma with edema—efficacy is controversial.
 IV. Side effects, precautions, toxicity
   A. Handle with care, wear gloves (percutaneous absorption—sulfurous breath). Keep container tightly closed—extremely hygroscopic.
   B. Topical
      1. Erythema (histamine release?) and skin irritation (drying effect)

TABLE 5-4. SELENIUM/VITAMIN E—PREPARATION AND DOSAGE

Preparations	Dose	Route	Frequency	Species
Seletoc inj.	1 ml/9 kg	IM, SQ (several sites)	72 hr	Dog
Seletoc caps	1 cap/9 kg	PO	72 hr	Dog

TABLE 5-5. DMSO—PREPARATIONS AND DOSAGE

Preparation		Dose	Route	Frequency
Domoso	(90%)	As appropriate (70% best)	Topical	8–12 hr
Rimso	(50%)	0.5–1.0 g/kg (10–20% soln)	IV	8 hr

2. Prolonged use—change in refractive index of lens of the eye. Slowly reversible.
3. Potentially teratogenic during first trimester
4. Will facilitate excessive absorption of concurrently applied agents which may be toxic, e.g., insecticides.
5. Odor on breath
   C. Intravenous
   1. Hemolysis if concentration greater than 20%
   2. Diuresis (often beneficial)
V. Preparations and dosage schedules—DMSO (see table 5-5)

SUGGESTED READINGS

Eyre P, Hanna CJ, Wells PW, McBeath DG: Equine immunology 3. Immunopharmacology—anti-inflammatory and hypersensitivity drugs. Equine Vet J 14:277, 1982

Flower RJ, Moncada S, Vane JR: Analgesic-antipyretics and anti-inflammatory agents; drugs employed in the treatment of gout. p. 682 In Gilman AG, Goodman LS, Gilman A (eds): The Pharmacological Basis of Therapeutics. 6th Ed. Macmillan, New York, 1980

Jacob S, Herschler R, Knowles R: Proceedings of a symposium on dimethyl sulfoxide, Vet Med/Sm Anim Clin 77(3):365, 1982

Majno G, Coltran RS, Kaufman N (eds): Current Topics in Inflammation and Infection. Williams and Wilkins, Baltimore, London, 1982

Metz SA: Anti-inflammatory agents as inhibitors of prostaglandin synthesis in man. Med Clin N Am 65(4):713, 1981

Nelson AM, Conn DL: Glucocorticoids in rheumatic disease. Mayo Clin Proc 55:758, 1980

Ryan GB, Majno G: Acute inflammation. Am J Pathol 86(1):185, 1977

Samuelsson B: Leukotrienes: mediators of immediate hypersensitivity reactions and inflammation. Science 220:568, 1983

Short CR, Beadle RE: Pharmacology of antiarthritic drugs. Vet Clin N Am 8(3):401, 1978

Snow DH: Anti-inflammatory agents. p. 391. In Bogan JA, Lees P, Yoxall AT (eds): Pharmacological Basis of Large Animal Medicine. Blackwell Scientific Publications, Oxford, London, Edinburgh, Boston and Melbourne, 1983

6

Immunologic Disorders

Arthur I. Hurvitz, D.V.M.
Judith Johnessee, D.V.M.

INTRODUCTION

MECHANISMS OF IMMUNOLOGIC INJURY

Type I: Anaphylaxis

  I. Immune reactant: immunoglobulin E (IgE)
 II. Mediators:
    A. Histamine
    B. Slow-reacting substance of anaphylaxis
    C. Eosinophilic chemotactic factor of anaphylaxis
III. Effector Cell
    A. Mast cell
    B. Basophil
 IV. Pathologic mechanism
    A. Degranulation and release of vasoactive amines
    B. Vasodilators and edema
    C. Bronchoconstriction
    D. Splanchnic pooling and shock
  V. Species-specific target organ
    A. Dog: liver and viscera
    B. Cat: lungs

Type II. Cytotoxic

  I. Immune reactant: immunoglobulin G (IgG), immunoglobulin M (IgM)
 II. Mediator: complement
III. Effector cell: macrophage
 IV. Pathologic mechanism
    A. Cell lysis

   B. Phagocytosis

   C. Antibody-dependent cell-mediated cytotoxicity

V. Examples

   A. Autoimmune hemolytic anemia

   B. Autoimmune thrombocytopenia

   C. Pemphigus

Type III: Immune Complex

  I. Immune reactant: IgG, IgM

 II. Mediator: complement

III. Effector cell: polymorphonuclear neutrophilic granulocyte (PMN)

IV. Pathologic mechanism: release of lysosomal enzymes from PMN infiltrate

 V. Examples

   A. Arthus reaction

   B. Immune complex glomerulonephritis

   C. Systemic lupus erythematosus (SLE)

   D. Rheumatoid arthritis

   E. Vasculitis

Type IV: Cell-Mediated or Delayed Hypersensitivity

  I. Immune reactant: T lymphocyte

 II. Mediator: lymphokines

III. Effector cell: macrophage

IV. Pathologic mechanism

   A. Chronic inflammation

   B. Granuloma formation

 V. Examples

   A. Allergic contact dermatitis

   B. Cancer immunosurveillance

   C. Arthropod hypersensitivity

PRINCIPLES OF THERAPEUTICS

Glucocorticoids

I. Mechanisms by which glucocorticoids influence immunologic injury

   A. Glucocorticoids have little direct effect on specific immune phenomena; they act primarily by inhibiting the inflammatory response.

   B. Effect on macrophage function

      1. Suppress proliferation

      2. Alter expression of receptors

      3. Depress phagocytosis

4. Depress cytotoxic activity

5. Suppress initiation of immune response

6. Depress enzyme secretion

C. Decrease vascular permeability

D. Decrease release of vasoactive amines

E. Block clearance of immune complexes by reticuloendothelial cells

F. Decrease serum complement levels

G. Redistribute leukocytes

H. Stabilize plasma membranes

I. Significant suppression of antibody formation is not generally seen, although suppression of autoantibody formation is occasionally seen.

II. Dosage recommendations

A. Intermediate-acting glucocorticoids such as prednisone or prednisolone are preferred.

B. Prednisone must be biotransformed to prednisolone in the liver. In the absence of liver disease, prednisone may be preferred on the basis of cost.

C. Initial doses are 1–3 mg/kg prednisone divided BID to TID in dogs. Cats may require twice this dosage.

D. Equivalent doses of other glucocorticoids may be used but steroid preparations with short half-lives and low sodium retention are preferred (see Table 6-1).

III. Side effects

A. Side effects with immunosuppressive dosage develop rapidly but resolve as the dose is tapered.

B. Most side effects are not life threatening (with the exception of pancreatitis or gastrointestinal bleeding) but may seriously inconvenience or alarm the owner.

TABLE 6-1. GLUCOCORTICLIDS

Glucocorticoid	Relative Glucocorticoid Potency	Relative Mineralocorticoid Potency	Tissue Half-life[a] (hr)
Hydrocortisone	1	+ +	8–12
Triamcinalone	3	0	12–36 (depending upon preparation)
Prednisolone, prednisone	4	+	12–36
Methylprednisolone	5	0	12–36
Dexamethasone	29	0	35–54

[a] Depends upon formulation. Acetonide, acetate, diacetate, and tebulate esters are poorly water soluble and form sustained-release deposits.

C. Side effects must be weighed against disease severity. Life-threatening diseases may justify temporary side effects of a relatively severe nature.
D. Signs often seen
    1. Profound polydipsia, polyuria, and polyphagia
    2. Behavioral changes (depression, sleepiness, temperament changes)
    3. Panting
    4. Diarrhea
    5. Gastrointestinal bleeding (cimetidine may be protective)
    6. Muscle weakness and wasting or myopathy (more common with fluorinated glucocorticoids)
    7. Hepatopathy: elevated serum alkaline phosphatase (SAP), hepatomegaly
    8. Iatrogenic Cushing's syndrome with or without calcinosis cutis and concurrent secondary adrenocortical insufficiency due to hypothalamic-pituitary-adrenal (HPA) axis suppression
    9. Growth retardation in young animals
    10. Pancreatitis
    11. Diabetes mellitus
E. Cats
    1. Are quite resistant to the side effects of glucocorticoids
    2. Rarely develop any of the above side effects except HPA suppression and retarded hair growth.
    3. Elevated SAP levels not seen
    4. Recommendations for immunosuppressive glucocorticoid regimens
       a) Use high doses initially until clinical improvement or remission is well established.
       b) Glucocorticoids should be given for several months after remission is achieved. Exacerbations more likely to occur if the taper is too rapid.
       c) Dose should be tapered by about 25% every 3–4 weeks while carefully monitoring disease status.
       d) Treatment of most systemic immune-mediated diseases cannot be switched to alternate-day regimens early in the course of the disease. Alternate-day therapy may be possible after several months of a slow taper.
       e) Prednisone or prednisolone is suitable for alternate-day therapy to minimize HPA suppression. Dexamethasone must be given every 4 days to prevent HPA suppression and therefore is not as suitable as prednisone for maintenance therapy.
       f) Glucocorticoids must not be discontinued abruptly even if signs of iatrogenic hyperadrenocorticism are present because underlying HPA suppression can result in an adrenal crisis.
       g) Occasional animals may respond to dexamethasone when prednisone is ineffective.

        h) Dogs on once daily or alternate-day therapy should be dosed in the morning; cats should be dosed in the evening.

        i) Many animals can be tapered off steroids completely; judge each animal individually.

    5. Prophylactic antibiotics should not routinely be used. Specific therapy should be instituted if infection occurs.

    6. If the immunologic disease is not adequately controlled by glucocorticoids alone, or the side effects are unacceptable, other therapeutic modalities should be added as alternatives or adjunctive therapy.

Immunosuppressant Agents

  I. The cytotoxic drugs usually used are the alkylating agents cyclophosphamide (Cytoxan), melphalan (Alkeran), and chlorambucil (Leukeran), and the purine analog azathioprine (Imuran).

  II. Mechanisms of action

    A. Immunosuppressant agents decrease antibody formation and decrease the number of leukocytes.

    B. They do not alter reticuloendothelial cell clearance of immune complexes and they should be used in conjunction with corticosteroids.

  III. Cyclophosphamide

    A. Give orally for 4 consecutive days out of 7 for up to 3 weeks.

    B. White blood cell count should be monitored closely for drug-related leukopenia.

    C. Hemorrhagic cystitis is rarely seen with this protocol, but increasing water consumption and encouraging frequent urination reduces risk.

    D. Doses employed are 1.5 mg/kg for dogs greater than 25 kg, 2.2 mg/kg for dogs 5–25 kg, and 2.5 mg/kg daily for dogs and cats under 5 kg.

    E. Alternatively, a once-weekly IV dose of 7 mg/kg may be given.

  IV. Azathioprine

    A. This drug is less immunosuppressive but has fewer side effects.

    B. It is given once daily at a dose of 2.2 mg/kg, orally.

    C. The white cell count should be monitored closely.

  V. If the white blood cell count falls to 5,000–7,000 cells/mm^3, the doses of both azathioprine and cyclophosphamide should be reduced by one fourth. If the white blood cell count drops below 5,000 cells/mm^3, both drugs should be discontinued until the leukopenia resolves.

  VI. Chlorambucil and melphalan

    A. These potent immunosuppressive agents are generally restricted to use in plasma cell dyscrasias.

    B. Bone marrow suppression is possible, although these drugs tend to be less toxic than cyclophosphamide.

    C. Therapeutic regimens are discussed in the section on diseases of immunoproliferation.
VII. Vinca alkaloids
    A. Vincristine and vinblastine have been shown to cause dose-related thrombocytosis due to increased megakaryopoiesis. The mechanism by which this effect is achieved is unknown, but appears to be dose-related.
    B. Because of this effect, the vinca alkaloids are particularly useful in the treatment of immune-mediated thrombocytopenia. The immunosuppressive effect of these compounds is minor.
    C. The dose of vincristine employed is 0.01–0.025 mg/kg IV given once every 4–7 days. A maximum dose of 1.5 mg should not be exceeded in giant breed dogs. The dose of vinblastine is 0.05 mg/kg IV once every 7 days.
    D. Corticosteroids are used concurrently to depress reticuloendothelial system removal of antibody-labeled target cells.

Splenectomy

  I. The spleen is a major site of antibody production, although postsplenectomy some of this function may be assumed by other organs.
 II. Due to the slow rate of flow through the sinusoids, the local high antibody levels, and the large number of macrophages present, the spleen is the major site of removal of antibody-labeled target cells.
III. Splenectomy is less efficacious in IgM-mediated disease where antibody-labeled target cells are removed primarily in the liver. Whether enough decrement in IgM production occurs postsplenectomy to make it a useful adjunct for managing IgM-mediated disease in unknown.

Plasmapheresis, Lymphoplasmapheresis, and Immunoadsorption

  I. Plasma exchange may selectively or nonselectively remove immunoreactants depending upon the technique used. Immunosuppressive drugs nonselectively suppress antibody production and take longer to become effective.
 II. These new techniques are of benefit in crisis situations.
III. They appear to induce changes in the immunoregulatory system unrelated to simple removal of immunoreactants.

Remission-Inducing Agents

 I. Aurothioglucose (Solganol)
    A. Mechanism of action is unknown.

  B. Signs of toxicity include:
  1. Lesions of mucous membranes
  2. Blood dyscrasias (thrombocytopenia, anemia, leukopenia, aplastic anemia)
  3. Proximal tubular damage
  4. Encephalitis
  5. Neuritis
  6. Hepatitis
  C. Dosage: 1 mg/kg IM once a week
II. Penicillamine
  A. Chelates copper, mercury, and lead and promotes excretion in urine. Inhibits pyridoxol-dependent enzymes.
  B. Toxic reactions
  1. Skin eruptions
  2. Blood dyscrasias (eosinophilia, thrombocytopenia)
  3. Gastrointestinal signs (anorexia, vomiting)
  4. Nephrotoxicity
  C. Mechanism of action in immune-mediated disease is unclear

DISEASES OF IMMUNOPROLIFERATION

MONOCLONAL GAMMOPATHIES

Multiple Myeloma

  I. Diagnosis requires fulfillment of two of the following four criteria
  A. Radiographic evidence of osteolytic bone lesions.
  B. A diagnostic bone marrow aspirate
  C. Demonstration of production of a homogeneous monoclonal immunoglobulin or polypeptide subunit (M component) other than IgM.
  D. Bence Jones proteinuria. Bence Jones proteins are free light-chains which appear in the urine and occasionally serum. They are not detected on a routine urine dipstick test for protein. The heat precipitation test or electrophoresis of the urine is more reliable.
  II. Clinical signs are referable to proliferating plasma cells or to the products of these cells.
  A. Clinical signs caused by proliferating plasma cells
  1. Anemia may be caused by bone marrow infiltration by plasma cells, or by blood loss secondary to bleeding diatheses.
  2. Bone lesions may be of two types: diffuse osteoporosis which may lead to pathologic fractures, or punched-out osteolytic lesions.
  3. Recurrent infection. Although there is a total increase in globulins, most of this represents an increase in the M component. There is a

functional decrease in immunoglobulins, leading to immunoincompetence. Bone marrow infiltration may result in granulocytopenia and increased susceptibility to infection.

B. Clinical signs related to products of proliferating cells (see table 6-2)

    1. Renal failure. Excretion of Bence Jones proteins causes tubular damage leading to renal failure. This is complicated by additional extrarenal factors such as hypercalcemia, anemia, hyperviscosity, coagulopathies, and hypovolemia. The use of iodinated contrast material may exacerbate the renal failure on the basis of hypovolemia and direct toxicity to the renal tubular cells.

    2. Bleeding and clotting disorders. Many of the myeloma proteins can interact with the various clotting factors, the vascular endothelium, and the platelet surface to cause bleeding diatheses. The combined effects of anoxia, clotting abnormalities and thrombocytopenia lead to a bleeding tendency.

    3. Hyperviscosity syndrome

        a) The serum viscosity is related to the size, shape, and concentration of the M component. It is usually associated with IgM (macroglobulinemia) but also occurs with polymeric immunoglobulin monoclonal gammopathies.

        b) The following clinical signs have been seen in dogs with hyperviscosity syndrome:

            (1) Bleeding diatheses

            (2) Retinopathy with dilated, sausage-shaped retinal vessels and retinal hemorrhages

            (3) Neurologic signs—dementia, depression, coma

            (4) Congestive heart failure (hypervolemia)

    4. Hypercalcemia. A serum calcium concentration greater than 12 mg/dl. Hypercalcemia may be seen in myeloma due to elaboration

TABLE 6-2. CLINICAL SIGNS RELATED TO PRODUCTS OF PROLIFERATING CELLS (PARANEOPLASTIC SYNDROMES)

Disorders that result from antibody activity of certain M components
Cold agglutinin disease
Autoimmune hemolytic anemia
Bleeding diathesis
Hyperlipidemia

Disorders that result from effects of certain physicochemical properties of M components
Hyperviscosity syndrome
Cryoglobulinemia
"Myeloma kidney"
Amyloidosis

Disorders that may result from release of other products of monoclonal neoplasms of B-cell origin
Antibody deficiency syndrome
Hypercalcemia

of osteoclast activating factor and possibly due to binding of calcium by IgG.

III. Treatment
  A. Antineoplastic therapy
    1. Chemotherapeutic agents
      a) Melphalan
         0.1 mg/kg PO SID for 10 days, then 0.05 mg/kg PO SID
      b) Prednisone
         0.5 mg/kg PO SID
      c) Cyclophosphamide can be used if resistance develops to melphalan: 1.0 mg/kg PO SID
    2. Surgical excision or radiation therapy is possible only for solitary lesions or areas of bony involvement where pain or spinal compression is clinically significant. Surgical manipulation of diseased bone is potentially dangerous and should be undertaken only after careful patient evaluation.
  B. Aims of therapy
    1. Clinical reduction in presenting signs (bone pain, lameness, lethargy, anorexia).
    2. Reduction in serum and Bence Jones proteins
      a) Aim for a 50% reduction in Bence Jones protein and serum M component.
      b) Due to a short half-life, a significant reduction in Bence Jones proteins is observed earlier than a decrease in serum proteins.
    3. Cats are often refractory to treatment and prognosis is poor.
  C. Care of concurrent problems
    1. Infection should be treated specifically and vigorously, based upon the results of culture and sensitivity testing.
    2. Hypercalcemia is a true medical emergency which, if untreated, leads to irreversible renal failure. Induce saline diuresis supplemented with furosemide (2–4 mg/kg TID) after hydration is adequate. As sodium and calcium compete for the same transport mechanism in the proximal tubule, this promotes intensive calciuresis. Prednisone (1–3 mg/kg divided TID) inhibits osteoclast activating factor secretion by some tumors, and may have a direct immunosuppressive effect on other lymphoid tumors.

Macroglobulinemia

  I. If the M component produced by the plasma cell dyscrasia is an IgM immunoglobulin, the disease is called *macroglobulinemia*.
 II. Clinical signs include plasma cell infiltration of the spleen, liver, and lymph nodes. Bone lysis is rare. Hyperviscosity syndrome and bleeding diatheses are common.

III. Antineoplastic therapy
   A. Chlorambucil
         0.2 mg/kg PO SID for 10 days, then 0.1 mg/kg PO SID
   B. Prednisone
         0.5 mg/kg PO SID
   C. Cyclophosphamide can be used if resistance develops to chlorambucil.
         1.0 mg/kg po SID

LYMPHOPROLIFERATIVE DISORDERS

M Components may be made in some functional B-cell neoplasms. In these cases, treatment should be directed against the underlying disease.

NONMYELOMATOUS MONOCLONAL GAMMOPATHY

I. This may be associated with another disease process (cirrhosis, chronic inflammatory disease), or with a neoplasm not normally known to produce immunoglobulins.
II. Benign monoclonal gammopathy
   A. This condition, in which a serum protein abnormality is noted in the absence of underlying disease or a plasma cell neoplasm, must be a diagnosis of exclusion which is continuously monitored.
   B. Suggested criteria for diagnosis are
      1. A concentration of M component not exceeding 3 g/100 ml
      2. The absence of Bence Jones proteinuria
      3. Normal immunoglobulin levels other than the M component
      4. Constant low concentrations of M component

IMMUNOHEMATOLOGY

IMMUNE-MEDIATED THROMBOCYTOPENIA

Platelet and Antibody Kinetics

I. Mechanisms of antibody production
   A. Autoantibodies may be formed to antigens present on the surface of platelet membranes (type II disease). Alternatively, the platelet surface antigens may be altered and no longer recognized as "self" by the host animal with consequent autoantibody production.
   B. Platelets are highly adsorbent and carry large numbers of foreign proteins on their surface. When the foreign protein serves as a hapten complexing with antigen on the platelet surface, antibody production is di-

rected toward this complex (type II disease). Antibody production ceases when the hapten is no longer present. Exogenous drug administration is the most common cause of this type of disease.

C. Preformed antigen-antibody complexes may become adsorbed to the sticky platelet surface (type III disease). When macrophages recognize and phagocytize the immune complexes, the platelet may be incidentally destroyed, causing thrombocytopenia.

II. F_c-receptors on the macrophages recognize the F_c-portion of the immune complex on the surface of the platelet. Once recognition has occurred, the macrophage phagocytizes the immune complex and destroys the platelet. Most antiplatelet antibodies are IgG and most antiplatelet antibody production occurs in the spleen. Due to local high antibody levels, slow flow through the sinusoids, and the presence of large numbers of macrophages, most platelets are removed in the spleen. In animals, most cases of immune-mediated thrombocytopenia are associated with splenomegaly.

Diagnosis

I. *Thrombocytopenia* is defined as a platelet count of less than 200,000 cells/mm^3, with clinically apparent bleeding at levels of less than 50,000 cells/mm^3.

II. Clinical signs
  A. Bleeding usually present as petechiae or ecchymoses, melena, epistaxis, hematuria, hyphema, or bleeding at venipuncture sites.
  B. Rarely, the presence of central nervous system (CNS) bleeding may be deduced from the association of seizures, coma, or other neurologic signs.
  C. Hemarthrosis, or bleeding into a major body cavity, is not a typical sign of thrombocytopenia.

III. Platelet production
  A. Production is usually adequate, as evidenced by megakaryopoiesis in a bone marrow aspirate or large young platelets on a peripheral smear.
  B. Rarely, antibodies to platelets have been suspected to cross-react with megakaryocytes, causing a nonregenerative thrombocytopenia. This must be a diagnosis of exclusion after all other causes of nonproduction, such as bone marrow infiltration by tumor or bone marrow suppression by tumor, drugs, or toxins have been eliminated.

IV. All known causes of thrombocytopenia must be excluded.
  A. Neoplasia commonly causes thrombocytopenia, either through consumption (hemangiosarcoma) or its suppressive effects on megakaryopoiesis (Sertoli cell tumor, lymphosarcoma).
  B. Infectious diseases causing thrombocytopenia are rare, being limited to *Ehrlichia* and a rare rickettsial organism reported in Florida. Usually, but not always, other signs of the disease are present. In unexplained cases, an *Ehrlichia* titer should be run.

   C. Sepsis has been seen associated with a low platelet count and clinically significant bleeding.
   D. The drug most commonly associated with thrombocytopenia in animals is estrogen, which causes thrombocytopenia, anemia, and terminally, complete bone marrow aplasia. Phenylbutazone, Styrid caracide (styrylpyridinium chloride—diethyl carbamizine citrate), and amphetamine have also been shown to induce antiplatelet-antibody formation. Any drug should be suspect and discontinued where possible.
 V. Platelet factor 3 test
   A. Platelets from normal subjects are incubated with serum from the affected animal. In the presence of antiplatelet antibody, the platelets are damaged and release platelet phospholipids, shortening the clotting time.
   B. The test is positive in the presence of specific antiplatelet antibody, and negative in drug-induced or antigen-antibody complex immune-mediated disease.
   C. If the thrombocytopenia is autoimmune in nature, other autoimmune diseases should be investigated.

Treatment

   I. Discontinue all drugs not absolutely critical to the welfare of the patient, or switch to an alternative therapy.
  II. Therapeutic guidelines:
   A. Aim for a complete remission through initial vigorous therapy, utilizing an individualized regimen based upon the clinical response and platelet count.
   B. PF-3 positive or true autoimmune thrombocytopenia may be much more difficult to control, and will probably require combination therapy with disease recurrence even with lifelong treatment.
   C. Recurrences of thrombocytopenia are often more difficult to manage and may require progressively more vigorous therapy.
   D. Although the ideal is to maintain a normal platelet count with the minimum amount of therapy, it is preferable in severe chronic refractory cases to maintain the platelet count at levels at which the animal is clinically normal, albeit thrombocytopenic, rather than risk the effects of high-dose, long-term corticosteroid and immunosuppressive treatment.
 III. Therapy
   A. Corticosteroids are the mainstay of therapy at the dosage recommended in the section on Principles of Therapeutics, above
   B. If the animal is nonresponsive or steroid toxicity is severe, adjunctive therapy with vinca alkaloids or splenectomy is added.
      1. Vincristine is effective and has a minimum of side effects.
      2. Splenectomy incurs the risk of anesthesia and may require several

whole blood or platelet transfusions. Nevertheless, it has been effective in producing long-term remissions or a marked reduction in adjunctive drug therapy. It may be performed as an elective procedure during a period of remission in chronic recurrent cases. If the animal is intact and can tolerate the additional surgery, ovariohysterectomy should be performed in conjunction with the splenectomy.

3. If splenectomy, steroids, and IV vincristine are ineffective, cytotoxic drugs may be added.

C. Animals that require such intensive combination chemotherapy have a poor prognosis.

IV. Transfusions
A. Give only as a life-saving measure.
B. Dogs and cats kept at cage rest are not transfused until the packed cell volume (PCV) falls to 10–15%, although fluids are given to prevent intravascular volume depletion and maintain renal status.
C. Evidence of renal or hepatic hypoxia may indicate the need for a transfusion at higher packed cell volumes (PCV).

V. Catheters should be placed in peripheral veins only, as bleeding around a jugular catheter may cause fatal airway compression.

VI. Antibiotics are not necessary except in documented cases of infection where therapy should be specific.

VII. Infection, vaccination, stress, surgery, estrus, and pregnancy may cause exacerbations of the disease, even in well-controlled animals. Killed vaccines should be used. Surgical procedures are safe as long as the platelet count is adequate to prevent bleeding, but steroids at immunosuppressive levels should be given before and after surgery to prevent disease exacerbation.

AUTOIMMUNE HEMOLYTIC ANEMIA

Antibody—Red Blood Cell Kinetics

I. Mechanisms of antibody formation
A. Autoimmune (type II disease)
B. Hapten-induced (type II disease)
C. Immune complex adsorption onto the red blood cell membrane (type III disease)

II. The same considerations regarding toxins, drugs, and neoplasia must be addressed in immune-mediated hemolytic anemia as in thrombocytopenia.

III. Red blood cells are usually removed extravascularly in the liver or spleen rather than by intravascular hemolysis. Whether the primary site of red blood cell removal is the liver or spleen depends upon the type and concentration of autoantibody.

A. Immunoglobulin G-coated cells are removed primarily by the spleen.
B. Immunoglobulin M-coated cells are removed primarily by the liver.

Diagnosis

I. Coombs' test
   A. A positive direct Coombs' test verifies the presence of antibodies and/or complement on the surface of the red cell.
   B. An indirect Coombs' test requires red blood cells from a donor of an identical blood group as the patient to prevent false-positive reactions to isoagglutinins. As it is difficult to match the red blood cell groups of dogs, this test is not recommended.
   C. False-positive Coombs' tests may result from transfusions.
   D. Negative Coombs' tests may be seen after glucocorticoid administration.
II. Anemia
   A. The anemia produced is strongly regenerative. Rarely, a Coombs'-positive anemia is seen that is nonregenerative and for which no other cause may be found. In these cases, autoimmune hemolytic anemia must be a diagnosis of exclusion after all other causes of nonproduction are eliminated.
   B. Spherocytosis and evidence of red blood cell production (anisocytosis, poikilocytosis, polychromatophilic red blood cells) are seen in the peripheral blood. The bone marrow response occurs about 4 days after the development of the anemia.
III. Agglutination
   A. Gross agglutination of red blood cells may be seen in an anticoagulant upon drawing the blood sample.
   B. In-saline agglutination differentiates agglutination from rouleau formation. Rouleau formation is dispersed when blood is diluted in saline, whereas agglutination will remain.

Clinical Syndromes

I. Auto-agglutinating
   A. Usually due to IgM antibody
   B. Types: determined by temperatures at which antibodies react with target cells
      1. Warm-reacting (in-saline agglutination)
         a) Causes severe anemia due to extravascular removal in liver and some intravascular hemolysis
         b) Extremely aggressive disease; prognosis is poor even with vigorous therapy
         c) High levels of glucocorticoids and cyclophosphamide should be started as initial therapy.

    2. Cold-reacting—cold agglutinin disease
        a) Seen as peripheral vascular occlusion due to agglutination of red
           blood cells in microvasculature of cooler sites
        b) Gangrene of tail, eartips, and toes is seen.
        c) Cold agglutinin titer must be greater than 1/64 to be significant, as
           cold agglutinins are formed in low levels in normal animals.
II. Nonagglutinating
    A. Most common form of the disease
    B. Caused by IgG antibody
    C. Red blood cells removed extravascularly, primarily by spleen
    D. Usually nonhemolytic

Treatment

  I. Transfusion
     A. Should be avoided except as a life-saving measure
     B. Affected animals are difficult to cross-match and the most compatible
        donor should be chosen to prevent a transfusion-induced hemolytic
        crisis.
     C. Considerations for transfusions are the same as outlined in the section
        on Thrombocytopenia, above.
 II. Drug therapy
     A. Corticosteroids are given at immunosuppressive doses. The PCV
        should rise or stabilize in 24 hours.
     B. If there is a poor response to steroids alone, adjunctive therapy such
        as splenectomy or cytotoxic drugs should be added.
     C. In animals with warm-reacting autoagglutination, or animals with ful-
        minant, aggressive disease, cytotoxic drugs should be started with ster-
        oids as initial therapy. Cyclophosphamide is usually used initially with
        azathioprine added in refractory cases.
     D. Response to cytotoxic therapy is not usually as dramatic as steroid
        response can be, and several weeks of therapy may be needed to raise
        the PCV to normal values.
III. Splenectomy
     A. Splenectomy may be of benefit in reducing the side effects of corti-
        costeroids and cytotoxic drugs by allowing reduction in dosage.
     B. Animals with severe disease may be poor surgical candidates for sple-
        nectomy, and therefore it may not be feasible in crisis situations. In
        these animals, the procedure may be performed as an elective when
        and if the disease is controlled.
     C. Splenectomy will not be as useful in IgM-mediated disease.
     D. Indications for splenectomy are chronic smouldering disease which is
        only partially responsive to drug therapy, and relapsing cases.
IV. Therapy guidelines:
     A. If the PCV stabilizes, therapy should be continued until the anemia

resolves, the reticulocyte count falls, and sound clinical remission is established.

  B. Cyclophosphamide and azathioprine may be discontinued after sound clinical remission is established and the animal observed for relapse.
  C. In spite of side effects, therapy should not be tapered rapidly. Guidelines for glucocorticoid therapy outlined in the section on Principles of Therapeutics, above should be followed.
  D. After several months of therapy, corticosteroids are tapered and may eventually be withdrawn entirely in some cases, and the animal carefully monitored for recurrence.
  E. The probability of disease recurrence cannot be deduced from initial disease severity.
  F. Any underlying or concomitant diseases should be treated appropriately.
 V. Autoimmune hemolytic anemia is exacerbated by infection, stress, surgery, vaccination, estrus, and pregnancy. The animal should be neutered and vaccinated with killed instead of live virus vaccines.

IMMUNE COMPLEX DISEASES

PATHOGENIC MECHANISM

   I. The mechanism common to all immune complex diseases is the deposition of circulating antigen-antibody complexes in vessel walls.
  II. With the fixation of complement and complement activation, neutrophils are chemotactically attracted to vessel walls and surrounding tissues.
 III. The neutrophils degranulate and release lysosomal enzymes which cause endothelial cell damage and increased vascular permeability.
  IV. Platelets aggregate and may cause vessel occlusion, thrombosis, and hemorrhage.
   V. Mononuclear cells move into the area and monocytes, lymphocytes, and plasma cells can be seen surrounding the vessel.

CLINICAL SIGNS

A variety of factors related to the immune complexes themselves determine the site of organ localization and the clinical signs associated with the disease. Clinical signs may include

   I. Glomerulonephritis
  II. Arthritis
 III. Dermatitis
  IV. Panniculitis
   V. Pleuritis
  VI. Pericarditis

VII. Serositis
VIII. Neuritis
 IX. Tissue ulceration and infarction
  X. Leukopenia, anemia, and thrombocytopenia

IMMUNE COMPLEX LEVELS

Although determination of circulating immune complex levels is now possible at some institutions, the levels must be correlated with clinical disease. Histopathologic evidence of vasculitis in conjunction with elevated immune complex levels and hypocomplementemia is strongly supportive of an immune complex etiology.

SYSTEMIC LUPUS ERYTHEMATOSUS

Diagnosis

 I. Diagnosis of SLE is supported by demonstration of antinuclear antibodies (ANA), antibodies to red blood cells, platelets, thyroglobulin, and immunoglobulin (rheumatoid factors). These may be present in any combination but most investigators require demonstration of a positive ANA (greater than 1:100) or naturally occurring lupus erythematosus (LE) cells in body tissues or fluids in conjunction with clinical signs.
 II. A diagnostic scheme has been proposed for canine SLE utilizing major and minor signs.
   A. Major signs include Coombs'-positive anemia, thrombocytopenia, leukopenia, glomerulonephritis, and musculoskeletal and dermatologic signs.
   B. Minor signs consist of fever, central nervous system (CNS) involvement, and pleuritis.
III. Clinical signs
   A. Glomerulonephritis
     1. 24-hour urine collection may demonstrate significant proteinuria (greater than 0.75 g albumin/24 hr) due to glomerulonephritis.
     2. Renal insufficiency and/or progression to the nephrotic syndrome are important sequelae to the glomerulonephritis.
     3. Histopathologic patterns of canine lupus nephritis have not been clearly defined.
   B. Polyarthropathy
     1. This is a nonerosive, nondeforming polyarthropathy which usually affects distal joints. Radiographs may show soft tissue swelling but no bony lesions. Occasionally, arthritis becomes erosive and clinical features overlap with that of canine rheumatoid arthritis.
     2. The synovial fluid cytology is characterized by sterile inflammation

with many neutrophils and some monocytes, plasma cells, and synovial cells. No bacteria are seen or cultured. Lupus erythematosus cells may be seen.

3. The polyarthropathy is primarily a tendosynovitis. Joint enlargement is due primarily to fibrosis of the joint capsule and synovial hypertrophy. Histopathologic examination reveals chronic, active inflammation of the joints and periarticular structures.

C. Polymyositis has been reported in several dogs. Electromyography and muscle biopsy verify the diagnosis. The muscle enzymes creatinine phosphokinase and aspartate aminotransferase [formerly serum glutamic oxaloacetic transaminase (SGOT)] may be elevated.

D. Autoimmune hemolytic anemia

E. Autoimmune thrombocytopenia

F. Systemic manifestations. Fever, anorexia, and malaise can be seen in SLE. The fever is nonantibiotic responsive but responds to high doses of glucocorticoids.

G. Cutaneous manifestations

1. Petechiae or purpura may be caused by thrombocytopenia or vasculitis. Ulcerative lesions due to vasculitis may be present on mucous membranes or skin.

2. Direct immunofluorescence reveals immunoglobulin and complement deposition along dermal-epidermal junctions.

3. Histopathologic examination reveals degeneration of the basal cell layers, disruption of the dermal-epidermal junctions, and a mononuclear cell infiltrate around vessels.

H. Neuritis—meningitis and myelopathy have been reported in dogs.

Treatment

I. Prednisone alone is effective in controlling clinical signs in some dogs. Most require continuous low-dose therapy given every other day.

II. If prednisone alone is ineffective in alleviating disease signs, a combination of prednisone and cyclophosphamide may be used, and azathioprine added if necessary. White blood cell counts should be monitored for drug-induced bone marrow suppression.

RHEUMATOID ARTHRITIS

Pathogenesis

I. Rheumatoid arthritis is characterized histologically by microvasculitis with associated inflammation.

II. Plasma constituents leak between endothelial cells. If this occurs in the synovium, the synovial lining cells proliferate and chronic granulation tis-

sue (pannus) encroaches on neighboring tissues like bone, tendon, cartilage, and periarticular tissues, and disrupts joint stability and function.
III. Continuous joint motion and weight-bearing contribute to tissue destruction. A severe, deforming degenerative arthritis ensues.

Immunopathogenic Mechanism

Because the cells involved in the tissue processes suggest an immune complex etiology, an underlying immunopathogenic mechanism has been sought.
I. Common to most cases of rheumatoid arthritis is the demonstration of rheumatoid factor (RhF).
II. Rheumatoid factor is commonly IgM (or, rarely, IgG) which has antibody activity against other immunoglobulins.
III. Rheumatoid factor-immunoglobulin complexes seem to be the underlying stimulus for the development of the microvasculitis.
IV. The initiating factor prompting development of RhF production is unknown.

Diagnosis

I. Although veterinary clinicians attempt to follow the guidelines which the American Rheumatism Association has established for the diagnosis of rheumatoid arthritis in people, many of the criteria are not applicable to animals. Subcutaneous nodules are not reported in dogs with the disease, and many of the clinical syndromes causing exclusion are not recognized in domestic animals.
II. Animals usually have a combination of the following signs:
   A. Depression, fever, and anorexia
   B. Joint swelling and lameness may involve one or several joints. Muscle wasting and decreased exercise tolerance is variable.
      1. Affected joints are usually distal, with carpi and tarsi most commonly affected.
      2. Early in the disease, joint thickening alone may be appreciated; as the disease progresses, crepitus and laxity advance to joint deformity and subluxation, instability, and chronic degenerative joint disease.
      3. Synovial fluid cytology is characterized by sterile inflammation with a preponderance of polymorphonuclear neutrophilic granulocytes (PMNs).
   C. Radiographic findings may be absent early in the disease but eventually bony demineralization develops with subchondral and juxtaarticular bone destruction. As the disease progresses, degenerative joint disease progresses to ankylosis of subluxation and collapse.
   D. Positive RhF
      1. In the absence of supportive signs, a positive RhF alone is not di-

agnostic. Because RhF is an antibody formed in response to immunoglobulin, it is present in many diseases.

2. Because rheumatoid arthritis is an immunologic disorder, other immunologic phenomena such as an ANA titer may be present. Indistinct clinical entities with several positive autoimmune phenomena are found (so-called overlap syndromes). These are difficult to fit into well-defined disease syndromes, but indicate that the underlying pathologic mechanism is immunologic.

3. Synovial biopsy shows villous proliferation of the synovium with plasma cell and lymphocyte infiltration. This has the highest diagnostic specificity for rheumatoid arthritis.

Treatment

I. Limit activity, as periods of intense exercise may aggravate clinical signs. Joint mobility may be preserved and muscle atrophy decreased by regular periods of controlled activity or joint manipulation.

II. Weight reduction may be desirable to reduce stress on joint tissues.

III. In severely deformed and painful joints, arthrodesis may be of benefit.

IV. Drug therapy

   A. Nonsteroidal antiinflammatory drugs (NSAID)

   1. The use of NSAIDs may be of benefit in reducing pain and inflammation and therefore encourage weight-bearing, but these drugs do little to retard progression of the underlying disease.

   2. Aspirin is the most widely used of these compounds—phenylbutazone, naproxen, indomethacin, and ibuprofen have also been used. *Naproxen and indomethacin have been associated with gastrointestinal hemorrhage when used at extrapolated human dosages.*

   3. Until further data on the pharmacokinetics of these drugs in animal species are available, buffered aspirin and aspirin-Maalox combinations may be the most rational choice. A dose of 10 mg/kg TID PO should provide therapeutic blood levels, but the dose may need to be adjusted to the individual patient.

   4. See Chapter 5.

   B. Glucocorticoids

   1. Like NSAIDs, systemic glucocorticoids do not alter the natural course of the underlying disease. They may, however, reduce severity of clinical signs in the patient which is rapidly deteriorating despite other therapy.

   2. The use of glucocorticoids should be restricted to short courses, as continuous therapy is often associated with osteoporosis and muscular atrophy as well as other signs of steroid toxicity.

   3. Prednisone is used at immunosuppressive dosages.

   4. Intraarticular glucocorticoid administration may be helpful in a few

well-chosen instances. It may help restore joint motion by alleviating pain and swelling, but may lead to infection or damage of articular structures. The benefit/risk ratio must be weighed in each instance.

C. Immunosuppressive agents
   1. Cyclophosphamide and azathioprine have been of value in reducing disease activity in animals which no longer benefited from oral or intraarticular glucocorticoids.
   2. Because complete clinical remissions have been achieved and progression of joint disease has been halted, early vigorous therapy utilizing a combination of prednisone, cyclophosphamide, and azathioprine has been advocated to prevent the development of disabling joint deformity. Early diagnosis, before significant joint damage has occurred, improves the prognosis.

D. Remission-inducing agents
   1. Aurothioglucose has been used in several instances where previous therapy with aspirin, prednisone, and phenylbutazone were ineffective. The dosage recommended is 1 mg/kg body weight, given once weekly by IM injection.
   2. Penicillamine has been used occasionally in some patients with rheumatoid arthritis and has resulted in some palliation of signs. The mechanism of action is unknown.

IMMUNE-MEDIATED OCCULT DIROFILARIASIS

Chronic pulmonary disease and heart failure may be caused by patent *Dirofilaria* infection in the absence of circulating microfilaremia due to the elaboration of an antimicrofilarial antibody.

PATHOGENESIS

 I. Antibodies are formed against microfilaria antigens.
II. As microfilaria are released from gravid females, they are coated with antibody and sequestered in the lungs.
III. Eosinophilic granulomatous pneumonia develops, causing pulmonary signs.

CLINICAL SIGNS

Clinical signs may be present in varying combinations and degrees of severity. Cardiac signs may be seen, but most clinical signs are referrable to the pulmonary involvement.

Pulmonary Signs

I. Increased interstitial infiltrate
II. Focal parenchymal lesions, most likely due to thromboembolism
III. Coughing
IV. Hemoptysis
V. Tachypnea

Cardiac Signs

I. Increased right apex beat
II. Split-second heart sounds
III. Increased central venous pressure
IV. Right-sided congestive heart failure
V. Right bundle branch block
VI. Right axis deviation
VII. Pulmonary knob
VIII. Right-sided heart enlargement

Systemic Signs

I. Fever
II. Shock
III. Weight loss
IV. Anorexia
V. Thromboembolism

CLINICAL PATHOLOGY

I. Tracheal wash contains a marked eosinophilic infiltrate. Secondary bacterial infection may occasionally be present.
II. Hyper-β-globulinemia is present on serum electrophoresis.
III. Antibody titers
    A. Types
        1. Indirect fluorescent antibody test (IFA) detects circulating antibodies to microfilaria.
        2. Enzyme-linked immunoassay (ELISA) test detects circulating antibodies to adult *Dirofilaria*.
    B. May be used to differentiate between immune-mediated occult dirofilariasis and other causes of occult infestation (prepatent infestation, infestation by only one sex, infestation by sterile worms)

TREATMENT

I. If significant respiratory signs due to eosinophilic infiltration of the lungs are present, prednisone should be instituted at immunosuppressive dosage until the pulmonary signs resolve.
II. Cardiac signs should be treated according to standard protocols, depending upon the severity of the involvement.
III. Treat the adult *Dirofilaria* infection with an approved adulticide according to standard available protocols (see Chapter 4).

MYASTHENIA GRAVIS

Myasthenia gravis is a neuromuscular disease characterized by (1) progressive weakness and fatiguability of voluntary muscles, (2) weakness which is aggravated by exercise, and (3) weakness which is ameliorated by anticholinesterase drugs.

TYPES

Congenital

I. Breeds affected
   A. Fox terrier
   B. Springer spaniel
   C. Jack Russell terrier
II. The defect is an intrinsic deficiency of the number of acetylcholine receptors on the postsynaptic membrane of of the neuromuscular junction. The mechanism of receptor deficiency is unknown, but is not autoimmune as it is in the acquired form. It is inherited in the Jack Russell terrier as an autosomal-recessive trait.

Acquired

I. Age at onset ranges from 7 weeks to 11 years and there is no breed or sex predisposition.
II. Pathogenesis
   A. Circulating autoantibodies to muscle acetylcholine receptors are demonstrable, and autoantibodies are found complexed to receptors in most affected animals.
   B. There is an absolute reduction in the number of muscle acetylcholine receptors.
   C. The level of autoantibody present correlates loosely with the clinical condition of the affected animal.

III. Clinical signs
  A. Episodic weakness is exacerbated by exercise and ameliorated by rest or acetylcholinesterase inhibitors.
  B. Megaesophagus is often seen in the acquired form due to the high proportion of striated muscle fibers in the canine esophagus. This may lead to the development of aspiration pneumonia.
  C. Change in the character of the bark, dysphagia, and drooling due to weakness of the pharyngeal and laryngeal muscles is a characteristic sign.
  D. Neurologic examination should be normal before collapse, with the exception of a possible Bell's palsy; lower motor neuron paresis of cranial and peripheral nerves may be seen during an attack.
IV. Diagnosis
  A. Electromyography
    1. Demonstration of decreased action potential amplitude during repetitive supramaximal stimulation (decremental response) is characteristic.
    2. The decremental response should be abolished by administration of acetylcholinesterase inhibitors.
  B. Pharmacologic challenge with acetylcholinesterase inhibitors
    1. Acetylcholinesterase inhibitors delay degradation of acetylcholine, thereby permitting more postsynaptic receptor stimulation and improving muscle strength.
    2. Administration of edrophonium chloride (Tensilon) at 1.1–2.2 mg/kg with a total dose range of 1–5 mg, should result in dramatic resolution of weakness within 10–30 seconds. Muscarinic side effects may be reversed if necessary with IV atropine (0.05 mg/kg).
V. Treatment
  A. Acetylcholinesterase inhibitors
    1. Most dogs are responsive to these drugs, but there is marked individuality in effective doses. Doses given below are suggested initial guidelines only; titrate doses to the patient.
    2. Drugs available
      a) Neostigmine methylsulfate (Prostigmin)
        (1) Less than 5 kg: 0.25 mg QID IM
        (2) Five to 25 kg: 0.25–0.5 mg QID IM
        (3) Greater than 25 kg: 0.5–0.75 mg QID IM
      b) Pyridostigmine bromide (Mestinon)
        (1) Less than 5 kg: 45 mg QID PO
        (2) Five to 25 kg: 45–90 mg QID PO
        (3) Greater than 25 kg: 90–135 mg QID PO
    3. Development of diarrhea or other muscarinic signs (salivation, urination, drooling) indicates the dose should be lowered by 25%. Treatment with atropine is usually not necessary.
    4. If overdosage of acetylcholinesterase inhibitors is severe, the con-

tinuous depolarization of the postsynaptic membrane may cause a cholinergic crisis with a generalized weakness which is difficult to differentiate from a myasthenic crisis. A test dose of edrophonium will differentiate between the two. A cholinergic crisis should be treated with atropine and temporary cessation of acetylcholinesterase inhibitors.

5. Animals with megaesophagus should be placed on injectable forms of the drugs until pills may be successfully swallowed.

6. Spontaneous remissions are possible and drug dosage may need to be lowered to prevent a cholinergic crisis. Owners can titrate the dose by watching for diarrhea.

B. Glucocorticoids appear to be efficacious as adjunctive therapy in dogs not responsive to acetylcholinesterase inhibitor therapy. Immunosuppressive dosages should be used.

C. Other therapeutic modalities occasionally used which may be of benefit in selected animals include azathioprine and immunoadsorption.

D. Treat accompanying conditions

1. Aspiration pneumonia is a frequent and life-threatening complication. Treatment should be specific and vigorous, based upon culture and sensitivity testing.

2. Megaesophagus. Dietary and feeding management may be necessary for the duration of the life of the animal. Feed and water in an upright or sitting position. Daily water requirements may be mixed into the food.

3. Anterior mediastinal masses. Thymomas are occasionally found associated with myasthenia gravis in the dog. As surgical excision in some cases appeared to ameliorate disease signs, anterior mediastinal masses should be investigated.

BULLOUS SKIN DISEASES

PEMPHIGUS GROUP

I. These are blistering diseases involving the skin and mucous membranes, caused by elaboration of antibodies against intercellular cement substance. The loss of intercellular bridges causes acantholysis (separation of epidermal cells from one another) and bulla formation. The site of acantholysis within the epidermis determines the nature of the observed lesion and the clinical picture of the disease. Forms seen in veterinary medicine include pemphigus vulgaris, foliaceus, vegetans, and erythematosus. Pemphigus foliaceus is the most common form in both the dog and the cat in our clinic.

II. Diagnosis requires demonstration of the classic histopathologic lesions of acantholysis and bulla formation with the results of direct immunofluorescence testing. Indirect immunofluorescence is generally unrewarding.

Normal skin will not show diagnostic changes, therefore, bullae must be biopsied, being careful to include perilesional tissue.

III. Treatment
   A. Glucocorticoids at immunosuppressive levels are started as initial therapy. Poor clinical response or unacceptable side effects should prompt addition of adjunctive therapy.
   B. Adjunctive therapy
      1. Cyclophosphamide
      2. Aurothioglucose
      3. Azathioprine
         a) This drug appears to be particularly effective as an induction agent in cats with pemphigus foliaceus. It should be given at a dose of 1 mg/kg every other day.
         b) Azathioprine is not suitable for chronic maintenance in cats due to drug-induced leukopenia.
   C. Spontaneous remissions are unlikely. Remissions due to therapy are possible but relapses are common. Most animals require chronic to chronic-intermittent therapy for life.

BULLOUS PEMPHIGOID

   I. In this disease, antibodies are formed against the basement membrane zone of the dermal-epidermal junction causing subepidermal cleft formation. Acantholysis is not present. Immunoglobulin, and often complement, can be demonstrated with direct immunofluorescence. Indirect immunofluorescence is generally unrewarding.
  II. Clinically, this disease looks much like pemphigus vulgaris, and histopathology and direct immunofluorescence are necessary to differentiate them.
 III. Treatment is as for the pemphigus group.

SUGGESTED READINGS

Hurvitz AI: Mechanisms of immune injury. J Am Vet Med Assoc 181:1080, 1982.

Hurvitz AI (ed): Hematology-oncology-immunology. p. 384. In Kirk RW (ed): Current Veterinary Therapy VIII. Philadelphia, WB Saunders Company, 1983.

Katz P, Fauci AS: Treatment of immune complex-mediated diseases: corticosteroids and cytotoxic agents. Clin Immunol Allergy 1:415, 1981.

MacEwen EC, Hurvitz AI: Diagnosis and management of monoclonal gammopathies. Vet Clin N AM 7:119, 1977.

Pederson NC, Halliwell R, Hurvitz AI: Basic and clinical immunology. p. 159. In Proceedings of the American Animal Hospital Association 46th Annu Meeting. 1979.

Scott DW, Manning TO, Smith BA, Lewis RM: Observations on the immunopathology and therapy of canine pemphigus and pemphigoid. J AM Vet Med Assoc 180:48, 1982.

7

Chemotherapy of Neoplastic Diseases

Robert C. Rosenthal, D.V.M.

CANCER AND CHEMOTHERAPY

THE SCOPE OF THE CANCER PROBLEM

I. Although it is difficult to define incidence and prevalence rates precisely for the neoplastic diseases of companion animals, more cancer cases are being diagnosed and treated than ever before.
II. Incidence rates may be rising with increased exposure to environmental pollution and chemical carcinogens. Prolonged life span related to the control of infectious disease, an improved nutritional plane, and better management of other disorders allows more pets to reach the "cancer age."
III. As dogs and cats assume an increasingly important psychological role in our society, knowledgeable and caring owners will be more aware of and responsive to their pets' medical needs. Clinicians will be called upon to deal with a significant number of cancer cases.

THE ROLE OF CHEMOTHERAPY

I. Historically, cancer has been considered a surgical disease. Today, multimodality therapy is becoming the rule.
II. Local therapies (surgery, radiation) may control the primary lesions grossly, but undetectable residual disease and micrometastatic disease is better managed by a systemic therapy such as chemotherapy or immunotherapy.
  A. To date, immunotherapy has not lived up to its theoretical promise.
  B. Chemotherapy remains the best method to control disseminated cancer.
III. There is, however, much to be learned regarding optimal combinations of drugs, scheduling, and the interplay of the various treatment modalities.

To evaluate the effect of chemotherapy in an undetectable disease is, of course, a vexing problem.

IV. There are a few tumors of veterinary importance which are quite responsive to chemotherapy and for which primary chemotherapy is entirely appropriate. (See section on Treatment of Specific Diseases, below)

CARE OF THE CANCER PATIENT

I. The quality of the patient's life is of utmost importance. The ability to deliver chemotherapy is limited not by the capacity to kill tumor cells, but rather by host toxicity.

A. Most owners are aware of possible toxic side effects of chemotherapy and will accept limited toxic reactions.

B. Euthanasia is an option clear in the minds of most owners and the veterinarian must be prepared to discuss that choice and advise the client.

II. The major dose-limiting toxicities in most veterinary chemotherapy protocols are hematologic and gastrointestinal, although others (sterile hemorrhagic cystitis, cardiomyopathy, dermatologic problems) cannot be ignored.

A. The clinician must be prepared to monitor toxicity and respond appropriately by withholding further therapy and providing measures specific for the toxicity in question.

B. Other important topics include nutrition in the cancer patient, the control of pain, and the paraneoplastic syndromes but are beyond the scope of this chapter. Refer to the list of suggested readings for further information.

III. Often very complex, but equally rewarding, the management of cancer patients is a challenge to the practitioner.

A. Consultation with a veterinary clinical oncologist can frequently answer many questions.

B. Referral may provide the opportunity for comprehensive diagnostic and therapeutic work beyond the scope of many practices.

IV. In the final analysis, the patient's quality of life as perceived by the owner will be used to measure the success of treatment. All the considerations mentioned above and the specifics to follow are important to achieve this end.

UNDERLYING PRINCIPLES

BIOLOGIC BASIS

I. Proliferative activity: neoplastic cells may be:

A. Permanently nondividing (end stage)

B. Temporarily nondividing with the potential to resume cell cycle activity

C. Actively cycling

II. The cell cycle: those neoplastic cells that are actively cycling pass through the same phases as do normal cycling cells.

A. M-phase: mitosis, active cell division, takes about 30–90 minutes in mammalian cells.

B. G_1 (gap one): a period of marked temporal variability, days to weeks, during which RNA and protein synthesis occur.

C. G_0 (gap zero): a resting, nonproliferating phase that cells may enter from G_1. Cells may or may not return to active cycling.

D. S-phase: a period of DNA synthesis which generally lasts for several hours.

E. G_2 (gap two): another period marked by RNA and protein synthesis preparing for mitosis, usually 6–8 hours long.

The successful completion of each cycle involves synthetic and divisional events which are subject to chemotherapeutic attack.

III. Differential growth rates: Gompertzian growth is a growth pattern characterized by an increased doubling time and a decreased growth fraction as a function of time. Neoplasms with such growth patterns will be more or less susceptible to various drugs at different times.

PHARMACOLOGIC BASIS

The efficacy of a chemotherapeutic agent is related to the product of its time of exposure and concentration at the site of the tumor, i.e., the effective contact time. This is influenced by pharmacologic factors which include:

I. Route of administration

II. Absorption

III. Biotransformation

IV. Distribution

V. Excretion

Drug resistance, interactions, and toxicities all affect the use of a single agent or combinations.

THE ROLE OF CHEMOTHERAPY

With the continuing development of anticancer drugs and a growing understanding of their appropriate use, chemotherapy will assume an increasingly important role in the management of neoplastic disease. The objectives of chemotherapy include:

I. Cure—often difficult to define clinically and in most cases not attainable

II. Palliation—providing systematic relief and temporary restoration of deteriorated function

III. Reduction of tumor mass to facilitate local therapies (surgery, radiation)

IV. Control of micrometastatic disease in the adjunct setting following other primary therapy

GUIDELINES FOR CHEMOTHERAPY

I. Establish a complete data base including a histologic diagnosis.
II. Assure owner compliance. A satisfying outcome depends on realistic expectations and continuous cooperation on the owner's part.
III. Know the drugs being used.
IV. Use established drugs and schedules for dogs and cats.
V. Monitor toxicity and modify therapy as necessary.
VI. Evaluate the response of the neoplasm.

PRINCIPLES OF COMBINATION CHEMOTHERAPY

The use of combinations of drugs has theoretical and practical advantages compared to the use of single agents. Recall that chemotherapy is limited not by the ability to kill neoplastic cells but rather by the associated toxicity to normal tissues. Also, the fraction of cells killed by one drug is independent of that killed by another drug. Thus, it is possible to design combination protocols which

I. Use drugs with known activity against a specific neoplasm.
II. Use drugs with different mechanisms of action to attack the cell cycle at various points (see table 7-1).
III. Use drugs with different toxicities to limit the adverse affects on any system.
IV. Use pulse therapy to allow normal cells to recover between therapies.

CHEMOTHERAPEUTIC AGENTS

COMMONLY USED DRUGS

Table 7-1 presents pertinent information regarding the anticancer drugs commonly employed in veterinary protocols. Note that only a few of these agents are incorporated in the recommendations in this section. The clinician should be thoroughly familiar with the drugs used. It is far better to have a sound understanding of a few drugs and protocols than a poor understanding of many. For information regarding drugs or malignancies not presented, consultation with a veterinary clinical oncologist is highly recommended.

EXPRESSION OF DRUG DOSE

In most instances, the drug has been expressed as /m^2 (meters squared, body surface area), a physiologically more accurate method of dose calculation than

TABLE 7-1. CHEMOTHERAPEUTIC AGENTS USED IN VETERINARY MEDICINE

Class/Name	Brand Name (Manufacturer)	Cell Cycle Specificity[a]	Possible Indications	Suggested Dosage	Toxicity
ALKYLATING AGENTS					
Cyclophosphamide	Cytoxan (Mead Johnson)	CCNS	Lymphoreticular neoplasms, mammary and lung carcinomas, miscellaneous sarcomas	50 mg/m^2 PO 4 days/week or 200 mg/m^2 IV weekly	Leucopenia, anemia, thrombocytopenia (less common); nausea, vomiting, sterile hemorrhagic cystitis
Chlorambucil	Leukeran (Burroughs Wellcome)	CCNS	Lymphoreticular neoplasms, chronic lymphocyte leukemia	2 mg/m^2 PO 2–4 days/week	Mild leucopenia, thrombocytopenia, anemia, nausea, vomiting (not common)
Nitrogen mustard	Mustragen (Merck, Sharp & Dohme)	CCNS	Lymphoreticular neoplasms	5 mg/m^2 IV	Leucopenia, thrombocytopenia, nausea, vomiting, anorexia
Triethylenethio-phosphoramide	Thiotepa (Lederle)	CCNS	Various carcinomas and sarcomas	9 mg/m^2 as a single dose or divided over 2–4 days (60 mg in 60 ml water for bladder instillation, 30 min/week)	Leucopenia, thrombocytopenia, anemia
Busulfan	Myleran (Burroughs Wellcome)	CCNS	Granulocytic leukemias, myeloproliferative disorders	3–4 mg/m^2 PO daily	Leucopenia, thrombocytopenia, anemia

(cont.)

Class/Name	Brand Name (Manufacturer)	Cell Cycle Specificity[a]	Possible Indications	Suggested Dosage	Toxicity
Melphalan	Alkeran (Burroughs Wellcome)	CCNS	Multiple myeloma, monoclonal gammopathies, lymphoreticular neoplasms	1.5 mg/m² PO for 7–10 days, repeat cycle every 3 weeks	Leucopenia, thrombocytopenia, anemia, anorexia, nausea, vomiting
Dacarbazine	DTIC (Dome)	CCNS	Malignant melanoma, various sarcomas	200 mg/m² IV for 5 days every 3 weeks	Leucopenia, thrombocytopenia, anemia, nausea, vomiting, diarrhea (often decreases with later cycles)
Lomustine	CeeNU (Bristol)	CCNS	Various carcinomas, lymphosarcoma	100 mg/m² PO every 6 weeks	Leucopenia, thrombocytopenia (both develop in 3–6 weeks), nausea, vomiting (transient)
ANTIMETABOLITES Methotrexate	Methotrexate (Lederle)	S	Lymphoreticular neoplasms, myeloproliferative disorders, various carcinomas and sarcomas	2.5 mg/m² PO daily	Leucopenia, thrombocytopenia, anemia, stomatitis, diarrhea, hepatopathy, renal tubular necrosis
6-Mercaptopurine	Purinethol (Burroughs Wellcome)	S	Lymphosarcoma, acute lymphocytic leukemia, granulocytic leukemia	50 mg/m² PO daily until response or toxicity	Leucopenia, nausea, vomiting, hepatopathy
5-Fluorouracil	Fluorouracil (Roche Laboratories)	S	Various carinomas and sarcomas	200 mg/m² IV weekly	Leucopenia, thrombocytopenia, anemia, anorexia, nausea, vomiting, diarrhea, stomatitis
	Efudex cream (Roche Laboratories)		Cutaneous tumors	Apply twice daily for 2–4 weeks	

Drug	Manufacturer	Specificity	Dose	Toxicity
Cytosine arabinoside	Cytosar-U (Upjohn)	S	100 mg/m² SQ or IV drip for 4 days	Leucopenia, thrombocytopenia, anemia, nausea, vomiting, anorexia
PLANT ALKALOIDS				
Vincristine	Oncovin (Eli Lilly)	M	0.5 mg/m² IV weekly	Peripheral neuropathy and paresthesia, constipation
Vinblastine	Velban (Eli Lilly)	M	2.5 mg/m² IV weekly	Leucopenia, nausea, vomiting
ANTIBIOTICS				
Doxorubicin	Adinamycin (Adria Laboratory)	CCNS	30 mg/m² IV every 3 weeks (do not exceed 240 mg/m² total)	Leucopenia, thrombocytopenia, nausea, vomiting, cardiac toxicity, reactions during administration
Actinomycin-D	Cosmegen (Merck, Sharp & Dohme)	CCNS	1.5 mg/m² IV weekly	Thrombocytopenia, leucopenia, stomatitis, proctitis, nausea, vomiting
Bleomycin	Blenoxane (Bristol Laboratories)	CCNS (G_1, S, and M)	10 mg/m² IV or SQ for 3–9 days, then 10 mg/m² IV weekly (do not exceed 200 mg/m² total)	Allergic reactions following administration, pulmonary fibrosis
HORMONES				
Prednisolone	—	NA	Vary widely depending on indication: 60 mg/m² PO daily–20 mg/m² PO every 48 hours	Hyperadrenocorticism, secondary adrenocortical insufficiency

(cont.)

TABLE 7-1. CHEMOTHERAPEUTIC AGENTS USED IN VETERINARY MEDICINE (*Continued*)

Class/Name	Brand Name (Manufacturer)	Cell Cycle Specificity[a]	Possible Indications	Suggested Dosage	Toxicity
Diethylstilbesterol	—	NA	Perianal adenomas, prostatic neoplasms (adjunctively)	1.1 mg/kg IM once (do not administer more than 25 mg) or 1 mg PO q72h	Bone marrow toxicity, feminization
MISCELLANEOUS					
L-Asparaginase	Elspar (Merck, Sharp & Dohme)	NA	Lymphoreticular neoplasms	20,000 U/m² IP weekly	Anaphylaxis, leucopenia
Mitotane	Lysodren (Calbio)	NA	Adrenocortical tumors	50 mg/kg PO daily to effect, then 50 mg/kg PO q7–14d PRN	Adenocortical insuffiency

Abbreviations: CCNS, cell-cycle-phase-nonspecific; CNS, central nervous system; M, M-phase-specific; NA, not applicable; S, S-phase-specific.

TABLE 7-2. CONVERSION TABLE OF WEIGHT IN KILOGRAMS TO BODY SURFACE AREA IN SQUARE METERS FOR DOGS

kg	m²	kg	m²
0.5	0.06	26.0	0.88
1.0	0.10	27.0	0.90
2.0	0.15	28.0	0.92
3.0	0.20	29.0	0.94
4.0	0.25	30.0	0.96
5.0	0.29	31.0	0.99
6.0	0.33	32.0	1.01
7.0	0.36	33.0	1.03
8.0	0.40	34.0	1.05
9.0	0.43	35.0	1.07
10.0	0.46	36.0	1.09
11.0	0.49	37.0	1.11
12.0	0.52	38.0	1.13
13.0	0.55	39.0	1.15
14.0	0.58	40.0	1.17
15.0	0.60	41.0	1.19
16.0	0.63	42.0	1.21
17.0	0.66	43.0	1.23
18.0	0.69	44.0	1.25
19.0	0.71	45.0	1.26
20.0	0.74	46.0	1.28
21.0	0.76	47.0	1.30
22.0	0.78	48.0	1.32
23.0	0.81	49.0	1.34
24.0	0.83	50.0	1.36
25.0	0.85	—	—

body weight. Table 7-2 is a conversion chart for dogs and is applicable for domestic cats as well.

TREATMENT OF SPECIFIC DISEASES

CANINE LYMPHOSARCOMA (LSA)

I. Objectives

Canine LSA must still be considered a terminal disease. To date, histologic grading by cell type has not been reliably correlated with prognosis.

Similarly, clinical staging has offered little to exact prognosis with the exception that substage (b) patients (severe systemic effects, hypercalcemia, and so forth) do less well than substage (a) patients (minimal systemic effects). The goal of therapy is to achieve a complete remission, freeing the patient of clinical signs and maintaining a high quality of life.

II. Recommended Therapy
  A. Multicentric form
    1. Week 1
      a) Cytosar arabinoside, 100 mg/m^2 slow IV drip or SQ, SID, days 1–4
      b) Prednisolone, 40 mg/m^2 PO, SID
      c) Cyclophosphamide, 50 mg/m^2 PO, SID, days 1–4
      d) Vincristine, 0.5 mg IV, day 1 only
    2. Weeks 2–8
      a) Prednisolone, 20 mg/m^2 SID every other day
      b) Cyclophosphamide and vincristine as in week 1
      c) If remission is attained after 8 weeks, a maintenance schedule of prednisolone, 20 mg/m^2 SID every other day, and chlorambucil, 2 mg/m^2 PO days 1–4 each week, is continued until relapse. At that time, a second 8-week induction substituting vinblastine for vincristine is begun. (Many protocols using other combinations have also been useful. The scope of this manual does not allow an exhaustive discussion of their merits.)
  B. Other anatomic presentations
      Renal, alimentary, central nervous system, and cutaneous LSA do not appear to be as responsive to therapy as the multicentric form. Other protocols may be more helpful, and a veterinary medical oncologist should be consulted.
III. Precautions
      During induction, the clinician should perform a complete blood count (CBC) and urinalysis prior to each week's therapy. If myelosuppression occurs [<4,000 white blood cells (WBC)/μL, <1,500 polymorphonuclear neutrophilic granulocyte (PMN)/μL], the cyclophosphamide should be eliminated for that week. After the bone marrow has recovered, cyclophosphamide can be reinstituted at 75% of the previous dose. If hematuria occurs, cyclophosphamide should be replaced by chlorambucil immediately. After the induction period, monitoring the hemogram should continue at 2- to 4-week intervals.
IV. Prognosis
      Untreated canine LSA patients generally do not survive more than 30–60 days. Combination chemotherapy, as outlined above, has resulted in remission induction in more than 70% of patients. Survival with a good quality of life has averaged approximately 10 months.

V. Comment

The "best" combination chemotherapy for canine LSA is not known. Several different protocols give similar results. This protocol is recommended for its minimal toxicity, efficacy, and modest cost.

FELINE LYMPHOSARCOMA

I. Objectives
    A. LSA represents a single manifestation of the many possible clinical presentations of the feline leukemia virus (FeLV). It is, in fact, only an infrequent end result compared to the occurrence of other proliferative, degenerative, and neoplastic diseases associated with FeLV infection. It is important to remember than no therapy has been proven capable of converting a cat from an FeLV-positive to an FeLV-negative status.
    B. The goal of therapy is to reduce the tumor mass and provide symptomatic relief. The continued presence of the FeLV warrants a thorough discussion with the owner of the patient's prognosis.
II. Recommended Therapy
    A. Anterior mediastinal and multicentric forms
        1. Induction
            An 8-week induction regimen as for canine LSA (see above) is employed. Cats must be monitored closely for myelosuppression, but seem to have fewer problems with cyclophosphamide-induced sterile hemorrhagic cystitis.
        2. Postinduction
            Cats should continue to receive prednisolone, 20 mg/m^2 PO SID every other day. They should then receive eight more cycles of vincristine and cyclophosphamide at biweekly intervals. This is followed by a third course of eight cycles of vincristine and cyclophosphamide at triweekly intervals. The entire course of therapy is 48 weeks, after which all drugs are discontinued.
    B. Other anatomic presentations
        As with canine LSA, other forms respond less well. Other protocols may offer better responses. A veterinary medical oncologist should be consulted.
III. Prognosis
    Cats with anterior mediastinal LSA often have rapid and remarkable responses, particularly in conjunction with thoracocentesis. Overall, however, a smaller proportion of feline than canine patients will attain a complete remission. As a general guideline, only about 30% will survive more than 16 weeks. Among those that complete the 48 weeks of therapy, 2- to 4-year survivals are reported.

MAST CELL TUMORS (MCT)

I. Objectives·
    Mast cell tumors demonstrate a wide range of biological behavior. His-
    topathologic grading by the Bostock classification aids in prognosis of can-
    ine MCT; feline cutaneous MCT is often very aggressive and usually re-
    sponds poorly to therapy. The objective of chemotherapy is the control of
    recurrent and/or disseminated disease. Solitary MCT is a surgical problem.
    Wide (3 cm) margins should be planned. If surgical margins are not free
    of mast cell infiltration histopathologically, adjunctive radiation or chem-
    otherapy is indicated.
II. Recommended Therapy
    A. Canine MCT—recurrent or disseminated disease
       Prednisolone as a single agent appears to be as efficacious as other
       more costly and toxic drugs alone or in combination.
       1. 60 mg/m^2 SID for 2 weeks followed by
       2. 30 mg/m^2 SID for 2 weeks followed by
       3. 30 mg/m^2 SID every other day for 5 months, then taper off.
    B. Feline MCT—cutaneous and visceral forms
       Cats have responded poorly to various chemotherapies for cutaneous
       MCT. Visceral mastocytosis marked by splenomegaly responds well
       to splenectomy alone. Response to therapy is poor when mastocytemia
       and symptoms recur.
III. Precautions
    A. The rapid destruction of MCTs releases vasoactive amines. In the face
       of any gastrointestinal signs or a large tumor burden, the use of the H$_2$-
       blocker cimetidine (Tagamet) is indicated at 5–10 mg/kg TID.
    B. It is imperative to monitor these patients for signs of corticosteroid
       excess, although most patients show less polyuria/polydipsia after 2–
       4 weeks.
IV. Prognosis
    A. Canine MCT
       Prognosis is related to histopathologic grading. Many dogs will have
       a good initial response but the tumor may recur at 4–5 months in spite
       of therapy. Among those patients completing 6 months of therapy, later
       recurrences are often very aggressive and unresponsive to further ther-
       apy.
    B. Feline MCT
       Usually responds poorly to chemotherapy

TRANSMISSIBLE VENEREAL TUMOR (TVT)

I. Objectives
    Cure is a realistic goal in the chemotherapy of TVT. Surgical intervention
    is probably necessary only to eliminate masses which physically interfere

with normal function to a degree requiring immediate attention. Metastatic sites respond well to chemotherapy.
II. Recommended Therapy
   Vincristine, 0.5 mg/m² IV every 7 days until there is no evidence of disease. This usually requires only four to six treatments, but more may be necessary.
III. Precautions
   Although vincristine is not strongly myelosuppressive, the CBC should be monitored prior to each treatment. If myelosuppression does occur, therapy should not be given until normal numbers of WBC and neutrophils return. Subtle signs of peripheral neuropathy may also be noted but are rarely dose-limiting in dogs. Vincristine may cause constipation.
IV. Prognosis
   The prognosis for complete elimination of TVT with vincristine therapy is excellent.

MULTIPLE MYELOMA

I. Objectives
   Reduction in osseous pain, palliation of signs associated with hyperviscosity, return toward normal serum protein patterns, and elimination of Bence-Jones proteinuria along with a generally improved attitude in the patient are realistic goals.
II. Recommended therapy
   Melphalan, 1.5 mg/m² PO daily for 7–10 days; repeat every 3 weeks, indefinitely.
III. Precautions
   The major dose-limiting toxicity of melphalan is leucopenia. The CBC should be monitored prior to beginning each cycle of therapy. Patients with multiple myeloma are very susceptible to infection. Sepsis should be treated promptly, but prophylactic antibiotics are not warranted. The use of IV catheters should be avoided.
IV. Prognosis
   Remission rates of over 70% have been reported with median survivals of 11 months.

OTHER NEOPLASTIC DISEASES

There are, of course, many other neoplastic diseases for which the role of chemotherapy is not well defined nor protocols well developed. Canine and feline mammary gland tumors, osteosarcoma, hemangiosarcoma, prostatic carcinoma, squamous cell carcinoma, pancreatic carcinoma, and other less frequently encountered diseases have not proven particularly amenable to routine chemotherapy. Many new drugs, combinations, and schedules are under investigation. Consultation with and referral to a veterinary clinical oncologist may help define the most appropriate therapy. Prostatic and perianal neoplasms may benefit from hormonal therapy [diethylstilbestrol 1.1 mg/kg once IM (not to exceed a total dose of 25 mg) or 1 mg PO every 72 hours] as an adjunct to surgery.

SUGGESTED READINGS

Barton CL: The diagnosis and management of canine lymphosarcoma. Proc Am An Hosp Assn 345, 1983.

Brown ND: Paraneoplastic disorders of humans, dogs and cats. J Am An Hosp Assn 17(6):911, 1981.

Crow SE: Cancer cachexia. Comp Contin Ed Pract Vet 3(4):681, 1981.

Pedersen NC, Madewell BR: Feline leukemia virus disease complex. In Kirk RW (ed): Current Veterinary Therapy. Vol. 7. WB Saunders, Philadelphia, 1980.

Rosenthal RC: Hormones in cancer therapy. Vet Clin N Am 12(1):67, 1982.

Rosenthal RC: Chemotherapy. In Slatter D (ed): Textbook of Small Animal Surgery. WB Saunders, Philadelphia, 1984 (in press).

Tams TR, Macy DW: Canine mast cell tumors. Compend Contin Ed Pract Vet 3(10):869, 1981.

8

Anemia and Bleeding Disorders

Bernard F. Feldman, D.V.M.

GENERAL FEATURES OF ANEMIA

INTRODUCTION

Anemia is a common problem in primary care practice. Because anemia is a sign of underlying disease and usually not a primary disease itself, the veterinary clinician must diligently search for a cause before considering therapy. The diagnostic evaluation of anemia is complicated by a wide range of possible causes and the large number of diagnostic tests and procedures available. Nonetheless, most patients have a readily detectable illness and evaluations may often be accomplished without hospital admission.

DEFINITION

Anemia is defined in terms of mean hematocrit and hemoglobin concentration adjusted, in the case of young animals, for age. This definition is satisfactory when there is a normal plasma volume.

I. Hematocrit variation in young and adult animals
  A. Dogs
    1. Less than 12 weeks hematocrit is 30–40%
    2. Adult hematocrit is 37–55%
  B. Cats
    1. Less than 12 weeks hematocrit is 31–35%
    2. Adult hematocrit is 33–42%
II. The primary function of the erythrocyte is to provide a mode of transport for hemoglobin to deliver oxygen to the tissues.
  A. The physiologic consequences of anemia result from the associated total reduction of oxygen delivery capacity by the blood.
  B. Because this reduction, for whatever reason, generally results in a com-

pensatory expansion of blood volume, measurements of hemoglobin or of hematocrit very nearly reflect red blood cell (RBC) mass. Exceptions include

1. factitious anemia caused by increased plasma volume, as in late pregnancy.
2. masked anemia caused by decreased plasma volume, as in dehydration.
3. absence of anemia during the early period after hemorrhage and before compensatory expansion of plasma volume.

PATHOGENESIS

  I. Disordered erythropoiesis (bone marrow production)
 II. Blood loss
III. Hemolysis

HISTORY

  I. Predisposing factors
    A. Inadequate diet
    B. Drug or toxin exposure
 II. Impact of anemia on the patient.
    A. Explore for signs of anemia
    B. The age of the patient
    C. The presence of other disorders that limit cardiopulmonary compensation
    D. The rate of development of anemia
    E. The underlying cause, rather than the absolute concentration of the hematocrit

PHYSICAL EXAMINATION

    I. Examination of pulse and especially capillary refill time (CRT), allows assessment of the patient's blood volume.
   II. Examination of the skin, oronasopharynx, abdomen, vagina, and rectum and testing the feces and urine for blood helps to exclude active bleeding.
  III. Physical examination provides clues to the underlying cause.
  IV. Examination for signs of shock or congestive heart failure help to determine the patient's response to the anemia.
   V. Physical findings
    A. Mild anemia
      1. Dyspnea with slight exercise
      2. Increased listlessness
      3. Slight decrease in appetite
    B. Moderate anemia
      1. Marked exertional and nonexertional dyspnea

    2. Pounding pulse associated with increased cardiac output and decreased peripheral resistance

    3. Hypersensitivity to cold

    4. Pale mucous membranes

  C. Severe anemia

    1. Generalized weakness

    2. Syncope

    3. White mucous membranes

    4. Ataxia

    5. Systolic heart murmur due to decreased blood viscosity

VI. Cautions on physical examination

  A. The best areas for evaluating hemoglobin or hematocrit concentration are the conjunctivae and mucous membranes.

  B. Chronic anemia of sufficient severity to increase cardiac output is usually associated with an increase in stroke volume.

  C. The presence of tachycardia suggests volume depletion, heart disease, or increased tissue oxygen requirements due to inflammation.

BROAD GUIDELINES FOR THERAPY

  I. The primary cause must always be uncovered and addressed.

 II. Symptomatic therapy can include blood transfusion.

III. Packed red cells may be administered in situations devoid of hypovolemia.

IV. Iron preparations may be used as adjunctive therapy in chronic blood loss.

 V. Anabolic steroids (androgens) may be of help, after prolonged usage, in situations of abnormal erythropoiesis.

VI. Rest is always indicated.

DIFFERENTIAL DIAGNOSIS

  I. Capillary refill time is prolonged in both hypovolemia and circulatory disturbances.

 II. With uncomplicated anemia CRT is usually normal and low; even with serious anemia CRT is difficult to evaluate.

III. In circulatory disturbances and in hypovolemic shock the mucosae are bluish. Pulse is weak and fast and blood vessels are incompletely filled.

APPROACH TO DIAGNOSIS

ROUTINE DATA BASE APPROPRIATE IN THE
INITIAL EVALUATION OF ANEMIA

  I. Red blood cell count

 II. Hematocrit

   III. Hemoglobin
   IV. Total protein concentration
    V. Mean corpuscular volume (MCV)
   VI. Mean corpuscular hemoglobin concentration (MCHC)
  VII. Reticulocyte count
VIII. Leucocyte count
   IX. Examination of peripheral blood smear
    X. Platelet count

HEMATOCRIT AND HEMOGLOBIN
CONCENTRATION

    I. Anemia is present when hematocrit is consistently below 37% in adult dogs and 30% in adult cats.
   II. Variables that tend to increase the hematocrit
     A. Dehydration
     B. Prolonged tourniquet stasis
     C. Exposure to cold
     D. Increased muscular activity
  III. Variables that tend to decrease the hematocrit
     A. Volume overload
     B. Capillary tube leakage during centrifugation
     C. Automated techniques, i.e., calculated hematocrit
   IV. Mean corpuscular volume
     A. MCV = hematocrit divided by RBC [cubic micrometers or femtoliters (fl)]
     B. A measure of cell size which is more reproducible than the clinician's ability to detect subtle changes in size from examination of the peripheral blood smear
     C. Low MCV indicates microcytosis.
     D. High MCV indicates macrocytosis.
    V. Mean corpuscular hemoglobin (MCH)
     A. MCH = hemoglobin divided by RBC (in picograms)
     B. A measure of the average amount of hemoglobin in each individual cell
     C. A low MCH indicates hypochromia, microcytosis, or both.
     D. A high MCH is always seen with a high MCV.
   VI. Mean corpuscular hemoglobin concentration
     A. Mean corpuscular hemoglobin concentration = hemoglobin concentration divided by hematocrit (in grams per deciliter RBCs)
     B. A measure of concentration or percent hemoglobin in each cell
     C. A low MCHC indicates hypochromia.
     D. A high MCHC is seen only with prominent spherocytosis and reflects the RBC volume associated with decreased cell membrane.

VII. Rate of fall in hematocrit
- A. Total marrow shutdown in absence of hemorrhage or hemolysis results in a fall of hematocrit of 2–8%/week.
- B. A fall more rapid than this, in absence of change in plasma volume, indicates hemorrhage or hemolysis.

EXAMINATION OF PERIPHERAL BLOOD SMEAR

I. Red cell shape, color, and inclusions have diagnostic importance.
II. Common causes of various erythrocytic abnormalities
- A. Hypochromasia, microcytosis.
  1. Iron deficiency
  2. Chronic inflammation
- B. Macrocytosis
  1. Liver disease (central targeting)
  2. Reticulocytosis
  3. Some forms of leukemia
  4. Normal in some poodles
- C. Anisocytosis/poikilocytosis.
  1. Marked iron deficiency
  2. Microangiopathic hemolysis
  3. Leucoerythroblastosis
- D. Target cells
  1. Liver disease (rare)
  2. Postsplenectomy
  3. Artifact
  4. Reticulocytosis
- E. Spiculated RBCs
  1. Liver disease (rare)
  2. Renal disease (rare)
  3. Postsplenectomy
  4. Hypothroidism (rare)
  5. Microangiopathic hemolysis
- F. Teardrop cells
  Leucoerythroblastosis
- G. Howell-Jolly bodies
  1. Postsplenectomy
  2. Very responsive anemia
  3. Erythroleukemia
- H. Pappenheimer bodies
  1. Postsplenectomy
  2. Marked hemolysis
- I. Spherocytes
  Autoimmune hemolysis

   J. Heinz bodies.
      1. Methylene blue
      2. Acetaminophen
      3. Other oxidant drugs
III. Classification of anemia by erythrocyte morphology
   A. Microcytic, hypochromic
      1. Iron deficiency
      2. Chronic disease (some)
   B. Macrocytic anemia
      1. Megaloblastic (rare).
         a) Vitamin B_{12} and/or folate deficiency.
         b) Drug induced
         c) Myeloproliferative disease
      2. Nonmegaloblastic
         a) Accelerated erythropoiesis
            (1) Acute hemorrhage
            (2) Acute hemolysis
         b) Increased red cell membrane surface area
            (1) Postsplenectomy.
            (2) Chronic liver disease (rare)
         c) Marrow infiltration or failure
   B. Normocytic, normochromic
      1. Acute hemorrhage
      2. Acute hemolysis
      3. Endocrine-metabolic disorders
      4. Chronic disease (most)
      5. Renal disease
      6. Marrow infiltration or failure
      7. Chronic hemorrhage

RETICULOCYTE COUNT

Characterization

   I. Erythrocytes released into the circulation by the marrow
  II. Contain residual ribosomes
 III. Stain blue with Wright's or May-Grunwald-Giemsa stains

Counts

   I. Percentage of total erythrocyte count
      A. Normal is 0.5–2%
      B. Not an adequate measure of effective red cell production

II. Absolute reticulocyte count
   A. Number of reticulocytes released into the circulation daily
   B. Normal—75,000/mm^3
III. Corrected reticulocyte count (CRC)
   A. CRC = % reticulocytes × patient's hematocrit/mean normal hematocrit.
   B. Can be misleading index
      1. Assumes a 1-day survival of reticulocytes.
      2. In anemia, reticulocytes may have longer life span in circulation
IV. Reticulocyte production index (RPI)
   A. Applicable only to dogs.
   B. RPI = CRC divided by correction factor
   C. Correction factor for canine RPI (see table 8-1).
   D. Normal range 1–2
   E. Classification of anemia utilizing the RPI
      1. RPI less than 2
         a) Chronic blood loss
         b) Acute hemorrhage—first 2 or 3 days
         c) Anemia of inflammatory disease
         d) Decreased erythropoietin production
            (1) Renal disease
            (2) Endocrine disease
         e) Bone marrow disease
            (1) Aplasia
            (2) Leukemia
      2. RPI more than 2
         a) Hemolysis
         b) Acute hemorrhage response (occurs 3–6 days after blood loss)

EXAMINATION OF BONE MARROW ASPIRATE

   I. Performed concurrently with hemogram
  II. Time-consuming and requires experienced laboratory personnel

TABLE 8-1. CORRECTION FACTOR
FOR CANINE RETICULOCYTE
PRODUCTION

Hematocrit (%)	Correction Factor
45	1.0
35	1.5
25	2.0
15	2.5

III. Not useful in
    A. Iron deficiency anemia
    B. Anemia of renal failure
    C. Hemolytic anemia
IV. Indicated in suspected
    A. Occult hypochromic microcytic anemia
    B. Marrow infiltration

BONE MARROW BIOPSY INDICATED FOR

I. Pancytopenia
II. Neoplasia
III. Myelofibrosis
IV. Failure of bone marrow aspiration
V. Aplasia of one or more cell lines

MYELOID-ERYTHROID (M/E) RATIO

I. M/E ratio normally is 1–3.
II. Decreased with hemolytic anemias

ANEMIA WITH NORMAL RED CELL INDICES AND LOW RETICULOCYTE PRODUCTION INDEX

GENERAL COMMENTS

I. These anemias are the most common in clinical practice.
II. Before embarking on a diagnostic workup or considering possible etiologies make sure that the hematocrit and hemoglobin concentrations are reproducibly low and that volume overload is not the etiology.
III. Know the normals for your laboratory!
IV. In general, these anemias are not severe until the terminal state has been reached.

ANEMIA OF INFLAMMATORY DISEASE

I. This mild anemia is the most frequent anemia among hospitalized patients.
II. It has been associated with rheumatoid arthritis in humans, chronic infections, active collagen vascular disease [e.g., systemic lupus erythematosus (SLE)], and cancer.
III. Anemia usually develops within 2 months of the onset of illness. It is mild and is eclipsed by the manifestation of the underlying disease.

IV. Pathogenetic mechanisms
  A. Mild reduction in red cell survival
  B. Impaired bone marrow response to anemia
  C. Impaired mobilization of iron from iron stores
 V. Serum iron (SI) and total iron binding capacity (TIBC) are low. Bone
    marrow iron stores are normal or increased.
VI. Acute infections (viral, bacterial, and so on) will cause an immediate drop
    in SI. Acute infections or inflammation due to other causes will inhibit
    bone marrow response to any anemia such as bleeding or hemolysis.
VII. Therapy
  A. Treatment of the underlying problem must be achieved.
  B. Supplementation with iron, vitamin B_{12}, and so forth is useless.

CHRONIC RENAL INSUFFICIENCY

  I. Consistently accompanied by anemia
 II. Pathogenetic mechanism
  A. The most important mechanism is decreased production secondary to
     decreased erythropoietin.
  B. The usual hemolytic component is usually mild and a normal marrow
     could easily compensate for the change.
  C. Uremia also appears to inhibit marrow responsiveness.
  D. Uremia decreases RBC survival.
  E. Uremia decreases platelet function.
III. Laboratory findings
  A. Routine data include an extremely variable hematocrit.
  B. The RBC morphology is usually normal but burring of some RBCs has
     been reported.
  C. Mild thrombocytopenia is not unusual.
  D. Markedly depressed absolute lymphocyte counts, elevated serum fi-
     brinogen, and decreased total protein and albumin are hallmarks of the
     hemogram in renal failure.
IV. Therapy
  A. Reduce the azotemia.
  B. Androgen administration may increase the hematocrit 3–5%.
  C. If serum iron concentration is low, iron supplementation may be in-
     dicated. Experience, however, has indicated SI to be unreliable in di-
     agnosing iron deficiency in renal disease.
  D. Administration of packed RBCs may alleviate some of the signs as-
     sociated with the anemia.

HYPOENDROCRINE STATES

  I. Pituitary, thyroid, adrenal, and androgen deficiencies are associated with
     mild anemia and fatigue.

II. The mechanism appears to be decreased production secondary to decreased erythropoietin production. This is probably related to decreased peripheral oxygen requirements.

III. Therapy includes replacement with the proper hormone. This usually results in a slow rise in hematocrit which may not normalize for many months.

APLASTIC PANCYTOPENIA (AP)

I. Definition
   A. A disorder in which pancytopenia is associated with severe marrow hypoplasia that cannot be attributed to an ongoing systemic disease process
   B. Aplasia involving only erythropoiesis is referred to as *pure red cell aplasia (PRCA)*

II. Etiology
   A. Idiopathic
   B. Chemicals
      1. Industrial hydrocarbons; benzene solvents
      2. Chemotherapeutic agents
      3. Drugs
         a) Estrogen
         b) Chloramphenicol
         c) Anticonvulsants (phenytoin)
         d) Phenylbutazone
   C. Infections—Ehrlichiosis
   D. Myelophthisis or myelosclerosis
   E. Immunologic

III. Clinical signs
   A. Signs are related to the most deficient cell type.
   B. Most early cases of AP begin with thrombocytopenia followed by leukopenia and finally nonregenerative anemia.
   C. Patients with thrombocytopenia often have petechiae, ecchymosis, and mucosal bleeding.
   D. Fluctuating or persistent fever and infections may be noted.

IV. Differential diagnosis
   Dependent on finding depression of numbers of cells of cell lines and bone marrow aspirates without complete cellular maturation sequences. Bone marrow biopsy reveals myelophthisis, myelosclerosis, or simply absence of cell production foci.

V. Therapy
   A. All drugs and chemicals that the patient is currently receiving must be stopped or eliminated if an environmental problem.

B. Androgens have been successful in humans but have had limited success in animals.

C. Lithium citrate at 20 mg/kg daily, divided into three doses, in conjunction with normal corticosteroid dosages has been reported to be effective in one case.

D. Symptomatic handling of infections and anemia is usually feasible.

E. It is extremely difficult to continually treat thrombocytopenia and leukopenia.

F. When the marrow has normal cell maturation sequences but repeated hemograms reveal consistent aplasia suggestive of ineffective myelopoiesis, immunosuppressive drugs such as azathioprine (2 mg/kg, once daily) may be attempted.

PURE RED CELL APLASIA

I. General Comments

   A. Can be the first sign of aplastic pancytopenia

   B. Pure red cell aplasia may be caused by erythropoietin deficiency in chronic renal failure.

   C. Most patients with PRCA have causes difficult to ascertain by clinicians and thus are often given an idiopathic caption.

   D. Pure red cell aplasia has been noted in association with immune hemolytic anemia and therefore some success has been reported with immunosuppressive therapy.

II. Clinical signs

   A. Associated with the long duration of the process

   B. Patients are quieter and more listless for long periods.

   C. Most people report pica in their animals during later stages. This may be manifested by eating dirt or stones, or licking sidewalks.

III. Differential diagnosis

   Usually made easier by the severity of the problem (more severe than anemia of inflammatory disease), the absence of azotemia, and the chronic progression.

IV. Therapy

   A. Blood transfusions usually last a maximum of 3 weeks before transfusions must be repeated. It has been our practice to allow the hematocrit to drop below 15% before retransfusing the patient in order to stimulate production of erythropoietin.

   B. We have used androgens but have not had positive results directly attributable to these drugs.

   C. On occasion a surprisingly rapid response has been achieved with immunosuppressive therapy. This includes 2 mg/kg azathioprine and prednisone given mornings for 1–2 weeks. The dose is usually decreased to 1 mg/kg for each drug thereafter. The corticosteroid dosage is always tapered slowly even though the patient may display a positive response.

Marrow Infiltration

I. When extensive it is associated with leucoerythroblastosis. This includes marked variation in red cell morphology including teardrop-shaped red cells, nucleated RBCs, and a left shift to myelocytes in the white cell series seen on peripheral blood smears. Apparently the disrupted marrow releases blood cells early. Red cells so released contain cytoplasmic and nuclear fragments which are distorted during splenic passage and poikylocytes are formed.

II. Leucoerythroblastosis is *not* a sensitive indicator of bone involvement with metastatic cancer. Anemia is present in most cases.

HEMOLYSIS AND BLEEDING:

Anemia with a normal or slightly elevated MCV and an elevated RPI are indicative. Anemia caused by blood loss is usually quite evident. When the specific site of blood loss is not clear, the intestinal tract is almost always incriminated (occult blood loss) and the cause is usually ulceration or tumor. With acute blood loss associated with significant hemorrhage (more than 30% of blood volume lost) signs of severe anemia, despite modest decreases in hematocrit, will be evident. Decreases in total protein, albumin, and globulin makes the diagnosis of occult blood loss more evident.

Etiology of Hemolytic Anemia

I. Infection
   A. Bacterial: clostridial infections, streptococcal/colons infections, leptospirosis
   B. Viral: herpes virus
   C. Protozoal: babesiosis, hemobartonellosis
II. Chemicals
   A. Mothballs
   B. Onion
   C. Lead
   D. Ricin beans
   E. Many, many household preparations
III. Metabolic disturbances
   A. Hypophosphatemia after treatment of ketoacidosis
   B. Marked alkalosis

IV. Immunologic
   A. Idiopathic or true autoimmune disease
   B. Drug-induced
   C. Associated with lymphatic disorders including lymphoma
   D. Systemic lupus erythematosus
 V. Mechanical
   A. Microangiopathic
   B. Disseminated intravascular coagulation (DIC)
VI. Intrinsic red cell function or structure deficit
   A. Pyruvate kinase deficiency—Basenji
   B. Stomatocytosis-hemolytic anemia associated with chondrodysplasia—Alaskan Malamute
   C. Congenital feline porphyria

CLINICAL AND LABORATORY DIAGNOSIS

 I. Intravascular hemolysis occurs when RBC destruction occurs within the vascular space. Signs include
   A. Hemoglobinemia
   B. Hemoglobinuria
 II. Extravascular hemolysis
   A. Most hemolytic events occur extravascularly
   B. When destruction occurs primarily within phagocytic cells of the monocyte-macrophage system [reticuloendothelial system (RES)], diagnosis is more difficult as there is no hemoglobinemia or hemoglobinuria.
   C. There may be an elevation of indirect bilirubin but this is relatively insensitive and is dependent on the degree of hemolysis as well as the functional hepatic status.
   D. Urinary urobilinogen may be increased but the aforementioned statements about bilirubin hold for urinary urobilinogen.
   E. Peripheral smear changes include
      1. Spherocytosis
      2. Fragmentation
      3. Spiculated cells
      4. "Bite" or "blister" cells
      5. Heinz bodies within RBCs
III. Coombs' test
   A. Antibody-positive tests are for the most part immunoglobulin G (IgG) antibodies
   B. Complement may be present in many cases of antibody-induced hemolysis and may be present alone without identifiable antibody. Its presence implies the presence of antibody no longer on the red cell or presence in concentrations too low to detect.

    C. Our experience is that complement-positive, antibody-negative Coombs' tests must be carefully considered in the clinical context. We have noted many positive complement Coombs' tests in the absence of anemia and with diverse, though serious, inflammatory states.

IV. Warm or cold antibody

    A. Warm antibody is usually IgG. Some IgG antibodies fix complement. Specific Coombs' testing will reveal positive IgG alone, IgG plus C_3 positive or rarely, positive C_3 alone.

    B. Cold antibody is usually immunoglobulin M (IgM) and is identified by direct agglutination in test tubes, on glass microscope slides, or after 1 hour incubation in refrigerator.

AUTOIMMUNE HEMOLYSIS DUE TO WARM ANTIBODY

I. Idiopathic autoimmune hemolysis

    A. Patients are usually presented with signs of anemia and an enlarged spleen. Jaundice and fever are not common findings.

    B. Peripheral blood exhibits spherocytosis and an elevated reticulocyte count. (*Reticulocytopenia* may be present in some patients until after treatment, greatly confusing the diagnosis.)

    C. Severe autoimmune thrombocytopenia may be present as well (Evan's syndrome).

II. Secondary autoimmune hemolysis

    A. May be associated with viral illnesses or, on occasion, secondary to a drug such as penicillin.

    B. Chronic cases of secondary autoimmune hemolysis are seen in patients with SLE where hemolysis may precede the diagnosis by months or even years in lymphoproliferative disorders such as chronic lymphocytic leukemia or lymphoma and rarely with other malignancies or bacterial infections.

III. Therapy

    A. Self-limiting hemolysis is usually related to mycoplasma or viral infections.

    B. Conscious or unknowing discontinuation of drugs often results in recovery despite therapeutic clinical intervention.

    C. Warm antibody immune hemolysis often responds slowly, 1–3 weeks, to high doses of prednisone and azathioprine (2 mg/kg once daily, mornings, for each drug). The dose is then tapered slowly over several weeks or to a small daily or every other day dosage of 2.5–5 mg prednisone.

    D. *Splenectomy* should *always* be considered if the patient is refractory to therapy.

    E. In some canine cases, the disease is characterized by remissions and exacerbations over several years.

F. Secondary autoimmune hemolysis may be refractory to treatment and responds best to successful control of the underlying disease process.

AUTOIMMUNE HEMOLYSIS DUE TO COLD ANTIBODY

I. Primary cold agglutinin disease is rare and is associated with ischemia of the ears, nose, and toes. High concentrations of IgM may be noted on immunoelectrophoresis.
II. Most commonly, cold agglutinin hemolysis is seen *secondary* to mycoplasma or viral infections, SLE, or lymphoproliferative disease.
III. Therapy. Steroids and splenectomy are much less successful in cold agglutinin hemolysis although they should be attempted. Protection from cold is, of course, most helpful.

TRANSFUSION THERAPY

I. Transfusions may be necessary in some patients with immune hemolysis.
II. Though clinicians should avoid transfusion if possible, when necessary, transfusion with A⁻ blood may be accomplished with close observation of the patient.
III. Although survival of transfused red cells is shorter than normal, severe immediate intravascular transfusion reactions are uncommon, and improvement of the hematocrit usually results.
IV. Transfusions of fresh blood should be delivered over a 6- to 12-hour period.
V. The maximum amount of blood to be transfused should be *no more* than 20% of the total blood volume if a blood volume of 90 ml/kg is assumed.
VI. Packed RBCs are ideal for the anemic, normovolemic patient.

BABESIOSIS

ETIOLOGY

I. *B. canis* and, rarely, *B. gibsoni*
II. Babesiosis is seen in tropical and subtropical areas.
III. Transmitted through *Dermacentor* or *Rhipicephalus* ticks

PATHOGENESIS

I. The parasite lives and grows within the erythrocyte, eventually causing intravascular and extravascular hemolysis.
II. In heavy infections liver necrosis, caused by anoxia, can occur.

III. Other complications include DIC and extravascular hemolysis due to erythrocyte aggregation.

CLINICAL SIGNS

   I. Fever
  II. Listlessness
 III. Coffee colored- to port wine-colored urine.
  IV. Icterus can occur depending upon the degree of hepatic involvement.
   V. The mucous membranes may appear white.
  VI. Some patients have thrombocytopenia, weight loss, hepatosplenomegaly, and eventually proteinuria, uremia, leukopenia, and severe anemia.
 VII. Rarely, neurologic deficits may be observed.

DIFFERENTIAL DIAGNOSIS

   I. Immune hemolytic anemia or hemolytic anemias due to other reasons
  II. Leptospirosis
 III. Hepatobiliary disease such as infectious canine hepatitis
  IV. Due to the possible neurologic signs, distemper, Aujesky's disease, or rabies are often considered.

DIAGNOSIS

   I. Prepare blood smears from lightly centrifuged blood.
  II. The ideal cells to examine for the parasite are those red cells immediately below the buffy coat.

THERAPY

   I. One SQ injection of imidocarb diproprionate (Imizol)* 5 mg/kg is effective and also offers 3 weeks–1 month prophylaxis. The injection may be repeated once, 3 weeks after the first injection.
  II. *We do not recommend any other drugs.*

PROGNOSIS

   I. Dependent upon the degree and type of liver damage
  II. Chronic infections have been reported.
 III. In our experience, Imizol has been extremely effective in curing the disease.

---

* Imizol, Burroughs-Wellcome, London.

ANEMIA IN THE CAT—SPECIAL CONSIDERATIONS

I. Anemia in the cat is often seen at a more advanced stage than in the dog and occurs as a result of production disturbances, blood loss, and hemolysis.
II. Regenerative and nonregenerative anemia are diagnosed just as in the dog. It must be remembered, the regenerative response in the cat is usually less intense than in the dog. Nucleated red cells seem to appear more readily in peripheral blood without the same connotations they have in the dog.
III. Anemia is commonly associated with feline leukemia virus (FeLV), feline infectious peritonitis, or as a manifestation of myeloproliferative or lymphoproliferative disorders. Immune hemolytic anemia and anemia caused by blood loss are seen only occasionally clinically.
IV. Because of the quiet nature of the cat, more severe depression of the hematocrit and hemoglobin concentrations can occur before the typical signs of anemia (discussed under physical examination of the dog) may be observed.
V. Therapy must be directed toward the underlying problem in most cases.
VI. Cats have fewer drug or transfusion reactions than dogs.

FELINE INFECTIOUS ANEMIA

ETIOLOGY

I. *Hemobartonella* (Eperythrozoön) *felis* is a rickettsial-like organism.
II. *H. felis* may be observed on red cell membranes as a pleomorphic, multiple, coccoid organism 0.8–1 μm in size or as a rod-shaped form about 1.5 μm in length.
III. They are blue-black to purple in Wright's or May-Grunwald-Giemsa stains.

EPIDEMIOLOGY

Still not clear though severe stress and FeLV infections seem to be associated with its clinical presence.

TREATMENT

I. Among the antibiotics, only spiramycin in combination with chloramphenicol and metronidazole is recommended as ancillary therapy when respiratory or neurologic signs are manifest.
II. Penicillin, streptomycin, and oxytetracycline do not have activity against some forms of *H. felis* and may complicate the clinical signs.

III. Chlorpromazine 4–6 mg/kg IM followed by an 8-day course of oral chlor-
promazine (2–3 mg/kg once daily) has been reported to be successful.
   A. The IM injection is sometimes followed by agitation or transient com-
      atose states. Though this is not a permanent situation, care must be
      available.
   B. We suggest hospitalization during the first 24–48 hours of therapy and
      discussion of the complications of therapy with the owner.
   C. In theory at least, chlorpromazine reduces intestinal fluid loss by action
      on adenylate cyclase. This mechanism also seems to affect red cell
      permeability and perhaps facilitates detachment of *H. felis* from the
      red cell membrane.

HEINZ BODY ANEMIA IN CATS

DEFINITION AND DESCRIPTION

   I. A Heinz body [also called erythrocyte-refractile (ER) body] is an area of
      RBC membrane incorporated in a crystal of denatured (oxidized hemo-
      globin).
  II. Appears as a small refractile area on the margin of the cell stained with a
      Romanovsky-type stain
 III. The membrane protrudes very slightly.
  IV. Heinz bodies take up new methylene blue stain and thus are well visualized
      as dark round bodies which are larger and less densely stained than Howell-
      Jolly bodies

CAUSES OF HEINZ BODY FORMATION

   I. Methylene blue in urinary acidifiers
  II. B vitamin deficiencies have been speculated to induce Heinz body for-
      mation.
 III. Other oxidant drugs or toxins

ETIOLOGY OF HEINZ BODY-INDUCED ANEMIA

   I. Due to membrane damage to the RBC through intravascular hemolysis
  II. Splenic destruction of the Heinz body affected cell will result in extravas-
      cular hemolysis.

PATHOGENESIS

   I. Cats are perhaps more susceptible to Heinz body formation than other
      species due to increased numbers of sulfhydryl groups on their hemoglobin
      molecules.

II. FADH$_2$ is necessary as a cofactor in the enzymatic pathways required for regeneration of the reduced sulfhydryl groups. It has therefore been speculated that B vitamin deficiencies induced by prolonged anorexia may contribute to Heinz body formation.

III. B vitamin deficiency may help explain the observation that some cats develop Heinz body anemias without exposure to any toxins.

CLINICAL PRESENTATION

I. Depression

II. Anorexia

III. Pale mucous membranes

IV. Polypnea

V. Hemoglobinuria will be noted in intravascular hemolysis.

VI. It should be noted that Heinz bodies may be seen in cats that are clinically anemic, have normal padded cell volumes, and have as much as 50% of the red cells with Heinz bodies.

ROUTINE HEMOGRAM FINDINGS

I. Responsive anemia, that is, increased reticulocytes or polychromasia

II. Poikilocytes

DIFFERENTIAL DIAGNOSIS

I. Hemobartonellosis

II. Feline leukemia virus-associated anemia

III. Hemolytic anemia due to another etiology

THERAPY

I. Dependent on clinical presentations. In nonanemic cats with Heinz bodies, an extensive history should be taken to rule out exposure to oxidant drugs or toxins. These animals should be monitored carefully for the development of anemia.

II. Removal of cause

III. Supportive therapy

IV. Blood transfusion is dependent upon patient need rather than a specific red cell concentration.

V. The addition of B vitamins, according to manufacturer's directions, to IV fluids in anemic cats without exposure to toxins may be beneficial

This section was contributed by Dr. J. Kaufman, College of Veterinary Medicine, Colorado State University, Fort Collins, Colorado 80523.

BLEEDING DISORDERS

NORMAL PROCESS OF HEMOSTASIS

I. The function of the normal hemostatic mechanism is to prevent blood loss from intact vessels and to stop excessive bleeding from damaged vessels.

II. This is accomplished, in damaged vessels, by contriction of the blood vessel itself, the formation of a platelet plug, and the final stabilization of the platelet plug by blood coagulation proteins or factors.

  A. Vascular constriction is transient, lasting less than 1 minute.

  B. Platelets adhere to subendothelial connective tissue, release adenosine diphosphate (ADP), and then aggregate under the influence of ADP to form an unstable plug.

  C. The unstable plug is stabilized after a few minutes by fibrin, the final product of the blood coagulation process which consolidates the plug rendering it stable.

  D. Fibrin is then gradually digested by the fibrinolytic enzyme system and the defect in the vessel wall is covered by endothelium.

III. The process of blood coagulation occurs as a series of complex steps which terminate in the formation of a fibrin clot.

  A. Extrinsic pathway
    1. Tissue factor (III)
    2. Calcium (IV)
    3. Factor VII

  B. Intrinsic pathway.
    1. Factors XII and XI
    2. Factors IX and VIII
    3. Platelet phospholipid (platelet factor – 3; PF-3)
    4. Calcium (factor IV)

  C. Common pathway.
    1. Factors X and V.
    2. Platelet phospholipid (PF-3)
    3. Calcium (factor IV)
    4. Prothrombin (factor II)
    5. Fibronogen (factor I)

  D. Stabilization of fibrin.
    Factor XIII

PATHOGENESIS OF DEFECTIVE HEMOSTASIS

I. Vascular defects
  A. Structural
  B. Immune-mediated
  C. Inflammation

II. Platelet abnormalities—quantity
  A. Failure of production
  B. Reduced survival
  C. Increased loss due to splenic pooling
III. Platelet abnormalities—quality.
  A. Failure to adhere or release ADP
  B. Failure to aggregate
  C. Failure to make phospholipid available
IV. Coagulation defects.
  A. Absolute failure of synthesis
  B. Production of an abnormal molecule
  C. Excessive destruction
  D. Circulating inhibitors
 V. Excessive fibrinolysis

CLINICAL DIAGNOSIS OF BLEEDING DISORDERS

 I. Lesions
  A. *Petechiae* are small red spots representing blood extravasated from
     intact blood vessels due to abnormal permeability of these vessels.
     Petechiae also occur in thrombocytopenia and platelet function defects
     because platelets are required to maintain normal vascular integrity.
  B. Purpura results from confluent petechiae and is caused by the same
     abnormalities.
  C. Ecchymoses also are caused by the same abnormalities but are usually
     the result of trauma.
  D. A *hematoma* is a large bruise infiltrating SQ tissue and resulting from
     defects in the coagulation factor mechanism.
  E. Hemarthrosis, bleeding into joint space, is also seen in severe coagu-
     lation disorders such as hemophilia.
 II. Etiology
  A. Inherited or acquired.
    1. Acquired bleeding usually occurs in adult life, is generalized, is with-
       out a family history of bleeding, and bleeding has not occurred with
       previous trauma or surgery. It should be noted that a negative history
       does not completely exclude a hereditary disorder.
    2. Inherited bleeding disorders usually are manifest in younger animals
       during minor surgical procedures or during tooth loss. If a previous
       trauma or surgery was tolerated without excessive bleeding it is un-
       likely that the patient is suffering from an inherited bleeding disorder.
  B. Vascular, platelet, or coagulation defect
    1. Vascular-platelet defect
      a) Petechiae, superficial bruising

      b) Bleeding in skin and mucous membranes
      c) Bleeding is immediate after trauma.
    2. Coagulation defect
      a) Deep, spreading hemotoma
      b) Hemarthroses or retroperitoneal bleeding
      c) Bleeding is often recurrent and late, that is, it does not occur immediately after trauma.

LABORATORY DIAGNOSIS OF BLEEDING
DISORDERS

I. Testing for vascular or platelet disorders
  A. Bleeding time.
    1. The time required for bleeding to cease from incised SQ vessels
    2. This inexact test is best performed on a hairless area on the abdomen with template device or appropriately guarded scalpel blade.
    3. This test assesses the ability of the blood vessel to constrict and for platelets to form a plug. Thus, it tests for normal vascular integrity and adequacy, and platelet number and function.
  B. Platelet count
    1. Estimated by examining a well-distributed blood smear or by a direct platelet count. In a well-distributed blood smear, a normal dog will have approximately 12 platelets per oil immersion field. A normal cat may have as many as 20 platelets per oil immersion field.
    2. Platelet counts may be conducted in blood samples stored at refrigerator temperatures for up to 24 hours.
    3. Bleeding due to thrombocytopenia rarely occurs unless platelet counts are below 40,000/μL.
    4. The rapidity with which thrombocytopenia occurs certainly affects the time when bleeding will occur. The author has observed numerous patients with chronic sustained thrombocytopenia (less than 10,000/μL for longer than 1 year) without overt bleeding or untoward results. Several of these patients were splenectomized during this period without excessive bleeding.
II. Screening tests for coagulation disorders
  A. Activated partial thromboplastin time (APTT) tests for deficiencies in the intrinsic and common pathways [see Bleeding disorders, III, above]. Simplistically, APTT is prolonged in deficiencies of factors XII, XI, IX, VIII, X, V, II, and I. It is not prolonged with extrinsic factor (factor VII) deficits.
  B. Prothrombin time (PT) tests for deficiencies in the extrinsic and common pathway. Prothrombin time is prolonged in deficiencies of factors VII, X, V, II, and I. Deficits in the intrinsic pathway (factors XII, XI, IX, VIII) do not affect the PT.

C. Thrombin time (TT) tests for fibrinogen (factor I) quantity and quality. It bypasses all other factors above factor I. It also tests for thrombin inhibitors.

D. Fibrinogen quantitation is a valuable test. Elevation of fibrinogen is a nonspecific indicator of inflammation. Decrease in fibrinogen connotes use of this important protein and is associated with DIC.

E. Samples for APTT, PT, and TT assays are collected in citrate tubes with a ratio of one part citrate to nine parts blood. This ratio is critical and tests must be completed within 2 hours at room temperature or 12 hours at refrigerator temperature or the anticoagulated blood must be centrifuged and the plasma frozen for later assay.

Vascular Disorders

 I. Characterized by easy bruising and spontaneous bleeding
 II. The underlying abnormality can be caused by structurally weak vessels (hereditary, Ehlers-Danlos syndrome; acquired, Cushing's syndrome), or inflammatory or immune processes.
III. Bleeding is not usually severe, is mainly into the skin, and occurs immediately after trauma.
 IV. The inexact bleeding time is often prolonged in vascular disorders.
 V. Excessive aspirin usage may result in bruising.
 VI. Bacterial toxins and many drugs result in microthrombi and toxic damage to the vascular endothelium.

Hemophilia

 I. Hereditary condition
   A. Classic hemophilia (hemophilia A–F VIII) and Christmas disease (Hemophilia B–F IX) are sex-linked (x-chromosome) recessive hereditary problems, generally resulting in affected males and carrier females.
   B. Deficits in almost all the other coagulation factors have been reported but are rare.
 II. Signs
   A. Occurs in young animals
   B. Bleeding occurs often at the time of normal tooth growth progression and loss.
   C. Lameness may occur as the result of intraarticular bleeding.
   D. Bleeding into the tracheobronchial tree or mediastinum may cause severe respiratory problems.
   E. Uncontrollable bleeding despite correct and appropriate hemostatic measures during surgery
   F. Large SQ hematomas
III. Differential diagnosis includes bleeding due to other causes and Von Willebrand's disease (VWD)

IV. Diagnosis
    Prolonged APTT with normal PT.
 V. Therapy
    Fresh blood, fresh plasma, or cryoprecipitate
VI. Prognosis is dependent upon
    A. Consistent availability of A⁻ blood (hemophilia is difficult to control
       in large dogs)
    B. Extent and repeatability of articular bleeding, which is a crippling pro-
       cess.

VITAMIN K DEFICIENCY

  I. Etiology and pathogenesis
    A. Deficits of vitamin K caused by vitamin K antagonists, including cou-
       marin and coumarin-like drugs, cause the production of a normal but
       functionally inactive molecule.
    B. There is failure to carboxylate the terminal glutamic acid residues on
       the ends of the protein molecule.
    C. Factors II, VII, IX, and X are dependent upon vitamin K to become
       functional.
 II. Clinical signs
    A. Epistaxis.
    B. Gastrointestinal bleeding
    C. Bleeding around teeth
    D. Severe retroperitoneal bleeding
III. Differential diagnosis
    A. Hemophilia.
    B. Other causes of hemorrhagic diatheses
    C. Severe hepatobiliary disease
IV. Diagnosis
    A. Prolonged APTT, PT with normal platelet counts, and TT
    B. Early in the intoxication the PT will be prolonged (factor VII has a
       short half-life) while the APTT is normal. This is transient and usually
       lasts only 6–12 hours.
 V. Therapy
    A. Fresh plasma or fresh blood when bleeding is severe or involves a vital
       area.
    B. Vitamin K_1 preparations may be administered SQ or *orally* (*never* IM
       or IV). Dosage varies from 1 to 4 mg/kg/day. The dose is usually divided
       and given at 8- or 12-hour intervals.
    C. If the diagnosis of vitamin K deficiency is correct, screening coagulation
       tests will return to normal within 12–24 hours and certainly within 36
       hours with the higher dosage.
    D. Failure to correct the screening tests immediately or to stop obvious
       bleeding should result in patient reevaluation and correction of the di-
       agnosis.

E. Usually intoxications require a minimum of 5 days of therapy. With some of the newer vitamin K antagonists being marketed, therapy for as long as 3–8 weeks may be required.

Von Willebrand's Disease

I. Hereditary disorder
 A. Due to deficiency of factor VIII-related antigen (Von Willebrand's factor) and an associated platelet function defect
 B. It is generally considered to be transmitted as an autosomal-dominant trait and is transmitted to offspring regardless of sex.
 C. It should be noted that autosomal-dominant transmittance may not be completely correct.
II. Signs are similar to the hemophilias
III. Diagnosis
 A. Breed predilection
  1. Doberman pinschers
  2. Scottish terriers
  3. Golden retrievers.
  4. German shepherds
  5. Miniature pinschers
  6. Other breeds have also been involved.
 B. The diagnosis is dependent on finding a low quantity of factor VIII and factor VIII molecule [factor VIII-related antigen (F VIII RA; Von Willebrand's factor)] as well as abnormal platelet function.
 C. While the APTT is occasionally prolonged, this does not occur in most clinical cases. This latter finding greatly confuses the diagnosis.
IV. Therapy includes fresh plasma, fresh blood, or cryoprecipitate.
V. The disease in the Doberman breed is associated with hypothyroidism.

Disorders of Platelets

I. Congenital thrombocytopathy or thrombasthenia
 A. Observed in otterhounds, Basset hounds, Scottish terriers, and foxhounds
 B. It is a platelet functional defect and is diagnosed by tests designed to screen for such defects.
 C. See the present section on clinical and laboratory diagnosis of bleeding disorders.
II. Acquired thrombocytopathy
 A. Etiology
  1. Many drugs, including aspirin, isoniazid, phenylbutazone, promazine derivatives, sulfonamides, and nitrofurazone
  2. Uremia and myeloma will also cause platelet functional defects

    B. Prognosis

        Treatment is usually successful if the offending drug can be removed or the underlying uremia or myeloma can be treated.

III. Thrombocytopenia

    A. Signs have been discussed in the present section on clinical diagnosis of bleeding disorders

    B. Diagnosis—platelet count

    C. Differential diagnosis

        1. Decreased survival, sequestration

            a) Disseminated intravascular coagulation

            b) Sepsis

            c) Immune thrombocytopenia

            d) Hypersplenism

        2. Decreased production

            a) Myelophthisis

            b) Infection; after vaccinations

            c) Marrow depressing drugs

            d) Primary bone marrow disorder

        3. Ineffective production

            Immune thrombocytopenia

    D. Therapy.

        1. Dependent upon the exact mechanism

        2. If the mechanism is DIC the primary disorder must be treated.

        3. Sepsis is handled with appropriate antimicrobial agents after bacteriologic culture.

        4. Offending drugs are removed.

        5. Most clinical cases of thrombocytopenia are considered to have an immunologic origin.

            a) Immunosuppressive dosages of corticosteroids (1–2 mg/kg/day in the morning; as response is achieved dosage is gradually tapered) and azathioprine (1–2 mg/kg/day in the morning) are administered.

            b) Splenectomy in the vast majority of immune thrombocytopenias offers only transient relief (1–2 months) through elevation of the platelet count. However, relapse in postplenectomy patients seems to be more swiftly and effectively treated with immunosuppressive therapy.

IV. Thrombocytosis accompanied by clinical signs is often associated with iron deficiency or chronic myeloid leukemia.

DISSEMINATED INTRAVASCULAR COAGULATION

    I. General comments

        During the workup of a patient for a bleeding diathesis, evidence of abnormalities involving both coagulation and platelets suggests the presence of DIC, liver disease, or VWD.

II. Etiology of DIC
    A. Sepsis
    B. Pancreatitis
    C. Metastatic malignancy
    D. Shock
    E. Hemolysis
    F. Heat stroke
    G. Chronic active hepatitis
III. Pathogenesis
    A. Coagulation factors are consumed due to acute or chronic activation of hemostasis by exposure of subendothelial collagen, activation of coagulation factors and platelets (and thus consumption), and secondary activation of fibrinolysis.
    B. Circulating plasminogen is activated to the enzyme plasmin which digests fibrinogen and fibrin as well as coagulation factors.
    C. This results in the production of fibrin(ogen) degradation products (FDPs) which circulate until cleared by the liver. These products interfere with normal hemostasis and normal platelet function.
    D. Disseminated intravascular coagulopathy can occur acutely, subacutely, or chronically. Subacute or chronic DIC may be difficult to diagnose as laboratory tests will be only moderately abnormal.
IV. Diagnosis of acute DIC
    A. A primary disease associated with DIC
        1. Neoplasia
        2. Pancreatitis
        3. Heat stroke
        4. Severe hemolysis
        5. Heart worms
        6. Severe trauma
        7. Chronic active hepatitis
    B. Prolongation of the APTT, PT, and TT
    C. Thrombocytopenia
    D. Elevations of FDPs and poor clot formation (clot lyses when observed in vitro).
    E. Subacute DIC may simply decrease fibrinogen concentration and cause a mild thrombocytopenia and elevation of FDPs.
    F. Chronic DIC is difficult to diagnose accurately in private practice.
V. Treatment
    A. Alleviate primary cause.
    B. If the precipitating cause cannot be reversed rapidly and severe hemorrhages taking place a logical sequence of therapeutic maneuvers must be undertaken.
        1. Administration of low doses of aspirin (3 mg/kg, orally) once daily.
        2. Delivery of large quantities of isotonic IV fluids in an attempt to prevent stasis. This allows maximum activity of the monocyte-ma-

    crophage system in clearing activated factors, platelets, tumor em-
boli, and so forth, and restoring normal inhibitor activity.

3. Administration of heparinized fresh whole blood. Heparin (5,000 U/
500 ml blood) is added to warmed blood 30 minutes before transfusion. This activates antithrombin III, a major inhibitor of activated
coagulation factors. Fresh blood also supplies needed RBCs, platelets, and coagulation factors.

4. Alternatively, fresh blood may be administered IV, and heparin SQ.
An initial dose of 10–150 U/kg may be given. Heparin is administered
at 12-hour intervals.

5. Success in therapy and thus modification of therapy including heparin dosage will be manifest first by normalization of screening
coagulation tests (APTT, PT) and later by decrease in FDPs and
elevation of fibrinogen concentration.

6. Caution—administration of heparin cannot be abruptly stopped without having a "rebound effect." Heparin therapy must be tapered
through 48 hours. The SQ route is ideal for this period.

SUGGESTED READINGS

Lichtman, MA: Hematology and Oncology. Grune & Stratton, New York, 1980

Hoffbrand AV, Lewis SM: Postgraduate Hematology. 2nd Ed. Appleton-Century-
Crofts, New York, 1981.

Hillman RS, Finch CA: Red Cell Manual. Ed. 4. FA Davis, Philadelphia, 1974.

Jain NC, Zinkl J: Veterinary Clinics of North America Small Animal Practice—
Clinical Hematology, Vol. II, No. 2, WB Saunders, Philadelphia, 1981

9

Cardiovascular Diseases

Mark D. Kittleson, D.V.M.

PERICARDIAL DISEASE

GENERAL COMMENTS

 I. Effusion is generally present except in constrictive pericarditis and can be identified by radiography or echocardiography.
 II. Effective therapy is predicated on an accurate diagnosis
III. Diagnostic procedures
  A. Pericardiocentesis with culture and cytology of the fluid
  B. Pneumopericardiography may delineate masses within the pericardial sac. This procedure is contraindicated in effusive-constrictive pericarditis.
  C. Echocardiography
  D. Surgical exploration and biopsy is required for accurate diagnosis in some cases.

ACUTE PERICARDITIS

Etiology

 I. Numerous bacterial pathogens including actinomyces and nocardia
 II. Fungi are uncommon causes of pericarditis.
III. Trauma
IV. Uremia is a rare cause.
 V. Idiopathic

Clinical Signs

 I. Fever may or may not be present
 II. Leukocytosis can occur and is most common when a suppurative process is present.
III. Chest pain is variable and usually difficult to identify.

IV. Pericardial friction rubs and muffled heart sounds are common on auscultation.
 V. Signs of right heart failure may be present if intrapericardial pressures are high.

Diagnosis

   I. Pericardiocentesis with cytology and culture should be done.
  II. Appropriate bloodwork should be performed to rule out uremia as a cause and to document the systemic effects of the disease.
 III. If signs of right heart failure are present, central venous pressure (CVP) should be measured.

Medical Therapy

   I. General medical therapy
      A. Symptomatic therapy is aimed at relieving pain, if necessary, and at keeping the patient quiet.
      B. Pericardiocentesis
         1. Decreases intrapericardial pressure
         2. May be dangerous if adhesions and pockets of blood and exudate are present since bleeding may occur and result in tamponade.
  II. Bacterial pericarditis
      A. Specific therapy is predicated on the results of bacterial culture and sensitivity.
      B. Initial therapy pending laboratory results
         1. Oxacillin 10 mg/kg, q6h or
         2. Nafcillin 10 mg/kg, q6h, plus
         3. Gentamicin 4 mg/kg, q12h
      C. Nocardial pericarditis
         1. Trimethoprim/sulfadiazine 60 mg/kg, q12h for 30 days
         2. Folic acid supplementation to prevent suppression of erythropoiesis
      D. Surgical drainage in conjunction with medical treatment is advised.
 III. Mycotic pericarditis should be treated with amphotericin B and/or 5-fluorocytosine or ketoconazole (see chapter 3).
 IV. Idiopathic pericarditis.
      A. Characterized by a serosanguinous to sanguinous sterile effusion, usually with evidence of inflammation, that has no identifiable underlying cause
      B. Medical therapy may include pericardiocentesis (this may need to be repeated several times) and corticosteroid administration (systemic or intrapericardial).
      C. Recurrence of the effusion may occur when corticosteroid administration is discontinued.

V. Uremic pericarditis
  A. Control the uremia (see chapter 12).
  B. Systemic corticosteroid administration
  C. Intrapericardial triamcinolone hexacetonide (0.25 mg)

Surgical Therapy

  I. Objectives
   A. To create surgical drainage of the pericardial sac
   B. To remove the pericardial sac (pericardectomy)
   C. To visualize structures, obtain biopsies, and culture specimens.
 II. Pericardial drainage through a pericardial window
   A. Can be used in bacterial or fungal pericarditis but pericardectomy is preferred.
   B. Is used when idiopathic or uremic pericarditis is unresponsive to medical therapy
III. Pericardectomy
   A. Should be used in conjunction with medical therapy in bacterial or fungal pericarditis
   B. May be used to treat uremic or idiopathic pericarditis

CHRONIC PERICARDIAL EFFUSION

Etiology

   I. Right heart failure (transudate or modified transudate)
  II. Tumors—heart base, hemangiosarcoma, mesothelioma (modified transudate to pure blood)
 III. Left atrial tear (blood)
  IV. Bleeding disorder (blood)
   V. Trauma (blood)
  VI. Pericarditis (exudate, usually with a variable amount of blood)
 VII. Chylopericardium
VIII. Idiopathic (serosanguinous to hemorrhagic effusion usually with evidence of inflammation [see section above])
  IX. Pericardial cysts (same as tumors)

Clinical Signs

   I. Muffled heart sounds
  II. Jugular venous distension
 III. Ascites or other signs of right heart failure if the intrapericardial pressures are greater than 15–20 mmHg
  IV. Chest radiographs generally show an enlarged, rounded cardiac silhouette.

V. Electrocardiography may reveal small complexes and/or electrical alterans.
VI. A fluid space between visceral and parietal pericardium can be visualized on an echocardiogram.

Diagnosis

I. Pericardiocentesis and fluid analysis should generally be performed but oftentimes will not yield a specific diagnosis.
II. Pneumopericardiography may be done if a tumor is suspected.
III. Angiocardiography may aid in delineating masses that impinge on intracardiac structures.
IV. Two-dimensional echocardiography may identify masses within the pericardial sac.
V. Surgical exploration may be performed.

Medical Therapy

I. Treat the underlying disease process.
II. Pericardiocentesis
III. Administer diuretics if right heart failure is present
IV. Intracardiac tumors are usually well advanced at the time of diagnosis. Palliative pericardiocentesis may be beneficial in improving the quality of life. There are no reports of successful chemotherapy of this disease.

Surgical Therapy

I. Tumor removal is usually impossible because of the advanced nature of the disease but may be done in selected patients.
II. Pericardial windows or pericardectomy may be indicated in effusions unresponsive to medical therapy.
III. Repair of left atrial tears may be attempted in dogs stable enough to tolerate anesthesia and surgery.

EFFUSIVE-CONSTRICTIVE PERICARDITIS

I. Definition—an inflammatory process causing a thickened, incompliant pericardial sac along with pericardial effusion
II. Because of the very incompliant pericardium, small amounts of fluid in the pericardial sac can cause marked elevations in intrapericardial pressure.
III. The causes are most commonly idiopathic pericarditis and neoplastic involvement of the pericardial sac.
IV. Diagnosis
   A. Is oftentimes difficult

B. The hallmark is persistent evidence of cardiac constriction following pericardiocentesis.

C. On echocardiogram, effusion is present and the visceral and parietal pericardia move together.

V. Therapy

A. Aimed at the underlying disease process

B. Pericardectomy

CONSTRICTIVE PERICARDITIS

Etiology

I. Constrictive pericarditis occurs when the parietal or visceral pericardium is involved with an inflammatory process that results in scarring severe enough to cause cardiac constriction.

II. Acute pericarditis that has been allowed to become chronic.

Clinical Signs

I. Increased intraventricular diastolic pressures, especially on the right side, cause signs of backward heart failure (systemic venous congestion, ascites, and edema)

II. Signs of acute pericarditis may be present in early cases.

Therapy

I. Medical therapy is unsuccessful.

II. Surgical therapy consists of total pericardiectomy.

PERICARDIAL TAMPONADE

Definition

I. Elevated pressures within the pericardial sac high enough to impede right and/or left ventricular filling

II. Increased intraventricular diastolic pressures (usually first apparent in the right ventricle) are present and a decreased stroke volume may result, especially in acute tamponade.

Clinical Signs

I. Acute cardiac tamponade

A. Jugular venous pressure and CVP are elevated.

B. Compensatory tachycardia.

   C. Pulsus paradoxus (small pulse pressure on inspiration, larger pulse pressure on expiration) may be present.

   D. A decreased pulse pressure, and diminished intensity of the heart sounds are usually present.

   E. Cardiac output and systemic blood pressures may decrease.

II. Chronic cardiac tamponade

   A. Signs of right heart failure (ascites, peripheral edema, hepatic enlargement, and so forth) predominate.

   B. Cardiac output and systemic blood pressures are usually normal.

Etiology

  I. Acute tamponade can be due to trauma, left atrial tears, pericardiocentesis, and so forth.

II. Chronic tamponade occurs secondary to chronic effusions or pericardial constriction.

Diagnosis

  I. Acute tamponade

   A. Is usually based on clinical signs

   B. Emergency echocardiography and radiography may help.

II. Chronic tamponade

   A. Clinical signs

   B. Elevated CVP

   C. Other diagnostic procedures for pericardial effusion and constriction.

Therapy

  I. If the patient is deteriorating rapidly, emergency closed pericardiocentesis is necessary.

   A. Asepsis is maintained, if possible.

   B. The patient may be standing or in left lateral recumbency.

   C. An electrocardiograph is attached.

   D. A 21-gauge 1- to 1.5-in. needle is attached to an extension tube which is attached to a three-way stopcock and a syringe.

   E. A local anesthetic may be used.

   F. The needle is inserted in the right, fourth intercostal space at the costochondral junction.

   G. The needle is advanced slowly with intermittent, gentle suction.

   H. Fluid will be obtained when the needle enters the pericardial space. If the needle encounters myocardium, the moving muscle can be felt as a grating on the end of the needle or a premature ventricular depolarization may be seen on the electrocardiogram (ECG)

  I. If the right ventricular chamber is entered, blood that clots on standing will be obtained. Blood that does not clot is from hemorrhage into the pericardial or pleural spaces.
 II. If fluid cannot be obtained or if the patient is relatively stable, open drainage via thoracotomy is preferred.
III. Chronic cardiac tamponade is treated like chronic pericardial effusion.

MYOCARDIAL DISEASE

GENERAL COMMENTS

  I. Myocardial disease usually causes loss of myocardial contractility (myocardial failure) which, if severe enough, can result in heart failure.
 II. Myocardial failure may be due to primary myocardial diseases or secondary to chronic increases in myocardial workload.
III. The treatment of choice for myocardial failure is reversal of the depression in myocardial contractility, usually through the administration of positive inotropic agents.

ETIOLOGY

Primary diseases

   I. Viral myocarditis due to parvovirus
  II. Myocarditis due to other organisms
 III. Idiopathic myocarditis
  IV. Toxic cardiomyopathy (adriamycin, cobalt)
   V. Idiopathic congestive cardiomyopathy
  VI. Restrictive cardiomyopathy
 VII. Hypertrophic cardiomyopathy
     A. This is the exception to the rule in that cell death is not a prominent feature and cardiac contractility is not reduced.
     B. Instead myocardial hypertrophy and increased left ventricular stiffness are the prominent features.

Secondary Myocardial Failure

  I. Chronic valvular lesions
     A. Valvular stenosis
     B. Valvular regurgitation
 II. High cardiac output demand states
     A. Chronic thyrotoxicosis
     B. Chronic anemia
III. Chronic left-to-right shunts

VIRAL MYOCARDITIS

Etiology

I. Parvovirus in dogs
II. Possibly distemper virus in dogs

Clinical signs

I. Parvovirus usually infects neonatal puppies
   A. Produces a diffuse myocarditis which results in severe, acute heart failure and death at ages 3–8 weeks.
   B. Occasionally it will result in myocardial failure indistinguishable from congestive cardiomyopathy in adult dogs.
II. Distemper virus can cause myocarditis in gnotobiotic dogs infected at 5–7 days of age. It probably is not a clinically apparent problem.

Therapy

I. Supportive
II. Diuretic and dobutamine administration may be helpful (see section below).
III. If the myocarditis results in chronic myocardial failure, treatment should be the same as for congestive cardiomyopathy (see section below).

IDIOPATHIC ENDOMYOCARDITIS

General Comments

I. Etiology is unknown
II. Occurs in cats of all ages
III. The endocardium and myocardium are infiltrated with various white blood cells.

Clinical Signs

I. Congestive heart failure from myocardial failure and/or impaired ventricular filling.
   A. Pulmonary edema
   B. Poor peripheral perfusion
   C. Ascites, hydothorax, and so forth
II. Dysrhythmias
III. Systemic thromboembolism

Diagnosis

I. Clinical signs
II. Radiography and echocardiography

III. Definitive diagnosis is based on pathologic examination or endomyocardial biopsy

Therapy

I. The same as for congestive cardiomyopathy
II. Corticosteroid or immunosuppressive therapy may be indicated but is controversial in human medicine.
III. Aspirin prophylaxis for systemic thromboembolism (1.25 grains per cat every 2 to 3 days)

CONGESTIVE CARDIOMYOPATHY

Etiology

I. Unknown.
II. Many human cases are thought to be secondary to viral infections
III. In Syrian hamsters the disease is genetic and may be due to a primary defect in intracellular calcium transport or to constriction of arterioles within the myocardium.

Clinical Signs

I. Backward heart failure.
   A. Pulmonary edema with left ventricular failure.
   B. Ascites, hydrothorax (common in cats), peripheral edema with right ventricular failure.
II. Forward heart failure
   A. Low cardiac output resulting in inadequate tissue oxygen delivery
      1. Large arteriovenous oxygen difference
      2. Low venous oxygen tension (see section on Shock below)
   B. Pale mucous membranes and slow capillary refill time
III. Dysrhythmias
   A. Atrial fibrillation in large dogs
   B. Ventricular tachydysrhythmias are most common in Doberman pinschers and boxers.
   C. Atrial and ventricular tachydysrhythmias may be present in cats.
IV. Radiography.
   A. Generalized enlargement of the cardiac silhouette
   B. Edema and congestion
V. Echocardiography
   A. Dilated chambers
   B. Poor systolic wall motion
   C. Evidence of elevated diastolic intraventricular pressures (mitral valve "B" bump)
   D. Evidence of poor stroke volume (reduced systolic aortic root motion)

VI. Cardiac catheterization
  A. Is usually not indicated because of anesthetic risk and the ability to confirm the diagnosis by other means
  B. Increased atrial and diastolic intraventricular pressures
  C. Decreased stroke volume
  D. Cardiac output may be decreased.
  E. Mitral regurgitation may or may not be present.

Therapy

  I. Depends on the severity of clinical signs.
     A. Patients that have evidence of disease or cardiac dysfunction but who do not show clinical signs (class 1) do not require treatment.
     B. Patients that only show clinical signs of heart failure when they exercise (class 2) respond well to exercise restriction and possibly a low salt diet and diuretic administration.
     C. When clinical signs are present with normal activity (class 3) or at rest (class 4), a positive inotrope should be administered orally along with a diuretic and a low salt diet.
     D. When the patient does not respond to the above measures, vasodilators may be tried.
     E. When dealing with severe, life-threatening heart failure, IV dobutamine, diuretics, vasodilators, and oxygen administration should be utilized. Stressful situations (radiology, administration of oxygen by mask) should be avoided.
  II. Diuretics
     A. The diuretic most commonly used is furosemide.
        1. Chloride, and therefore sodium, resorption are blocked in the ascending loop of Henle.
        2. Venodilation may occur especially when administered IV.
        3. Half-life = 15 minutes
        4. Duration of effect is 2 hours after IV administration and 6 hours after oral administration.
        5. Peak effect occurs within 1–2 hours of oral administration and 30 minutes of IV administration.
        6. Dose is 2–4 mg/kg for chronic oral administration and up to 8 mg/kg for acute, short-term IV administration.
        7. Dosage frequency is from once every 2–3 days to every 6 hours for oral administration and as frequently as every hour for IV administration.
        8. Overdosage can result in dehydration, decreased cardiac output, and poor tissue oxygen delivery, hypokalemia, hyponatremia, and hypochloremic alkalosis.
     B. Thiazides
        1. May be used in patients with mild to moderate signs of heart failure.

    2. Decrease the permeability of the distal tubule to sodium and chloride.

    3. Are about 40–50% as potent as the loop diuretics in promoting sodium loss

    4. Dosage: hydrochlorothiazide—2–4 mg/kg BID PO; chlorothiazide–20–40 mg/kg PO; bendroflumethiazide—0.2–0.4 mg/kg PO.

    5. Can be administered along with the loop diuretics to promote additional sodium excretion in patients that are refractory to the administration of a single diuretic.

C. Spironolactone and triamterene

    1. Are used infrequently in veterinary medicine.

    2. Can be used to prevent excessive potassium loss caused by other diuretics

    3. Can be used in conjunction with other diuretics to promote diuresis in patients refractory to one diuretic.

    4. Spironolactone's peak effect occurs 2–3 days after starting therapy.

    5. Triamterene has an effect within 2 hours, a peak effect in 6–8 hours, and the effect lasts 12–16 hours.

    6. Dose for both triamterene and spironolactone is 2–4 mg/kg/day PO.

D. Diuretics decrease blood volume, decrease intraventricular diastolic blood volumes, and so decrease diastolic intraventricular and venous blood pressures. By doing so they decrease the rate of edema formation.

III. Low-salt diets (30–250 mg/100 g dry weight of food)

A. Should be used whenever diuretics are used, if possible.

B. Are not practical in all dogs because of low palatability.

C. Can be a prescription diet or home-cooked

    1. If clients wish to prepare home-cooked meals they can obtain booklets from a local American Heart Association chapter listing allowed and restricted foods.

    2. Commercial diets are extremely low in salt (10–30 mg/100 g)

    3. Salt substitutes using KC1 can be added to increase palatability and add potassium to the diet.

IV. The digitalis glycosides

A. Are used to increase myocardial contractility in class 3 and 4 patients when myocardial failure is present

B. Are also used to abolish supraventricular tachydysrhythmias and to slow the ventricular response to atrial flutter and fibrillation.

C. The cardiac glycosides increase myocardial contractility in normal and, to a variable degree, in failing myocardium.

    1. The percentage of patients with myocardial failure that respond to the digitalis glycosides is controversial in the human literature.

    2. The number that respond is probably variable depending on the severity and type of failure.

3. Approximately 40–50% of dogs with severe myocardial failure due to congestive cardiomyopathy respond to digoxin.
4. Dogs with congestive cardiomyopathy that have an increase in cardiac contractility after digoxin administration live longer than those dogs that do not (average survival time = 6 months for responders versus 6 weeks for nonresponders).

D. The increase in contractility is most likely caused by inhibition of Na^+-K^+ ATPase at the myocardial cell membrane.
1. This inhibition results in increased calcium ion influx into the cell.
2. Increased calcium concentration in a normal or mildly abnormal cell results in increased contractility.
3. Increased calcium concentration in a severely diseased cell can result in toxicity and dysrhythmia.

E. Antidysrhythmic effects
1. Digitalis increases vagal tone to the sinus node, atria, and atrioventricular node.
2. It also has direct effects, especially in the atrioventricular (AV) node where it slows conduction and prolongs the refractory period.
3. Improvement in myocardial blood flow and decrease in myocardial oxygen consumption may decrease myocardial irritability in patients that respond to digitalis.

F. Digoxin pharmacokinetics and dosage
1. Half-life in the dog is 24–36 hours and in the cat is controversial but is probably between 24 and 58 hours.
2. In the dog, tablets are 60% and the elixir is 75% absorbed from the gastrointestinal tract.
3. The dose in dogs is 0.22 mg/m² of body surface area given BID for tablets and 0.18 mg/m² given BID for the elixir (see chapter 7 for table of conversion of body weights to surface area).
4. In cats the dose is 0.01 mg/kg given once a day or divided BID for tablets (1/4 of 0.125 mg digoxin tablet every other day for cats weighing 2–3 kg; 1/4 tablet daily for cats weighing 4–5 kg; 1/4 tablet BID for cats weighing 6 or more kg). Cats dislike the taste of the elixir.
5. Therapeutic serum concentrations (1.0–2.5 ng/ml) are achieved within 24–72 hours with these doses. Loading dose schedules are not recommended for dogs or cats with myocardial failure.

G. Tincture of digitoxin (Foxalin) pharmacokinetics and dosage
1. Half-life is 8–12 hours in the dog and greater than 100 hours in the cat. Because of the long half-life in the cat, digitoxin is not used in this species.
2. Ninety percent is protein bound in serum so a high dose relative to digoxin is needed to maintain therapeutic serum concentrations.

3. Ninety-five to 100% is absorbed from the gastrointestinal tract.
4. Dose in the dog is 0.03–0.04 mg/kg BID to TID.
5. Digitalization (therapeutic serum concentrations between 15 and 35 ng/ml) is achieved within 16–24 hours when the drug is administered without a loading dose.
6. Foxalin is supplied in capsules too small to make dosing a large dog practical.

H. Signs of adequate digitilization
1. PR interval prolongation is an insensitive and nonspecific indicator. However, if it is noted during digitalization, other signs of digitalization or toxicity should be looked for carefully.
2. Clinical signs are improvement in perfusion (improved capillary refill time, increased venous oxygen tension) and decreased edema.
3. Improved hemodynamics in heart failure patients (increased cardiac output, decreased intraventricular diastolic blood pressures, improved indexes of left ventricular function on echocardiogram)
4. Slowing of the heart rate in patients with supraventricular tachy-dysrhythmias

I. Serum concentrations of a glycoside should be determined in patients that do not respond to its administration before increasing the dose and in patients exhibiting signs of toxicity (see chapter 22).
1. Low serum concentrations are associated with abnormal pharmacokinetics and necessitate an increased dose.
2. Therapeutic serum concentrations in an unresponsive patient suggest that the patient is refractory to the drug.
3. There is evidence to suggest that there is no benefit to increasing the serum concentration of digitalis within its therapeutic range. In other words, if the serum digoxin concentration is 1.5 ng/ml, increasing the dose to increase the serum concentration to 2.5 ng/ml will not increase contractility any further. It may slow heart rate further, however.
4. Serum samples should be collected 8 hours after the last dose of digitalis and sent to a local laboratory.

J. Factors that alter the dose of digitalis
1. Patients that have lost skeletal muscle mass need smaller dosages because skeletal muscle is a large storage depot for digitalis.
2. Patients with decreased glomerular filtration rates need smaller doses of digoxin since digoxin is excreted via glomerular filtration. Digitoxin is preferred in these patients.
3. Cardiac contractility does not increase as much with the digitalis glycosides in older dogs as in younger dogs.
4. Digoxin is poorly lipid soluble so lean body weight should be used to calculate doses for obese dogs.
5. Patients with hypokalemia, hypernatremia, and hypercalcemia re-

quire decreased doses of digoxin and digitoxin. Electrolyte abnormalities should be corrected whenever possible.

6. Hypothyroid and hyperthyroid patients require lesser amounts of digitalis.

7. Furosemide can decrease GFR by decreasing blood volume so digoxin dosages may need to be reduced when furosemide is being given concomitantly, especially when it is being given in high doses.

8. Quinidine decreases renal excretion of digoxin and displaces digoxin from skeletal muscle and probably myocardial binding sites. This will result in toxicity and may reduce efficacy.

9. Verapamil administration increases serum concentrations of digoxin in human patients.

10. Drugs that reduce hepatic microsomal enzyme activity (chloramphenicol, quinidine, quinine, tetracycline) decrease digoxin excretion and should be avoided. The barbiturates and phenylbutazone may enhance digoxin excretion by inducing hepatic microsomal enzymes.

11. Myocardial failure greatly enhances the sensitivity of the myocardium to the digitalis glycosides. Because of this, dogs or cats with severe myocardial failure should be digitalized very carefully. Loading doses of digoxin or digitoxin should be avoided. Since large dogs are commonly involved, a dose based on body surface area should always be used in this species rather than one based on body weight.

12. Hypoxemia enhances myocardial sensitivity to digitalis. Patients with pulmonary edema or pulmonary failure must be treated cautiously.

K. Digitalis toxicity

1. Should be avoided at all costs, especially in patients with severe myocardial failure, i.e., congestive cardiomyopathy.

2. Mild digitalis toxicity (anorexia, vomition) can usually be treated simply by discontinuing digitalis administration for 24 hours and reducing the dose.

3. Moderate to severe toxicity can produce various dysrhythmias. Ventricular dysrhythmias are the most serious and require vigorous therapy.

4. Lidocaine and phenytoin are the drugs of choice (see chapter 10). Propranolol may be beneficial. Procainamide is usually not as effective and quinidine and verapamil are contraindicated in this situation.

5. Hypokalemia potentiates digitalis intoxication and hinders the actions of antidysrhythmics. Potassium should be supplemented in all cases with serum concentrations <3.5 mEq/L.

6. Supraventricular tachydysrhythmias may respond to propranolol.

7. Bradydysrhythmias may respond to atropine.

V. Milrinone

A. This is an orally active experimental drug which increases contractility by a mechanism other than that attributed to either the digitalis glycosides or the sympathomimetics.

B. Its mechanism of action is unknown.

C. In the normal heart it can increase contractility up to 100% compared to 33% for the digitalis glycosides.

D. It is also a mild to moderate arteriolar dilator.

E. It has a wide therapeutic range, little toxicity, and is active after oral administration.

F. Half-life is approximately 2.0 hours in the dog.

G. Dose is 0.5 to 1.0 mg/kg given orally BID to QID.

H. Peak effect occurs within 1–2 hours after oral administration.

I. The only side effect of the drug noted to date is an occasional exacerbation of a ventricular dysrhythmia.

J. The drug appears to be effective in about 70–80% of dogs with severe myocardial failure compared to 40–50% for digoxin.

K. Dogs that respond to milrinone have an average survival of about 6 months.

VI. Vasodilators

A. Dogs or cats that are refractory to digitalis or milrinone usually have a very poor prognosis.

1. Vasodilators may improve clinical signs and the quality of life.

2. Vasodilators probably do not significantly prolong survival time in dogs with myocardial failure.

B. Vasodilators produce hemodynamic benefits by dilating systemic veins, systemic arterioles, or both.

C. Venodilators

1. Nitrates (nitroglycerin, isosorbide dinitrate) are the classic examples

2. Should be used when diuretics are no longer effective

3. Generally are not as effective as diuretics

4. Act by redistributing blood volume into the systemic venous system away from the central system. Intraventricular diastolic blood volumes and therefore pressures are reduced.

5. Dosage for nitroglycerin cream is 0.25–0.5 in. in small dogs up to 1.0 in. in large dogs.

6. Duration of effect is 3 hours in human patients.

7. Cream should be applied to a hairless area where the patient cannot lick (inside the pinna).

8. There have been no clinical studies reported to document the efficacy of nitroglycerin cream in the dog or cat.

   D. Hydralazine
      1. Is a pure arteriolar dilator.
      2. Decreases systemic vascular resistance, lowers systemic arterial blood pressure, and increases cardiac output
      3. See the section on mitral regurgitation for the pharmacodynamics and dosage schedules (section below).
   E. Prazosin
      1. Dilates both arterioles and veins by blocking α_1-adrenergic receptors and by inhibiting phosphodiesterase.
      2. Increases cardiac output and decreases congestion and edema in human patients.
      3. There are no reports of controlled clinical studies in veterinary medicine.
      4. Clinical benefit may occur when a total dose of 1 mg is given TID to dogs less than 15 kg. Larger dogs may respond to 2 mg TID.
      5. Hypotension is a possible side effect. Blood pressure should be monitored if the means are available.
      6. The dosage should be titrated, starting at a low dose and gradually increasing the dose until a response is seen.
   F. Captopril
      1. Inhibits the action of the angiotensin-converting enzyme, peptidyl dipeptidase
      2. Decreases circulating concentrations of angiotensin II and aldosterone
      3. The net result is arteriolar and venodilation and decreased renal salt and water retention.
      4. Studies of the pharmacodynamics of captopril have not been performed in veterinary medicine.
      5. A dose of 1–2 mg/kg orally TID may be successful in dogs with heart failure.
      6. The dose should be titrated.
      7. Hypotension can be produced. If severe, it can be treated with dopamine, usually at a constant infusion rate of 10 μg/kg/min or greater.
      8. The author has observed the development of renal failure in several dogs following captopril administration.
VII. Sympathomimetics
   A. Dobutamine
      1. Can be used to stabilize patients with signs of acute, severe heart failure.
      2. Increases contractility when administered IV without appreciably changing blood pressure or heart rate.
      3. Increases cardiac output and increases the percentage of flow to skeletal and cardiac muscle more than to other tissues.
      4. Half-life is 1–2 minutes so it must be given as constant infusion.

5. The infusion rate is 5–40 μg/kg/min. Table 9-1 can be used to determine the amount of dobutamine to add to a bottle of 5% dextrose in water to achieve a certain infusion rate.

B. Dopamine
   1. Similar features to dobutamine
   2. Dilates renal and splanchnic vasculature via stimulation of dopaminergic receptors.
   3. May cause venoconstriction in patients with chronic heart failure so should be used with caution in this situation.
   4. Constant infusion rate is 1–10 μg/kg/minute.

VIII. Aspirin
  A. All cats with congestive cardiomyopathy should receive 1.25 grains of aspirin every 2–3 days with (Ascriptin) or without (baby aspirin) antacid.
  B. It is administered to prevent thrombus formation in the left side of the heart and resultant systemic thromboembolism.

IX. Monitoring drug effects
  A. All patients receiving therapy for heart failure should be monitored to determine if the patient is responding.
  B. Dogs or cats with pulmonary edema should have serial chest radiographs to determine if the edema is clearing.
  C. Patients with right heart failure can have their CVP or abdominal size followed.
  D. If hypoperfusion (forward failure) is present, mucous membrane color or capillary refill time can be monitored.
    1. Determinations of mixed or jugular venous oxygen tensions are more objective and easier to interpret (see section on shock, patient monitoring, below)
    2. Treatment should be directed at keeping venous oxygen tension >35 mmHg.

TABLE 9-1. THE APPROXIMATE AMOUNT OF DRUG TO ADD TO 500 ml FLUID TO ACHIEVE A CERTAIN INFUSION RATE WHEN THE FLUID IS ADMINISTERED AT 2.2 ml/kg/hr

Add	To Achieve	Infusion Rate
15 mg		1 μg/kg/min
30 mg		2 μg/kg/min
45 mg		3 μg/kg/min
70 mg		5 μg/kg/min
140 mg		10 μg/kg/min
200 mg		15 μg/kg/min
270 mg		20 μg/kg/min
340 mg		25 μg/kg/min
410 mg		30 μg/kg/min
480 mg		35 μg/kg/min
550 mg		40 μg/kg/min

   3. Cardiac output can be monitored if the equipment and expertise
      are available.

DOXORUBICIN CARDIOTOXICITY

   Doxorubicin, a cancer chemotherapeutic agent, can cause myocardial de-
generation and necrosis leading to myocardial failure and dysrhythmias in the
dog.
   I. Signs may appear when cumulative doses >250 mg/m^2 of body surface
      area are reached.
  II. Dysrhythmias of many different types are more common than myocardial
      failure in the dog.
      A. Sudden death may occur.
      B. Therapy depends on the type of dysrhythmia (see Chapter 10).
 III. Therapy of myocardial failure is discussed in the section on congestive
      cardiomyopathy

RESTRICTIVE CARDIOMYOPATHY

   I. Is an uncommon disease of cats
  II. Is characterized by diastolic dysfunction and usually normal systolic func-
      tion
      A. The left ventricular chamber is stiffer (less compliant) than normal.
      B. Diastolic intraventricular pressures are increased causing edema
 III. Is caused by a disease that produces massive fibrosis of the endocardium
      or myocardium
  IV. Approximately 33% of cats with restrictive cardiomyopathy brought to
      necropsy have aortic thromboembolism so aspirin should be administered
      prophylactically.
   V. Is oftentimes refractory to medical management although diuretics and
      venodilators should be tried

HYPERTROPHIC CARDIOMYOPATHY

   I. Is characterized by concentric hypertrophy of the left ventricular myo-
      cardium in the absence of increased systolic intraventricular pressures
  II. Is most frequently recognized in the cat
 III. Produces an incompliant or stiff left ventricle which cannot fill properly
      A. The end-diastolic volume is normal or decreased and end-diastolic pres-
         sure is increased.
      B. If the end-diastolic volume is very small it may result in a less than
         normal stroke volume.
  IV. Contractility is normal but afterload (systolic myocardial wall stress) is less

than normal because of the thick wall so end-systolic volume is less than normal.

V. Massive hypertrophy and high velocity flow in the left ventricular outflow tract may produce obstruction to outflow, especially in the last half of systole.

VI. Therapy

A. Propranolol is the standard treatment.

1. It does not improve left ventricular compliance.

2. It may decrease the left ventricular outflow tract gradient if it is present.

a) The importance of the gradient in altering hemodynamics in human patients is controversial since it usually occurs late in systole.

b) The prevalence and importance of this gradient is unknown in cats.

3. Dose is 2.5–5.0 mg/cat BID to TID for cats weighing less than 6.0 kg and 5.0–7.5 mg/cat BID to TID for cats > 6.0 kg.

4. The therapeutic end-point is relief of clinical signs or abolition of dysrhythmias.

5. Propranolol may worsen myocardial failure in congestive cardiomyopathy so a definitive diagnosis must be made before its administration.

a) Echocardiography is the best means of differentiating hypertrophic from congestive cardiomyopathy because it is noninvasive and requires no anesthetic.

b) Nonselective venous angiography can also be used.

6. Propranolol also decreases platelet function which may help prevent systemic thromboembolism.

7. *Propranolol should not be used in cats with asthma, diabetes mellitus, atrioventricular block, sinoatrial block, sinus arrest, or acute systemic thromboembolism.*

B. Calcium channel blockers (verapamil, nifedipine)

1. Increase left ventricular compliance in human patients with hypertrophic cardiomyopathy

2. Also produce arteriolar dilation

a) Lowering blood pressure may increase the left ventricular outflow tract gradient.

b) May produce a decrease in cardiac output

3. Clinical response is variable in human patients.

4. Use is generally reserved for patients that are unresponsive to propranolol.

5. The use of calcium channel blockers has not been investigated in cats.

C. Aspirin should be given prophylactically.

SYSTEMIC ARTERIAL THROMBOEMBOLISM

General Comments

I. A common sequela to myocardial disease in the cat.
II. Thrombi probably form in the left atrium and/or ventricle.
III. Emboli most commonly lodge in the terminal aorta although embolization of many other regions of the body may occur.
IV. The embolus releases vasoactive substances that cause intense vasoconstriction distal to the region of embolization.
    A. Distal aortic embolization causes intense caudal limb pain, edematous musculature, flaccid paraparesis, lack of femoral pulses, and pale, cyanotic nail beds.
    B. Disseminated intravascular coagulation (DIC) may occur.

Diagnosis

I. Is confirmed with nonselective angiography
II. The type of underlying cardiac disease should always be determined prior to instituting therapy.
    A. Congestive or restrictive cardiomyopathy implies a poor prognosis and poor response to therapy.
    B. Cats with hypertrophic cardiomyopathy tolerate anesthesia and surgery better than cats with congestive cardiomyopathy.

Therapy

I. Surgical therapy may be attempted if clinical signs are present for less than 6 hours.
    A. Transabdominal aortotomy and clot removal
    B. Fogarty balloon-tipped catheters can be used from a transfemoral approach under local anesthesia.
        1. A femoral artery cutdown is performed and the catheter passed retrograde up the aorta beyond the thromboembolus.
        2. The balloon is inflated, and the embolus and any associated thrombus removed by withdrawing the catheter.
II. Medical treatment along with nursing care may result in recovery within 2 days to 7 weeks.
    A. Aspirin with an antacid (Ascriptin) is administered every other day at a dose of 1.25 grains (1/4 of a 5-grain tablet). This should continue indefinitely.
    B. The underlying heart disease should be stabilized, if possible.
    C. Prolonged physical therapy and nursing care is required. A dedicated and forewarned owner is needed to accomplish a satisfactory outcome.
    D. Minidose heparin therapy may help further decrease further thrombus formation in the heart and around the existing embolus.

E. An arteriolar dilator may help decrease the vasoconstriction distal to the thromboembolus and aid in establishing collateral circulation.

VALVULAR DISEASE

CHRONIC MITRAL VALVE FIBROSIS

General Comments

I. Is the most commonly diagnosed valvular abnormality in the dog.
II. Affects small-breed dogs and oftentimes causes signs of heart failure in dogs >8 years old.
III. The valvular lesion creates a defect between the left ventricle and left atrium during systole which results in systolic regurgitant blood flow into the left atrium.
IV. The disease is progressive so the size of the mitral valve orifice increases with time.
V. Heart failure is usually caused by massive regurgitant flow causing left atrial and secondary left ventricular volume overload.
    A. The overload causes increased diastolic blood pressures within the left ventricle, increased systolic and diastolic pressures in the left atrium and pulmonary capillaries, and pulmonary edema.
    B. Regurgitant fractions are >80% in dogs with signs of severe heart failure.
    C. Myocardial function is usually normal or only mildly depressed.

Diagnosis

I. Auscultation of typical murmur
II. Radiographic evidence of left atrial and ventricular enlargement
III. Echocardiographic evidence of left atrial and ventricular enlargement along with exaggerated systolic movement of the septum and free wall
IV. Cardiac catheterization

Medical Therapy of Chronic Mitral Regurgitation

I. Patients that have a murmur but no signs of heart failure (class 1) are not treated. There is no medical therapy that will slow the progression of the disease.
II. When a dog only shows signs of heart failure with heavy exercise (class 2), heavy exercise should be discontinued. When lesser amounts of exercise produce coughing or dyspnea, diuretics may be administered.

III. When signs become evident with normal activity (class 3) or at rest (class 4) and there is evidence of pulmonary edema, pulmonary congestion, or left atrial compression of the left mainstem bronchus, diuretic therapy should be initiated (see section above).
  A. A low salt diet should be instituted along with the diuretic, if possible.
  B. The dosage of the diuretic should be adjusted so that clinical signs are controlled.
  C. Overzealous diuretic administration should be avoided.
IV. Hydralazine
  A. Should be administered when the patient becomes refractory to diuretics.
    1. Refractory means that the patient has pulmonary edema despite maximal use of diuretics.
    2. Usually perfusion is poor and the venous oxygen tension is low at this time.
  B. Hydralazine increases forward blood flow into the aorta and decreases regurgitant blood flow into the left atrium.
    1. It reduces systemic arterial blood pressure by decreasing systemic vascular resistance and increasing aortic compliance.
    2. This decreases left ventricular systolic pressure and reduces the pressure gradient between the left ventricle and the left atrium, reducing systolic regurgitant blood flow. Left atrial pressures decrease and pulmonary edema resolves.
    3. The improved aortic flow and the lessened regurgitant flow result in a decrease in left ventricular end-diastolic volume which decreases the size of the mitral valve annulus. This decreases regurgitant flow further.
    4. Forward flow into the aorta is favored by the reduction in aortic blood pressure so cardiac output increases.
  C. Titration of dose
    1. Obtain a baseline chest radiograph, venous oxygen tension, or capillary refill time, and systemic arterial blood pressure, if possible.
    2. Administer 1 mg/kg hydralazine orally.
    3. Repeat blood pressure in 1 hour. If blood pressure is not available, repeat venous oxygen tension in 3 hours. If blood gases cannot be obtained, reassess the patient's clinical status (mucous membrane color, chest radiographs) 6–24 hours later.
    4. If the mean arterial blood pressure is <80 mmHg or has decreased 15–20 mmHg; if the venous oxygen tension was <35mmHg and is now >35 mmHg; or if the mucous membrane color and capillary refill time or the chest radiographs have improved, do not administer any more drug. Repeat the 1 mg/kg dose every 12 hours.
    5. If a response is not identified, either administer another 1 mg/kg dose, if the last dose was given less than 10 hours ago or administer a 2 mg/kg dose if it has been longer than 10 hours.

6. This is repeated until a response is identified.
7. The total dose needed to produce an effect is administered every 12 hours.
8. A total dose of 3 mg/kg given every 12 hours should not be exceded.
9. If hypotension results from hydralazine administration, perfusion to the brain, kidneys, and heart may be compromised. The patient may appear weak from poor brain perfusion. Severe hypotension may result in renal injury and renal failure. Severe hypotension should be treated with dopamine at infusion rates of 10 μg/kg/min or greater.

V. The digitalis glycosides
   A. Are used when dogs are refractory to diuretics and hydralazine or when supraventricular tachydysrhythmias are present.
      1. Hydralazine oftentimes induces a sinus tachycardia.
      2. Heart rates >180 beats/min should be controlled with digitalis and/or propranolol.
   B. Are safer to use in dogs with chronic mitral valve fibrosis since myocardial failure is usually not severe so life-threatening dysrhythmias are more difficult to produce. The increase in contractility may induce rupture of the chordae tendineae.

VI. Milrinone
   A. Arteriolar dilation and increased contractility produced by this drug may improve the hemodynamics of mitral regurgitation.
   B. No controlled clinical studies have been performed but preliminary findings suggest that milrinone is beneficial in heart failure secondary to mitral regurgitation.
   C. The increase in contractility may cause the chordae tendineae to rupture.

Medical Therapy of Acute Heart Failure due to Mitral Regurgitation

I. Acute cardiac emergencies due to mitral regurgitation may be due to acute rupture of chordae tendineae or to chronic mitral fibrosis that has not been treated or has been treated inappropriately.
II. Intensive therapy is required to maintain life.
III. Most dogs that die from acute, life-threatening heart failure do so because of severe pulmonary edema.
IV. Cardiac output may also be inadequate resulting in pale mucous membranes, poor capillary refill, and a low venous oxygen tension.
V. Stress should be avoided.
   A. Following an initial cursory examination the patient should be placed in a cage.
   B. *Additional stress or excitement from handling oftentimes results in death.*
   C. Procedures that require restraint (taking chest radiographs, placing

indwelling catheters, administration of oxygen by mask, and so forth), should be postponed until the patient is stabilized.

VI. If pulmonary edema fluid is emanating from the mouth and/or nostrils, the patient's rear quarters may be gently elevated and the patient gently shaken. This will help remove accumulations of fluid in the large airways. IF THE PATIENT RESISTS OR BECOMES EXCITED, DO NOT CONTINUE.

VII. Furosemide (4–8 mg/kg IM or IV)
   A. The IV route is preferred if it is not unduly stressful.
   B. Repeat up to every hour. Try to avoid overdosing since hypoperfusion and electrolyte abnormalities may result.

VIII. Vasodilators can be lifesaving.
   A. Nitroprusside is the vasodilator of choice if blood pressure can be monitored and an IV catheter placed.
      1. Infusion rates for dogs are 1–5 µg/kg/min.
      2. Mean systemic blood pressure should not be decreased below 70 mmHg.
   B. Hydralazine can also be utilized in this situation. The same titration schedule outlined in section on Medical Therapy of Chronic Mitral Regurgitation, III, C, above can be used but titration can start with a 2 mg/kg dose.

IX. IV dobutamine may also be helpful, administered at an infusion rate of 5–20 µg/kg/minute.

MITRAL REGURGITATION SECONDARY TO OTHER DISEASE PROCESSES

Other Causes

I. Congestive cardiomyopathy
   A. Secondary to left ventricular and mitral annular dilatation
   B. Secondary to papillary muscle dysfunction
II. Hypertrophic cardiomyopathy.
   A. Systolic anterior motion of the mitral valve
      1. High-velocity flow in the left ventricular outflow tract draws the anterior mitral valve leaflet into the outflow tract.
      2. Creates an incompetent valve
   B. Abnormal papillary muscle orientation

Therapy

I. Congestive cardiomyopathy patients with mitral regurgitation may respond better to arteriolar dilators than those without.
II. Propranolol may alleviate systolic anterior motion of the mitral valve in hypertrophic cardiomyopathy.

TRICUSPID REGURGITATION

I. Congenital tricuspid regurgitation in the dog
   A. Causes.
      1. Tricuspid valve dysplasia
      2. Ebstein's anomaly.
         a) Ventral displacement of the tricuspid valve.
         b) Large "sail-like" leaflets.
   B. May cause right-sided heart failure, usually when the dog is a young to middle-aged adult.
   C. Medical therapy consists of a low salt diet, diuretic administration, and possibly digitalis or milrinone.
   D. Mechanical removal of ascites may be needed.
   E. Surgical valve replacement is not indicated.
II. Acquired tricuspid regurgitation
   A. Is usually due to chronic tricuspid valve fibrosis.
   B. Usually accompanies mitral valve fibrosis.
   C. Usually does not cause clinical signs unless pulmonary hypertension is also present.
      1. Pulmonary hypertension can be due to chronic upper or lower respiratory failure.
      2. Pulmonary hypertension can also occur secondary to chronic mitral regurgitation and left heart failure.
   D. Treatment is the same as for congenital tricuspid regurgitation.

AORTIC REGURGITATION

Etiology

I. Bacterial endocarditis
II. In association with subvalvular aortic stenosis in the dog

Pathophysiology

I. A variable volume of blood leaks from the aorta back into the left ventricle during diastole.
II. This along with salt and water retention produces a left ventricular volume overload (increased left ventricular end-diastolic volume).
III. The volume overload helps the ventricle to increase its stroke volume to compensate for the loss in forward stroke volume caused by the regurgitant leak.
IV. Heart failure occurs when the regurgitant leak is so severe that it overwhelms the ability of the left ventricle to accommodate the increased diastolic blood volume and overwhelms the systolic compensatory mechanisms or when myocardial failure occurs.

Therapy

I. Depends on the clinical signs of the patient
II. Diuretics and a low salt diet are used to control signs of edema.
III. Milrinone or digitalis are used to treat myocardial failure.
IV. Hydralazine decreases the amount of regurgitation and so improves forward blood flow and decreases intraventricular diastolic pressure.

AORTIC STENOSIS

Etiology

I. Congenital lesion in the dog and cat
II. Is usually a subvalvular lesion
III. Is inherited in the Newfoundland breed

Pathophysiology

I. Aortic stenosis creates an impedance to left ventricular outflow.
II. The increased impedance forces the left ventricle to increase intraventricular pressure.
III. The left ventricle generates new sarcomeres in parallel to offset the increased afterload creating concentric left ventricular hypertrophy to decrease left ventricular afterload (systolic myocardial wall stress).
IV. Heart failure can be due to severe stenosis and/or myocardial failure.
V. Myocardial failure may develop over time with moderate to severe aortic stenosis.
   A. Myocardial failure may occur secondary to prolonged inadequate myocardial oxygenation.
   B. Myocardial oxygen requirements are elevated because of increased afterload and prolonged ejection times.
   C. Myocardial oxygen transport is decreased because of concentric hypertrophy and impaired coronary blood flow.
VI. The concentric hypertrophy makes the left ventricle stiffer than normal in diastole, creating higher diastolic pressures for normal diastolic volumes.
VII. When myocardial failure occurs, the poor contractility along with the increased impedance to aortic flow results in a decrease in cardiac output. The combination of severely increased afterload and poor contractility cannot be compensated for adequately, resulting in a more rapidly spiraling downward course, a poor prognosis, and a short survival time.

Diagnosis

I. Auscultation, chest radiographs, and echocardiography can establish the diagnosis.

II. Cardiac catheterization should be performed to establish the site of the lesion and to assess the severity of the stenosis.

Therapy

I. Surgical correction
   A. Dogs should be less than 6 months old.
   B. If cardiopulmonary bypass is used, dogs must be larger than 15 kg.
   C. If the peak systolic pressure gradient across the obstruction is greater than 100 mmHg, surgical correction is necessary.
   D. If the gradient is between 50 and 100 mmHg, surgery is indicated if the dog is showing clinical signs of heart disease.
   E. Surgical techniques include resection of the subvalvular stenotic band with cardiopulmonary bypass, valved conduit implantation and valvulotomy through a closed left ventriculotomy.
II. Medical therapy
   A. Dogs with subvalvular aortic stenosis are prone to ventricular dysrhythmias, syncope, and sudden death.
      1. The treatment of ventricular dysrhythmias is outlined in chapter 10.
      2. Propranolol can be administered prophylactically in an attempt to prevent sudden death.
   B. Dogs with aortic pressure gradients greater than 50 mmHg, evidence of concentric hypertrophy on echocardiogram, or ST segment depression on electrocardiogram should be treated with propranolol (1–2 mg/kg BID to TID).
   C. Myocardial failure should be treated with a positive inotropic agent such as milrinone or a digitalis glycoside.

PULMONIC STENOSIS

General Comments

I. Congenital lesion
II. Usually is a combination of valvular and subvalvular stenosis (pulmonary valve dysplasia)

Pathophysiology

I. Increased right ventricular systolic pressures produce concentric hypertrophy of the right ventricular myocardium.
II. Severe stenosis generally results in death due to myocardial failure or dysrhythmias before middle age if surgical correction is not performed.

Diagnosis

I. Can usually be established with auscultation, chest radiographs, and echocardiography.

II. Cardiac catheterization is used to define the site of the lesion and to assess severity.

Therapy

I. Surgical correction
   A. Should be performed if systolic pressure in the right ventricle is greater than 70 mmHg in the young animal, greater than 100 mmHg in the mature animal, or if clinical signs referable to the lesion are present.
   B. Can be accomplished via inflow occlusion-pulmonary arterotomy, patch graft technique, and valvulotomy
II. Medical therapy
   A. If heart failure occurs, central venous pressure increases and ascites and/or peripheral edema occur.
   B. Myocardial failure is probably present so long-term treatment with positive inotropic agents (milrinone, digitalis) is indicated.
   C. Ascites and edema are controlled with diuretics and a low salt diet.
   D. Captopril may be beneficial for controlling edema if the patient is refractory to diuretics.

LEFT-TO-RIGHT SHUNTS

GENERAL COMMENTS

I. Left-to-right shunts occur as congenital defects in the dog and cat.
II. They are caused by intra- or extracardiac defects that result in communication between the systemic and pulmonary circulations but do not cause cyanosis.
III. They result in a volume overload of the portions of the circulation involved in the shunt.
IV. The volume overload can cause signs of heart failure by itself or can cause secondary cardiovascular problems such as myocardial failure and pulmonary hypertension which can also result in signs of heart failure.

ATRIAL SEPTAL DEFECT

General Comments

I. An uncommonly diagnosed congenital defect in small animals
II. It is more commonly diagnosed in combination with other defects as in endocardial cushion defects.

Pathophysiology

  I. It creates a shunt between the left and right atria.
 II. It results in a volume overload of the right atrium and ventricle and the pulmonary vasculature.
III. The magnitude of the shunt flow depends on the size of the defect and the relative impedances of the right and left circulations.

Diagnosis

  I. May be suggested by auscultation and chest radiographs.
 II. Echocardiography reveals a dilated right ventricle.
III. Confirmation of the diagnosis and an assessment of severity can be obtained with cardiac catheterization.

Therapy

  I. Isolated atrial septal defects oftentimes never result in clinical disease.
 II. Surgical intervention is logical only if the defect is large and if it causes signs of heart failure.

    A. Only one case of surgical correction has been reported in the veterinary literature.

    B. Correction requires open heart surgery.

III. Medical management is aimed at relieving the signs of right heart failure.

    A. Diuretics and a low salt diet are generally adequate.

    B. Milrinone or the digitalis glycosides may be indicated in the later stages of heart failure if myocardial failure ensues.

    C. Physical removal of ascitic fluid may be required in refractory cases.

VENTRICULAR SEPTAL DEFECTS

General Comments

  I. Congenital defects
 II. May occur in any region of the ventricular septum but are most commonly located just below the aortic valve, high in the ventricular septum

Pathophysiology

  I. These defects allow blood to flow from the left to the right ventricle and result in volume overload of the left atrium and ventricle, the pulmonary vasculature, and, to a variable degree, the right ventricle.
 II. Clinically significant defects produce pulmonary to systemic flow ratios >2.5/1.
III. Severe shunts can cause signs of left heart failure by themselves.

IV. Myocardial failure is only present about 1/3 of the time in infants with ventricular septal defects (VSDs) and severe heart failure.

Diagnosis

I. Is suggested by auscultation and chest radiographs
II. May be confirmed by contrast echocardiography
III. Cardiac catheterization is used to establish the diagnosis and assess shunt severity.

Therapy

I. Surgical
  A. Banding of the pulmonary artery if the shunt is severe
    1. This increases impedance to right ventricular outflow.
    2. This increases right ventricular pressure and decreases shunt flow.
  B. Surgical correction of the defect can be accomplished with cardiopulmonary bypass and open heart surgery if the dog is large enough (usually >15 kg).
II. Medical therapy
  A. Arteriolar dilators such as hydralazine decrease the impedance to left ventricular outflow, reduce left ventricular systolic pressure, and reduce shunt flow.
  B. Infants with myocardial failure and some infants without myocardial failure respond clinically to digoxin administration.
    1. The response of infants without myocardial failure suggests some noninotropic mechanism for the action of digitalis.
    2. Until more is known about the state of the myocardium in veterinary patients with ventricular septal defects, milrinone or digitalis should be used in dogs or cats with signs of heart failure due to VSDs.
  C. Diuretics and a low salt diet should be used to treat pulmonary edema.

ENDOCARDIAL CUSHION DEFECTS

General Comments

I. Are the most common congenital heart defect in the cat
II. Various combinations of atrial septal defect (ostium primum), ventricular septal defect, and tricuspid and mitral regurgitation
III. Create left-to-right shunts and AV valvular regurgitation.

Diagnosis

I. Is suggested by auscultation, chest radiographs, and echocardiogram.
II. Is usually confirmed with nonselective venous angiography but can be confirmed with cardiac catheterization

Therapy

I. Pulmonary artery banding may be helpful if clinical signs are due to left-to-right shunts.
II. Hydralazine reduces left-to-right shunting and mitral regurgitation.
    A. Hydralazine dose must be titrated initially to identify an effective dose.
    B. In the cat the initial dose should be 2.5 mg which can be titrated up to 7.5 mg BID in an adult cat.
    C. An effective dose may decrease pulmonary edema, improve mucous membrane color and capillary refill time, increase venous oxygen tension, and lessen the intensity of the murmur(s).

PATENT DUCTUS ARTERIOSUS (PDA)

General Comments

I. Congenital defect
II. Inherited in the miniature poodle and probably in other breeds
III. Most prevalent in females

Pathophysiology

I. Creates a volume overload of the left ventricle, proximal aorta, pulmonary circulation, and left atrium.
II. Signs of heart failure in the young dog are most likely due to severe volume overload of the left ventricle.
III. Heart failure in the adult dog with longstanding, unrecognized PDA is due to severe myocardial failure.

Diagnosis

I. Can usually be confirmed by auscultation and chest radiographs.
II. Nonselective angiography and cardiac catheterization may be needed infrequently to confirm the diagnosis.

Therapy

I. Surgical closure is recommended as soon as the defect is recognized.
II. Diuretic administration is indicated prior to surgery if pulmonary edema is present.
III. Older dogs with PDA and heart failure should be treated the same as a dog with congestive cardiomyopathy and the ductus should be ligated.

RIGHT-TO-LEFT SHUNTS

GENERAL COMMENTS

   I. Right-to-left shunts occur when impedance to pulmonary blood flow is high and a communication is present between the systemic and pulmonary circulations.
   II. Decreased pulmonary blood flow is usually present.
   III. Tetralogy of Fallot and patent ductus arteriosus with pulmonary hypertension are the most common causes in veterinary medicine.
   IV. Other causes include common truncus arteriosus, transposition of the great arteries, and VSD with pulmonic stenosis or pulmonary hypertension.

TETRALOGY OF FALLOT

General Comments

   I. Congenital defect
   II. Inherited in the Keeshound

Pathophysiology

   I. Right-to-left shunt through a VSD occurs because of pulmonic stenosis and overriding aorta.
   II. This results in systemic hypoxemia because of venous blood flowing into the systemic circuit and reduced pulmonary blood flow.
   III. Polycythemia occurs secondary to the hypoxemia.
   IV. The hypoxemia and polycythemia cause cyanosis.
   V. Severe polycythemia increases resistance to blood flow which, in combination with the hypoxemia, can cause poor cerebral oxygen delivery and signs of central nervous system (CNS) dysfunction.

Diagnosis

   I. Clinical signs, auscultation, chest radiographs, and echocardiography suggest the diagnosis.
   II. Diagnosis is confirmed by cardiac catheterization.
   III. Severity can be reasonably assessed by measuring systemic oxygen tension and saturation and hemoglobin concentration or packed cell volume (PCV).

Therapy

   I. If cyanosis and/or polycythemia are present, propranolol (1–2 mg/kg BID to TID) can be administered in an attempt to reduce any subvalvular systolic pressure gradient due to muscular obstruction of the right ventricular outflow tract.

II. If polycythemia is severe [packed cell volume (PCV) >70%] or clinical signs attributable to polycythemia are present, phlebotomy should be performed.

The amount of blood to be withdrawn should be calculated.

A. As an example, start with a dog with a PCV of 75%.

B. The PCV to be achieved must be chosen (60% is reasonable).

C. Divide the desired PCV by the dog's original PCV and subtract from 100% ($100\% - \dfrac{60}{75} = 20\%$ in this case) and multiply that value by the dog's total blood volume (8% × body weight in grams = milliliters of blood) to determine the volume of blood to withdraw.

D. During the phlebotomy infuse a volume of isotonic fluid equal to two to three times the amount of blood withdrawn.

III. Surgical palliation can be used to control clinical signs.

A. Palliative surgical procedures anastomose a systemic artery to a pulmonary artery to increase pulmonary blood flow.

B. The Blalock technique creates an end-to-side anastomosis of the left subclavian artery to the pulmonary artery.

C. The Potts technique is a side-to-side anastomosis of the aorta and pulmonary artery.

D. Surgical correction of the defects requires cardiopulmonary bypass and open heart surgery.

RIGHT-TO-LEFT SHUNTING PATENT DUCTUS ARTERIOSUS

Etiology

I. Persistance of fetal circulation because of continued high pulmonary vascular resistance after birth.

II. Prolonged elevations in pulmonary blood flow and proximal pulmonary arterial pressure resulting in pulmonary vasoconstriction and pulmonary arteriolar disease and degeneration.

Pathophysiology

The pathophysiology is similar to tetralogy of Fallot except cyanosis is usually confined to the caudal regions of the body because the shunt occurs after the arteries to the cranial regions have already exited.

Diagnosis

Diagnosis is based on clinical signs, chest radiographs, echocardiography, and cardiac catheterization.

Therapy

   I. Surgical closure of the PDA is generally contraindicated because patients usually die in the postoperative period.
  II. Phlebotomy is used to control signs of polycythemia.

HEARTWORM DISEASE

ETIOLOGY

   I. Infestation of the right heart and pulmonary arteries with adult *Dirofilaria immitus*
  II. Systemic reactions to circulating microfilaria

PATHOPHYSIOLOGY

   I. Adult worms cause disease in the pulmonary arteries.
     A. Endarteritis and pulmonary embolization create an increase in pulmonary impedance by decreasing the caliber of the pulmonary arteries, decreasing the compliance of the pulmonary arteries, and reducing the total number of arteries available for blood flow.
     B. Pulmonary hypertension results which increases right ventricular afterload which can lead to right ventricular hypertrophy, dilation, and failure.
  II. Allergic reactions to the adult worms and microfilaria can result in secondary disease.
     A. Allergic pneumonitis can result in mild to severe pulmonary dysfunction.
     B. Immune complex glomerulonephritis can be produced leading to proteinuria and possibly hypoalbuminemia and renal failure.
     C. Hypergammaglobulinemia can oftentimes be identified in those patients exhibiting signs of an allergic response to their disease.

DIAGNOSIS

   I. Examination for circulating microfilaria
  II. Chest radiographs and determinations for circulating heartworm antibodies in those cases in which microfilaria are not present (occult heartworm disease)

Pretreatment Evaluation

I. Chest radiographs to assess cardiac and pulmonary abnormalities and to establish a baseline from which posttreatment films can be compared.
II. A complete blood count to detect anemia, inflammatory response, and eosinophilia.
III. Renal function tests and urinalysis to detect renal failure, proteinuria, and urinary tract infection
IV. Serum concentrations of hepatic enzymes may be evaluated.
   A. Mild elevations do not preclude arsenical therapy.
   B. Moderate or severe increases in serum glutamic pyruvic transaminase (SGPT) or serum alkaline phosphatase should prompt further hepatic evaluation if the dog is not in right heart failure and if corticosteroids have not been administered.
V. Dogs with occult heartworm disease should be evaluated closely before treatment.
   A. Special attention should be paid to evaluating the lungs.
      1. Pulmonary changes may be due to pulmonary artery embolization, allergic pneumonitis, or secondary bacterial pneumonia.
      2. If moderate to severe disease is present, and if the dog is not severely dyspneic, transtracheal wash, or bronchoscopy can be performed to obtain material for cytologic exam and bacterial culture.
      3. If predominately eosinophils are obtained, an allergic pneumonitis is most likely present and prednisone (1 mg/kg BID) can be administered.
      4. If bacteria are cultured, an antibiotic should be chosen, based on antibiotic sensitivity of the organism, and therapy initiated.
      5. A nonseptic, noneosinophilic exudate may be identified with a pulmonary embolus.
   B. Several urine samples should be evaluated for evidence of proteinuria. If identified, protein loss should be quantified before treatment.
   C. Serum globulin concentrations should be analyzed.
VI. Dogs with heart failure must also be evaluated carefully and treated for heart failure before adulticide therapy.
   A. Determinations of central venous pressure should be obtained (normal is <11 cm H_2O).
   B. The dog should receive a minimum of 7 days of cage rest before adulticide therapy.
   C. Aspirin (10 mg/kg/day) should be administered.
   D. Furosemide and a low salt diet can be used to reduce the central venous pressure, ascites, and peripheral edema.
   E. Milrinone can be administered to increase the contractility if the right ventricular myocardium.

 F. Digoxin administration does not appear to be beneficial.

 G. Heart failure therapy can oftentimes be discontinued 4–8 weeks after adulticide therapy.

Treatment for Killing Adult Heartworms (Adulticide Therapy)

 I. Thiacetarsemide sodium administration

  A. Dose is 2.2 mg/kg (0.22 ml/kg of a standard 10 mg/ml solution) given BID for 2 days.

  B. Other dosage schedules are either less effective or more toxic.

  C. The drug should be given via a winged infusion set or indwelling intravenous catheter to avoid extravasation of the drug.

   1. Extravasation should be treated by infiltrating the area with isotonic saline and dexamethasone.

   2. Topical dimethyl sulfoxide (DMSO) may also be applied.

  D. Concomitant administration of vitamin C, methionine, choline, or corticosteroids is unnecessary.

   1. Corticosteroid administration may decrease the number of worms killed.

   2. A meal should be given prior to each injection to insure that the dog is not anorectic. If severe anorexia or vomition occur, the drug administration should stop.

 II. Levamisole

  A. The number of adult worms killed is highly variable (0–100%).

  B. The drug is not recommended as an adulticide.

Side Effects of Thiacetarsemide Administration

 I. Anorexia and vomition are common.

  A. Usually they are benign signs and do not necessitate discontinuation of treatment.

  B. If vomition is severe, persistent, or associated with depression, icterus, or azotemia, drug administration should be stopped.

  C. After the drug is stopped, appropriate laboratory work should be performed and supportive therapy given.

 II. Elevations in SGPT and alkaline phosphatase are common but do not necessitate discontinuation of therapy unless hepatic failure is also present.

 III. Treatment should be stopped if hepatic failure occurs.

  A. Earliest evidence may be an increase in bilirubinuria.

  B. Severe bilirubinuria or icterus necessitates discontinuation of therapy.

  C. Thiacetarsemide administration should be tried again in 4 weeks. Complications usually do not reoccur at this time.

  D. Abnormal sulfobromophthalein (BSP) retention probably does not occur with thiacetasamide.

IV. Azotemia may occur during adulticide therapy.
   A. It is usually prerenal and due to vomiting, anorexia, and dehydration.
   B. Renal failure is an uncommon side effect of thiacetarsemide in dogs with no preexisting renal insufficiency.
   C. Renal failure is a contraindication to the use of an arsenical.

Adverse Effects Following Adulticide Therapy

I. Pulmonary embolization with dead worms occurs from 2 days to 3 weeks after the administration of thiacetarsemide
   A. Patients should be confined indoors, usually at home, and any vigorous activity or excitement should be avoided.
   B. Clinical signs of embolization range from no signs to severe pulmonary failure.
   C. Mild coughing may be treated solely with cage rest.
   D. Moderate coughing or mild dyspnea may be treated at home with confinement and corticosteroids.
   E. Severe coughing or dyspnea requires hospitalization along with antibiotic and corticosteroid administration.
      1. Chest radiographs should be monitored.
      2. Arterial blood gases can be monitored.
      3. Oxygen should be administered, preferably via an oxygen cage, if the arterial oxygen tension is <50 mmHg, if dyspnea is severe, or if the patient is cyanotic.
      4. If the dog does not respond to initial therapy, a transtracheal wash or bronchoscopy should be performed to obtain material for cytology abd bacterial culture.
II. Disseminated intravascular coagulation may develop. It suggests a poor to grave prognosis.
III. Right ventricular failure may develop and should be treated as outlined above.

Microfilaricide Therapy

Should begin 4–6 weeks after adulticide therapy.
I. Dithiazanine is the drug of choice.
   A. Initial dose is 8–10 mg/kg for 7 days and a blood sample is rechecked for microfilaria.
   B. If microfilaria are still present, the dose is increased to 12–14 mg/kg for 7–10 days.
   C. Vomition and diarrhea are the most common side effects.
   D. The medication is a purple dye which produces an indelible stain in cloth.

II. Levamisole hydrochloride may be used to kill microfilaria if dithiazanine is not effective. The drug is not approved for use in dogs by the FDA.
   A. Dose is 11 mg/kg administered as a single dose after a small meal for 7 days.
   B. If microfilaria are still present after 7 days, the same dose can be administered for another 5 days. The dose should not be increased.
   C. Vomition is the most common side effect.
      1. If severe, further dosing may be impossible
      2. Smaller doses may be tried but are usually less effective.
      3. Centrally acting antiemetics may be tried but with caution since vomition may be an early indication of CNS toxicity.
   D. Panting, shaking, and agitation are the most common signs of CNS toxicity.
      1. Drug withdrawal will usually solve the problem.
      2. Rarely, more severe signs will develop.
III. Ivermectin is another drug used as a microfilaricide that is not approved for use in dogs by the FDA.
   A. The dose in dogs is 0.05–0.2 mg/kg administered as a single dose orally.
   B. The preferred preparation is the bovine worming product (Ivomec®). It is supplied as a 1% (10 mg/ml) solution in propylene glycol which is used parenterally in cattle.
   C. The drug should not be given to collies or collie-crosses due to reports of fatal reactions in this breed. All dogs should be observed closely following ivermectin administration.
   D. Microfilaria exams are performed weekly after ivermectin administration.
      1. If the exam is negative heartworm prophylatis is initiated.
      2. If the exam is still positive 3 weeks after ivermectin administration, the initial dose can be repeated.
IV. If microfilaria are not killed by recommended doses of dithiazanine, levamisole or ivermectin, adulticide therapy may be repeated.

Heartworm Prophylaxis

I. Dogs in endemic areas should be tested for microfilaremia and placed on diethylcarbamazine (DEC) for prophylaxis if microfilaria are not present.
   A. In northern climates dogs should be tested each spring before starting DEC, and DEC administration should be stopped in December.
   B. In southern climates, DEC should be given year round.
   C. Dogs that have been treated for adult heartworms should be placed on DEC after all of the microfilaria have been killed.
   D. Dose is 5.5–6.5 mg/kg given once daily.
II. If DEC is administered to microfilaremic dogs an immediate hypersensitivity reaction may occur resulting in anaphylactic shock and death.

The Vena Caval Syndrome

  I. Most commonly seen in warmer climates
 II. Is generally associated with a massive (>100) worm burden
III. The only effective treatment is surgical removal of the worms.
  A. An elongated forceps is passed down the jugular vein into the anterior vena cava and right atrium.
  B. Worms are removed until six successive passes have failed to identify any worms.
 IV. Supportive therapy includes fluids, antibiotics, and corticosteroids.
  V. After recovery, thiacetarsemide should be administered to kill the remaining worms.

INFECTIVE ENDOCARDITIS

GENERAL COMMENTS

  I. Is oftentimes difficult to diagnose and to treat
 II. Before initiating therapy a strong attempt should be made to make a definitive diagnosis and to identify the causative organism.
III. The course of the disease depends on the aggressiveness of the organism, the stage of the disease, and the ability to identify and to eliminate the organism.
 IV. The organisms most commonly reside on the aortic and mitral valves in dogs and cats.
  V. The organisms either cause valvular destruction or vegetative lesions that produce septic emboli or interfere with valvular function.

CLINICAL SIGNS

Acute Bacterial Endocarditis

  I. Patients are usually acutely ill, have high-grade fevers, evidence of embolic disease, and may or may not have a murmur.
 II. If a murmur is not present at presentation, it may develop during the course of hospitalization.

Subacute Bacterial Endocarditis

  I. Patients generally have low-grade or recurrent fevers.
 II. They may or may not have murmurs and have usually been ill for some period of time.
III. They may have signs related to embolic disease.
 IV. They may present because of organ dysfunction from chronic embolization or from chronic immunologic disease.

Therapy

Acute Bacterial Endocarditis

I. Blood cultures (two to three within the first 2–6 hours) should be taken before antibiotics are administered.
II. Urine cultures may be helpful in identifying the organism present in the bloodstream.
III. Antibiotic therapy should not be withheld until culture results are obtained.
   A. An antibiotic may be chosen based on culture results of a previous infection or based on the history of an infection in a certain region of the body.
   B. If there is no present or historical infection, antibiotic treatment must be empirical (a combination of a penicillinase resistant penicillin and an aminoglycoside, e.g., oxacillin plus gentamicin, is appropriate).

Subacute Bacterial Endocarditis

I. Blood cultures should be collected immediately from a febrile patient.
II. In cases that have recurrent fevers, blood cultures should be taken during a febrile episode, preferably while the animal's temperature is rising.
III. At least three to four samples, for aerobic and anaerobic culture, should be taken over 24 hours.
IV. In most cases antibiotic therapy can be withheld until blood culture results are obtained.
V. An appropriate antibiotic should then be administered.
VI. If an organism cannot be identified from blood or urine culture, a combination of a penicillinase-resistant penicillin and gentamicin should be administered.
VII. If this combination is not successful, a cephalosporin or a combination of trimethoprim and a sulfonamide may be tried.

Antibiotics (see chapter 3)

In order for an antibiotic to be effective in bacterial endocarditis it should be:
I. Bactericidal
II. Able to penetrate fibrin
III. Continued for at least 4–6 weeks
IV. Antibiotic therapy of bacterial endocarditis is most effective when the antibiotic is administered parenterally.
V. IV boluses are preferred over IV infusions which are preferred over IM injections.

Corticosteroids

Corticosteroids are absolutely contraindicated in patients in which the possibility of bacterial endocarditis exists as the outcome of such treatment is usually fatal.

SYSTEMIC HYPERTENSION

GENERAL COMMENTS

I. Essential hypertension is rare in the dog and cat.
II. Hypertension secondary to renal failure is probably relatively common in small animals although it is usually not recognized.
III. Hyperadrenocorticism also causes systemic hypertension in the dog.
IV. If hypertension is recognized, blood pressure control should be attempted.
   A. Prolonged hypertension can produce vascular damage, myocardial hypertrophy, further renal damage, and myocardial failure.
   B. In patients with mitral regurgitation, hypertension increases the severity of regurgitation.

PATHOPHYSIOLOGY

I. In people, renal hypertension is usually due to an increase in blood volume.
II. In some patients a major component of the disease is an increase in peripheral vascular resistance, usually associated with elevations in plasma renin activity.
III. The cause of hypertension in hyperadrenocorticism is thought to be multifactorial, including volume expansion, increased production of angiotensin II, and increased sensitivity of vascular smooth muscle to vasoactive agents.

THERAPY

I. The treatment of renal hypertension has not been studied in canine patients so recommendations are based on experimental studies in the dog and clinical experience in man.
   A. Dietary sodium restriction and diuretics are the mainstays of therapy.
      1. Thiazides may be effective if the serum creatinine concentration is less than 2.5 mg/dl.
      2. If it is greater than 2.5 mg/dl in human patients, furosemide, oftentimes in high doses, is required.
   B. Patients that are resistant to the above treatment may be given propranolol (0.5–2.0 mg/kg BID to TID) along with diuretics.
   C. The vasodilators hydralazine and captopril can be used if the patient is unresponsive to diuretics and propranolol.

  D. Captopril may be especially effective in patients with elevated plasma
     renin concentrations.
 II. Hypertension secondary to hyperadrenocorticism is treated by correcting
     the underlying disease.
     A. The same measures used to treat renal hypertension can be used.
     B. Diuretics that cause potassium loss should be used with caution.
III. Essential hypertension is treated the same as renal hypertension.

PULMONARY HYPERTENSION

ETIOLOGY

  I. Is usually caused by heartworm disease or chronic respiratory disease in
     the dog.
 II. Pulmonary hypertension secondary to chronic respiratory disease can be
     due to chronic hypoxemia with or without hypercarbia, causing pulmonary
     vasoconstriction or obliteration of capillaries and small pulmonary arteries.
III. Obliteration of pulmonary vasculature is common in interstitial pulmonary
     fibrosis in people.

THERAPY

  I. Treatment of heartworm disease has already been discussed.
 II. When the inciting cause is pulmonary disease, treatment is aimed at the
     underlying disease.
     A. Successful reduction of pulmonary artery pressures is usually associ-
        ated with an increase in arterial oxygen tension.
     B. Chronic oxygen administration is successful in human patients but usu-
        ally impractical in the dog.
III. Hydralazine is a potentially useful drug.
     A. It decreases pulmonary artery pressures in some cases in people.
     B. If used in a dog, pulmonary and systemic arterial blood pressures should
        be monitored to document efficacy and to avoid systemic hypotension.
 IV. Phentolamine, diazoxide, prazosin, and isoproterenol have been reported
     to be successful in selected cases in the human literature.

PULMONARY THROMBOEMBOLISM

GENERAL COMMENTS

  I. This is an uncommon cause of acute pulmonary hypertension in the dog.
 II. It may occur in postoperative patients or spontaneously in dogs with hy-
     peradrenocorticism, hypothyroidism, or glomerulopathies.

III. Patients are usually presented for acute respiratory distress. Diagnosis should be confirmed by angiography prior to therapy.

THERAPY

I. Heparin should be administered.
   A. Initial dose is 200–225 mg/kg followed by 75–125 mg/kg every 4 hours for the first 24 hours followed by boluses of 60–80 mg/kg every 6 hours.
   B. The activated partial thromboplastin time (APTT) should be prolonged to 1.5–2.5 times the baseline value.
II. After APTT prolongation is achieved, oral administration of crystalline warfarin sodium can begin.
   A. An initial dose of 0.2 mg/kg once daily is administered.
   B. After that, doses from 0.05 to 0.1 mg/kg can be given once daily.
   C. The prothrombin time should be prolonged 1.5–2.5 times the baseline value.
   D. When this happens, heparin administration can be discontinued.
   E. Warfarin administration should continue, until the pulmonary arteries are angiographically normal.
III. If bleeding develops the administration of anticoagulants should be stopped. Fresh plasma or blood may be given. Vitamin K_1 will help reverse the effects of warfarin.

SHOCK

PATHOPHYSIOLOGY AND CLINICAL SIGNS

I. Shock is a syndrome brought about by inadequate tissue perfusion.
II. Inadequate blood flow results in cellular hypoxia with resultant cell injury, dysfunction, and death.
III. Poor perfusion also results in inadequate transport of other nutrients to the cells and inadequate removal of metabolic by-products from the cellular environment.
IV. Poor perfusion is recognized clinically, in the more common forms of shock, as a prolonged capillary refill time and poor mucous membrane color.
V. The mixed venous oxygen tension is decreased when perfusion is inadequate.
VI. Arterial blood pressure may be low.
   A. Poor cerebral blood flow occurs when arterial blood pressures de-

crease below 60–70 mmHg and oftentimes causes alterations in consciousness.
  B. Hypotension also results in oliguria.
VII. Metabolic acidosis may be present.

PATIENT MONITORING DURING SHOCK

  I. Blood gas evaluation is highly desirable in any shock patient.
    A. Analysis of blood pH, partial pressure of carbon dioxide, and bicarbonate concentration by a blood gas analyzer is preferred but measurements of only bicarbonate by an Oxford titrator or total carbon dioxide by an Harleco apparatus may be substituted.
    B. If the pH is <7.20 or if the bicarbonate concentration is <12 mEq/L, bicarbonate replacement should be considered.
      1. If the base deficit is known, the formula, base deficit × 0.3 × kg body weight, can be used to calculate the amount of bicarbonate to administer.
      2. If only bicarbonate concentration is known, the bicarbonate deficit (26 − blood bicarbonate concentration) can be substituted for base deficit.
    C. The clinical status of the patient determines how rapidly bicarbonate is replaced.
      1. Only in emergency situations should sodium bicarbonate be given as an IV bolus.
      2. In most shock patients sodium bicarbonate should be added to 1/2 strength saline and 1/2 the total dose administered over 30 minutes to an hour.
      3. At that time the acid-base balance should be rechecked and appropriate changes in therapy made.
      4. Sodium bicarbonate is extremely hypertonic so it should not be added to isotonic solutions.
      5. Even in emergency situations overzealous bolusing of bicarbonate must be avoided since marked hypernatremia, hyperosmolality, and brain damage may occur.
      6. Patients with heart failure should not receive sodium bicarbonate and those patients with cardiac disease should receive it with extreme caution.
      7. Trihydroxymethylaminomethane (TRIS) (0.4 × base deficit × kg body weight = mEq of TRIS) may be substituted.
  II. If blood gas analysis is not available, a clinical judgement of the severity of shock must be made.
    A. The judgement should be based on the severity and duration of clinical signs.
      1. Patients classified as mild can receive 1 mEq/kg of sodium bicarbonate over 2–3 hours.

    2. Patients with moderate signs may receive 2–3 mEq/kg over 2–3 hours.

    3. Severe, prolonged shock can be treated with up to 3–4 mEq/kg over 1–2 hours.

  B. If the patient is not responding or if additional bicarbonate administration is anticipated, every effort to obtain a blood gas determination should be made.

III. When large volumes of fluid are being administered to a shock patient, measurements of CVP or pulmonary capillary wedge pressure (PCWP) are desirable.

  A. The CVP is measured easily by placing a long polyethylene catheter into the anterior vena cava or right atrium via the jugular vein.

    1. The catheter is attached to a manometer filled with fluid via a three-way stopcock.

    2. The manometer is opened to the catheter and the fluid level allowed to stabilize and read as the height of the fluid column above the right atrium.

  B. The measurement of PCWP requires the placement of a catheter within the pulmonary artery.

    1. A Swan-Ganz flow-directed catheter is generally used.

    2. Placement requires an experienced person and facilities for image intensification and/or pressure recording.

IV. Mixed venous oxygen tension is a direct indicator of the adequacy of total tissue oxygenation.

  A. When oxygen delivery to the tissues decreases below an adequate level due to poor blood flow, hypoxemia, or anemia, the venous effluent has a lowered oxygen tension or pressure.

  B. In shock, other than septic shock, or in heart failure, poor tissue blood flow results in poor tissue oxygenation and a decreased mixed venous oxygen tension.

  C. Measurement of mixed venous blood requires sampling from the pulmonary artery which may be impossible

    1. Sampling from the right atrium via a jugular catheter is a good substitute.

    2. Sampling from the anterior vena cava or jugular vein only measures the adequacy of oxygen delivery to the upper regions of the body but sampling is more practical.

  D. Normal = 35–45 mmHg.

    1. When <30 mmHg, therapeutic intervention is advised.

    2. When <20 mmHg, oxygen tension at the ends of capillaries is inadequate to maintain oxygen diffusion into cells. Anaerobic metabolism predominates, lactic acid is produced, and cells die.

V. Systemic arterial blood pressure is a poor index of tissue perfusion and cardiac output.

  A. It is the major determinant of cerebral, myocardial, and renal blood flow so it is useful to monitor during patient evaluation and therapy.

B. Invasive monitoring via an indwelling arterial catheter is preferred since peripheral vasoconstriction is present in shock and noninvasive determinations of blood pressure may be inaccurate.

C. Mean arterial blood pressure should be maintained above 60–70 mmHg to insure adequate flow to the aforementioned critical vascular beds.
   1. Fluid therapy is the treatment of choice to increase blood pressure.
   2. Dopamine and dobutamine may be used in unresponsive patients.
   3. Vasopressors are generally contraindicated and should be used only if all other measures fail.

VI. Urine output should be monitored in most patients in shock.
   A. An indwelling urinary catheter should be placed aseptically and a closed collection system should be maintained.
   B. Effective therapy should result in urine flow rates of 0.5–1.0 ml/kg/hr or greater.

THERAPY

I. Hypovolemic shock
   A. The primary treatment is rapid replacement of fluid volume (90 ml/kg within 30 minutes is a safe limit for a dog if heart failure or oliguric renal failure is not present; 60 ml/kg is the limit in cats) with an isotonic crystalloid fluid, such as lactated Ringer's solution or isotonic saline solution.
   B. If the PCV is below 20%, whole blood or packed red cell replacement is indicated.
   C. If the total plasma protein is <3.0 g/dl after fluid therapy, the administration of plasma or a colloid solution (dextran 70) is indicated.
   D. If there is any question of the patient's ability to tolerate the fluid volume, CVP or PCWP should be monitored. The CVP should be maintained below 15 cm H_2O and the PCWP below 18 mmHg.
   E. Glucocorticoid administration is controversial but its short-term use poses little risk and the potential benefits greatly outweigh any potential harm.
      1. Prednisolone sodium succinate (35 mg/kg) is recommended.
      2. Dexamethasone has very slow cellular uptake (>3 hours) and is not recommended as an initial agent for improving survival in shock.

II. Cardiogenic shock (a decrease in forward cardiac output caused by a cardiac disease severe enough to produce tissue hypoxia)
   A. If cardiac function can be assessed, appropriate therapy should be administered.
   B. If cardiac function cannot be assessed IV fluids should be administered and if no response is seen or if fluid overload occurs, dopamine or dobutamine should be administered.
   C. If a patient with known cardiovascular disease is presented, acutely decompensated and in shock, dobutamine should be administered and

the patient treated the same as outlined in the section on Valvular Disease.

1. Fluids should be administered with extreme caution or not at all.
2. If fluids are administered, 5% dextrose in water or half-strength saline are preferred and serum electrolyte concentrations should be monitored.

III. Septic Shock
   A. The initial stage of gram-negative sepsis may be characterized by pyrexia, vasodilation, an increased cardiac output, and an elevated venous oxygen tension (>45 mmHg in the author's experience).
   B. Later in the course, cardiac output decreases, vasoconstriction occurs, and venous oxygen tension decreases.
   C. Blood cultures and cultures of exudate should be obtained before therapy.
   D. Antibiotic therapy must be started immediately after culture so the antibiotic selection is usually empirical.
      1. Gentamicin is frequently the drug of choice when gram-negative sepsis is suspected.
      2. Penicillinase-resistant penicillins should be used when the probability of a gram-positive organism is suspected.
   E. Specific treatment of the underlying disease is mandatory for survival.
   F. Large volumes of fluid are needed to maintain vascular volume.
   G. Glucocorticoids are of no benefit and may be harmful to patients with septic shock.
   H. Dopamine (1–10 μg/kg/minute) may be beneficial if the response to fluid administration is poor.

IV. Anaphylactic shock (see chapter 6)
   A. Anaphylactic shock usually occurs after exposure to an environmental antigen (e.g., a beesting) or to a drug (e.g., DEC, vaccines, local anesthetics, BSP, iodinated contrast materials).
   B. Cardiovascular collapse and/or respiratory distress occur peracutely.
      1. Respiratory distress may be due to laryngeal edema, bronchospasm, or both.
      2. Death can occur within minutes.
   C. Epinephrine is the drug of choice; 1.0 ml of a 1:1,000 solution should be diluted in 10 ml of saline (1:10,000 solution) and 1 ml/10 kg should be administered IV or IM. This may be repeated every 5–15 minutes.
   D. Endotracheal intubation or tracheostomy may be required.
   E. IV fluids should be administered as rapidly as possible.
   F. Aminophylline may be given for bronchospasm.
   G. An antihistaminic should be administered to prevent relapse.

ACUTE HEART FAILURE THERAPY

I. Acute heart failure is treated according to the type of cardiac failure that exists.

   A. If myocardial failure is present, positive inotropic agents (dobutamine, milrinone) should be administered (see Section on Myocardial Disease, above). Vasodilators (nitroprusside, hydralazine) may also be beneficial.
   B. If a severe volume overload is present due to valvular regurgitation or left-to-right shunts, diuretics and arteriolar dilators (hydralazine) can be used (see section on Valvular Disease, above).
II. If an assessment of cardiovascular function cannot be made because of lack of equipment or time, therapeutic decisions should be based on clinical signs.
   A. Patients that have only evidence of peripheral hypoperfusion (prolonged capillary refill time, poor mucous membrane color, low venous oxygen tension) should initially be treated with IV fluid administration.
      1. Central venous pressure or PCWP should be monitored (see the present section on Shock, above).
      2. If fluid overload occurs and the patient has not responded, fluid administration should be discontinued and dobutamine, dopamine, milrinone (see section on Myocardial Disease, above) or vasodilators administered.
   B. Patients with only pulmonary edema should be treated in the same way as patients with acute mitral regurgitation (see section on Valvular Disease, above).
      1. Diuretics are standard therapy.
      2. If mitral valve regurgitation or a left-to-right shunt is present, hydralazine administration is usually beneficial.
      3. If hypoperfusion occurs, dopamine, dobutamine, or milrinone may be administered.
   C. If both hypoperfusion and pulmonary edema are present, diuretics, arteriolar dilators, and positive inotropic agents are indicated.

SUGGESTED READINGS

Braunwald E: Clinical manifestations of heart failure. p. 493. In Braunwald E (ed): Heart Disease: A Textbook of Cardiovascular Medicine. WB Saunders, Philadelphia, 1980

Braunwald E: Pathophysiology of heart failure. p. 453. In Braunwald E (ed): Heart Disease: A Textbook of Cardiovascular Medicine. WB Saunders, Philadelphia, 1980.

Burns MG: Pulmonary thromboembolism. p. 257. In Kirk RW (ed): Current Veterinary Therapy. Vol. 8. WB Saunders, Philadelphia, 1983.

Calvert CA, Rawlings CA: Diagnosis and management of canine heartworm disease. p. 348. In Kirk RW (ed): Current Veterinary Therapy. Vol. 8. WB Saunders, Philadelphia, 1983.

Fox PR: Feline myocardial diseases. p. 337. In Kirk RW (ed): Current Veterinary Therapy. Vol. 8. WB Saunders, Philadelphia, 1983.

Kittleson MD: Concepts and therapeutic strategies in the management of heart failure. p. 279. In Kirk RW (ed): Current Veterinary Therapy. Vol. 8. WB Saunders, Philadelphia, 1983.

Kittleson MD: Drugs used in the management of heart failure. p. 285. In Kirk RW (ed): Current Veterinary Therapy. Vol. 8. WB Saunders, Philadelphia, 1983.

Kittleson MD, Eyster GE, Olivier NB, Anderson LK: Oral hydralazine therapy for chronic mitral regurgitation in the dog. J Am Vet Med Assoc 182:1205, 1983.

Kittleson MD, Hamlin RL: Hydralazine pharmacodynamics in the dog. Am J Vet Res 44:1501, 1983.

Smith TW, Braunwald E: The management of heart failure. p. 509. In Braunwald E (ed): Heart Disease: A Textbook of Cardiovascular Medicine. WB Saunders, Philadelphia, 1980.

Sprung CL, Caralis PV, Marcial EH, et al: The effects of high-dose corticosteroids in patients with septic shock. A prospective, controlled study. N Engl J Med 311:1137, 1984.

10

Cardiac Dysrhythmias

Jeff R. Wilcke, D.V.M.

The management of cardiac dysrhythmias is a formidable challenge to the practicing veterinarian. Knowledge of the basic pathophysiology of dysrhythmias and pharmacotherapeutics of antidysrhythmic drugs has increased dramatically in recent years. Clinical correlates for basic electrophysiologic mechanisms are, however, difficult to derive and useful pharmacokinetic information about many drugs used in veterinary patients is lacking. As a consequence, specific drug therapy for cardiac dysrhythmias has remained empirical.

Emphasis in this chapter is on the correction of underlying cardiac and noncardiac abnormalities, specific drug therapy, and the clinical pharmacology of the antidysrhythmic drugs used in small animal practice.

PREMATURE ECTOPIC BEATS

SUPRAVENTRICULAR PREMATURE CONTRACTIONS

I. Definition

Supraventricular premature contractions (SPC) arise from cardiac tissue above the ventricles, including the area of the sinoatrial (SA) node, right and left atria, atrioventricular (AV) node, and junctional tissue. Electrocardiographically they are seen as premature P waves of abnormal configuration (less so as the ectopic focus nears the SA node) (Fig. 10-1). P Waves may be absent if the rhythm is nodal or junctional.

II. Associated disease

Generally SPCs are associated with atrial disease such as atrial dilatation and atrial myocarditis. Junctional premature contractions may also result from drug intoxication (including digitalis), excessive vagal tone, and AV node irritability.

III. Clinical signs

Animals are usually asymptomatic although syncope and paroxysmal weakness may occur.

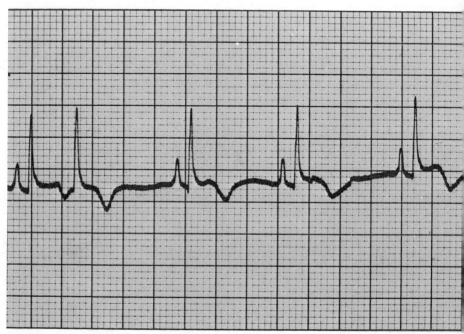

Fig. 10-1. Supraventricular Premature Contraction. The second beat from the left is a typical APC. The P wave is obscured by the preceding T-wave. The QRS complex and T wave of the APC appear normal. Paper speed = 25 mm/sec. Sensitivity: 1 cm = 1 mv. Lead II. (Reprinted with permission from Pyle, RL: Tachyarrhythmia. pp 381–388. In Kirk RW (ed): Current Veterinary Therapy VII. WB Saunders, Philadelphia, 1980).

IV. Treatment

Isolated and infrequent SPCs do not require therapy. Therapeutic digitalization is indicated for patients with concurrent congestive heart failure.

VENTRICULAR PREMATURE CONTRACTIONS

I. Definition

Ectopic foci which arise distal to the bundle of His and result in ventricular contraction are ventricular premature contractions (VPCs). Their electrocardiographic appearance may vary from fairly normal QRS complexes without associated P waves (near the bundle of His) to wide bizarre complexes (more distal) (Fig. 10-2).

II. Disease associations

Ventricular premature contractions are seen in association with cardiovascular disease, drug intoxication (including digitalis), anxiety, stress, and cardiac manipulation during cardiac catheterization and surgery.

III. Clinical signs

Isolated VPCs rarely result in clinical signs. Multiple VPCs may cause weakness, syncope, and occasionally seizure-like signs.

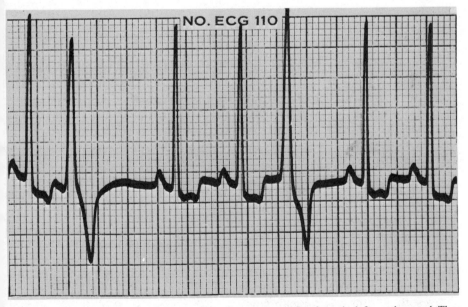

Fig. 10-2. Ventricular Premature Contractions. Beats two and five from the left are abnormal. They occur prematurely and are followed by a pause. The QRST complexes appear bizarre when compared with the beats originating in the sino-atrial node. In the normal beats there is P wave prolongation (P mitrale), S-T segment depression, and high amplitude T waves. Paper speed = 25 mm/sec. Sensitivity: 1/2 cm = 1 mv. Lead II. (Reprinted with permission from Pyle RL: Tachyarrhythmia. pp 381–388. In Kirk RW (ed): Current Veterinary Therapy VII. WB Saunders, Philadelphia, 1980).

IV. Treatment
   A. Drug intoxication
      Withdraw the offending agent. In the specific case of cardiac gly-coside intoxication, the glycoside should be withheld until electrocar-diographic evidence of toxicity abates. Digitalis may then be reinsti-tuted at a lower total daily dose.
   B. Antiarrhythmics
      Lidocaine should be considered the drug of first choice. Procain-amide, quinidine, disopyramide, and aprindine can be used for lido-caine-resistant VPCs. Phenytoin is particularly effective for cardiac glycoside-induced VPCs. The use of antidysrhythmic agents that are negative inotropes (quinidine, disopyramide, and to a lesser extent pro-cainamide) is discouraged in the presence of congestive heart failure.
   C. Cardiac glycosides
      Cardiac glycosides may be beneficial in the treatment of VPCs as-sociated with congestive heart failure. Close clinical supervision and electrocardiographic monitoring are necessary.

TACHYCARDIA

Supraventricular Tachycardia

   I. Definition
      Two forms of supraventricular tachycardia are recognized. Sinus tach-ycardia arises from the normal pacemaker within the sinus node while atrial tachycardia is generated by one or more ectopic foci within the atria. The two can be differentiated electrocardiographically (Fig. 10-3). The former gives P waves of normal configuration and the latter gives abnormal or changing P waves. In either event the heart rate is generally in excess of 180 beats/min.
  II. Disease associations
      Supraventricular tachycardias are associated with pain, fever, anxiety, congestive heart failure, hyperthyroidism, electric shock, and drug intox-ication (i.e., anticholinergic overdose).
 III. Clinical signs
      Clinical signs are generally compatible with the underlying disease state.
  IV. Treatment
      Physiologic tachycardia associated with pain or anxiety requires no spe-cific therapy. Therapeutic intervention is necessary only for tachycardia resulting from specific pathology.
      A. Vagal maneuvers
         Carotid sinus or direct ocular pressure will usually result in temporary remission of the tachycardia.
      B. Vasopressors
         α-Adrenergic agonists such as phenylephrine or methoxamine can be

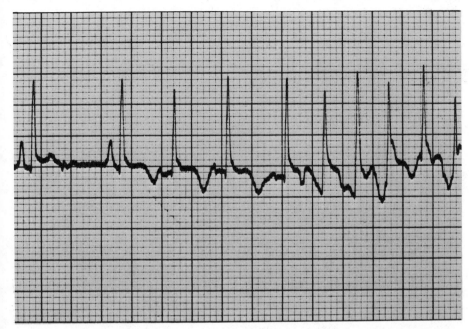

Fig. 10-3. Supraventricular tachycardia. The first two beats from the left are normal. The third beat is premature, with the P wave partially obscured by the preceding T wave. The last six complexes are part of a paroxysmal atrial tachycardia with a rate of 300/minute. Paper speed = 25 mm/sec. Sensitivity: 1 cm = 1 mv. Lead II. (Reprinted with permission from Pyle RL: Tachyarrhythmia. pp 381–388. In Kirk RW (ed): Current Veterinary Therapy VII. WB Saunders, Philadelphia, 1980).

used to elevate blood pressure and reflexly increase vagal tone on a short-term basis.

C. Cardiac glycosides

Therapeutic digitalization is indicated for supraventricular tachycardia associated with congestive heart failure. Its effects slow the heart rate by delaying AV conduction and improving the contractile performance of the myocardium. Compensatory sympathetic stimulation of heart rate is subsequently diminished (see Chapter 9).

VENTRICULAR TACHYCARDIA

I. Definition

Ventricular tachycardia (VT) is generated by an impulse arising within the ventricular myocardium at a rate greater than that of the coexisting sinus node pacemaker. As with ventricular premature contractions, the QRS complexes may vary from fairly normal to wide and bizarre (Fig. 10-4). P Waves may or may not be discernible. Ventricular tachycardia should be considered a serious and possibly profibrillatory rhythm.

II. Associated disease

Ventricular tachycardia may be associated with a wide variety of cardiac pathologies, including myocarditis, advanced congestive heart failure (myocardial anoxia), electrolyte disturbances (especially hypokalemia), hypoxia, endocarditis, heartworm disease, and advanced congenital defects.

III. Clinical signs

Clinical signs can include: dyspnea, weakness, collapse, and seizure-like disorders. Pulse deficits are common and poor peripheral perfusion may be evident.

IV. Treatment

A. Underlying disorders

Drugs (particularly cardioactive drugs) being used at the time VT is documented should be discontinued until the cause of the dysrhythmia is determined. Systemic hypoxia can be corrected with appropriate oxygen therapy. Potassium chloride, at a rate not to exceed 0.5 mEq/kg/hr should be administered if hypokalemia exists. Sodium bicarbonate therapy (see chapter 2) can be instituted if metabolic acidosis has been documented.

B. Positive Inotropes

Therapeutic digitalization can be useful in the management of VT

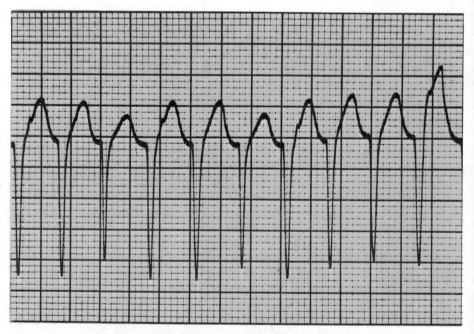

Fig. 10-4. Ventricular tachycardia. There are rapid (200/minute), regular; and bizarre-appearing QRST complexes. Paper speed = 25 mm/sec. Sensitivity 1 cm = 1 mv. Lead II. (Reprinted with permission from Pyle RL: Tachyarrhythmia. pp 381–388. In Kirk RW (ed): Current Veterinary Therapy VII. WB Saunders, Philadelphia, 1980).

associated with congestive heart failure. Close clinical supervision and electrocardiographic monitoring are indicated. Recently, dobutamine (see chapter 9) has emerged as a potential drug of choice for short-term inotropic support in congestive heart failure, particularly in the presence of ventricular dysrhythmias.

C. Antidysrhythmia agents

Lidocaine, procainamide, quinidine, and phenytoin are considered to be the drugs of choice (in decreasing order of preference). Lidocaine and phenytoin are thought to be particularly useful for the management of cardiac glycoside-induced VT. Newer antidysrhythmic agents such as disopyramide, encainide, tocainide, and verapamil appear to be useful although clinical documentation is sparse.

D. Direct-current cardioversion

Direct current countershock can be used to terminate VT. It is probably best to avoid this modality unless the defibrillator automatically synchronizes its discharge with the cardiac cycle. Failure to do so can result in ventricular fibrillation.

ATRIAL FIBRILLATION

I. Definition

Atrial fibrillation is defined as an absence of synchronized atrial contraction. Normal atrial P waves are replaced by undulating F waves on the electrocardiogram (Fig. 10-5).

II. Associated disease

Atrial fibrillation in the dog and cat should be considered a sign of serious and advanced heart disease. It is generally associated with significant enlargement of one or both atria, and occurs primarily in large to giant breed dogs (particularly males).

III. Clinical signs

In most cases atrial fibrillation is associated with signs consistent with congestive heart failure.

IV. Treatment

Atrial fibrillation is rarely treated as an isolated clinical entity. As it is generally associated with congestive heart failure, treatment for atrial fibrillation becomes part of an overall management scheme. The primary therapeutic objective is to decrease the ventricular rate. Termination of atrial fibrillation is, in the authors experience, coincidental with improved cardiac function.

A. Cardiac glycosides

Digitalis slows the ventricular rate through both vagal and extravagal mechanisms. The net therapeutic effects are to slow AV conduction, increase atrial frequency (lessens the potential for ventricular following), and increase contractile performance.

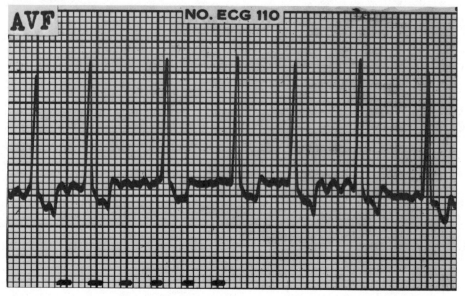

Fig. 10-5. Atrial fibrillation. The ECG is characterized by a rapid and irregular R-R interval, absence of P waves, and presence of fibrillation (f) waves. Heart rate = 140/minute. Paper speed = 25 mm/sec. Sensitivity: 1 cm = 1 mv. Lead II. (Reprinted with permission from Pyle RL: Tachyarrhythmia. pp 381–388. In Kirk RW (ed): Current Veterinary Therapy VII. WB Saunders, Philadelphia, 1980).

B. β_1-Adrenergic blockade

If digitalization fails to reduce the ventricular rate sufficiently, orally administered propranolol may be effective. The negative inotropic potential of β_1-adrenergic blockade should be considered if propranolol is used without prior therapeutic digitalization. Pure β_1-adrenergic blocking drugs such as practolol and atenolol have not received sufficient therapeutic evaluation to comment on their potential use.

C. Antiarrhythmics

Quinidine may be used to convert atrial fibrillation to normal sinus rhythm. Paradoxically, quinidine's vagolytic effects may actually lead to dangerous increases in ventricular rate by enhancing AV conduction. This effect is prevented by prior therapeutic digitalization which (by vagal mechanisms) delays AV conduction. Other antidysrhythmics, such as disopyramide and procainamide can be considered and offer the same potential risks and benefits as does quinidine. The success rate for conversion of atrial fibrillation to normal sinus rhythm is low and quite variable among authors. In severe heart failure, the negative inotropic effects of active antiarrhythmics preclude their use. Therapy should be directed at improved ventricular function and reduced ventricular rate.

The place of verapamil and other slow calcium-channel blockers is yet to be established in veterinary medicine.

I. Definition

Ventricular fibrillation is characterized by a complete lack of well-defined QRS complexes and an absence of coordinated ventricular contraction.

II. Associated disease

Ventricular fibrillation is seen as the terminal dysrhythmia in a wide variety of cardiac and noncardiac diseases.

III. Clinical signs

Signs seen with ventricular failure characterize cardiovascular collapse. Hemodynamically, ventricular fibrillation is equivalent to cardiac arrest.

IV. Treatment

Ventricular fibrillation, like cardiac arrest, is a true medical emergency. Therapy must be instituted immediately if there is to be any chance for success.

A. Airway

Endotracheal intubation to insure delivery of oxygen must be performed first. Artificial ventilation by mouth, Ambu bag, or mechanical respirator is instituted. If available, 100% oxygen administered at a rate of 140 ml/kg/min is helpful.

B. Cardiac massage

A sharp blow to the precordium is made and followed by external message. If external massage does not produce a palpable peripheral pulse, internal message via thoracotomy can be considered. Effective cardiac massage is essential for delivery of oxygen and emergency drugs to the myocardium; removal of metabolic waste and maintenance of vital organ function.

C. Adrenergic agents

β_1-Adrenergic stimulation, a property shared by epinephrine, isoproterenol, norepinephrine, and dopamine results in increased excitability of conductive tissue. Epinephrine is the preferred drug in this situation as it possesses α-adrenergic activity (which isoproterenol lacks). α-Adrenergic stimulation increases peripheral resistance necessary to enhance myocardial blood flow during resuscitation and can result in a coarsening of the fibrillatory pattern. Unlike norepinephrine, epinephrine stimulates β_2-receptors. This β_2-stimulation may be important in the post-resuscitation period in order to prevent reflex bradycardia and to enhance blood flow to vital organs.

D. DC countershock

Cardiopulmonary resuscitation (CPR), ventilation, and emergency drugs are a prelude to definitive therapy for ventricular fibrillation. As in atrial fibrillation, direct current countershock causes depolarization of the entire myocardium. If successful, control is resumed by a single pacemaker somewhere within the myocardium.

E. Chemical defibrillation

If an electrical defibrillator is unavailable, chemical defibrillation can be attempted. Acetylcholine (6 mg/kg) and potassium chloride (1 mEq/kg) are administered by intracardiac injection. As with DC countershock the entire myocardium is depolarized. Cardiopulmonary resuscitation is continued until spontaneous ventricular rhythm occurs. While this method has gained experimental support, clinical use needs to be evaluated.

BRADYARRHYTHMIAS

SINUS BRADYCARDIA

I. Definition

Sinus bradycardia is recognized by normal QRS complexes in either sinus rhythm or sinus arrhythmia at a heart rate of less than 70 beats/min.

II. Associated disease

Sinus bradycardia is generally recognized in large or giant breed dogs, and athletic or highly trained animals. It is generally not a sign of significant disease.

III. Clinical signs

Sinus bradycardia is not usually accompanied by clinical signs. Occasionally patients may manifest weakness, syncope, or lethargy.

IV. Treatment

Treatment of this condition is generally unnecessary in the absence of clinical signs. If clinical signs are apparent, treatment is the same as for other forms of bradycardia (see below).

SINOATRIAL ARREST

I. Definition

Sinoatrial arrest (SA) is said to occur when the next regularly scheduled atrial depolarization does not occur. Electrocardiographically it is characterized by an absence of an expected P wave and its accompanying QRS-T complex. Generally the PP interval will be at least twice that of the dominant PP interval. At times AV nodal or Purkinje tissue temporarily assumes dominance and junctional or ventricular escape beats result.

II. Associated disease

Sinoatrial arrest is seen in association with excessive vagal stimulation, digitalis, quinidine, and other drug intoxications. Occasionally this rhythm is documented along with atrial pathology such as enlargement or fibrosis. Sinoatrial arrest arrest can be seen unaccompanied by detectable primary disease, particularly in brachycephalic breeds.

III. Clinical signs

Clinical signs that occur include weakness, ataxia, or syncope.

IV. Treatment
  It is unnecessary to treat SA arrest not associated with clinical signs.
  A. Underlying causes
    Electrolyte imbalances should be corrected as indicated following evaluation of serum electrolyte concentrations. Treatment for cerebral edema may be indicated if excessive vagal tone is associated with intracranial trauma or disease.
  B. Adrenergic drugs
    Epinephrine, isoproterenol, or dopamine can be used to support heart rate and speed AV conduction.
  C. Anticholinergics
    Atropine and atropine-like drugs (glycopyrrolate) may be beneficial. They are definitely indicated as preoperative medications if SA arrest exists. Successful (long-term management of SA arrest has been accomplished with oral prochlorperazine and prochlorperazine in combination with isopropramide).

ATRIOVENTRICULAR BLOCK

I. Definition
  A partial delay or complete obstruction to impulse conduction from the atria to the ventricles defines AV block. The severity or completeness of the block is subdivided into first, second, and third degree.
  A. First degree
    The PR interval is greater than 0.13 seconds and each P wave is followed by an associated QRS complex.
  B. Second degree
    The PR interval increases progressively until a QRS complex is dropped (type I, Wenkenbach phenomenon) or the PR interval remains unchanged and an occasional QRS complex is dropped (type II. Mobitz) (Fig. 10-6).
  C. Third degree
    The atrial rate is rapid and unassociated with QRS complexes. By definition, the ventricular rate is less than 40 (Fig. 10-7).
II. Associated disease
  Cardiac disease such as enlarged atria, fibrosis of the atria or junctional tissue, congenital defects, invasive endocarditis, trauma, and heartworm disease can be associated with varying degrees of AV blockade. Septicemia, toxemia, excessive vagal discharge, hypoxia, and hyperkalemia are possible causes. Atrioventricular block is occasionally seen in brachycephalic breeds unassociated with other disease.
III. Clinical signs
  A. First degree
    Signs usually do not occur unless associated with cardiac glycoside intoxication.

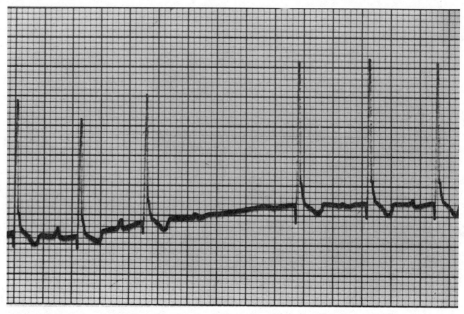

Fig. 10-6. Second-degree heart block. P-R intervals are prolonged. The third P wave from the left is not conducted. HR = 85. Paper speed = 25 mm/sec. Sensitivity: 1 cm = 1 mv. Lead II. (Reprinted with permission from Pyle RL: Tachyarrhythmia. pp 381–388. In Kirk RW (ed): Current Veterinary Therapy VII. WB Saunders, Philadelphia, 1980).

    B. Second degree

        Weakness or syncope can occur as well as signs associated with cardiac glycoside intoxication. Other signs are auscultatory.

    C. Third degree (and severe second degree)

        Exercise intolerance, listlessness, and panting are common. Syncopal episodes may occur with or without provocative exercise (Stokes-Adams seizures).

IV. Treatment

    A. Underlying causes

        Discontinue cardiac glycoside therapy until signs abate. Electrolyte and blood gas abnormalities should be managed appropriately (see chapter 2).

    B. Anticholingergics

        Atropine and atropine-like drugs may give temporary remission of the heartblock. They are definitely indicated as preanesthetic agents in these patients.

    C. Adrenergics

        β_1-adrenergic stimulation increases AV conduction velocity and enhances ventricular excitability. Isoproterenol can be administered IV, IM, SQ, and orally to achieve a heart rate of 80–120 beats/min.

    D. Mechanical pacemaker

        Dogs with severe unresponsive AV block may require cardiac pacing

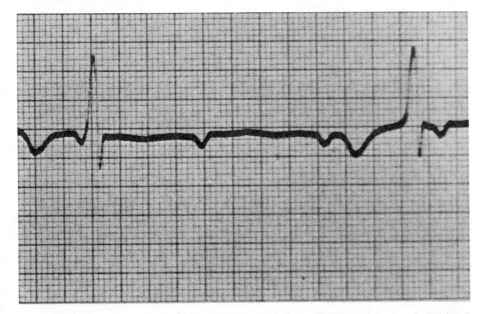

Fig. 10-7. Third-degree (complete) heart block. The P waves and QRST complexes are not related to each other. Heart Rate = 38/minute. Paper speed = 25 mm/sec. Sensitivity: 1 cm = 1 mv. Lead II. (Reprinted with permission from Pyle RL: Tachyarrhythmia. pp 381–388. In Kirk RW (ed): Current Veterinary Therapy VII. WB Saunders, Philadelphia, 1980).

for remission of clinical signs. Intracardiac pacing by implantable, permanent electronic pacemakers has been successful in a limited number of patients.

ANTIDYSRHYTHMIC DRUGS

Electrophysiologic effects of this group of drugs are compared in Table 10-1.

QUINIDINE

I. Routes of administration

IV, IM, and oral routes can be used. Severe hypotension can result from rapid IV administration. Experience with slow-release forms of oral quinidine is sparse in veterinary medicine.

II. Dosage

Dosage recommendations provisional. Orally 6–20 mg/kg q6H; IM 2–12 mg/kg q6h; IV 1–10 mg/kg q 2–4h. Inconsistent dosage recommendations make quinidine difficult to use and more difficult to assess in terms of effectiveness in patients.

III. Metabolism and excretion

Considerable metabolism occurs although up to 40% may be excreted unchanged. Extensive protein binding occurs.

IV. Toxicity

Hypotension occurs (particularly by IV route). Conduction depression may produce AV block. Myocardial contractility is depressed which results in decreased cardiac output. Vagolytic effect can produce dangerous acceleration of the ventricular rate if supraventricular tachycardia exists.

V. Drug interactions
  A. Quinidine increases the concentration of concurrently administered cardiac glycosides in blood.
  B. Antacids which increase urinary pH increase resorption and hence plasma concentrations of quinidine.
  C. Quinidine enhances the hypoprothrombinemia produced by oral anticoagulants.
  D. Barbiturates enhance quinidine metabolism and decrease plasma concentrations.
  E. The coadministration of skeletal muscle relaxants or aminoglycoside antibiotics may result in excessive neuromuscular junction blockade.
  F. Quinidine is a potent inhibitor of hepatic microsomal enzymes.

PROCAINAMIDE

I. Routes of administration
  Oral, IM, and IV routes are suitable.
II. Dosage
  A. Orally as much as 6 mg/kg q3h can be given.
  B. Intravenous boluses of 6 to 8 mg/kg followed by 10–40 µg/kg/min constant intravenous infusion.
  C. Intramuscularly dose recommendations range from 8 to 10 mg/kg q3–6h.
III. Metabolism and excretion
  The specifics of metabolism in the dog are not well worked out. N acetylprocainamide produced in human patients (and associated with immunologic side effects) is not produced by the dog.
IV. Toxicity
  A. Hypotension can be severe following rapid IV injection.
  B. Depression of myocardial conduction and contractility may result in decreased cardiac output.
  C. Vagolytic effect can produce rapid ventricular rates in the presence of supraventricular tachycardia.
  D. May induce production of antinuclear antibody (ANA).
V. Drug interactions
  None are reported.

DISOPYRAMIDE

I. Routes of administration
  Disopyramide for oral administration is the only form currently available.

TABLE 10-1. ELECTROPHYSIOLOGIC EFFECTS

	Conduction Velocity			Automaticity		Action Potential		
	Atrium	AV Node	Ventricle	Atrium	Ventricle	Action Potential Duration	Absolute Refractory Period	Relative Refractory Period
Quinidine, procainamide, disopyramide, aprindine	↓	↓[a]	↓	↓	↓	↑	↑	↑
Lidocaine, nexilitine, tocainide, encainide	↓[b]	0	0	↓[b]	↓	↓	↓	↓
Phenytoin	↓	↑[c]	↑[c]	0	↓	↓	↓	↓
Propranolol	↓	↓	0	↓	↓	↓[d]	↑[d]	↑[d]
Verapamil	0	↓	0	↓	0 or ↓	0	0	0
Potassium	0	↓	↓	↓	↓	↓	↓	↓
Cardiac glycosides	↑[e]	↓	0[e]	↑	↑	↓	↓	↓
Atropine	↓	↑	0	↑	0	∫	∫	∫
β-Adrenergics	↑	↑[g]	↑	↑	↑	↓	↓	↓

[a] Vagolytic—may decrease heart block, especially with atrial tachyarrhythmias.
[b] At high concentrations.
[c] Particularly in abnormal fibers.
[d] Blocks adrenergic-induced decreases.
[e] Decreased with toxic doses.
[f] Increased in the atrium, decreased in AV node.
[g] Reflex decrease (vagus) may result.

II. Dosage
    7–30 mg/kg q2h.
III. Metabolism and excretion
    High clearance rate implies significant metabolism although critical stud-
    ies are lacking.
IV. Toxicity
    A. Hypotension can occur.
    B. Depression of myocardial contractility may result in decreased cardiac
       output.
    C. Disopyramide is *absolutely contraindicated* with preexisting congestive
       heart failure.
    D. Vagolytic effect can produce dangerous acceleration of ventricular rate
       if supraventricular tachycardia is present.
V. Drug interactions
    Coadministration of disopyramide may increase the amount of oral an-
    ticoagulants needed to produce a desired change in clotting function.

APRINDINE

I. Routes of administration
    IV and oral routes are useful. Oral bioavailability is good.
II. Dosage—1–2 mg/kg q8h orally. May be increased 1 mg/kg q8h after 24
    hours until effect is noted. Constant IV infusions at a rate of 100 µg/kg/min
    have been utilized.
III. Metabolism and excretion
    Hepatic metabolism predominates. Renal elimination is minimal. An ac-
    tive metabolite is usually present at concentrations equal to or greater than
    those for aprindine.
IV. Toxicity
    Dose-related dizziness, ataxia, anxiety, seizures, nausea, and diarrhea
    have been described.
V. Drug interactions
    Have not been reported

LIDOCAINE

I. Routes of administration
    A. IV—bolus administration fairly safe. Constant infusion necessary to
       maintain effective concentrations.
    B. IM—doses must be given q1–2h to maintain effect. Intramuscular form
       (100 mg/ml) decreases the otherwise excessive volume that must be
       given. Clinical evaluation of this route has not been completed in dogs.

II. Dosage
   A. IV—4 mg/kg bolus STAT and begin simultaneous 50 µg/kg/min constant infusion. Bolus may need to be repeated if no effect (4 mg/kg) occurs or if effect is lost (2 mg/kg) during infusion equillibration period. Final infusion rate may vary from 25 to 100 µg/kg/min depending upon severity of the rhythm disturbance and concurrent disease or drug therapy.
   B. IM—6 mg/kg every 1 1/2 hours produces similar average plasma concentration to a 50 µg/kg/min constant IV infusion. Peak and trough plasma concentrations make management difficult.
III. Metabolism and excretion
   Extensive metabolism and rapid liver extraction results in high clearance. Pronounced first-pass effect gives poor oral availability and excess toxicity. Certain active metabolites contribute to effect and toxicity.
IV. Toxicity
   A. Neurologic signs include depression, muscle tremors, and convulsions. Convulsions can be controlled with diazepam (gives enhanced antiarrhythmic activity) or phenobarbital and a reduction in rate of administration.
   B. Nausea and vomiting may occur (often transient).
   C. The cardiovascular effects are minimal in healthy heart although lidocaine may potentiate disease-induced deficiencies in automaticity, contractility, and AV conduction.
V. Drug Interactions
   The clearance of lidocaine is reduced when the following treatments are coadministered: propranolol, pentobarbital, and gaseous anesthesia (reduced liver blood flow), and chloramphenicol or quinidine (reduced metabolism). The result can be as much as a five-fold increase in serum lidocaine concentrations at any given administration rate.

MEXILITINE, TOCAINIDE, ENCAINIDE

I. Routes of administration
   Oral
II. Dose
   Tocainide 50–100 mg/kg q12h
III. Metabolism and excretion
   Steric hindrance to metabolism and attendant decrease in first-pass elimination are the major advantages of this group. Hepatic metabolism still predominates as route of elimination. Most have a prolonged half-life as compared to lidocaine.
IV. Toxicity
   As for lidocaine
V. Drug interactions
   Have not been reported

PHENYTOIN

I. Routes of administration

Oral or IV administration is recommended. IM use is discouraged due to low systemic availability. Oral absorption is slow, incomplete, and may be dose-dependent. Rapid IV injection is not recommended as the propylene glycol vehicle is cardiodepressant.

II. Dosage

Dog—oral—30 mg/kg q8h. IV—10 mg/kg q8h; cat—oral 2–3 mg/kg q24h.

III. Metabolism and excretion

Metabolism by microsomal enzymes is rapid. While the potential for dose-dependent elimination rates (saturation) exists it does not seem to occur at therapeutic doses.

IV. Toxicity

Postural ataxia and hypermetric gaits are seen at high serum concentrations.

V. Drug interactions

The coadministration of chloramphenicol increases serum phenytoin concentrations by as much as 20%. Barbiturates acutely decrease phenytoin clearance by competitive inhibition of metabolism. Long-term enzyme induction will result in decreased serum concentrations of both.

PROPRANOLOL

I. Routes of administration

Oral and IV routes are employed. Oral availability limited although this route is successfully employed.

II. Dosage

IV—0.5–1.5 mg/kg (to effect as needed). Oral 5–40 mg q6h. First-pass effect; hence, doses are reduced after the first dose.

III. Metabolism and excretion

Hepatic metabolism is extensive, renal elimination is insignificant.

IV. Toxicity

Propranolol blocks the sympathetic component of the compensatory mechanisms of congestive heart failure. Therefore it should be used with caution in heart failure patients. Propranolol *is contraindicated* in the presence of supraventricular bradycardia or AV block. It may promote bronchospasm if chronic obstructive pulmonary disease or bronchial asthma exist.

V. Drug interactions

A. Propranolol decreases the clearance of drugs dependent upon liver blood flow (see Lidocaine, above).

B. Antacids decrease the oral absorption of propranolol.

C. Barbiturates increase its metabolism by inducing microsomal enzymes.
D. Excessive α-agonist activity may result if epinephrine or drugs resulting in endogenous epinephrine release (clonidine) are used.

VERAPAMIL

I. Routes of administration
    IV only
II. Dosage
    Suitable dosage rates for verapamil in veterinary patients have not been determined.
III. Metabolism and excretion
    Clearance is high. Substantial first-pass elimination may limit oral availability.
IV. Toxicity
    Depression of contractility may lead to decreased cardiac output. Hypotension, third-degree AV block, nodal rhythms, and asystole are seen with overdosage in humans.
V. Drug interactions
    Interactions have not been commonly reported although additive depression of conduction and contractility with other antiarrhythmics can be expected.

PHARMACOKINETICS (Table 10-2)

TABLE 10-2. PHARMACOKINETICS

Antidysrhythmic Drug	Vd (L/kg)	CL_T (L/kg/hr)	$T_{1/2}$ (hr)	Therapeutic Range
		Dog		
Quinidine	2.9	0.36	5.6	3–5 µg/ml
Procainamide	2.1	0.75	2.0	4–10 µg/ml
Disopyramide	3.0	1.50	1.2	3–8 µg/ml
Lidocaine	4.5	2.40	0.9	2–6 µg/ml
Phenytoin	1.2	0.24	3.3	10–16 µg/ml
Tocainide	1.7	0.25	4.7	6–10 µg/ml
Propranolol	3.3–6.5	2.04–4.2	1.1	40–120 µg/ml
Verapamil	4.5	0.39	0.8	?
		Cat		
Phenytoin	?	Low	24	10–16 µg/ml
Quinidine	2.22	0.89	1.9	3–5 g/ml

Vd–apparent specific volume of distribution; CL_T–total body clearance

ACKNOWLEDGMENT

The author wishes to thank Dr. R.L. Pyle VMD, MS, Diplomate ACVIM, for providing the figures used in this chapter.

SUGGESTED READINGS

Adams HR: Antiarrhythmic agents. p 458. In Booth NH, MacDonald LE (eds): Veterinary Pharmacology and Therapeutics. Iowa State University Press, Ames, 1982

Bolton GR: Handbook of Canine Electrocardiography. WB Saunders, Philadelphia, 1975

Kumana C, Hamer J: Anti-arrhythmic Drugs. p. 44. In Hamer J (Ed): Drugs for Heart Disease. Year Book Medical Publishers, Inc., Chicago, 1979

Lucchesi BR: Antiarrhythmic drugs. In Antonaccio MJ (ed): Cardiovascular Pharmacology. Raven Press, New York, 1977

Tilley LP: Feline cardiac arrhythmias. Vet Clin No Am 7:273, 1977

Tilley LP, Gompf RE: Feline electrocardiography. Vet Clin No Am 7:257, 1977

11

Respiratory Diseases
Philip Roudebush D.V.M.

INFECTIOUS RESPIRATORY DISEASE

CANINE INFECTIOUS TRACHEOBRONCHITIS

General Comments

Canine infectious tracheobronchitis is a highly contagious respiratory disease of dogs which is characterized by coughing. The common name given to this condition is "kennel cough," but this name is no more specific than the terms "common cold" or "flu" in humans. This condition is usually recognized in younger animals of all canine breeds and often occurs in local epizootics because of its highly contagious nature.

Etiologic Agents

I. Viruses
   A. Until the early 1960s canine distemper virus was thought to be the only viral cause of infectious canine respiratory disease. Canine distemper is a multisystemic infection of which respiratory signs are a portion of the disease complex.
   B. Canine parainfluenza virus is the most frequently isolated viral agent from dogs with infectious tracheobronchitis.
   C. Canine adenovirus type 2 was the first viral agent other than canine distemper virus associated with canine infectious respiratory disease, and is also a common pathogen.
   D. Canine herpesvirus and reoviruses have been isolated from dogs with respiratory disease, but their overall contribution to the infectious respiratory disease complex is minor.
II. Bacteria
   A. The role of mycoplasmas in canine infectious tracheobronchitis remains undetermined, since the induction of respiratory disease in dogs using *Mycoplasma* spp. alone has not been accomplished. *Mycoplasma* spp.

infections may exacerbate other viral and bacterial respiratory infections.

B. *Bordetella bronchiseptica* actively colonizes and attaches to cilia of the tracheobronchial and nasal mucosa. Bordetellosis may be a primary disease or may commonly be associated with a primary viral infection.

Clinical Syndromes

I. General characteristics
   A. Infectious tracheobronchitis in dogs usually causes exhaustive paroxysmal coughing, nonproductive or productive retching, fever, tonsilitis, pharyngitis, rhinitis, anorexia, and depression.
   B. A cough is easily elicited upon tracheal palpation.
II. Mild uncomplicated tracheobronchitis
   A. The patient is bright, alert, afebrile, and has little or no nasal discharge.
   B. The respiratory rate, tonsils, and pharynx appear normal.
   C. A nonproductive cough is easily elicited upon tracheal palpation.
   D. Breath sounds are normal to increased in intensity with no crackles or wheezes.
III. Severe complicated tracheobronchitis
   A. The patient is febrile, mildly to moderately depressed, and may be anorectic.
   B. There are signs of a productive painful cough with frequent gagging and retching.
   C. Nasal discharge, tonsilitis, and pharyngitis may be present.
   D. The respiratory rate is increased and breath sounds are increased in intensity.
   E. Coarse crackles (rales) may be ausculted.

Treatment

I. Antibacterials
   A. Severe complicated tracheobronchitis
      1. Antibacterials are best chosen based on known susceptibility patterns of bacterial pathogens.
      2. Such susceptibility patterns can be determined by culturing the offending pathogen via transtracheal washing, or consulting established susceptibility patterns (Table 11-1).
      3. Chloramphenicol (50 mg/kg q8h PO)
      4. Tetracycline (20 mg/kg q8h PO)
      5. Kanamycin (5 mg/kg q12h IM)
      6. Gentamicin (1–1.5 mg/kg q8h IM)
   B. Mild uncomplicated tracheobronchitis is usually a primary viral infection and rarely warrants antibacterial therapy.

TABLE 11-1. ANTIBACTERIAL
SUSCEPTIBILITY PATTERNS OF
BORDETELLA BRONCHISEPTICA ISOLATES

Drug	Resistance (%)
Ampicillin	57
Cephaloridine	79
Chloramphenicol	0
Gentamicin	0
Kanamycin	0
Nitrofurantoin	96
Streptomycin	96
Sulfachlorpyridazine	80
Tetracycline	0
Trimethoprim/sulfa	89
Triple sulfa	81

II. Antitussives
   A. The primary clinical sign associated with tracheobronchitis is a paroxysmal cough.
   B. The objective of antitussive therapy is to decrease the frequency and severity of the cough without the concomitant impairment of evacuation of bronchopulmonary secretions.
   C. Peripherally acting antitussives include mucosal anesthetics, and mucokinetic agents such as expectorants, hydrating agents, demulcents, and bronchodilators. Bronchodilators are the most commonly used peripherally acting antitussives. They are found in proprietary antitussive mixtures but are often effective when used by themselves. The commonly used bronchodilators and their dosage are listed in Table 11-2.
   D. Centrally acting antitussives
      1. Narcotic antitussives are drugs with powerful analgesic, sedative, and psychic properties which have a strong tendency to produce addiction in humans. These drugs act to depress the cough center's sensitivity to afferent stimuli and decrease a patient's perception of peripheral irritation. Morphine, codeine, and hydrocodone are the most commonly used narcotic antitussives in dogs. Dosages are given in Table 11-2.
      2. Nonnarcotic centrally acting antitussives are available which have fewer side effects than narcotics but have equivalent potency. Dextromethorphan, butorphanol, and noscapine are opioids which are frequently used in dogs. Dosages are listed in Table 11-2.

TABLE 11-2. DOSAGE OF BRONCHODILATORS, NARCOTIC, AND NONNARCOTIC CENTRALLY ACTING ANTITUSSIVES IN THE DOG

Generic Name	Trade Name	Dosage
	Bronchodilators	
Theophylline	Many	5–7 mg/kg q8h PO
Aminophylline	Many	10 mg/kg q8h PO; cat: 5 mg/kg q12h PO
Oxtriphylline	Brondecon Choledyl	10–15 mg/kg q8h PO
Methoxyphenamine	Orthoxicol syrup	0.5–1 mg/kg q8h PO
Ephedrine	Ephedrine sulfate syrup	5–15 mg q8h PO
	Narcotics	
Morphine	Many	0.1 mg/kg q6–12h inj. SQ
Codeine	Codeine sulfate Robitussin A-C Many others	1–2 mg/kg q4–8h PO
Hydrocodone	Dicodid Codone Hycodan	2.5–10mg q6–12h PO not to exceed 0.5–1 mg/kg
	Nonnarcotic centrally acting drugs	
Dextromethorphan	Dextromethorphan USP Cheracol syrup Many others	1–2 mg/kg q6–8h PO
Butorphanol	Torbutrol Stadol	0.05–0.10 mg/kg q6–12h inj. SQ
Noscapine	Vetinol	0.5–1 mg/kg q6–8h PO

E. Proprietary antitussive mixtures include the previously mentioned antitussives in various combinations. Combinations of antihistamines, expectorants, nonnarcotic centrally acting drugs, and bronchodilators are often marketed as single antitussive products. There is no evidence that such combinations are any more effective than single antitussive drugs, and they frequently constitute irrational mixtures.

III. Vaporization/nebulization

   A. Humidification or vaporization should be used in conjunction with long-term administration of dry gases (oxygen cage, anesthetics) to avoid respiratory mucosal dehydration.

   B. Nebulization is the addition of particulate water to a gas (aerosol) the goal of which is to deposit water and/or medication on the mucosal surface of airways so as to relieve bronchospasm, decrease mucosal edema, and mobilize retained secretions.

      1. The simplest form of nebulization, which can be performed by clients, is placing the dog in a "steamy" bathroom.

      2. Sophisticated nebulizers are available which can produce a uniform

aerosol to improve deposition in lower airways, but the use of therapeutic aerosols remains controversial because in most cases no conclusive evidence for their efficacy exists.

IV. Supportive care

The anorectic, dehydrated patient should receive adequate nutritional and fluid therapy. Many times this type of holistic care is overlooked while attempting merely to control clinical signs such as coughing (see chapter 1).

FELINE INFECTIOUS RESPIRATORY DISEASE COMPLEX

General Comments

There are few syndromes quite as confusing to the cat owner or to the veterinarian as the feline infectious respiratory diseases. Until recently, the feline respiratory diseases were all lumped as "pneumonitis" by cat owner and veterinarian alike. Only lately have the viruses, bacterial agents, and their clinical signs been characterized well enough to permit even tentative differential diagnosis.

Clinical Syndromes Associated with Specific Etiologic Agents

I. Feline chlamydia
   A. Pneumonitis, the disease which was a few years ago the "garbage can" diagnosis made on all cats with respiratory disease, is caused by *Chlamydia psittaci*. This obligate intracellular bacterial organism is a cat-adapted strain of the same organism that causes psittacosis in birds.
   B. Clinical signs include unilateral or bilateral conjunctivitis. The severity of the inflammatory process will vary between eyes; that is, both eyes may not be similarly affected. Blepharospasm, chemosis, serous to mucopurulent ocular discharge, anorexia, fever, and lethargy may develop but are not consistent clinical findings. "Pneumonitis" is a misnomer because chlamydia causes only mild focal interstitial lung lesions with no clinical signs of pneumonia.

II. Feline reovirus
   A. The signs are so mild in cats with reovirus infection that many clients will not even seek veterinary assistance.
   B. Clinical signs include photophobia and a mild serous ocular discharge.
   C. Cats rarely show other manifestations of reovirus infection.

III. Feline calicivirus
   A. Feline calicivirus has special affinity for the lung and oral mucosa, while the upper respiratory tract and conjunctiva are minimally affected.

    B. Clinical signs usually include dyspnea due to pneumonia and severe
       ulceration on the tongue, hard palate, philtrum, nostrils, gums, and
       nasal mucosa. Anorexia, fever, and salivation accompany these lesions.
    C. Numerous pathogenic strains exist, so the disease process varies from
       mild to severe among cats.
IV. Feline herpesvirus
    A. Herpesvirus has a predilection for the upper respiratory tract and con-
       junctiva. Thus, the name for the disease condition caused by herpes-
       virus is *rhinotracheitis*.
    B. Cats will present with a moderate fever, anorexia, dyspnea, salivation,
       coughing, paroxysmal sneezing, and severe mucopurulent nasal and
       ocular discharge.
    C. Pneumonia and severe ulcerative stomatitis are very unusual in feline
       herpesvirus infection.
    D. Small punctate glossal and pharyngeal ulcers may occur but are less
       frequent than ulceration seen in calicivirus infection.

Treatment

   Treatment of all the feline infectious respiratory diseases is by necessity
supportive and relates to the clinical signs of the individual patient. Supportive
measures differ widely among veterinarians, but an outline of specific care is
given here.
  I. Antibacterial therapy
    A. Broad-spectrum antibiotics are probably indicated in most cats to elim-
       inate secondary bacterial pathogens.
    B. Ampicillin (10–20 mg/kg q8–12h PO or parenteral)
    C. Amoxicillin (10 mg/kg q12–24h PO or parenteral)
    D. Chloramphenicol (20–50 mg/kg q12h PO)
    E. Tetracycline (20 mg/kg q8h PO) antibiotic of choice for *C. psittaci* in-
       fection
    F. Cephalexin (15 mg/kg q12h PO)
 II. Ocular care (see chapter 18)
    A. Conjunctivitis
      1. Apply a broad-spectrum antibiotic ophthalmic ointment four to six
         times daily.
      2. Tetracycline ointment (Terramycin ophthalmic ointment) should be
         used in suspected chlamydial infections.
      3. The eye should be gently cleansed before each treatment and as often
         as necessary to prevent readherrence of the lids by dried exudate.
    B. Keratitis
      1. Keratitis is more difficult to treat than the other ocular manifestations
         of feline herpesvirus infections because of the persistence of virus
         deep in the tissue.

2. 0.5% idoxuridine ointment (Stoxil)
3. 3% vidarabrine ointment (Vira-A)
4. 1% trifluridine solution (Viroptic)
5. Acycloquanosine (Zovirax).
6. These products should be used frequently (every 2–3 hours) during the day until reepitheliazation occurs and then for 2 additional weeks.
7. Antiviral drugs may also be helpful in chronic persistent conjunctivitis.
C. Corticosteroids are contraindicated in the topical treatment of most cases of conjunctivitis and superficial keratitis. However, they may have application in treatment of deep stromal herpetic keratitis.
III. Nebulization by means of a room vaporizer or steamy bathroom will help mobilize secretions in the clogged nasal passages and soothe irritated mucous membranes.
IV. Nasal decongestants
A. Their use in cats with copious serous nasal discharge seems indicated.
B. Use the topical pediatric preparations of
1. 0.25% phenylephrine (Neo-Synephrine)
2. 0.025% oxymethazoline (Afrin)
C. These preparations are probably contraindicated in cats with thick tenaceous mucopurulent discharges, since the exudate may become more viscous and difficult to expel.
V. Nutritional/fluid therapy
A. Cats generally die from the effects of dehydration and anorexia.
B. The feline appetite is influenced to a great extent by the odor of food so that, with edema of the nasal mucosa, cats lose the sense of smell and often become anorectic, lose weight, and become dehydrated.
C. Oral hyperalimentation using nasogastric intubation or a pharyngostomy tube often will mean the difference between life and death in a severely affected cat.
D. Fluids should be given IV, SQ, or via the pharyngostomy tube.
VI. Supportive care
A. Patience and tender loving care
B. Best supplied by the owner who can clean the eyes and nares several times daily, provide periodic nebulization, and give assurance to the cat.
C. Good nursing care is often underestimated in the recovery of the feline patient.

Disinfectants

Disinfectants are used extensively to reduce or eliminate pathogenic microorganisms from the environment (see chapter 1 and Table 11-3).

TABLE 11-3. DISINFECTANT ACTIVITY AGAINST FELINE VIRUSES

Virucides	Recommended Dilution	Activity				
		FPV	FCV	FHV	FIP	RV
Alcohols						
Methyl alcohol	70%	−	−	+ +	NT	NT
Ethyl alcohol	70%	−	+	NT	NT	+ +
Isopropyl alcohol	70%	−	±	NT	NT	NT
Coal and wood tars						
Hexachlorophene	3%	NT	−	NT	NT	NT
Pine oil	1:180	NT	−	NT	NT	NT
Iodines						
Betadine (Povidone iodine) Wescodyne	UD	±	+ +	+ +	NT	+ +
Phenolics						
Lysol solution	1:32	−	+ +	+ +	−	±
Lysol spray	UD	−	±	+ +	−	±
One-Stroke Environ	1:256	±	+ +	+ +	NT	NT
Quaternary ammonium compounds (cationic detergents)						
Roccal-D	1:200	−	−	+ +	NT	+
Zephiran (Benzalkonium chloride)	1:750	NT	NT	NT	+ +	+
Soaps (anionic detergents)		−	±	+ +	NT	NT
Miscellaneous						
Bleach (sodium hypochlorite)	1:30	+ +	+ +	+ +	NT	+ +
Formaldehyde	4%	+ +	+ +	+ +	+ +	+ +
Glutaraldehyde	2%	+ +	+ +	+ +	NT	NT
Nolvasan (chlorhexidine)	1:128	−	−	+ +	+ +	+ +
Hydrogen peroxide	3%	+	+	NT	NT	NT

Abbreviations: FCV, feline calicivirus; FHV, feline herpesvirus; FIP, feline infectious peritonitis; FPV, feline parvovirus; NT, not tested; RV, rabies virus; UD, undiluted; −, no virucidal activity; ±, minimum activity; +, mild activity; + +, good virucidal activity.

BACTERIAL PNEUMONIA

Definitions

  I. Pneumonia—inflammation of the lungs
 II. Pneumonitis—not strictly defined; applied to inflammatory lesions which are characterized by cellular infiltration and proliferation in alveolar septa or interstitium (interstitial pneumonia) rather than exudation
III. Alveolitis—inflammation of the lung distal to the terminal bronchiole
 IV. Bronchopneumonia—lobular exudative pneumonia which is an extension of bronchiolitis; site of initial inflammation is the terminal bronchi or bronchiolar-alveolar junction where it spreads endobronchially into alveoli, peribronchially to pulmonary parenchyma, and to other lobes through airways and lymphatics

V. Bacterial pneumonia—fully developed inflammatory process in lung parenchyma in response to virulent bacterial infection

Physical Findings

I. Patients with bacterial pneumonia are usually febrile, depressed, and restless.
II. They show chest wall pain or discomfort, cough, dyspnea with accentuated abdominal breathing, orthopnea, mucopurulent nasal discharge, and anorexia.
III. Lung sounds are increased in intensity and rough in character with crackles (rales).

Etiopathogenesis

I. Etiology
   A. Aerobic and anaerobic bacteria
   B. Viruses
   C. Fungi
   D. Protozoa
   E. Helminths
   F. Allergic or hypersensitivity reaction
   G. Aspiration of gastric contents or other foreign material
II. Routes of infection
   A. Penetrating chest wounds
   B. Hematogenous spread to the lung
   C. Aspiration of nasopharyngeal contents and inhalation of aerosol droplets
III. Pathogenesis
   A. Pneumonia is most commonly caused by aerogenous spread or aspiration of a bacterial or viral pathogen.
   B. Infection depends on the complex interplay of size of the inoculum and virulence of the organism on the one hand versus resistance of the host on the other.
   C. Pneumonia causes interference with gas diffusion, increased airway resistance, decreased pulmonary compliance, ventilation-perfusion mismatches, loss of lung volume due to surfactant destruction, hypoxemia, and septicemia.

Treatment

I. Adequate hydration
   A. Adequate fluid intake must be insured and supplemented with parenteral fluids, if necessary, to maintain volume.
   B. See chapter 2.

II. Antibacterials
   A. The most important criterion for selection of an antibiotic is identifi-
      cation of an organism. This can be accomplished based on cytology,
      Gram's stain and culture of sputum, nasal discharge, transtracheal
      washing, percutaneous lung aspirate, pleural effusion, or blood. Spe-
      cific antibacterial therapy is based on the bacterial agent and antibac-
      terial susceptibility pattern (see chapter 3).
   B. It is commonly necessary to predict the most likely organism and treat
      empirically.
      1. Anaerobic organisms are most commonly found in lung abscesses,
         and pneumonia associated with aspiration of food, gastric contents,
         or foreign bodies and are best treated with penicillin or clindamycin
         (5–10 mg/kg q12h).
      2. Aerobic bacterial pneumonia is caused by a wide variety of organ-
         isms so that empiric antibacterial therapy should be wide-spectrum
         in nature, e.g., cephalothin (10–15 mg/kg q6h IV), ampicillin (5–10
         mg/kg q6h IV), or potassium penicillin G (40,000 U/kg q6h IV) com-
         bined with aminoglycosides such as kanamycin (5 mg/kg q8h IM) or
         gentamicin (1–1.5 mg/kg q8h IM).
III. Bronchodilators
   A. Bronchospasm and wheezing often accompany inflammatory lung con-
      ditions so bronchodilator therapy may be beneficial.
   B. See Table 11-1 for dosage.
IV. Oxygen
   A. Supplemental oxygen is extremely important during the early hypox-
      emic crisis of pneumonia.
   B. Supply 100% oxygen via face mask or oxygen cage for short-term ther-
      apy and 40–50% oxygen via oxygen cage for long-term therapy of more
      than several hours.
 V. Secretion removal
   A. Secretion removal includes the use of mucolytics, expectorants, ne-
      bulization, and physiotherapy.
   B. See the section on treatment of tracheobronchitis for a discussion of
      nebulization.

A Poor Prognosis is Associated with

   I. Aspiration of gastric contents
  II. Profound hypoxemia
 III. Primary versus secondary pneumonia (preexisting condition)
  IV. Senescence
   V. Documented bacteremia
  VI. Leukopenia
 VII. Certain etiologic agents (gram-negative bacillary pneumonia)
VIII. Pleural effusion/pneumothorax

IX. Involvement of over two lung lobes on radiographs
X. Duration and degree of involvement (chronic anatomic changes)

SYSTEMIC MYCOTIC INFECTIONS

Clinical Syndromes

I. Cryptococcosis
 A. *Cryptococcus neoformans* has a predilection for the upper respiratory tract, central nervous system (CNS), eye, and skin.
 B. Lesions and clinical signs
   1. Chronic rhinitis/sinusitis
   2. Nasopharyngeal granuloma
   3. Granulomatous chorioretinitis
   4. Fluctuant cutaneous swellings or ulcerated cutaneous granulomas
   5. Various CNS signs depending on the location of the lesion
II. Coccidioidomycosis
 A. *Coccidioides immitis* has a predilection for lungs, skin, bone, CNS, and eye; may disseminate to a wide number of other visceral organs.
 B. Lesions and clinical signs include
   1. Fever
   2. Malaise
   3. Granulomatous pneumonia with chronic cough or dyspnea
   4. Hilar lymphadenopathy
   5. Cutaneous granulomas or draining cutaneous lesions
   6. Granulomatous panuveitis
   7. Disseminated visceral granulomas
III. Histoplasmosis
 A. *Histoplasma capsulatum* has a predilection for lungs, intestinal tract, lymph nodes; it may disseminate to other visceral organs and bone marrow.
 B. Lesions and clinical signs include
   1. Fever
   2. Malaise
   3. Granulomatous pneumonia with chronic cough or dyspnea
   4. Hilar lymphadenopathy
   5. Peripheral lymphadenopathy
   6. Chronic diarrhea and disseminated visceral granulomas
   7. Osseous, cutaneous, and ocular involvement is rare compared to other systemic mycotic infections.
IV. Blastomycosis
 A. *Blastomyces dermatitidis* has a predilection for lungs, lymph nodes, skin, bone, CNS, eye, and the male genital tract.
 B. Lesions and clinical signs include
   1. Granulomatous pneumonia

2. Lymphadenopathy
3. Draining cutaneous lesions
4. Destructive bone lesions with lameness
5. Granulomatous uveitis and retinitis
6. Prostatitis
7. Orchitis
8. Encephalitis/meningitis
9. Dissemination may cause granulomas in a wide variety of other organs.

Treatment

I. Flucytosine (5-fluorocytosine)
   A. Synthetic oral antimycotic agent which is most effective in treating yeast-type infections such as cryptococcosis
   B. Antifungal properties result from its conversion to 5-fluorouracil in yeast cells. This inhibits both RNA and DNA synthesis in the yeast cell, but mammalian cells are spared.
   C. Well absorbed from the gastrointestinal tract
   D. Best used in combination with amphotericin B for treatment of cryptococcosis
   E. Supplied as Flucytosine in 250- and 500-mg tablets.
   F. Dosage: 25–38 mg/kg q6h PO
   G. Side effects
      1. Rapid drug resistance by organisms
      2. Gastrointestinal disturbances
      3. Cutaneous eruption and rash
      4. Leucopenia
      5. Thrombocytopenia
      6. Hepatotoxicity
      7. Teratogenicity
II. Amphotericin B
   A. Polyene antibiotic with broad-spectrum antifungal activity which routinely inhibits *Histoplasma, Blastomyces, Coccidiodes, Cryptococcus*, and other fungal/yeast species
   B. Binds to sterol moieties of the fungal cell membrane and disrupts the cell wall with resultant cell lysis
   C. Insoluble in water and poorly absorbed orally so a colloidal suspension is routinely given IV
   D. Amphotericin B is supplied as a sterile lypholized powder providing 50 mg active ingredient per vial. Each vial is reconstituted by adding 10 cc sterile water to achieve a concentration of 5 mg/ml. The reconstituted preparation can be kept for 1 week in the dark, when refrigerated.
   E. The recommended dose is diluted for IV infusion in 5% dextrose in water (NOT in electrolyte solutions such as saline or lactated Ringer's) to achieve a dilution of at least 0.1 mg/ml.

F. The total dose of amphotericin B that will consistently provide a cure is not precisely known for a given patient or for a given fungal infection; nor is the tolerable daily dose of amphotericin B predictable.

G. Dosage schedule
  1. 0.25 mg/kg diluted in 5% dextrose in water given IV over 5–10 min for first two treatments.
  2. If the patient tolerates this dose, give 0.5–1.0 mg/kg/treatment, until a total cumulative dose of 7.0–12.0 mg/kg is achieved. Higher cumulative doses and longer treatment schedules may be needed for disseminated visceral and osseous infections, and in many forms of coccidiomycosis.
  3. Give treatments two to three times weekly.
  4. Monitor blood urea nitrogen (BUN) and/or creatinine prior to each treatment and discontinue therapy if BUN is 60–75 mg%.
  5. During treatment it is best to keep a flow chart. The following information is recorded the day of each treatment
    a) Date
    b) BUN
    c) Daily dosage
    d) Accumulated dose
  6. Concurrent use of large volumes of fluids, sodium bicarbonate, mannitol, or heparin has been advocated to decrease toxic side effects, but the use of these agents is not based on detailed clinical studies. Mannitol (0.5–1 g/kg IV bolus) is most often used just before each treatment or can be used as the diluting substance for daily administration.

H. Side effects
  1. Thrombophlebitis
  2. Fever
  3. Vomition
  4. Nephrotoxicity

III. Ketoconazole
  A. Synthetic imidazole derivative with broad-spectrum antifungal activity against *Cryptococcus, Blastomyces, Histoplasma, Coccidiodes, Candida, Aspergillus*, dermatophytes, and others
  B. Only limited efficacy data are available for animal patients with systemic mycotic infections.
  C. Ketoconazole impairs the synthesis of ergosterol which alters cell membrane permeability and leads to cell death.
  D. Ketoconazole is water soluble and well absorbed from the gastrointestinal tract.
  E. Supplied as Ketoconazole in 200-mg tablets
  F. Dosage
    1. 5–10 mg/kg q8–12h PO with food for 2–6 months or until all clinical and ancillary tests indicate that active infection has subsided.
    2. Monitor hemogram and liver enzymes monthly during therapy.

G. Adverse effects
   1. Hepatopathy (elevated liver enzymes)
   2. Anorexia
   3. Vomiting
   4. Change in color of hair coat
   5. Teratogenicity

Parasitic Infections

General Comments

I. The dog and cat are often infected by parasites that reproduce in the air passages and pulmonary parenchyma.
II. The severity of clinical manifestations due to these parasitic infections is quite variable and ranges from asymptomatic to fatal infections.
III. This broad range of clinical syndromes depends largely on
   A. The number of organisms that infect the respiratory tract
   B. The site of predilection within the respiratory system
   C. The nature of the host's response to the presence of the parasite.

Clinical Syndromes Associated with Specific Parasites

I. *Filaroides osleri*
   A. This slender worm forms eosinophilic granulomatous nodules in the distal trachea and tracheal bifurcation; these nodules may extend into the mainstem and lobar bronchi of dogs.
   B. Clinical signs are usually seen in younger dogs and include
      1. Dyspnea
      2. Wheezing
      3. Anorexia
      4. Weight loss
      5. Chronic paroxysmal cough unresponsive to all forms of symptomatic therapy
   C. Diagnosis is accomplished by finding the embryonated ova in a transtracheal washing or finding larva in direct fecal smears.
II. *Capillaria aerophila*
   A. The "fox lungworm" is a slender worm which infects the trachea and bronchi of wild carnivores, dogs, and cats.
   B. Infections are often asymptomatic but may cause chronic coughing and occasional periods of dyspnea, respiratory distress, anorexia, and weight loss.
   C. Infection is confirmed by finding characteristic oval, pale-yellow eggs with bipolar plugs in transtracheal washings or fecal flotations.

III. *Aelurostrongylus abstrussus*
  A. The domestic cat is the only known domestic host for this worm which resides in the respiratory bronchiole, alveolar ducts, and alveoli.
  B. Infection is often asymptomatic but may cause a chronic nonproductive cough, dyspnea, fever, anorexia, and lethargy.
  C. Diagnosis is confirmed by finding characteristic first-stage larva in a transtracheal washing or in direct fecal smear.
IV. *Paragonimus kellicotti*
  A. This digenetic fluke forms fibrous cysts in the lungs of many different wild carnivores and domestic dogs and cats.
  B. Typical clinical signs of paragonimiasis include a chronic productive cough, respiratory distress, acute dyspnea associated with spontaneous pneumothorax, hemoptysis, excessive salivation, lethargy, anorexia, and weight loss.
  C. Diagnosis is confirmed by finding characteristic pneumatocysts on thoracic radiographs or identifying single operculated eggs in transtracheal washing or fecal flotation/sedimentation.

Treatment

  I. Levamisole
  A. Therapy with levamisole has been used safely to eliminate *Filaroides* infections in dogs, *Aelurostrongylus* in cats, and *Capillaria* in both dogs and cats.
  B. Canine dosage: 7–12 mg/kg q24h PO (treat 3–7 days for *Capillaria* and 20–45 days for *Filaroides*). Feline dosage: 25 mg/kg q48h PO for 10–14 days.
  C. Side effects: salivation, emesis, diarrhea, restless behavior, other CNS signs
  II. Thiabendazole
  A. Therapy with thiabendazole has been used safely in canine *Filaroides* infections.
  B. Canine dosage: 30–70 mg/kg divided q12h in food for 20–45 days.
  C. Side effects: severe emesis; because high initial dosages are poorly tolerated, thiabendazole should be introduced gradually.
  III. Fenbendazole
  A. Most commonly used for paragonimiasis but probably has good efficacy against all the respiratory parasites.
  B. Canine and feline dosage: 25 mg/kg q12h PO × 5–8 days, or 50 mg/kg q12h PO × 3 days, or longer if infection persists.
  C. Side effects: none established or reported
  IV. Albendazole
  A. Albendazole has shown good efficacy against *Capillaria* and *Paragonimus* but further efficacy studies are needed.

    B. Canine and feline dosage: 25 mg/kg q12h × 5–10 days, or longer if infection persists.

    C. Side effects: none established or reported

  V. Ivermectin

    A. Ivermectin has shown good efficacy against *Capillaria* but further efficacy studies are needed.

    B. Canine dosage: 0.2 mg/kg PO.

    C. Side effects: none established.

UPPER AIRWAY DISEASE

NASAL AND PARANASAL SINUS DISEASE

General Comments

  I. Clinical signs associated with nasal and paranasal sinus disease include

    A. Sneezing

    B. Noisy sonorous or snuffling sounds

    C. Coughing with gagging or retching

    D. Mouth breathing

    E. Facial deformity

    F. Pawing at the face or nose

    G. Nasal discharge

    H. Epistaxis

    I. Ocular discharge

    J. In general, sneezing is usually associated with a lesion or discharge in the rostral one-half of the nose and snorting/gagging is associated with a lesion or discharge in the caudal one-half of the nose.

  II. Paranasal sinus disease rarely occurs by itself but usually represents the extension of a disease process from the nasal cavity to the sinus.

Acute Nasal Diseases

  I. Viral bacterial rhinitis

    A. Viral rhinitis is usually associated with viral upper respiratory infection in the cat (feline rhinotracheitis).

    B. Bacterial rhinitis is rarely a primary disease but occurs secondary to trauma, foreign material, tumors, and viral or bacterial lower respiratory tract infections such as pneumonia.

    C. Treatment

      1. In most patients the signs of nasal congestion and rhinitis are temporary and may improve without treatment. Persistent or recurring signs require drug therapy for a limited period of time.

      2. Antibacterials

        a) Ampicillin (10–20 mg/kg q8–12h PO or parenteral)

      b) Amoxicillin (10 mg/kg q12–24h PO or parenteral)

      c) Chloramphenicol (20–50 mg/kg q8–12h PO)

      d) Tetracycline (20 mg/kg q8h PO)

      e) Cephalexin (15 mg/kg q12h PO)

  3. Nebulization will help mobilize secretions in the clogged nasal passages and soothe irritated mucous membranes.

  4. Nasal decongestants

      a) The use of sympathomimetic nasal decongestants in patients with copious serous nasal discharge seems indicated.

      b) 0.25% phenylephrine (Neo-Synephrine)

      c) 0.025% oxymethazoline (Afrin)

      d) Nasal decongestants are contraindicated in patients with thick tenaceous mucopurulent nasal discharges since the exudate may become more viscous and difficult to expel.

      e) Chronic treatment with nasal decongestants is undesirable since it may actually perpetuate the clinical signs.

      f) Extreme cases of viral rhinitis demand more vigorous measures. Systemic antihistaminics or combined sympathomimetic-antihistaminic products may help alleviate these signs. Commonly used products include diphenhydramine (Benadryl) 2–4 mg/kg q12h PO and chlorpheniramine 2–8 mg q12h PO. Numerous combination preparations are available for topical or oral use in man as both over-the-counter and prescription products. A few veterinary products are also available.

  5. Good nursing care, adequate hydration, and nutritional support are important in the recovery of severely affected patients.

II. Allergic rhinitis

  A. Allergic rhinitis is a rarely or poorly documented disease in domestic animals when compared to the common "hay fever" in humans.

  B. Topical or oral nasal decongestants, and antihistaminics offer the best relief.

III. Foreign material rhinitis

  A. Both discrete foreign bodies and food particles are very irritating to the sensitive nasal mucosa and incite clinical signs of violent sneezing, pawing at the nose and face, and mucopurulent nasal discharge.

  B. Foreign bodies usually are composed of plant material such as grass blades, weed awns, and foxtails.

  C. Food particles usually enter the nose via a cleft palate, oronasal fistula, or regurgitation retrograde through the nose.

  D. Treatment

    1. Foreign bodies are best removed retrograde with forceps, during exploratory rhinotomy, or by vigorous nasal flushing. General anesthesia is often required for diagnosis and treatment because the nasal mucosa is so sensitive.

    2. Food particles are best removed by vigorous flushing and correction of the underlying problem.

3. Rhinitis usually resolves without further treatment once the offending foreign material is removed.

IV. Traumatic epistaxis

A. Epistaxis is most commonly associated with blunt trauma to the nose and head such as from a motor vehicle accident.

B. Other causes of epistaxis include

1. Nasal tumor
2. Foreign body
3. Bleeding diathesis (thrombocytopenia, ehrlichiosis, Von Willebrand's disease)
4. Mycotic rhinitis
5. Other severe inflammatory nasal lesions.

C. Treatment

1. Enforced cage rest
2. Sedation

Epistaxis may stimulate violent sneezing which potentiates the bleeding and prevents normal hemostasis. Tranquilization often inhibits these sneezing reflexes and allows normal hemostasis to proceed. Phenothiazine derivatives may worsen hemorrhage by dilating the mucosal arteries.

3. Epinephrine flush

A dilute (1:50,000) solution of epinephrine can be used as a nasal flush to constrict mucosal vessels and inhibit bleeding. This can be done in the anesthetized or awake animal.

4. Nasal packs

The external nares, nasal cavity, and nasopharynx can be packed with gauze in the anesthetized patient to help initiate and maintain hemostasis. This should not be attempted in the unanesthetized patient since the nasal packs will usually promote violent sneezing and exacerbate the problem.

5. Rhinotomy

When epistaxis is uncontrollable and the problem becomes life threatening then a blood transfusion and exploratory rhinotomy are indicated. Vessels can be ligated or packed, or an underlying problem can be identified as the cause of the epistaxis. A complete hemostatic laboratory profile (platelet count, bleeding time, prothrombin time (PT), activated partial thromboplastin time (APTT), or activated clotting time) should be performed prior to surgery to rule out hemostatic disorders.

V. Reverse sneeze

A. Definition

The name given to the syndrome commonly seen in dogs with clinical signs of recurrent episodes of violent inspiratory difficulty lasting 15–60 seconds. These episodes occur in paroxysms and are associated with noisy nasal and pharyngeal sounds and puffing of the cheeks. The exact cause is not known although epiglottal entrapment, postnasal drip, or nasopharyngeal spasm are suspected.

B. Treatment

   1. Physiotherapy

      Many owners report that rubbing the neck, pulling the tongue, blowing in the nose, beating on the chest, or other physical manuvers will stop the episode.

   2. Nasal decongestants

      Some dogs seem to obtain symptomatic relief from the use of oral decongestant drugs. A combination of triprolidine and pseudoephedrine (Actifed; $\frac{1}{4}$–1 tablet per dog q12h) seems beneficial to some but not all dogs. Other decongestants can also be tried, e.g., ephedrine (2 mg/kg q12h) or phenylpropanolamine (3 mg/kg q12h).

Chronic Nasal Disease

I. Feline rhinitis/frontal sinusitis

  A. This syndrome is often called the "chronic snuffler" because the clinical signs in cats include chronic snorting and snuffling-type of breathing with purulent nasal discharge and sneezing.

  B. Rhinitis and frontal sinusitis is a sequela to feline upper respiratory infection in young cats with severe nasal mucosa and turbinate destruction and secondary bacterial infection is common.

  C. Check the feline leukemia virus status of these patients. Many of the young cats with this syndrome are feline leukemia virus-positive which may influence their response to treatment.

  D. Treatment

    1. Treatment is often frustrating because the underlying pathogenesis of the disease syndrome is poorly understood and many of these patients fail to respond to all forms of symptomatic therapy.

    2. Nasal flush

      The nasal cavity can be vigorously flushed with saline and/or antibiotic solutions to remove the exudate and inhibit bacterial growth.

    3. Antibacterials

      Broad-spectrum antibiotics are used for prolonged periods of time (2–4 months) following bacterial culture and susceptibility testing.

    4. Nasal decongestants

      These may be helpful in individual cats but can also exacerbate the problem by drying the exudate.

    5. Rhinotomy

      Surgical turbinectomy and sinus trephination may be helpful to establish drainage of these areas and remove inspissated pockets of exudate. Nasal flushing and systemic antibacterials can be used subsequent to surgical intervention.

II. Mycotic rhinitis
   A. General comments
       Fungal growth and subsequent inflammation occur commonly in the nasal cavity and frontal sinuses of both the dog and cat. Nasal aspergillosis (*Aspergillus fumigatus*) has been reported in the dog while nasal penicilliosis (*Penicillium* spp.) and nasal cryptococcosis (*Cryptococcus neoformans*) have been reported in both the dog and cat. Aspergillosis is more common in dogs while cryptococcosis is considered the most common feline systemic mycotic infection.
   B. Clinical syndromes
     1. Canine nasal aspergillosis/penicilliosis
       a) Wide age range of 1–15 years old for infection
       b) Brachycephalic breeds are underrepresented while dolichocephalic breeds (especially collie and German shepherd) are overrepresented.
       c) One study indicated that 19% of dogs with mycotic rhinitis had prior nasal or head trauma.
       d) Clinical signs include chronic unilateral or bilateral nasal discharge which is mucoid, hemorrhagic, or serosanguinous in nature. Sneezing or snorting may accompany the discharge. Severe cases have softening of bones over the nasal cavity or frontal sinus.
       e) Fever or systemic signs are unusual.
       f) Diagnosis is confirmed by nasal culture, serology, radiography, rhinoscopy, nasal biopsy, or exploratory rhinotomy.
     2. Feline nasal cryptococcosis
       a) Similar clinical findings as other nasal mycotic infections although a distinct granuloma may be visualized
       b) Cats with nasal cryptococcosis are often feline leukemia virus-positive.
   C. Treatment
     1. General comments
       a) Medical management is successful in early cases of mycotic rhinitis before extensive anatomic changes have occured.
       b) In severe cases surgical management followed by medical therapy is necessary.
     2. Systemic medical management
       a) Thiabendazole 20 mg/kg/day PO × 6–8 weeks
       b) Ketoconazole 10–30 mg/kg/day PO with food × 6–8 weeks. See section above on treatment of systemic mycotic infections for more details.
     3. Surgical management
       Unilateral or bilateral turbinectomy plus frontal sinus trephination followed by nasal flush for 5–10 days through indwelling nasal or sinus catheters

4. Local antifungal treatment

Nasal flush with povidone-iodine solution (1:10 dilution with water) daily following surgical placement of indwelling nasal or sinus catheters.

III. Post-traumatic nasal disease

A. General comments

Nasal and paranasal sinus diseases are common as sequela to facial and head trauma. The thin facial bones covering the nasal cavity and frontal sinuses are easily damaged and this may lead to several types of syndromes.

B. Disease syndromes and treatment

1. Sequestration of nasal bone fragments

a) When traumatic incidents cause extensive nasal damage the bone fragments lose their vascular supply with subsequent sequestration. These sequestra serve as a nidus for infection and a chronic bacterial rhinitis ensues.

b) Treatment includes an exploratory rhinotomy to remove the sequestra and vigorous flushing of the nasal cavity. Broad-spectrum antibacterial therapy will control the secondary bacterial rhinitis.

2. Traumatic frontal mucocoele

a) Trauma to the caudal nasal cavity and frontal sinuses will cause a noninfectious mucocoele to form. The traumatic incident causes obstruction to the opening between the frontal sinus and nasal cavity (frontal sinus ostium) and multiple fractures of the facial bones over the frontal sinus. Mucus which is normally produced in the frontal sinus and drains into the nasal cavity via the ostium will then accumulate in the sinus. Because of the facial bone fractures, the mucus accumulation causes a soft fluctuant swelling to arise dorsal to the orbit in the area of the frontal sinus.

b) Treatment includes opening the frontal sinus to remove the excess mucus and establishing drainage of mucus from the frontal sinus to the nasal cavity.

IV. Nasal neoplasia

A. General comments

Canine nasal and paranasal sinus tumors represent 1% of all canine tumors but are less frequent in the cat. These tumors are malignant in 80% of the cases with 60–75% of these malignant tumors being carcinomas. Nasal tumors are most prevalent in older mesocephalic and dolichocephalic canine breeds. These tumors cause morbidity and mortality due to local invasion and destruction, not by metastasis. Clinical signs include all signs associated with nasal disease including chronic unilateral or bilateral nasal discharge, epistaxis, snorting and gagging, coughing, sneezing, facial deformity, ocular discharge, and mouth breathing.

B. Treatment

1. A method of early diagnosis for nasal tumors which would allow treatment to improve survival time significantly is not available at present. Treatment of nasal tumors is generally unsatisfactory because of the advanced state of the disease at the time of diagnosis and the complex anatomy of the region involved.
2. Treatment modalities include surgery, chemotherapy, radiation therapy, or a combination of these regimes.
   a) Rhinotomy with tumor excision and turbinectomy will provide temporary relief for nasal obstruction but does not prolong the patient's life expectancy when compared to no therapy at all.
   b) Chemotherapy and radiation therapy alone are usually not successful because of the large tumor cell burden which must be eliminated.
   c) The most promising therapeutic regimen includes surgical debulking of the tumor mass in the nasal cavity or sinus followed by orthovoltage or cobalt radiation. This type of therapy is generally not available to the practicing veterinarian except on a referral basis to an institutional hospital.

PHARYNGITIS

General Comments

I. Primary pharyngitis is uncommon but may occur concurrently with tonsilitis.
II. Pharyngitis is usually a secondary problem as part of a widespread oral or systemic disease. Pharyngitis often accompanies viral or bacterial upper respiratory tract infections, pharyngeal foreign bodies, and retropharyngeal abscesses.

Treatment

I. Treat any underlying diseases such as removal of foreign bodies or surgical drainage of abscesses.
II. Broad-spectrum antibacterial therapy for 7–14 days

TONSILITIS

General Comments

I. Tonsilitis is usually bilateral but may occasionally occur as a unilateral disease when a foreign body is trapped in the tonsillar crypt.
II. Primary tonsilitis usually occurs in young, small breed dogs which exhibit clinical signs of malaise, gagging cough with retching, fever, and inappetence. Inspection will often reveal a bright-red tonsil with an associated

pharyngitis. Punctate hemorrhages on the tonsil itself and purulent exudate in the tonsillar crypt may also be visible. The tonsil will be friable and easily bleeds upon manipulation. Tonsilitis is not always associated with gross enlargement of the tonsil; in fact, the benign appearance of the tonsil in some cases may be in sharp contrast to the severity of the clinical signs.

III. Tonsilitis most commonly occurs secondary to a preexisting disease process. Primary diseases which are commonly associated with a secondary tonsilitis include chronic vomiting or regurgitation, tracheobronchitis, and nasopharyngeal irritation due to rhinitis. Tonsilitis is often the most obvious clinical finding but the astute veterinarian must always look for preexisting problems causing the inflammatory process.

Treatment

I. Inflamed swollen tonsils are not an absolute indication for treatment. Elimination of preexisting problems will usually result in resolution of the tonsilitis.

II. If clinical signs are severe or persist, then broad-spectrum antibacterial therapy for 10–14 days should be considered.

III. Tonsillectomy is indicated when
   A. Primary tonsilitis is a recurrent problem
   B. Hyperplastic tonsils protrude from the crypts causing mechanical interference to breathing and swallowing

BRACHYCEPHALIC RESPIRATORY DISTRESS COMPLEX

General Comments

I. Brachycephalic respiratory distress complex is a syndrome of airway obstruction involving the entire nasal-pharyngeal-tracheal region in various ages of the brachycephalic breeds such as English bulldog, boxer, Boston terrier, pug, Pekinese, and Shiz-tsu.

II. Lesions involve the entire upper airway; the foreshortened nasal cavity results in reduced airspace and increased respiratory efforts raise the negative pressure in the pharynx and larynx which leads to further problems. A concomitant tracheal hypoplasia also contributes to the distress in some dogs (see Tracheal Disease).

III. Lesions include
   A. Stenotic nares
   B. Elongated soft palate
   C. Laryngeal disease
      1. Everted laryngeal saccules (swollen, edematous, or fibrotic)
      2. Laryngeal collapse (arytenoid cartilages and aryepiglottic folds collapse medially and ventrally)
   D. Hypoplastic trachea

IV. Clinical signs include snuffling, snorting, and snoring-type respiratory pattern; these signs progress to severe dyspnea, mouth breathing, exercise intolerance, cyanosis, and collapse.

Treatment

   I. Surgical correction
      A. Partial excision of the nasal alae
      B. Excision of the excess soft palate
      C. Excision of laryngeal saccules
      D. Partial laryngectomy
   II. Client education is important.
      A. Repair of the stenotic nares and elongated soft palate should be encouraged as an elective procedure while the dog is young and free of complicating laryngeal disease.
      B. This type of surgery can often be performed along with other elective procedures such as ovariohysterectomy.
      C. Anesthesia for the surgical procedures is a critical step in patient management and should be approached with caution.
         1. Affected animals should be placed in an oxygen chamber for 15–20 minutes before induction.
         2. Anesthesia is best induced with IV barbiturates and the patient quickly intubated for maintenance with inhalant agents.
         3. Endotracheal intubation can be difficult in English bulldogs because of congenital tracheal hypoplasia.

LARYNGEAL DISEASE

Laryngitis

   I. Laryngitis usually occurs as part of a widespread viral or bacterial respiratory infection such as canine tracheobronchitis or feline rhinotracheitis. Other common causes of acute laryngitis are trauma to the larynx during endotracheal intubation and prolonged barking.
   II. Treatment
      A. Treatment is aimed at the coexisting infectious problem.
      B. Coughing or gagging due to endotracheal tube trauma is best controlled with antibiotic and/or corticosteroid therapy.
      C. Laryngitis due to overuse of the vocal apparatus is best treated with vocal rest.

Laryngeal Masses

   I. Laryngeal polyps and tumors are uncommon but cause a change in voice and later an airway obstruction.

II. Endoscopic removal of polyps is easily performed using laryngeal cup forceps. Endolaryngeal surgical excision is recommended for laryngeal tumors although this is not curative for malignant tumors which require adjuvant therapy.

Laryngeal Paralysis

I. Laryngeal paralysis occurs as an acquired disease in older large or giant breed dogs and as a congenital disease in Bouviers, Siberian huskies, and racing sled dogs.
II. Paralysis may occur as unilateral or bilateral lesions. Unilateral lesions cause few clinical signs in a dog at rest but signs may be accentuated under working conditions.
III. Severely affected dogs in acute respiratory distress will require immediate endotracheal intubation or tracheotomy. Surgical correction includes arytenoid lateralization or partial laryngectomy.

Laryngeal Edema

I. Laryngeal edema occurs in brachycephalic dogs due to excessive panting caused by excitement or hyperthermia. The lesions associated with brachycephalic respiratory distress complex contribute to the panting problem.
II. Sublingual and pharyngeal edema may occur concurrently and contribute to the respiratory distress.
III. May occur in drug-induced hypersensitivity reactions
IV. Treatment
  A. Calm dog with enforced cage rest and/or tranquilization.
  B. Cool dog.
  C. Corticosteroids
    1. Prednisolone 1.0 mg/kg IM
    2. Dexamethasone 0.25 mg/kg IV or IM
  D. Tracheotomy if signs are life threatening
  E. Epinephrine (1:10,000) administered IV or IM for immediate hypersensitive reactions.

AIRWAY DISEASE

TRACHEAL DISEASE

General Comments

I. The trachea is a flexible connective tissue tube lined by respiratory mucosa which has three basic functions
  A. Conduit for movement of air from oropharynx to major airways of the lung

B. Transport foreign materials and mucus to be expelled
C. Flexible tube to allow movement of the airway and neck
II. Tracheal disease usually causes a cough, dyspnea, production of abnormal secretions, or noisy breathing.

Disease Syndromes and Treatment

I. Tracheitis
    A. Inflammation of tracheal epithelial lining with the major clinical sign of coughing.
    B. Classification
        1. Canine infectious tracheobronchitis (see section on infectious diseases)
        2. Feline infectious respiratory disease complex (see section on infectious diseases)
        3. Parasitic tracheitis (see section on parasitic diseases)
        4. Chronic hyperplastic tracheitis
           a) Rare condition seen in dogs older than 10 years
           b) Lesions are multiple nodular proliferations of fibrous granulation tissue or papillomas of chronically inflamed fibrous lamina propria.
           c) Symptomatic antitussive and corticosteroid therapy is recommended.
II. Congenital tracheal hypoplasia
    A. Definition: a congenital defect primarily recognized in young brachycephalic breeds resulting in inadequate or defective growth of all tracheal rings and/or main stem bronchi
    B. Signalment
        1. Usually recognized in young brachycephalic breeds, especially English bulldogs and bull mastiffs
        2. A slightly different form of tracheal hypoplasia than that seen in the brachycephalic breeds has been described in young basset hounds and may occasionally be seen in other breeds.
    C. Lesions
        1. The cartilaginous tracheal rings are found to be closed dorsally causing a decreased diameter in the trachea, or the cartilaginous rings will actually overlap.
        2. Associated lesions include tracheitis and bronchopneumonia.
        3. In most patients this lesion is part of the brachycephalic respiratory disease complex.
    D. Clinical signs include
        1. Lethargy
        2. Moist cough
        3. Diminished exercise tolerance and various degrees of dyspnea
        4. These chief complaints often include a history of a brachycephalic

animal less than 1 year of age which suffers chronic respiratory distress with exacerbations of severe upper respiratory tract infections and bronchopneumonia.

5. The veterinarian often sees the condition after the animal has been treated several times for an upper respiratory tract infection.

E. Treatment

1. Therapy for bronchopneumonia (see section on treatment of pneumonias)

2. In client education it is important to emphasize that there is nothing that can be done for the primary lesion and that recurrent bouts of bronchopneumonia may be common.

3. Prognosis is guarded since severely affected animals often succumb to severe pneumonia.

III. Segmental tracheal stenosis

A. A clinical condition characterized by a respiratory distress syndrome, stridorous respiratory sounds, dyspnea, and cyanosis which is usually iatrogenic or posttraumatic in origin.

B. The syndrome may be recognized in any breed or age of small animal after routine use of a cuffed endotracheal tube or cuffed tracheotomy tube during a surgical procedure. It is recognized in all breeds of cats as a posttraumatic problem.

C. In the more common iatrogenic form, lesions consist of a segmental tracheal stenosis characterized as a circumferential cicatrix and dense fibrous granulation tissue with possible cartilage ring necrosis. In cats there is a fractured tracheal cartilage with resultant callus formation and herniation of tracheal mucosa. Exuberant circumferential scar tissue or web-like cicatrization frequently occurs.

D. Human subjects with segmental tracheal stenosis will present with weakness, diminished exercise tolerance, dyspnea, inability to clear throat, and a cough (usually seen within 90 days of extubation). Clinical signs in the dog and cat include severe inspiratory or expiratory dyspnea of acute onset, coughing, cyanosis, stridorous breathing, exercise intolerance, and extreme respiratory distress.

E. Etiology—angulation of the tube end against the tracheal wall and the tracheotomy stoma may produce a localized stenotic lesion. Cuffed tubes promote stenosis by two methods

1. Overinflation of cuff causes ischemic necrosis of tracheal mucosa or deeper tracheal structures. The initial lesions are an acute superficial tracheitis with fibrin deposits. This may lead to ulceration of the tracheal mucosa often with pseudomembrane production over the ulceration. Ulceration may be deep enough to expose tracheal cartilages. Stenosis is the end-stage of healing in this process.

2. Sterilization with ethylene oxide and improper poststerilization airing; ethylene oxide reacts with tissue fluid to form ethylene glycol and ethylene chlorohydrin which are irritating chemicals.

  F. Treatment
    1. Endoscopic debridement
    2. Segmental tracheal resection and anastomosis
 IV. Tracheal obstruction
  A. Tracheal obstruction is characterized by
    1. Harsh wheezing or sonorous tracheobronchial breathing
    2. Sudden onset of productive or nonproductive coughing which is worse after exercise
    3. Severe dyspnea with cyanosis and collapse
    4. Exercise intolerance
    5. Paroxysmal panting
    6. Foamy hemorrhagic fluid expelled from the mouth
    7. No relief with symptomatic therapy
    8. Stridor is ausculted over the trachea and thorax.
  B. Extrinsic obstruction
    1. Thyroid tumor
    2. Mandibular or retropharyngeal lymphadenopathy
    3. Peritracheal abscesses or cysts
    4. Cranial mediastinal mass
    5. Esophageal tumor or granuloma
    6. Hilar lymphadenopathy
    7. Heart base tumor
  C. Intrinsic obstruction
    1. Laryngeal tumor
    2. Laryngeal paralysis
    3. Tracheal foreign body
     a) Safety pins
     b) Plant material
     c) Rocks
     d) Marbles
     e) Dry dog food
     f) Endotracheal tube
    4. Tracheal tumors
     a) Primary and metastatic tracheal tumors are uncommon.
     b) The most common tracheal tumor has been termed a tracheal osteochondral dysplasia or osteochondroma. This tumor involves the ossification centers developing adjacent to the growth plate of the tracheal rings; probably better classified as a developmental abnormality of cartilaginous origin. Theoretically they should stop growing at skeletal maturity; usually seen causing signs in young dogs less than 1 year old.
  D. Treatment
    1. Extrinsic obstruction is relieved by excision or appropriate treatment of the extrinsic lesions.
    2. Tracheal foreign bodies are best removed retrograde through the mouth with an endoscope. Surgical removal is also possible.

      3. Tracheal tumors require segmental tracheal excision and anastomosis. Tracheal osteochondral dysplasia carries a good prognosis since it is classified as a developmental abnormality and thus will not recur.

V. Tracheal trauma
    A. Lacerations or punctures of the trachea usually occur as fight wounds. Air escapes from the tracheal lesion and enters the SQ tissue of the neck.
    B. The cervical tissue appears swollen and SQ emphysema is generally recognized by the crepitus of the animal's skin. Further complications include SQ emphysema over the entire body and/or pneumomediastinum.
    C. Treatment
        1. If SQ air collection is regressing and there are no signs of respiratory distress, cage rest is recommended and the emphysema is allowed to regress by slow resorption.
        2. If the condition worsens because of continued air leakage despite cage rest, surgical intervention and closure of the laceration site is essential.

VI. Tracheal collapse
    A. Tracheal collapse is a term used to describe two poorly defined syndromes which can result in clinical signs of coughing and respiratory distress in mature toy and miniature breeds.
        1. Cervical tracheal collapse: syndrome of coughing, inspiratory dyspnea, and stridor associated with structural abnormalities of the extrathoracic tracheal cartilages.
        2. Intrathoracic tracheal collapse: syndrome of intermittent coughing episodes and expiratory stridor initiated by tracheal irritation due to exaggerated dynamic airway compression occurring on both normal expiration and cough.
        3. Both problems may occur simultaneously in the same animal.
    B. The disease is usually recognized in middle-aged and older miniature and toy breeds such as the Chihuahua, Pomeranian, Yorkshire terrier, and miniature or toy poodle.
    C. History
        1. Respiratory distress syndrome
        2. Major complaint of a chronic harsh cough and attacks of dyspnea which are exacerbated when the dog is excited, barks, eats, or drinks
        3. The coughing is generally paroxysmal in nature and is initially sporadic but gradually becomes more frequent and severe.
        4. The cough often is described as a "goose honk" sound.
    D. Clinical signs
        1. A dry, hacking, occasionally productive, cough is often accompanied by inspiratory or expiratory stridor and dyspnea. Inspiratory stridor and dyspnea accompany cervical or thoracic inlet collapse while expiratory problems accompany intrathoracic collapse.

   2. There are varying degrees of cyanosis and dyspnea depending on the location and severity of the collapse.
   3. Usually afebrile
   4. Marked sinus arrythmia
   5. Normal to increased breath sounds
   6. Open-mouth breathing
   7. Signs often worse in hot, humid weather
   8. Dogs may either be obese or cachectic.
E. Lesions
   1. elongated, pendulous, or flaccid dorsal soft tissue tracheal structures (trachealis muscle)
   2. chondromalacia or weakening and malformation of the cartilaginous tracheal rings (dorsoventral flattening)
   3. Secondary tracheitis, bronchitis, squamous metaplasia of tracheal epithelium, and glandular hypersecretion are often present.
F. Pathophysiology
   1. The etiology and pathophysiology of cervical and intrathoracic tracheal collapse are poorly defined.
      a) It is likely that conformational peculiarities for which the affected breeds have been selectively bred, may uniquely predispose them to the development of tracheal collapse in late life.
      b) No specific hereditary pattern for the disease and no structural or functional congenital defects of the trachea have been identified.
   2. The progression of concurrent upper airway disease or obstructive lung disease with resultant changes in respiratory mechanics, may be a necessary component of these syndromes.
      a) Elastic fibers play an important role in maintaining large airway stability at physiologic transmural pressures.
      b) Repeated localized inflammatory insults, as in chronic bronchitis, may lead to a morphologic alteration in the elastic and muscular tissue of the membranous portions of the trachea.
      c) The membranous portion of the trachea then becomes pliable and elongated, and is invaginated into the airway lumen during normal expiration or coughing.
   3. Chronic bronchitis or other obstructive lung diseases may also lead to increased intrapulmonary airway resistance. Forced exhalation or coughing in the presence of this increased resistance applies excessive transmural pressure on the major extrapulmonary bronchi which could lead to their collapse.
G. Clinical management
   1. Client education is important!
      a) These patients will always have some signs of coughing.
      b) The client must realize that therapy will hopefully lessen the frequency and severity of coughing but will probably never completely cure the coughing.

2. Medical management is beneficial in early or mild cases but only palliative at best in more severe cases.
   a) Enforced rest
   b) Decrease situations in which dog barks.
   c) Use harness instead of a leash for restraint.
   d) Reduce animal's weight if obese.
   e) Long-term bronchodilator therapy (See Table 11-2.)
   f) Centrally acting antitussives, antibacterials, and corticosteroids can be used on a short-term basis to help control the patient with a severe exacerbation of clinical signs.
3. Various surgical procedures have been devised to correct the anatomic lesions but these should be reserved for the most severe patients which fail to respond to more conservative forms of management.

CHRONIC OBSTRUCTIVE PULMONARY DISEASE

Canine Chronic Bronchitis

I. A condition clinically manifested by coughing which is caused by excessive mucus secretion in the bronchial tree, and is initiated by many different respiratory irritants

II. Chronic bronchitis is usually recognized in small-sized breeds (terriers, miniature poodle, Corgi) of middle to late age; however, a younger animal may be affected.

III. Clinical signs include a chronic hacking cough with retching and phlegm production at the end of the coughing spell.

IV. There is usually a gradual insidious onset with a long duration and progressive course. The owner seeks veterinary assistance during an exacerbation of a problem which has been present for many months to years.

V. Lesions
   A. Excessive accumulation of mucus in the tracheobronchial tree with thickened and hyperemic bronchial mucosa.
   B. Histopathologic lesions
      1. Chronic peribronchial inflammatory infiltrate
      2. Proliferation of epithelial goblet cells
      3. Hypertrophy and increased activity of the submucosal tubuloalveolar glands
      4. Metaplasia of respiratory epithelium
   C. The end result is overproduction and increased viscosity of mucus with bronchiectasis in more severely affected animals.

VI. Etiology
   A. Tobacco smoke
   B. Air pollutants
   C. Infection
   D. Allergic reactions
   E. Other

VII. Treatment
   A. Client education
      1. The condition is controllable but rarely curable.
      2. The client must realize that therapy will lessen the frequency and severity of the cough but will never completely eliminate the coughing.
   B. Avoid irritating inhalants such as smoke, dusty environment, and climatic extremes.
   C. Facilitate bronchial drainage with humidification or aerosol therapy plus mild exercise and postural drainage.
   D. Avoid strenuous exercise which leads to open-mouth breathing.
   E. Control bacterial involvement with broad-spectrum antibiotics such as chloramphenicol (50 mg/kg q8h PO), tetracycline (20 mg/kg q8h PO), or gentamicin (1–1.5 mg/kg q8h IM).
   F. Control allergic or other underlying etiopathogenic factors.
      1. Chronic allergic bronchitis is associated with large numbers of eosinophils in the bronchial secretions and does not have a bacterial component.
      2. Prednisolone 1–2 mg/kg/day is started with bronchodilators.
      3. The prednisolone dosage is slowly reduced over several weeks and the bronchodilators are continued.
   G. Long-term use of bronchodilators is the cornerstone of therapy in chronic bronchitis. Bronchodilators should be continued indefinitely or used intensively during exacerbation of signs. (See Table 11-2 for drugs and dosage.)
   H. Avoid antitussive therapy except in exhaustive coughs. Centrally acting antitussives should be avoided because they tend to cause sequestration and drying of secretions in the airways.

Feline Bronchial Asthma (Feline Allergic Bronchitis)

   I. Feline bronchial asthma is an acute or chronic obstructive bronchospastic disorder of cats caused by heightened reactivity of the tracheobronchial tree to multiple irritants. This disease resembles extrinsic or allergic bronchial asthma in humans.
  II. All breeds of cats may be affected—there is no age or sex predilection.
 III. Clinical signs
   A. Acute syndrome—acute onset of severe dyspnea, tachycardia, accentuated or forceful expiration, anxiety, wheezing, gagging, cyanosis, and preferance for a sitting to a sternal position.
   B. Chronic syndrome—moderate to severe paroxysmal dry hacking cough with wheezing
  IV. Physical examination
   A. Respiratory distress syndrome as outlined under Clinical Signs above
   B. Easily elicited cough by tracheal palpation

C. Increased intensity of normal breath sounds and diffuse wheezes which
   are often worse after eliciting a cough

V. Etiopathogenesis

A. Lesions of reversible airway obstruction
   1. Hypertrophy and constriction of bronchial smooth muscles
   2. Arterial muscle hypertrophy
   3. Bronchial mucosal edema
   4. Bronchial obstruction by mucus plugs
   5. Eosinophilic infiltration
   6. Hyperplasia of bronchial mucosal glands with increased secretion

B. Specific causes of these lesions are unknown or poorly understood but
   allergic or immediate hypersensitivity reactions are proposed.

VI. Treatment

A. Therapy is flexible due to the variety of clinical presentations from the
   acute syndrome of "status asthmaticus" to chronic coughing. The acute
   syndrome requires more aggressive therapy.

B. Oxygen therapy (50–100% oxygen in oxygen cage)

C. Corticosteroids
   1. Acute syndrome—prednisolone 2 mg/kg IM or dexamethasone 0.5–
      1.0 mg/kg IV or IM
   2. Chronic syndrome
      Prednisolone 1 mg/kg every 24–48h PO or repositol methylpred-
      nisolone (DepoMedrol) 20 mg every 2–6 weeks IM.

D. Secretion removal
   Bronchial suctioning may be needed to remove the copious quantities
   of mucus.

E. Antihistaminics
   Chlorpheniramine 2–4 mg q12h PO or diphenhydramine 2–4 mg/kg
   q12–24h PO can be used in the chronic syndrome to control coughing.

F. Bronchodilators
   Aminophylline 5 mg/kg q12h PO for short-term management of the
   acute syndrome or long-term management of chronic coughing.

G. Control the environment and avoid precipitating factors.
   1. Dusty cat litter should be avoided. Replace litter with clean sand or
      sift litter to remove the dust.
   2. Avoid rooms where owners or friends are using tobacco heavily.
      Smoke causes exacerbation of clinical signs.

PLEURAL DISEASES

PLEURAL EFFUSION

Definitions

I. Pleural effusion
   Presence of increased amounts of fluid of any kind within pleural space;
   usually accompanies a large number of disease processes.

II. Hydrothorax

Term used in the broad sense to include any pleural effusion with a low fibrin and cell content (transudate, modified transudate).

III. Pyothorax; empyema

Effusions of purulent fluid with high fibrin and neutrophil content

IV. Hemothorax

Accumulation of blood in the pleural space.

V. Chylothorax

Accumulation of intestinal lymph (chyle) in the pleural space (high percentage of chylomicrons and triglycerides, low in cholesterol)

VI. Pseudochylothorax; chyloid or chyloform effusion

Presence of milky effusions in the pleural space which contains a high percentage of cholesterol or protein-lecithin compounds

Classification of Pleural Effusions

I. General comments
  A. Detection of pleural effusions does not imply a definite diagnosis since many diseases can have a pleural effusion as part of their syndrome.
  B. Pleural effusions are best characterized by the clinicopathologic properties of the pleural fluid itself.
  C. A list of rule-outs can then be generated for each pattern of pleural effusion.

II. Pure transudates
  A. Characteristics

    Clear, low viscosity, pale amber to no color, specific gravity <1.020, total protein <2.5 g/dl, low cell count (<1,000/mm^3) consisting of nondegenerate neutrophils, mononuclear cells, and red blood cells (RBC)

  B. Pathophysiology

    Hypoalbuminemia causes decreased colloid osmotic pressure which allows fluid to move out of both parietal and visceral pleura into the pleural space which overloads the capacity of the lymphatic system.

  C. Rule-outs
    1. Hypoalbuminemia (hepatic cirrhosis, protein-losing enteropathy, protein-losing nephropathy)
    2. Early congestive heart failure
    3. Pulmonary edema

III. Inflammatory (exudate)
  A. Characteristics

    Opaque, high viscosity, variable color, specific gravity >1.020, total protein >3.0 g/dl (pleural fluid protein: serum total protein >0.5), variable to high cell count (>30,000/mm^3) consisting of degenerate neutrophils with or without visible organisms

B. Pathophysiology

Inflamed capillary walls allow protein, cells, and fluid to leak into pleural space with subsequent increase in intrapleural colloid osmotic pressure; efficiency of lymphatic drainage is also reduced by thickening and inflammation of pleural membranes

C. Rule-outs

1. Septic inflammation (penetrating thoracic wound)
2. Ruptured esophagus
3. Mediastinitis
4. Pneumonia
5. Peritonitis, bacterial or mycotic pleuritis
6. Nonseptic inflammation (systemic lupus erythematosus)

IV. Obstructive (modified transudate)

A. Characteristics

Translucent, variable color, usually yellow to pink (serosanguinous), specific gravity 1.020–1.030, total protein 2.5–5.0 g/dl, moderate total cell count (1,000–20,000/mm^3)

B. Pathophysiology

Increased venous and lymphatic hydrostatic pressure with changes in capillary membrane permeability causes increased fluid and cells in the pleural space.

C. Rule-outs

1. Right-sided or generalized cardiac failure
2. Thoracic neoplasms
3. Diaphragmatic hernias
4. Pulmonary edema
5. Lung lobe torsion

V. Hemorrhagic

A. Characteristics

Recent—appears in all respects like peripheral blood and may clot; long-standing—aging erythrocytes and leukocytes, no platelets seen, macrophages with phagocytized erthrocytes and will not clot

B. Pathophysiology

Hemorrhage into pleural space from trauma, eroded vessel, or coagulopathy

C. Rule-outs

1. Fractured rib
2. Pulmonary contusion
3. Hemangiosarcoma
4. Dicoumarol toxicosis
5. Hemophilia
6. Diaphragmatic hernia with ruptured spleen or liver

VI. Chylous

A. Characteristics

Milky-white to tan or pinkish color, turbid, odorless, total protein

2.0–6.0 g/dl, total cell count less than 20,000/mm^3 with predominantly lymphocytes but may have increased cell count and nondegenerate neutrophils if chylous effusion is long-standing; fat globules stain with Sudan III; clears if shaken with ether

B. Pseudochylous or chyloform effusion
   Same gross appearance but fat globules do not stain with Sudan III and does not clear with ether.

C. Pathophysiology
   Obstruction or disruption of chyle flow in thoracic duct with subsequent accumulation in pleural space.

D. Rule-outs
   1. Chylous
      a) Congenital (Afghan)
      b) Traumatic surgical (postoperative pulmonary lobectomy)
      c) Traumatic nonsurgical (coughing, diaphragmatic hernia)
      d) Nontraumatic (heart base tumors, other intrathoracic neoplasms, lung lobe torsion)
   2. Pseudochylous
      a) Chronic congestive heart failure
      b) Intrathoracic lymphosarcoma

VII. Neoplastic
   A. Characteristics
      1. Any of the pleural fluids classified above can arise from an intrathoracic neoplastic process.
      2. The effusion will often contain cells which meet the cytologic criteria for malignancy.
         a) Large cellular size
         b) Marked anisocytosis
         c) High nuclear/cytoplasmic ratio
         d) Aberrant cellular shape
         e) Large nucleoli and/or multiple nucleoli
         f) Abnormal nuclear chromatin pattern and basophilic cytoplasm
   B. Pathogenesis
      Similar to the processes described above
   C. Rule-outs
      Common intrathoracic neoplasms which produce pleural effusions include
      1. Lymphosarcoma
      2. Bronchioloalveolar carcinoma
      3. Mesothelioma
      4. Hemangiosarcoma
      5. Heart base tumors

VIII. Pyogranulomatous
   A. Characteristics
      Translucent to clear, high viscosity, golden color, specific gravity

1.030, total protein 4.0–9.0 g/dl, low cell count (around 5,000/mm³) consisting of lymphocytes, mesothelial cells, and nondegenerate neutrophils

B. Pathophysiology

Pyogranulomatous pleuritis with subsequent exudation of protein-rich fluid into pleural space

C. Rule-outs

Effusive feline infectious peritonitis

Treatment

I. General comments

A. The first principle in treatment of pleural effusion is identifying the underlying disease process that is causing the effusion.

B. Symptomatic therapy outlined below will give temporary relief of clinical signs in the severely affected patient but will not resolve the underlying cause of the effusion.

II. Thoracocentesis

A. Thoracocentesis is usually performed to obtain a fluid specimen for analysis and classification of the effusion.

B. Occasionally thoracocentesis must be performed as an emergency procedure to relieve respiratory distress before other diagnostic tests are performed.

C. Procedure

1. The site of thoracocentesis is best determined after reviewing the thoracic radiographs.

2. If pleural fluid is diffuse or the patient is in respiratory distress, then the seventh or eighth intercostal space is used.

3. The puncture site should be clipped, prepped with an appropriate germicidal solution, and infiltrated with lidocaine.

4. The key to successful thoracocentesis and a comfortable patient is the adequate use of a local anesthetic.

5. Trauma to neurovascular structures can be avoided by advancing the needle or catheter through the chest wall on the cranial edge of the rib.

D. Precautions

1. Many patients with pleural effusion have compromised cardiopulmonary function and care must be taken in restraining or positioning the patient for radiography or thoracocentesis.

2. The patient frequently struggles when restrained in lateral recumbency but usually tolerates a standing or sternal position.

III. Chest tube drainage

A. A more aggressive approach is needed in cases where large amounts of pleural fluid accumulate quickly or lavage of the pleural space is required. A tube inserted into the pleural space and maintained there will allow pleural fluid to be withdrawn several times daily without the need for multiple thoracocentesis.

  B. Special thoracic catheters are manufactured for this purpose although Silastic tubing or any soft large-bore catheter will function well.

  C. The catheter is usually inserted into the pleural space at the level of the seventh to ninth intercostal space.

  D. The catheter should be carefully sutured and bandaged in place.

  E. Animals with chest tubes should be monitored closely since fatal pneumothorax can occur if the catheter becomes open to the atmosphere.

IV. Antibacterial therapy

  A. Only used where an infectious cause for the pleural effusion is identified or suspected. Both aerobic and anaerobic bacterial cultures should be performed on inflammatory effusions since pure anaerobic and mixed aerobic-anaerobic infections are common.

  B. Systemic and local antibacterial therapy is best determined based on culture and cytology results. Many cases of pyothorax are caused by *Actinomyces* spp., *Nocardia* spp., *Pasteurella* spp., and anaerobic bacteria. The antibacterials of choice in these cases are:

    1. Procaine penicillin G (20,000 U/kg q12h IM)

    2. Ampicillin (10 mg/kg q6–8h IM or PO)

    3. Trimethoprim-sulfadiazine (30 mg/kg q12h PO or SQ)

    4. Trimethoprim-sulfadiazine is the antibacterial of choice in *Nocardia* spp. infections at a dose of 60 mg/kg, q12h for 30–45 days. Folic acid must be supplemented to prevent suppression of erythropoiesis.

    5. Culture of organisms other than the ones listed above may dictate the use of other antibacterial agents.

V. Diuretics

  A. Furosemide (2–4 mg/kg q6–12h PO or IM)

  B. Hydrochlorothiazide (2–4 mg/kg q12h PO)

  C. Best used in cases with transudative or modified transudative effusions

  D. Congestive right heart failure is a common cause of pleural effusion and the use of diuretics in management of these patients is often beneficial.

  E. Effusion due to hypoproteinemia should be treated with colloid replacement rather than diuretic drugs.

VI. Restricted-fat diet

  A. Conservative management of chylothorax through dietary modification and pleural drainage should be attempted prior to surgery.

  B. Limiting oral fat should theoretically reduce the amount of chyle produced.

  C. Recommended diets include a commercially available veterinary reducing diet (prescription diet R/D) or, better yet, a homemade low-fat, high-quality protein diet supplemented with medium-chained triglycerides.

    D. The chylothorax may take several weeks to resolve with this form of management.

    E. Those patients which do not respond should be approached as surgical candidates for thoracic duct ligation.

VII. Surgery

    A. Exploratory thoracotomy can be used as both a diagnostic and therapeutic procedure. Surgical exploration of the thoracic cavity is necessary in those patients in which a diagnosis has not been achieved through noninvasive means.

    B. Common causes of pleural effusion which can be repaired during thoracotomy include diaphragmatic hernia, thoracic duct rupture, esophageal rupture, and lung lobe torsion.

PNEUMOTHORAX

General Comments

    I. Pneumothorax is the most common pleural space disease of dogs and cats because of the high incidence of thoracic trauma.

  II. Lung puncture due to penetrating thoracic wounds or fractured ribs, and lung rupture associated with blunt thoracic trauma are all common.

 III. Clinical signs include tachypnea or dyspnea with efforts to maintain a sitting position or sternal recumbency.

 IV. Tension pneumothorax occurs due to a one-way valve effect with flaps of tissue in the lung or chest wall. Air enters the pleural space but is unable to exit. The intrapleural pressure exceeds atomspheric pressure and quickly leads to a life-threatening situation which requires emergency treatment.

Treatment

    I. Most cases of pneumothorax respond to conservative management of enforced cage rest. Thoracocentesis and removal of the air is not indicated when the patient is stable and respiratory distress is not evident. The air is slowly reabsorbed over several days to weeks.

  II. Thoracocentesis and pleural drainage of air is indicated when the patient shows moderate or severe respiratory distress. Intermittent thoracocentesis with needle or catheter, three-way stopcock, and large syringe is most practical.

 III. Constant removal of air through a chest tube fitted with a water trap or Heimlich valve is needed when large volumes of air are removed from the pleural space. Continuous pleural drainage using a constant negative pressure suction system has also been advocated.

 IV. Exploratory thoracotomy is indicated when massive pneumothorax occurs or if the patient can not be stabilized with the more conservative efforts described above. Large lacerations of the lung and rupture of large airways will not heal with conservative management and require surgical intervention.

LOWER AIRWAY DISEASES

PULMONARY EDEMA

General Comments

Pulmonary edema is the excessive accumulation of liquid and solute in extravascular spaces and tissues of the lung.

Pathogenesis

I. Increased pulmonary capillary pressure (cardiogenic) associated with congestive left heart failure or overinfusion of IV fluids.
II. Increased microvascular permeability (noncardiogenic)
   A. Septicemia
   B. Endotoxemia
   C. Seizures
   D. Head trauma
   E. Hemorrhagic shock
   F. Microembolism
   G. Oxygen toxicity
   H. Smoke inhalation
   I. Electric shock
   J. Heat stroke
   K. Envenomation

Clinical Signs

  I. Tachypnea
 II. Dyspnea
III. Coughing with foamy or blood-tinged phlegm
IV. Cyanosis
 V. Diffuse fine to coarse crackles (rales) during auscultation

Treatment (see table 11-4.)

I. The first therapeutic decision is clinical evaluation of the severity of the pulmonary edema. Acute fulminating alveolar edema is life threatening and requires immediate intensive therapy while subacute or chronic forms may be treated after further diagnostic evaluation.

TABLE 11-4. SUMMARY OF THERAPEUTIC STRATEGIES FOR PULMONARY EDEMA

	Enforced Rest	Oxygen	Artificial Ventilation	Furosemide	Aminophyllin	Morphine	Phlebotomy/ Tourniquets	Vasodilators	Corticosteroids
Mild cardiogenic	+			+					
Severe acute cardiogenic	+	+	±	+	+	±	±	+	
Mild noncardiogenic	+	+		+					+
Progressive severe noncardiogenic	+	+	+	+	+				+

II. Noncardiogenic edema

    A. There is no specific treatment that will reverse the endothelial injury seen in cases of noncardiogenic edema. Pharmacologic doses of corticosteroids (methylprednisolone sodium succinate 30 mg/kg IV, prednisolone sodium succinate 35 mg/kg IV, or dexamethasone 6 mg/kg IV) and general supportive care are recommended. There is evidence that corticosteroids may aid in preventing endothelial damage but little evidence that corticosteroids restore injured endothelium to normal.

    B. General supportive care such as circulatory support and artificial ventilation is important because regeneration and repair of the injured endothelium will occur with time.

    C. Lowering pulmonary capillary pressure in patients with noncardiogenic edema is just as important as patients with cardiogenic edema. All the therapeutic measures listed in the section on Cardiogenic Edema, below can be used in the noncardiogenic patient.

III. Cardiogenic edema

    A. Cardiogenic pulmonary edema due to congestive left heart failure is the most common form in dogs and cats. Therapy is aimed at improving oxygenation and increasing tissue perfusion by decreasing pulmonary capillary pressure.

    B. Precipitating factors such as IV fluid overload or cardiac arrythmias should be identified and appropriately treated.

    C. Oxygen supplied via a face mask or cage should be started at a 100% concentration and then reduced to 40–50% concentration after several hours. Intermittent positive pressure ventilation may be needed in some patients.

    D. Furosemide is the diuretic of choice for management of patients with acute fulminant pulmonary edema (1–2 mg/kg q4–6h IV or IM). Furosemide (2–4 mg/kg q8–12h PO) or hydrochlorothiazide (2–4 mg/kg q12h PO) can be used for long-term oral therapy once the patient is stabilized.

    E. Aminophylline (10 mg/kg q8–12h PO or very slowly IV) may be helpful in reducing the bronchoconstriction associated with pulmonary edema.

    F. Morphine provides relief of anxiety (air hunger), mild depression of respiratory centers (changes respiratory character from violent movements to slow deep respirations), and dilates splanchic vasculature to redistribute blood away from the lung. The patient can be given small doses (0.1 mg/kg every 2–3 minutes IV) until dyspnea and anxiety are reduced, or a SQ dose of 0.25 mg/kg can be used.

    G. Excessive foaming of edema fluid in the airways can be managed by intubation and suctioning, or nebulization of a 20% ethanol solution into the airways. If USP ethanol is unavailable, vodka can be suitably diluted and nebulized.

    H. Rotating tourniquets on three extremities or phlebotomy (6–10 cc blood/kg) can be used to reduce venous return.

    I. Vasodilators have not been studied extensively in patients with pulmonary edema but would be expected to offer many benefits in cardiogenic edema. Venodilators redistribute blood away from the lungs by increasing venous capacitance while arteriodilators unload the left ventricle by decreasing arterial resistance (see chapter 9).

1. Nitroglycerin 2% ointment (Nitrol, Nito-BID)
   $\frac{1}{4}$–$\frac{3}{4}$ in. q4–8h on skin
2. Hydralazine (Apresoline)
   a) Dog 0.5–3.0 mg/kg q12h PO
   b) Cat 2.5–10.0 mg total dose q12h PO
3. Prazosin (Minipress)
   1–2 mg q8–12h PO (DO NOT use in cats or dogs less than 5 kg)
4. It is best to start with a low dose and titrate to effect. Nitroglycerin ointment appears best in acute left heart failure while the other oral vasodilators are more effective for long-term management.

PULMONARY EMBOLISM AND THROMBOEMBOLISM

General Comments

I. Pulmonary thromboembolism is obstruction of the pulmonary vasculature by clot material originating at some distant site in the body.
II. Showers of clot fragments usually settle in the capillaries and small diameter pulmonary vessels. Fat, vegetative matter, and parasites may also cause pulmonary embolism.
III. Pulmonary embolism is not well recognized in veterinary medicine and its overall incidence is unknown.
IV. It has been described in association with
   A. Endocarditis
   B. Heartworm infection
   C. Hypothyroidism
   D. Hyperadrenalcorticism
   E. Renal amyloidosis
   F. A postoperative complication
IV. The most common clinical sign is an acute onset of severe dyspnea in a patient with a normal thoracic radiograph. The dyspnea is unresponsive to oxygen, diuretics, cage rest, and other conventional modes of symptomatic therapy.
V. In some patients there will be radiographic evidence of pulmonary hemorrhage or infarction, and right-sided cardiomegaly (cor pulmonale).
VI. Arterial blood gas analysis will confirm hypoxemia ($Pa_{O_2} < 80$ mmHg).

Treatment

I. Enforced cage rest
II. Oxygen should be delivered as a 40–50% concentration in a cage environment.

III. Bronchodilators (aminophylline 10 mg/kg q8h PO)
IV. Antithrombotic therapy
    A. Aspirin (10 mg/kg/day) inhibits platelet function and has been advocated in the pulmonary arterial changes seen with heartworm disease. Do not use aspirin concurrently with heparin or warfarin.
    B. Heparin
        1. Dosage
            Dog—500 U/kg q8h SQ, cat 250–375 U/kg q8h SQ inhibits the reactions that lead to clotting by augmenting thrombin inactivation, thus preventing fibrinogen conversin to fibrin.
        2. The dose should be adjusted by frequently monitoring the APTT (activated partial thromboplastin time) to identify the dose that leads to a 1.5 to 2.5-fold rise in baseline or normal values. Thus, if the APTT is normally 12 seconds, the clinician would adjust the heparin dose to achieve an APTT of 18–30 seconds.
        3. The doses given above have been shown to achieve this level of anticoagulation in normal dogs and cats.
    C. Coumarin derivatives
        1. Warfarin sodium (0.2 mg/kg PO once daily then 0.05–0.1 mg/kg PO once daily) should also be adjusted to the dosage necessary to achieve a 1.5 to 2.5-fold elevation of the PT (prothrombin time). Parenteral heparin is used initially but can be stopped once the appropriate oral warfarin dosage is established.
        2. If the APTT or PT exceed 2.5 times the normal or baseline values, the dose of the anticoagulant should be reduced.
        3. If bleeding develops then all anticoagulants should be stopped and appropriate blood replacement or vitamin K therapy initiated promptly. Heparin therapy is the leading cause of drug-related complications in hospitalized humans and the use of heparin in animal patients should be approached with caution and careful monitoring. Heparin is rapidly destroyed in the body but the effects may be antagonized by the administration of protamine.

BRADYPNEA

General Comments

  I. *Bradypnea* is an abnormal slowness of breathing.
 II. This commonly occurs in anesthesia and other drug-induced depressions of the central respiratory centers, and in neonatal asphyxia.
III. Indications for use of respiratory stimulants are to stimulate respiration during and after general anesthesia, to speed awakening after anesthesia, and to initiate or stimulate respiration in neonatal animals following dystocia or cesarean section.

Treatment

I. Establish an open airway.
II. Doxapram hydrochloride (Dopram-V)
    A. Barbiturate anesthesia canine and feline (5 mg/kg IV)
    B. Inhalation anesthesia canine and feline (1 mg/kg IV)
    C. Neonatal canine 1–5 mg SQ, sublingually or via umbilical vein
    D. Neonatal feline 1–2 mg SQ, sublingually
III. Artificial ventilation if necessary

SUGGESTED READINGS

Burns MG: Pulmonary thromboembolism. p. 257. In Kirk RW (ed): Current Veterinary Therapy VIII. WB Saunders, Philadelphia, 1983

Lourenco RV, Cotromanes E: Clinical aerosols. II. Therapeutic aerosols. Arch Intern Med 142:2299, 1982

McKiernan BC: Principles of aerosol therapy—applications in the canine. p. 110. In Proceedings of Illinois Veterinary Respiratory Symposium, Champaign, IL, 1978

McKiernan BC: Lower respiratory tract disease. p. 760. In Ettinger SJ (ed): Textbook of Veterinary Internal Medicine. 2nd Ed. WB Saunders, Philadelphia, 1983

Moise SN, Spaulding GL: Feline bronchial asthma: pathogenesis, pathophysiology, diagnostic and therapeutic considerations. Compend Contin Ed Pract Vet 3:1091, 1981

Nasisse MP: Manifestations, diagnosis and treatment of ocular herpesvirus infection in the cat. Compend Contin Ed Pract Vet 4:962, 1982

Roudebush P: Antitussive therapy in small companion animals. J Am Vet Med Assoc 180:1105, 1982

Thayer GW, Robinson SK: Bacterial bronchopneumonia in the dog: A review of 42 cases. J Am Anim Hosp Assoc 20:731, 1984

Webb-Johnson DC, Andrews JL: Bronchodilator therapy (first part) N Engl J Med 297:476, 1977

Webb-Johnson DC, Andrews JL: Bronchodilator therapy (second part). N Engl J Med 297:758, 1977

Ziment I: Respiratory Pharmacology and Therapeutics. WB Saunders, Philadelphia, 1978

12

Diseases of the Urinary Tract

David J. Polzin, D.V.M.
Carl A. Osborne, D.V.M.

RENAL DISEASES

MANAGEMENT OF THE ACUTE UREMIC CRISIS

Definition

I. Acute uremic crisis is the polysystemic clinical syndrome which occurs as a result of diminished renal function.
II. Patients with acute uremic crisis may be anuric, oliguric or nonoliguric.

Etiopathogenesis

I. An acute uremic crisis may result from prerenal, postrenal, or acute and/or chronic parenchymal renal disorders, or various combinations of these causes.
II. Acute parenchymal failure may result from a variety of causes which may be broadly classified as: acute tubular necrosis or miscellaneous diseases.
   A. Acute tubular necrosis (ATN) is defined as an acute, potentially reversible decrease in renal function occurring as a result of ischemic or toxic injury to the kidneys.
   B. Other specific diseases which may result in acute parenchymal renal failure (not ATN) include:
      1. Glomerulonephritis
      2. Vasculitis
      3. Hypercalcemia
      4. Acute, diffuse pyelonephritis
      5. Acute arterial occlusion
      6. Renal venous occlusion
      7. Leptospirosis
III. Chronic parenchymal renal failure may result from any long-standing renal disease which affects the function of the majority of nephrons of both

333

TABLE 12-1. COMPARISON OF PRERENAL AZOTEMIA, ACUTE PARENCHYMAL RENAL FAILURE, CHRONIC PARENCHYMAL RENAL FAILURE, AND POSTRENAL AZOTEMIA

Data	Prerenal Azotemia	Acute Parenchymal Renal Failure	Chronic Parenchymal Renal Failure	Postrenal Azotemia
BUN	↑	↑	↑	↑
Serum Creatinine	↑	↑	↑	↑
Serum Phosphorus	N,↑	↑	↑	↑
Serum Calcium	N	↓,N,↑	↓,N,↑	N
Serum Sodium	N (↑)(↓)	↓,N,↑	N	N
Serum Potassium	N	N,↑	N	N,↑
Serum Chloride	N	↓,N,↑	N,↑	N
Blood Bicarbonate	↓,N	↓,N	↓,N	↓,N
Urine Specific Gravity	>1.030** >1.035***	<1.030** <1.035***	<1.030** <1.035***	*
Urine Sodium†	<10 mEq/L	>25 mEq/L	>25 mEq/L	*
FE$_{na}$†	<1.0	>1.0	>1.0	*
Urine/Serum Creatinine	>20	<5	<5	*
Urine Output	↓(N)	↓,N,↑	↑,(↓,N)	↓(N,↑)
PCV	N,↑	N,↑(↓)	↓,(N)	N
Previous History of Polyuria/Polydipsia	0	0	+(0)	0(+)
Previous History of Oliguria/Anuria	+(0)	+/0	+(0)	+(0)
Previous History of Uremic Symptoms	0	0	+/0	0
Debilitation	0	0	+/0	0
Renal Osteodystrophy	0	0	+/0	0
Renal Size	N	N,↑	↓,N,↑	N,↑

↑ = increased, N = normal range, ↓ = decreased
( ) = uncommon, * = no specific values characteristic of the condition
0 = absent, + = present
** = canine
*** = feline
† = extrapolated from data in human beings

kidneys including: immune-mediated disorders, amyloidosis, congenital renal diseases, hypercalcemia, ischemia, nephrotoxins, neoplasia, urinary obstruction, and infection.

IV. Commonly, acute uremic crisis encompasses a combination of prerenal, postrenal, and parenchymal renal causes. Factors which may permit differentiation of prerenal azotemia, postrenal azotemia, acute parenchymal renal failure, and chronic parenchymal renal failure are summarized in table 12-1.

Clinical and Laboratory Findings

I. Clinical manifestations typical of acute uremic crisis include:
  A. Anorexia
  B. Vomiting

    C. Depression

    D. Lethargy

    E. Scleral injection

    F. Oral ulcerations or erosions

    G. Altered urine output (increased or decreased)

II. Laboratory abnormalities typical of acute uremic crisis include:

    A. Azotemia

    B. Hyperkalemia

    C. Metabolic acidosis

    D. Hyperphosphatemia

    E. Reduced urine concentrating capacity

Diagnosis

  I. A presumptive diagnosis of acute uremic crisis is based on clinical signs and detection of azotemia.

 II. Prerenal azotemia should be considered as a possible cause or complication in all patients with acute uremic crisis.

    A. Detection of azotemia in the presence of adequate urine concentrating ability (specific gravity of 1.030 in dogs and 1.035 in cats) indicates a prerenal cause for the azotemia.

    B. A prerenal cause or component of azotemia should be suspected when clinical evidence suggests that decreased renal perfusion may be occurring as a result of actual hypovolemia (e.g., dehydration), functional hypovolemia (e.g. shock), or decreased cardiac output (e.g. cardiac failure).

    C. Rapid correction of oliguria or azotemia after rehydration of the patient suggests that a prerenal disorder is the cause or a complication of the uremic crisis and the prerenal component has been partially or fully corrected.

III. Postrenal failure should be suspected in patients with anuria or abnormal micturition patterns (e.g., dysuria, stranguria).

IV. Parenchymal renal failure is suggested by concomitant azotemia and reduced urine concentrating ability.

Treatment of Acute Uremic Crisis

  I. Samples should be obtained for baseline data and a diagnostic and therapeutic flow sheet should be initiated.

    A. Baseline data should include: body weight, urine output, fluid intake, assessment of hydration, pulse rate, mucous membrane color, capillary refill time, respiratory rate, body temperature, blood pressure (if available), drugs administered, PCV, total plasma proteins, BUN, serum creatinine, sodium, potassium, chloride, bicarbonate, calcium, and phosphorus concentrations.

    B. Progress of the disease and response to therapy should be monitored by reevaluation of appropriate data at intervals determined by the condition of the patient.

II. Rehydrate the patient with an appropriate fluid solution (usually lactated Ringer's solution), via an aseptically placed intravenous catheter.

    A. The volume of fluid required in ml = % dehydration × body weight in kilograms × 1000.

    B. Total rehydrating fluid dose should be administered with care during the initial 2 to 6 hours of therapy unless the patient has known cardiac disease or demonstrates intolerance to fluid administration (e.g. pulmonary edema). Fluid must be administered more rapidly if the patient is in shock.

    C. Proper selection of fluid is based on knowledge of deficits and excesses in water, electrolytes and acid-base balance (see Chapter 2).

    D. It may be desirable to induce a state of mild overhydration (1 to 3 percent of body weight) in patients that have normal cardiopulmonary function.

III. Determine urine production rate; however, do *not* catheterize (urinary) a patient suspected of renal failure unless absolutely essential.

    A. Patients with renal failure are unusually susceptible to urinary tract infections, particularly when oliguric.

    B. Infection is a major cause of morbidity and mortality in patients with renal failure.

    C. Urine output can generally be determined by serial "free-catch" urine collections or with the aid of a metabolism cage. Crude estimation of urine production rate can be made by serial palpation, radiographs, or sonographs of the bladder.

    D. When urinary catheterization is deemed necessary, intermittent urinary catheterization is preferred to placement of an indwelling catheter because intermittent catheterization is usually associated with a lower incidence of urinary tract infection.

    E. When indwelling urinary catheters are used, closed drainage systems should be used to reduce the risk of infection.

IV. Correct life-threatening electrolyte disturbances

    A. Specific treatment for hyperkalemia should be initiated if serious cardiotoxicity is evident.

        1. Intravenous administration of sodium bicarbonate ($NaHCO_3$) will drive K^+ intracellularly.

            a) If the patient has metabolic acidosis, the dose of $NaHCO_3$ in mEq = 0.3 × body weight (kg) × bicarbonate deficit (give $\frac{1}{2}$ the calculated dose as a slow IV bolus and give the remaining $\frac{1}{2}$ dose in fluids over 4–6 hours).

            b) If the patient is not acidotic, $NaHCO_3$ may still be effective in correcting hyperkalemia when given at a dose of 0.5 to 1.0 mEq/kg body weight IV.

      c) Effects of $NaHCO_3$ occur within minutes and may last up to several hours.

  2. Calcium gluconate (10% solution) may be administered intravenously over 10 to 20 minutes during ECG monitoring in a dose sufficient to correct ECG abnormalities (approximately 0.5 to 1.0 ml/kg body weight).

     a) Calcium is a specific antagonist of hyperkalemic cardiotoxicity.

     b) Calcium therapy is indicated for severe hyperkalemia (serum K^+ concentration > 8.0 mEq/L).

     c) Calcium therapy rapidly corrects arrhythmias, but the effect is very transient (10 to 15 minutes).

  3. Intravenous administration of glucose (20% solution) at a dose of 0.5 to 1.0 gm/kg body weight with or without insulin will transfer extracellular potassium ions intracellularly, thereby reducing plasma potassium concentrations.

     a) Addition of insulin probably offers little benefit over effects of glucose alone.

     b) If insulin is used, it should be added at a rate of 1 unit of regular insulin for each 3 grams of glucose.

     c) Effects of glucose (and insulin) are rapid in onset and may last for several hours.

B. Metabolic acidosis

  1. Intravenous $NaHCO_3$ may be given at a dose in mEq = 0.3 × body weight (kg) × bicarbonate deficit.

     a) Give ½ the calculated dose as a slow IV bolus.

     b) Give the remaining ½ dose in fluids over 4 to 6 hours.

     c) Determine blood bicarbonate or total CO_2 concentration after 6 hours to assess response to therapy.

     d) Reformulate therapy for metabolic acidosis based on serial determinations of blood bicarbonate concentration.

     e) Metabolic acidosis should generally be corrected over 24 to 48 hours.

  2. After correcting the initial metabolic acidosis, maintenance therapy of metabolic acidosis may be achieved with oral $NaHCO_3$ or by addition of $NaHCO_3$ to daily maintenance fluids.

     a) Daily dosage of $NaHCO_3$ is based on response to therapy.

     b) Response to therapy is determined by monitoring blood bicarbonate concentrations.

  3. Potential adverse effects of $NaHCO_3$ therapy include metabolic alkalosis, sodium overload, and hypertension.

C. Hypocalcemia

  1. Calcium gluconate (10% solution) may be administered to effect by slow intravenous infusion over a period of 10 to 20 minutes at an approximate dose of 0.5 to 1.5 ml/kg body weight for treatment of hypocalcemic tetany.

    a) Alternatively, calcium chloride (10% solution) may be used at a dose of approximately 0.2 to 0.5 ml/kg body weight.

    b) Excessively rapid infusion rate may induce restlessness, vomiting, or cardiac arrest.

2. Calcium therapy is usually required only for patients exhibiting clinical signs of hypocalcemia (muscle tremors, convulsions, muscle spasms, stiffness, ataxia).

3. CAUTION—*infusion of calcium salts to patients with hyperphosphatemia may lead to renal and other soft tissue mineralization.*

4. Rapid alkalinization of patients with asymptomatic hypocalcemia may further reduce blood ionized calcium concentrations and result in clinical signs of hypocalcemia.

V. Attempt to convert the patient from oliguria to nonoliguria

  A. Replace fluid deficit (see II above).

  B. If fluid therapy alone fails to convert the patient from oliguria to nonoliguria, consider administration of furosemide (Lasix) with dopamine (Intropin).

    1. Furosemide should be administered intravenously at a dose of 2 mg/kg body weight.

    2. Dopamine should be administered by intravenous infusion at a dose of 2 to 5 μg/kg body weight/minute (see chapter 9).

      a) Dopamine is indicated because it may increase renal blood flow and glomerular filtration rate as a result of renal vasodilation induced by its beta-adrenergic action.

      b) Dopamine should be diluted in lactated Ringer's solution in water (50 mg of dopamine in 500 ml of solution yields a concentration of 100 ug/ml).

    3. If substantial diuresis does not result from this therapy, furosemide may be administered at a higher dose.

      a) If no substantial diuresis ensues within 1 hour, repeat furosemide at a dose of 4 mg/kg body weight IV; dose may be increased to 6 mg/kg body weight if no response occurs with double dosage.

      b) If diuresis ensues, furosemide may be continued every 8 hours as needed to support diuresis.

      c) Potential adverse effects of furosemide include: electrolyte depletion (particularly hypokalemia; sometimes hypocalcemia), dehydration, hypotension, gastrointestinal upsets, ototoxicity, hematologic reactions, restlessness, and weakness.

      d) The dose of dopamine may be increased to 10 to 20 μg/kg body weight/minute.

      e) At higher dose rates, dopamine may cause tachycardia and other cardiac arrhythmias and vasoconstriction.

  C. Although we prefer to use the combination of furosemide and dopamine, several alterative therapies may be attempted in order to initiate diuresis.

1. Mannitol (20 or 25% solution) may be administered at a dose of 0.25 to 0.5 gm/kg body weight intravenously over 5 to 10 minutes.
   a) Hypertonic dextrose (20% solution) may be used in lieu of mannitol at a dose of 25 to 65 ml/kg body weight given IV over 15 to 20 minutes.
   b) If substantial diuresis ensues, administration of mannitol can be repeated every 4 to 6 hours or administered as a maintenance infusion (8 to 10% solution) during the initial 12 to 24 hours of treatment.
2. Furosemide may be administered without dopamine.
   a) Dose of furosemide in section V.B above.
   b) Furosemide may be used in combination with mannitol.
D. If oliguria cannot be converted to nonoliguria, 3 options are available:
   1. Dialysis
   2. Nondialytic medical management
   3. Some combination of these 2 therapeutic modalities.
   4. The decision to use dialysis is not based on failure to convert oliguria to nonoliguria, but rather on the occurrence of: (1) intractable hyperkalemia, (2) development or persistence of severe clinical signs of uremia, (3) intractable metabolic acidosis, or (4) severe overhydration.
   5. Methods and procedures for dialysis therapy are discussed elsewhere.
VI. Nondialytic medical management of the oliguric patient.
A. Maintenance of fluid and electrolyte balance
   1. Proper maintenance of fluid and electrolyte balance depends upon careful monitoring.
      a) We recommend that body weight, urine output, fluid intake, clinical hydration status, PCV, TPP, BUN, serum creatinine, sodium, potassium, and chloride concentrations be monitored at least daily during the uremic crisis.
      b) Complete blood count, routine urinalysis, serum calcium, phosphate, and bicarbonate (or total CO_2) concentrations should be monitored as needed.
   2. Fluid balance is maintained by balancing total fluid intake with total fluid losses (''ins and outs'').
      a) Total fluid intake should equal insensible fluid losses (about 20 to 25 ml/kg body weight/day) plus total urine output. Insensible losses should be replaced with 5% dextrose in water. Urinary losses should be replaced with balanced electrolyte solutions (e.g. lactated Ringer's solution).
      b) Accuracy of estimates of fluid loss may be determined by monitoring body weight, PCV, TPP, and assessment of hydration.
         (1) Anorectic dogs sustain losses in body weight of about 0.5 to 1.0 percent of body weight daily due to tissue catabolism (or 0.1 to 0.3 kg per 1000 calories required).

(2) Fluid intake should be adjusted according to changes in body weight and hydration status.

c) Serious overhydration resulting in respiratory compromise or other adverse effects may be treated by peritoneal dialysis with hypertonic dextrose solutions.

3. Subacute therapy of hyperkalemia

a) Sodium polystyrene sulfonate (Kayexalate) may be administered orally at a dose of 2 grams/kg body weight given 3 times daily in combination with 5 to 10 ml of 70% sorbitol. Potential adverse effects include: gastric irritation, vomiting, anorexia, constipation, diarrhea, hypokalemia, hypocalcemia, and sodium overload.

b) Furosemide may be effective in enhancing renal excretion of potassium even when oliguria persists.

4. Subacute therapy of metabolic acidosis

a) Oral or intravenous $NaHCO_3$ may be indicated (consult the section of this chapter on acute management of metabolic acidosis).

b) The dosage of $NaHCO_3$ is based on response to therapy; the goal is a blood bicarbonate concentration between 18 and 24 mEq/L.

B. Control of uremic manifestations

1. Reduced protein diets may be beneficial once the patient can tolerate oral intake.

a) Approximately 8 to 12 percent of the total calories should be protein (approximately 1.3 to 2.0 gm of protein/kg body weight/day) for adult dogs and approximately 12 to 20 percent of the total calories should be protein (approximately 2.1 to 3.8 gm of protein /kg body weight/day) for adult cats.

b) Calorie intake should be adjusted to maintain stable body weight (approximately 70 to 110 Kcal/kg body weight/day for dogs, and approximately 70 to 80 Kcal/kg body weight/day for cats).

2. Cimetidine (Tagamet) is indicated for treatment of uremic hemorrhagic gastritis.

a) Cimetidine reduces gastric acid secretion by competitively inhibiting the action of histamine and gastrin at H_2-histamine receptors on gastric parietal cells. It may also exert a centrally-mediated antiemetic effect.

b) Cimetidine is supplied as tablets (200 to 300 mg), oral liquid (300 mg/tsp), and injectable solution (150 mg/ml).

c) The initial recommended intravenous dose for uremic dogs is 10 mg/kg body weight followed by 5 mg/kg body weight given IV every 12 hours.

d) After uremic gastritis has been controlled and oral medication can be tolerated, cimetidine may be administered orally at a dose of 5 mg/kg body weight twice daily for up to 2 to 3 weeks for control of uremic gastritis; thereafter the same dose may be given once daily for 2 to 3 more weeks.

e) Doses recommended for cats are one-half the canine dose.

f) Adverse effects associated with the use of cimetidine have not been reported in dogs or cats; however, adverse effects recognized in human beings include: decreased white blood cell counts, thrombocytopenia, aplastic anemia, pyrexia, interstitial nephritis, renal failure, hepatitis, pancreatitis, arthralgia, myalgia, somnolence, transient diarrhea, and drug interaction due to inhibition of hepatic microsomal enzymes.

VII. Nondialytic management of the nonoliguric patient.

A. In general, management of fluid and electrolyte balance is easier in the nonoliguric patient than in the oliguric patient, hence the desire to convert the oliguric patient to nonoliguric.

B. Management of the nonoliguric patient is identical to that of the oliguric patient except that inappropriate therapy is more likely to be associated with deficits (e.g., dehydration, hypokalemia) rather than excesses.

C. Despite the fact that the patient is nonoliguric, dialysis may still be necessary to control fluid and electrolyte balance and uremic manifestations.

D. Intensive diuresis may be indicated in patients with polyuric renal failure when correction of volume depletion does not promptly reduce the magnitude of azotemia and alleviate clinical signs of uremia.

1. The purpose of intensive diuresis is to enhance the excretion of nitrogenous and non-nitrogenous waste products (uremic toxins) by that quantity contained in the additional urine flow induced by the diuretics.

2. Intensive diuresis may be induced by administration of osmotic diuretics (20% dextrose or mannitol solutions) or furosemide.

3. Serious fluid and electrolye imbalances may result from failure to carefully monitor patient response and adjust therapy accordingly.

4. Hypertonic dextrose may be used to induce intensive diuresis as follows:

a) Administer 20% dextrose solution IV at a total dose of 25 to 65 ml/kg at an initial rate of 2 to 10 ml per minute for 10 to 20 minutes; then adjust infusion rate so that the remainder of the fluid is administered over a 4 to 6 hour interval.

b) If administration of hypertonic dextrose solution does not induce adequate diuresis, overhydration and hyperosmolality will occur and may be associated with pulmonary edema; therefore, some assessment of response to diuretic therapy must be made in order to assure safety of continuing the technique.

(1) Test urine for glucose to assure that sufficient glucose has been given to exceed the renal threshold and that anuria does not exist.

(2) Urinary flow rate may be determined using indwelling or intermittent urinary catheterization; if urinary flow rate does

not approximate or exceed the rate of fluid administration by the time one-half of the calculated dose of hypertonic dextrose has been administered, overhydration may result and the procedure should be discontinued.

(3) Because urinary catheterization may increase the possibility of urinary tract infection and subsequent complications, it may be possible to avoid urinary catheterization in patients known to be polyuric by assessing urine production rate by noninvasive means described earlier and by carefully monitoring the patient for clinical evidence of overhydration and pulmonary edema.

c) After administration of the calculated dose of 20% dextrose solution and induction of adequate diuresis, lactated Ringer's solution (3 to 5% of body weight) is administered over a 4 to 6 hour interval.

d) Two or three cycles of administration of hypertonic dextrose solution followed by lactated Ringer's solution are administered during each 24 hour period.

e) Fluid input and urinary output are measured so that reasonable balance is maintained.

f) After 24 hours, the patient is reevaluated by physical examination, assessment of alertness, activity, and appetite, BUN concentration, and body weight (minimum); blood electrolytes (sodium, potassium, chloride) and an assessment of acid-base status are also desirable.

g) If necessary, the entire procedure is repeated. Generally, response to therapy, as indicated by a decrease in BUN concentration and improvement in clinical condition, will occur within 2 to 4 days.

5. Furosemide may be used to induce diuresis at a dose of 2 mg/kg body weight given every 8 hours.

a) The patient must be carefully monitored for evidence of dehydration and electrolyte imbalance, especially hypokalemia.

b) Adequate replacement fluids should be given throughout the period of diuresis to maintain hydration (total volume of fluids administered should equal insensible losses plus urinary losses).

CONSERVATIVE MEDICAL MANAGEMENT OF
RENAL FAILURE

Definitions and Indications

I. Conservative medical management of renal failure encompasses symptomatic, supportive and preventive therapy, primarily of patients with chronic renal failure and is not designed to modify or eliminate the primary cause

of the renal disease. The importance of determining an etiologic/pathologic diagnosis and formulating specific therapy should not be overlooked.
II. Conservative medical management is indicated for patients that are *not* anorectic or vomiting.

Treatment

I. Avoid stress

Unnecessary stress which might precipitate a uremic crisis by inducing dehydration or enhancing catabolism should be avoided, including: (1) changes in environment, (2) pregnancy, (3) unnecessary hospitalization, (4) anesthesia, or (5) surgery.

II. Free access to water

The patient should have free access to fresh, clear water at all times in order to prevent dehydration. Avoid adulterating the water source with chemicals, drugs or food additives.

III. Dietary therapy

Reduced protein diets are beneficial in reducing retention of nitrogenous and non-nitrogenous metabolic waste products and in ameliorating some of the clinical signs of uremia.

A. Dietary protein requirements of uremic patients probably vary; therefore, protein intake should be individualized for each patient.

1. Dogs

We currently recommend that approximately 8 to 12 percent of the total calories consumed should be protein (approximately 1.3 to 2.0 gm of high biological value protein/kg body weight/day) for adult dogs.

2. Cats

We currently recommend that approximately 12 to 20 percent of the total calories consumed should be protein (approximately 2.1 to 3.8 gm of high biological value protein/kg body weight/day) for adult cats.

B. If evidence of protein malnutrition (hypoalbuminemia, anemia, weight loss, or loss of body tissue mass) occurs, dietary protein should gradually be increased until these abnormalities are corrected.

C. If necessary to control clinical signs of uremia, dietary protein intake may be reduced below the ranges specified above. However, a compromise between protein malnutrition and control of uremic manifestations may be necessary.

D. Calorie intake should be adjusted to maintain stable body weight.

1. Provide approximately 70 to 110 Kcal/kg body weight/day for dogs.
2. Provide approximately 70 to 80 Kcal/kg body weight/day for cats.

E. Uremic dogs, especially those with inappetence or intermittent emesis, should be given several smaller meals daily rather than one large meal in order to enhance food consumption.

IV. Sodium intake

Routine sodium chloride supplementation is probably unjustified in most patients with renal failure because it may lead to volume overload and hypertension.

A. Most dogs with chronic renal failure are able to adapt to a wide range of sodium intakes and do not require NaCl supplements. However, dogs that are unable to adapt to normal or reduced sodium intake and develop evidence of hypovolemia when fed such diets (so-called "salt-waters") may require dietary salt supplementation).

B. Dietary sodium intake may be reduced from "normal" (i.e., levels found in most commercial dog foods) in dogs with congestive heart failure, nephrotic syndrome, or hypertension.

C. All adjustments in dietary salt intake must be made gradually (over 10 to 14 days) in patients with renal failure so that the kidneys have adequate time to adapt to the altered NaCl intake. The goal is to avoid inducing hypovolemia or hypervolemia.

V. Sodium bicarbonate therapy

Sodium bicarbonate therapy is indicated for therapy of metabolic acidosis associated with renal failure.

A. The dose of $NaHCO_3$ should be individualized to the patient's needs.

1. The suggested initial dose of $NaHCO_3$ is 8 to 12 mg/kg body weight given every 8 hours. Subsequent dosage should be according to response of the patient.

2. The goal is to attain a blood bicarbonate (or total CO_2) concentration between 18 and 24 mEq/L.

3. Blood bicarbonate (or total CO_2) concentration should be monitored at appropriate intervals to assess adequacy of therapy so that dose may be adjusted.

4. Urinary pH may be used as a guide to dosage of $NaHCO_3$; however, this method is substantially inferior to evaluation of blood bicarbonate concentration.

a) Uremic dogs that consistently have a urinary pH of 5.5 or lower may have metabolic acidosis of sufficient magnitude to warrant therapy.

b) A sufficient quantity of $NaHCO_3$ should be given to maintain urinary pH between 6.5 and 7.0.

c) During $NaHCO_3$ therapy, urinary pH values of 7.5 or greater suggest overdosage of $NaHCO_3$; urinary pH values of 6.0 or less suggest inadequate dosing of $NaHCO_3$.

B. Sodium bicarbonate is not an innocuous drug and must be used judiciously.

1. Avoid inducing metabolic alkalosis.

2. Use caution in administering sodium containing drugs to patients with congestive heart failure, nephrotic syndrome, hypertension, oliguria, or volume overload. Calcium carbonate or calcium lactate may be used as substitute drugs in such patients.

3. Because rapid correction of acidemia may decrease the concentration of ionized calcium and result in hypocalcemic tetany, acidemia should be corrected slowly in patients with severe hypocalcemia.

VI. Vitamin Supplementation

Water soluble vitamin (B and C) supplements have been recommended for dogs and cats with renal failure because of inadequate intake associated with decreased appetite and the possibility of impaired renal tubular reabsorption in polyuric animals.

A. The minimum daily requirements of B and C vitamins have not been determined for uremic animals. Therefore, it is recommended that a single high potency capsule containing B-complex vitamins and vitamin C be given daily.

B. Avoid multivitamin preparations containing vitamins A and D because of potential adverse effects on calcium-phosphorus balance.

VII. Anabolic steroids

Anabolic steroids have been recommended primarily for the treatment of anemia in patients with chronic renal failure.

A. Anabolic steroids may also be of value in promoting positive nitrogen balance (anabolism) and calcium deposition in bones.

B. The efficacy of anabolic steroids in treatment of anemia of chronic renal failure in dogs and cats has not been documented.

C. While differences in efficacy between various drugs have been proposed, there is no consensus on optimum drugs or dosages. Two products which have been recommended are:

1. Testoserone propionate (Oreton) should be given orally at a dose of 10 to 15 mg per day.

2. Nandrolone decanoate (Deca-Durabolin) should be given at a dose of 1.0 to 1.5 mg/kg body weight once weekly by intramuscular injection

3. Both of these products are postulated to be of benefit in treatment of the anemia of chronic renal failure by directly stimulating red cell precursors in bone marrow, increasing renal production of erythropoietin, and increasing red blood cell 2,3-diphosphoglycerate production.

D. Anabolic steroids may require 2 to 3 months of treatment to achieve beneficial effects.

E. Adverse effects of anabolic steroids which have been reported in human beings include: hepatotoxicity; nausea; suppression of some clotting factors (II, V, VII, and X) and bleeding in patients receiving concomitant anticoagulant therapy; and retention of sodium, chloride, water, potassium, calcium, and inorganic phosphates.

VIII. Therapy of hyperphosphatemia

Hyperphosphatemia may be minimized by maintaining body fluid balance, feeding reduced protein/phosphorus diets, oral administration of phosphorus binding agents, and/or some combination of these treatments.

A. We prefer to utilize reduced protein/phosphorus diets in properly hydrated patients. We recommend supplementation with phosphorus-binding agents only when diet alone fails to adequately control hyperphosphatemia.

B. Available oral phosphate-binding agents include aluminum hydroxide (Amphojel Tablets and Suspension, Dialume Capsules), aluminum carbonate (Basaljel Tablets, Capsules, and Suspension), and aluminum oxide (Alterna GEL Suspension).

   1. The dose of intestinal phosphate binding agents must be individualized.

   2. Capsules and liquid suspensions are generally preferred over tablets because their contents can be mixed with food and are more likely to be dispersed throughout ingesta.

      a) Although normalization of blood parathyroid hormone PTH activity is the optimum goal, a more practical goal is to reduce fasting serum phosphorus concentrations to normal (3.0 to 5.0 mg/dl).

      b) If reduced protein diets fail to reduce fasting serum phosphorus concentrations to the desired level, oral administration of phosphate-binding agents with or immediately after meals at an initial dose of 30 to 90 mg/kg body weight/day is recommended.

      c) Serum phosphorus concentration should be evaluated at 10 to 14-day intervals until the proper dose of phosphate binding agent is determined.

      d) Constipation, a possible side effect of therapy, may require treatment with laxatives. (See chapter 1)

IX. Treatment of hypocalcemia

Treatment of hypocalcemia in chronic renal failure consists of control of hyperphosphatemia, oral administration of calcium supplements, and vitamin D therapy. Consult reference material for information on treatment of hypocalcemia.

X. Use of corticosteroids, antibiotics, diuretics, and other drugs likely to be associated with nephrotoxicity or adverse reactions should be limited to specific therapy where expected benefits exceed potential risks.

Monitoring Response

I. Adequacy and appropriateness of therapy can be determined only by re-evaluation of patients at appropriate intervals.

II. In addition to evaluation of the owner's impression of therapeutic response and results of a physical examination including assessment of hydration and body weight, certain laboratory evaluations should be performed, including: serum urea nitrogen, creatinine, albumin, phosphorus, and calcium concentrations, packed cell volume, and blood bicarbonate (or total CO_2) concentration.

GLOMERULAR DISEASES AND THE NEPHROTIC SYNDROME

Definitions

I. The terms glomerulonephropathy and glomerulonephritis, with various qualifying prefixes (proliferative, membranous, membranoproliferative, and others), are used to describe a heterogenous collection of renal disorders in which glomeruli are the sole or predominant tissue involved. Persistent proteinuria is the hallmark of canine and feline glomerulonephropathies; renal failure and/or the nephrotic syndrome may also occur.

II. Renal amyloidosis is a condition wherein amyloid (a group of biochemically unique fibrillar proteins) is deposited in the kidneys. In dogs, renal deposition of amyloid occurs primarily in glomeruli, whereas in cats deposition of amyloid often occurs primarily in the medullary interstitium.

III. The nephrotic syndrome is a condition in which urinary protein losses are great enough to result in hypoalbuminemia. Edema, hypertension, lipidemia (hypercholesterolemia), blood clotting abnormalities, and lipiduria may also occur in patients with the nephrotic syndrome.

Etiopathogenesis

I. Glomerulonephropathies (GN) are often the result of immune-mediated injury to glomeruli.

  A. Immune-mediated GN may occur as the result of immune-complexes being deposited in or near the glomerular basement membrane (immune-complex GN), or immunologic reactions directed against the glomerular basement membrane (anti-GBM GN).

  B. Etiologies precipitating immune-mediated reactions in dogs and cats with GN have not been fully elucidated. Diseases which have been implicated in GN in dogs and cats include: neoplasia, systemic lupus erythematosus (SLE), infectious canine hepatitis, feline leukemia virus infection, canine heartworm disease, pyometra, and bacterial sepsis.

II. Amyloidosis causes renal dysfunction and destruction of glomerular architecture as the result of its physical presence in the kidneys. It has been subdivided into classes which differ as to apparent etiologic basis and chemical structure:

  A. Secondary or reactive systemic amyloidosis occurs in association with a variety of chronic suppurative, granulomatous, neoplastic, or inflammatory diseases.

  B. Primary amyloidosis, also termed immunoglobulin-associated amyloi-

dosis, occurs in patients without discernible pre-existing illness. In man, multiple myeloma may be associated with this type of amyloid.
C. A possible form of heredofamilial amyloidosis has been reported in Abyssinian cats.
D. Localized amyloidosis may occur in a variety of organs including the kidneys and the pancreatic islets of Langerhans.
III. Nephrotic syndrome may occur in association with any glomerular disorder which results in sufficient magnitude of proteinuria to cause hypoalbuminemia. Edema and coagulopathies are the most important clinical consequences of the nephrotic syndrome.

Clinical Signs

I. Clinical signs of GN and renal amyloidosis are nonspecific and nonlocalizing. Many animals are asymptomatic unless proteinuria becomes marked or renal failure ensues. When present, clinical signs may include:
A. Anorexia
B. Weakness
C. Listlessness
D. Depression
E. Weight loss (often profound)
F. Peripheral, dependent, or facial edema
G. Ascites
H. Pleural effusion
I. Clinical signs of uremia (consult the section of this chapter on the acute uremic crisis)
J. Signs related to thromboembolism
II. Renal size may be increased, normal, or decreased as determined by abdominal palpation or radiographic procedures.
A. Amyloidosis and acute GN may often be associated with normal to increased renal size.
B. Chronic GN may be associated with reduced renal size.

Diagnosis

I. Glomerulopathy should be suspected in all patients with persistent proteinuria unassociated with hematuria or pyuria.
A. Proteinuria may result from hemorrhage or inflammation originating from anywhere in the urinary tract, pyrexia, congestive heart failure, or glomerular disease.
B. Persistent moderate to severe proteinuria not associated with pyuria or hematuria is strong evidence for glomerular disease. Concomitant hypoalbuminemia provides support for the conclusion that persistent proteinuria is of glomerular origin.
C. The magnitude of proteinuria should be assessed by determining 24-

hour urinary protein loss. Normal 24-hour protein excretion in dogs should not exceed 0.5 gram.

II. Confirmation of immune-mediated GN or renal amyloidosis requires renal biopsy. Light microscopy will usually allow differentiation of immune-mediated GN from renal amyloidosis. Differentiation of various forms of GN (e.g., anti-GBM GN vs immune complex GN) requires electron microscopy and/or immunofluorescent microscopy.

III. When glomerular disease is suspected or proved, possible underlying etiologies should be sought, including:
   A. Neoplasia
   B. Systemic lupus erythematosus or other immune-mediated diseases
   C. Heartworm disease (canine)
   D. Feline leukemia virus infection
   E. Pyometra
   F. Bacterial endocarditis
   G. Chronic sepsis
   H. Other infectious or inflammatory conditions
   I. Toxins such as mercury

Specific Therapy for GN

I. Current therapeutic measures for GN in dogs and cats are empirical, frequently ineffective, and often potentially hazardous. Caution must be used in selecting potentially harmful drugs for treating patients with GN because the prognosis is not so uniformly poor in all animals that just any type of treatment is warranted.

II. Formulation of specific therapy for GN is based on:
   A. Removal of antigens
   B. Modification of immunologic disturbances
   C. Inhibition of inflammation
   D. Inhibition of coagulation

III. The most logical and possibly most effective form of therapy for GN is identification and elimination of the source of antigenic stimulation (e.g. *Dirofilaria immitis*, pyometra, bacterial endocarditis, or generalized sepsis).
   A. Unfortunately, in most cases it is difficult or impossible to identify and eliminate the antigen.
   B. Basic genetic and immunologic aberrations play an important role in the susceptibility of animals to immune-mediated glomerular disease and also influence the intensity and duration of glomerular lesions. Although elimination of antigens may result in temporary remission of the disease, long-term control and prevention may require manipulations that correct the predisposition to formation of biologically active immune reactants. Unfortuantely, nothing is known about immunologi-

cally specific forms of therapy or modification of host factors that predispose to immunologic damage.

IV. Corticosteroids and immunosuppressive drugs (e.g., cyclophosphamide and azathioprine) may be considered in the treatment of immune-mediated GN.

   A. These drugs are used with the expectation that they will inhibit production of pathogenic antibodies, interfere with factors that favor localization of immune complexes in the glomerular capillary walls, or suppress the inflammatory response thought to be initiated by antigen-antibody-complement reactions.

   B. Safety and efficacy of corticosteroid and immunosuppressive therapy of GN in dogs and cats has not been critically evaluated.

      1. Corticosteroids and immunosuppressive drugs may aggravate GN in some cases by creating a greater excess of antigen resulting in more biologically-active immune complexes and/or impairing clearance of circulating immune complexes by the mononuclear phagocytic system.

      2. Most studies have revealed that corticosteroid therapy is of "limited benefit" in treatment of immune-mediated GN in human beings.

      3. Serious complications of corticosteroid therapy in patients with GN may include:

         a) Induction or exacerbation of uremic signs resulting from the protein-catabolic effects of glucocorticoids

         b) Thromboembolic phenomena

         c) Steroid myopathy

         d) Gastrointestinal ulcerations

         e) Infection

         f) Suppression of hypothalamic- pituitary-adrenal axis

         g) Behavioral alterations

         h) Pancreatitis

      4. Serious complications of immunosuppressive drug therapy may include:

         a) Bone marrow toxicity

         b) Infection

         c) Gastrointestinal toxicity

         d) Hemorrhagic cystitis (cyclophosphamide)

   C. A therapeutic trial with corticosteroids and/or immunosuppressive drugs may be considered when:

      1. There is strong evidence that GN is immune-mediated based on results of renal biopsy and immunologic studies.

      2. The probability of inducing serious complications resulting from therapy is not unduly great.

      3. Results of renal biopsy indicate that glomerular lesions may be reversible.

   D. A therapeutic trial of corticosteroids may be initiated by giving prednisolone (or prednisone) orally at a dose of 0.5 to 1.0 mg/kg every 12 hours for the first 2 to 4 weeks of treatment.

1. Thereafter, dosage should be changed to 1.0 to 2.0 mg/kg given orally every other morning.
2. Response to therapy should be assessed by serial (we suggest monthly) evaluation of renal function (serum creatinine and urea nitrogen concentrations and/or endogenous creatinine clearance studies), serum albumin concentration, and magnitude of proteinuria.
3. If corticosteroid therapy is associated with complete remission or considerable improvement in renal function, serum albumin concentration, and/or proteinuria, the dose of prednisolone may be gradually tapered over the subsequent 8 weeks to 0.5 mg/kg given orally every other morning.
    a) Therapy may be cautiously discontinued at this time if the patient remains in complete remission.
    b) Continued therapy at this dose may be advisable for patients with partial improvement so long as therapy continues to sustain partial response.
    c) Relapses following partial or complete remission should be treated by returning to the original dosage schedule.
4. If after 8 weeks of treatment, renal function has deteriorated or little or no improvement in proteinuria has occurred, continued corticosteroid therapy is not recommended. The drug should be gradually withdrawn over the subsequent 4 weeks.
5. Dosage of prednisolone should be rapidly reduced if serious complications of corticosteroid therapy occur.

E. Administration of a combination of immunosuppressive drugs with prednisolone may be considered in patients that respond poorly to steroids alone or have rapidly progressive GN.
1. Use of such drug combinations in human patients with various forms of GN has generally not been very successful.
2. Efficacy of combination immunosuppressive therapy in treatment of canine and feline GN has not been critically evaluated. Dosage recommendations are extrapolated from recommendations for use of these drugs for other immune-mediated disorders.
    a) Cyclophosphamide (Cytoxan) may be given at the dose of 1.5 mg/kg PO daily for dogs greater than 25 kg, 2.0 mg/kg PO daily for dogs 5 to 25 kg, and 2.5 mg/kg PO daily for dogs under 5 kg and cats. Cyclophosphamide should be given for 4 consecutive days of each week followed by 3 days with no drug given. Alternatively, cyclophosphamide may be given at the previously mentioned dose on an alternate-day basis.
    b) Chlorambucil (Leukeran) may be given at a dose of approximately 0.07 mg/kg PO once daily for animals between 15 and 30 kg body

weight. Smaller dogs should be given 0.08 mg/kg and larger dogs 0.06 mg/kg PO once daily. Once remission is achieved, the drug may be given at the previously mentioned dosage every other day.

    c) Azathioprine (Imuran) may be given at a dose of approximately 2.0 mg/kg PO once daily. Once remission is achieved, the drug may be given at this same dose every other day. Prednisolone and azathioprine should be given on alternate days at this time.

F. Anticoagulant and antiplatelet drugs have been used with some success in treatment of certain forms of GN in human beings.

    1. There is evidence that activation of the coagulation system resulting in fibrin deposition in glomerular capillaries may contribute to development of some forms of GN.

    2. Safety and efficacy of anticoagulant and antiplatelet drugs in treatment of GN in dogs and cats has not been evaluated. Recommendations concerning use of these drugs awaits results of controlled clinical trials.

Specific Therapy of Renal Amyloidosis

I. There is no proven, specific treatment for renal amyloidosis.

II. Renal amyloidosis usually progresses inexorably to renal failure.

III. Patients with secondary or reactive systemic amyloidosis may respond to removal of the underlying disease process (e.g., chronic inflammatory, granulomatous, or neoplastic disease); however, it appears unlikely that removal of the predisposing cause would result in resolution of renal lesions once the renal disease has progressed sufficiently to result in uremia.

IV. Because of the consistently poor prognosis and the possibility that an occult immunocyte dyscrasia or multiple myeloma may be the cause of renal amyloidosis, a therapeutic trial with cytotoxic drugs (singly or in combination) may be indicated for patients with primary or immunoglobin-associated amyloidosis.

    A. Melphalan (Alkeran) may be administered orally at a dose of 1.5 mg/M^2 once daily for 7 to 10 days. Therapy should then be withheld for 2 to 3 weeks.

    B. Cyclophosphamide may be administered as described above in the section on specific treatment of GN.

V. *Corticosteroid therapy has been shown to be of no benefit and may be harmful to patients with renal amyloidosis.*

Symptomatic and Supportive Therapy

I. The following recommendations should be considered for patients that are proteinuric:

    A. If proteinuria is substantial, a diet with sufficient quantity of high quality protein should be fed to help compensate for urinary protein losses.

    B. Administer B-complex vitamins orally.

    C. Administer anabolic steroids to promote positive nitrogen balance. Consult the section of this chapter on conservative medical management of renal failure for additional information.

    D. Provide unlimited access to water.

    E. Monitor serum urea nitrogen, creatinine, and albumin concentrations.

II. The following recommendations should be considered for patients that are edematous (in addition to recommendations for proteinuria):

    A. Avoid unnecessary stress-inducing factors which may compromise renal function or promote catabolism (e.g. hospitalization, boarding, etc.)

    B. Diuretic therapy may be indicated for patients with moderate to severe edema. Cosmetic treatment of mild edema is not advocated because of an associated reduction in vascular volume.

       1. Furosemide (Lasix) is the diuretic of choice for acute relief of edema associated with the nephrotic syndrome. Dosage is 2–4 mg/kg given PO, IV, or IM 1 to 4 times daily until edema resolves.

       2. After therapeutic resolution of edema, furosemide dose may be gradually reduced to alternate day therapy. If alternate day therapy maintains the patient edema-free for a trial period of 2 weeks, the dose may be further reduced to once every third day for 2 weeks. If the patient still remains free of edema, furosemide can be discontinued. When chronic diuretic therapy is necessary to prevent recurrence of edema, the lowest dose which maintains the patient free of edema should be used.

       3. Excessive diuertic therapy may cause fluid and electrolyte (sodium and potassium) depletion and compromise renal function. Diuresis-induced fluid and electrolyte depletion may be prevented by proper control of diuretic dosage and replacement therapy with fluids and electrolytes when necessary.

       4. Depending on the biological behavior of the underlying cause of the nephrotic syndrome, control of edema may necessitate administration of low doses of oral diuretics for the life of the patient.

    C. Low-sodium diets may be considered in conjunction with, or in lieu of, chronic diuretic therapy for long-term management of edema. Reduced sodium diets minimize retention of sodium and fluid and thereby minimize edema formation.

    D. Repeated paracentesis for elimination of ascites should be avoided because it may deplete the patient of fluids and metabolites.

    E. *Use caution in administering sodium containing drugs.* Consider use of alternate drugs which do not contain sodium, if available, (e.g. calcium lactate instead of sodium bicarbonate).

III. For information on symptomatic and supportive treatment of uremia in patients with glomerular diseases, consult the section of this chapter on renal failure.

HYPERCALCEMIC NEPHROPATHY

Definition

Primary renal failure resulting from increased blood ionized calcium concentration is termed hypercalcemic nephropathy.

Etiopathogenesis

I. Hypercalcemic nephropathy may result from any cause of elevated blood ionized calcium including:
  A. Cancer-associated hypercalcemia
     1. Lymphosarcoma (particularly the thymic form)
     2. Perirectal adenocarcinoma arising from the glands of the anal sacs
     3. Testicular interstitial cell tumors
     4. Carcinomas of the mammary gland, stomach, thyroid gland, and lung
  B. Primary hyperparathyroidism
  C. Hypervitaminosis
  D. Septic osteomyelitis
II. Cancer associated hypercalcemia is the most common cause of hypercalcemic nephropathy in dogs.

Clinical Signs

I. Urinary signs of hypercalcemic nephropathy may include:
  A. Polyuria/polydipsia
  B. Decreased urine concentrating ability
  C. Azotemia
  D. Clinical signs of uremia
II. Nonrenal clinical signs of hypercalcemia include:
  A. Anorexia
  B. Weakness
  C. Vomiting
  D. Neurologic signs ranging from depression to stupor to coma

Diagnosis

I. Tentative diagnosis of hypercalcemic nephropathy is based on demonstrating renal dysfunction (decreased renal concentrating ability, azotemia, uremia, etc.) concurrent with hypercalcemia.

II. Primary renal failure which is not the result of hypercalcemic nephropathy may occasionally result in hypercalcemia up to approximately 15 mg/dl.

III. Differentiation of hypercalcemic nephropathy from primary renal failure with secondary hypercalcemia:

    A. When a cause for hypercalcemia other than primary renal failure is identified, and no other cause for primary renal failure is identified, hypercalcemic nephropathy is presumed to be present.

    B. When no identifiable cause for hypercalcemia other than primary renal failure is found and total serum calcium concentration does not exceed approximately 15 mg/dl, hypercalcemia is likely to be secondary to primary renal failure.

Treatment

I. Renal failure with secondary hypercalcemia

    A. The pathogenesis and clinical significance of hypercalcemia secondary to primary renal failure is unknown.

    B. It appears that hypercalcemia secondary to renal failure does not in most cases require the aggressive therapy recommended for hypercalcemic nephropathy. Therapy should be directed at management of renal secondary hyperparathyroidism (consult the section of this chapter entitled "Conservative Medical Management of Renal Failure").

    C. *Dietary supplementations of calcium and vitamin D are contraindicated in patients with hypercalcemia.*

II. Hypercalcemic nephropathy

    A. Hypercalcemic nephropathy may be reversible if hypercalcemia is corrected before irreversible renal damage occurs. Development of irreversible renal lesions depends on the magnitude and duration of hypercalcemia and the severity of renal damage. Treatment of hypercalcemic nephropathy involves correction of hypercalcemia and treatment of the clinical and laboratory abnormalities associated with renal failure and the acute uremic crisis. Consult the sections of this chapter entitled "Conservative Management of Renal Failure" and "Management of the Acute Uremic Crisis" for additional information on these subjects.

    B. Dehydration should be corrected by administration of an appropriate dose of 0.9% sodium chloride solution (dose of 0.9% NaCl in ml = % dehydration × body weight in kg × 1000). Sodium chloride solution is indicated because it promotes calciuresis and contains no calcium. Because administration of 0.9% NaCl solution may induce substantial kaliuresis, potassium supplementation may be required to prevent hypokalemia which may potentiate the harmful cardiac effects of hypercalcemia.

    C. If a treatable cause of hypercalcemia has been identified (e.g. lymphosarcoma, septic osteomyelitis, etc.), specific treatment directed at the underlying disease process should be initiated as soon as possible.

D. Furosemide is indicated to induce calciuresis. It should be administered at an initial bolus dose of 5 mg/kg followed by a maintenance infusion of 5 mg/kg/hour. The patient should be well hydrated before initiating this therapy. Normal hydration must be maintained by replacing urinary losses by intravenous administration of equal volumes of potassium-supplemented 0.9% NaCl solution. It appears that the ability of furosemide to reduce serum calcium concentrations is limited to a reduction of about 3 mg/dl. *Thiazide diuretics should be avoided because they may decrease urinary excretion of calcium.*

E. Glucocorticoids may be of value in decreasing serum calcium concentrations in some patients because they limit bone resorption, decrease intestinal calcium absorption, and enhance renal calcium excretion. However, decreases in serum calcium concentration induced by glucocorticoid therapy are small unless hypercalcemia results from a neoplastic process which is responsive to glucocorticoid therapy (e.g. lymphosarcoma). In such cases reduction in serum calcium concentration apparently results from the antineoplastic actions of the drug. Prednisone or prednisolone may be used at a dose of 1.1 mg/kg given every 12 hours.

F. Sodium bicarbonate solution (1 mEq/ml) may be administered intravenously at a dose of 0.5 to 1.0 mEq/kg for emergency treatment of hypercalcemic crisis. Sodium bicarbonate decreases ionized calcium concentration by increasing the relative portion of calcium which is protein-bound and less harmful. Total serum calcium concentration is not altered by administration of sodium bicarbonate.

G. Synthetic calcitonin solution (Calcimar) may be considered for temporary treatment of hypercalcemia. Doses are not available for dogs and cats, but synthetic calcitonin administered at a dose of 4 to 8 I.U./kg every 12 hours is reported to be effective in treatment of hypercalcemia resulting from excessive osteoclast activity in human patients. Calcitonin acts by decreasing osteoclastic activity and by decreasing formation of new osteoclasts. Maximal reduction of hypercalcemia in people is about 3 mg/dl and occurs 4 to 12 hours after injection.

H. If other methods have failed to reduce serum calcium concentration, peritoneal dialysis with calcium-free dialysis solutions may be considered.

NEPHROGENIC DIABETES INSIPIDUS (DI)

Definition

I. For a discussion of pituitary (central) diabetes insipidus see chapter 19.
II. Nephrogenic diabetes insipidus refers to a large group of physiologic, pharmacologic, and pathologic conditions in which the kidney fails to concen-

trate urine in spite of physiologic or supraphysiologic circulating concentrations of antidiuretic hormone (ADH).

Etiopathogenesis

I. Nephrogenic DI results from structural or functional abnormalities that alter ADH-induced cell membrane permeability to water in the distal renal tubules and collecting ducts.
II. Acquired nephrogenic DI may result from:
  A. Chronic generalized renal failure
  B. Renal diseases in which the renal tubules and collecting ducts are primarily involved
  C. Hypercalcemia
  D. Hypokalemia
  E. Hyperadrenocorticism
  F. Hypoadrenocorticism
  G. Hepatic failure (cirrhosis)
  H. Pyometra
  I. Certain drug toxicities
    1. Lithium carbonate
    2. Methoxyflurane
    3. Demeclocycline
    4. Alpha-adrenergic agents

Clinical Signs

I. Clinical signs in dogs with congenital nephrogenic DI may include:
  A. Insatiable polydipsia and voluminous polyuria
  B. Nocturia
  C. Formation of colorless urine
  D. Extreme enlargement of the urinary bladder detected by palpation
  E. Pot-bellied appearance due to bladder enlargement
II. Clinical signs in patients with acquired nephrogenic DI are highly variable.
  A. Polyuria and polydipsia are consistent findings, but in general, the magnitude of polyuria with acquired nephrogenic DI is much less than with congenital nephrogenic DI or pituitary DI.
  B. Other clinical signs, if any, are usually related to the disease process underlying the acquired nephrogenic DI.

Diagnosis

I. Congenital nephrogenic DI should be suspected in patients with a history of massive polyuria and polydipsia (urine volume is 5 to 20 times normal) and formation of hypotonic urine since they were immature. Otherwise these patients are usually clinically normal. Diagnosis of congenital ne-

phrogenic DI is based on the following findings:
A. Routine urinalysis usually reveals no abnormalities except a urine specific gravity between 1.001 and 1.007 (Uosm = 50 to 300).
B. Serum osmolality values may be slightly above normal.
C. Renal and hepatic function are normal and other causes of acquired nephrogenic DI may be ruled out by history and/or laboratory examination.
D. Patients with congenital nephrogenic DI fail to concentrate urine in response to water deprivation, partial water deprivation, saline loading, or ADH administration.
II. Acquired nephrogenic DI should be suspected in patients with polyuria, polydipsia, and formation of hypotonic urine.
A. Presumptive diagnosis of acquired nephrogenic DI and its underlying etiology may often be determined from the history, physical examination, and preliminary laboratory evaluations.
1. Preliminary laboratory evaluations should include: a complete blood count, serum urea nitrogen, creatinine, sodium, potassium, chloride, and calcium concentrations; serum alanine aminotransferase and alkaline phosphatase activities; routine urinalysis.
2. Additional studies may be necessary to confirm certain causes of acquired nephrogenic DI.
a) Determination of endogenous creatinine clearance rate may be required to confirm early renal failure.
b) ACTH response testing may be required to confirm hypoadrenocorticism or hyperadrenocorticism.
B. Confirmation of acquired nephrogenic DI is based on demonstrating the patient's inability to concentrate urine after water deprivation, partial water deprivation, saline loading, or ADH administration. However, a diagnosis of acquired nephrogenic DI does not usually require extensive studies to evaluate renal concentration as part of the diagnostic evaluation.

Treatment of Nephrogenic DI

I. The only effective means of controlling the polyuria of congenital nephrogenic DI is administration of chlorothiazide combined with a salt-restricted diet.
A. This therapy may reduce polyuria by 50 to 85 percent.
B. Chlorothiazide produces a mild negative salt balance, thereby contracting extracellular fluid volume and stimulating enhanced proximal renal tubular reabsorption of sodium, chloride, and water. The net effect is to substantially reduce the volume of fluid delivered to the distal renal tubules and collecting ducts. Thus, less urine is available for elimination (even though it is still dilute and relatively large in volume).
C. The recommended dose of chlorothiazide is 20 to 40 mg per kg given every 12 hours.

    D. A low-sodium diet should be fed in concert with administration of chlo-
rothiazide to maximize its effect.

II. Therapy for patients with acquired nephrogenic DI is directed toward eliminating or modifying the cause of the underlying disease (i.e. renal failure,
hypercalcemia, hyperadrenocorticism).

DISEASES OF THE UPPER AND LOWER URINARY TRACT

URINARY TRACT INFECTIONS

Definitions

    I. Urinary tract infection (UTI) encompasses a wide variety of clinical en-
tities whose common denominator is microbial invasion of any of the
urinary tract's components.

   II. Although pyelonephritis, cystitis, and urethritis are used commonly as
general terms, they each refer to localized UTI that has the potential to
affect the entire urinary tract. The entire system is at risk of invasion once
any of its parts becomes colonized with bacteria.

  III. Acute uncomplicated urinary tract infections are defined as those acute
(previously untreated) cases in which no underlying structural or functional abnormalities of the urinary tract altering host-defense mechanisms
can be defined.

  IV. Recurrent urinary tract infections are those which recur following withdrawal of therapy.

   V. Candiduria refers to UTI of any portion of the urinary tract caused by
Candida.

  VI. Relapses refer to recurrence of the same species (and serologic strain) of
microorganisms within several weeks of the date of cessation of therapy.
Relapses may result from use of inappropriate antimicrobial drugs, inadequate or inappropriate administration of medication, failure to eliminate predisposing causes, deep-seated infections inaccessible to the action
of antimicrobial drugs, or emergence of drug-resistant pathogens.

 VII. Reinfections represent recurrent infections caused by a different pathogen
from that causing the previous infection. Reinfections indicate failure to
eliminate predisposing causes (Table 12-2), presence of multiple pathogens
in which only sensitive pathogens were eliminated by therapy, iatrogenic
infection during follow-up procedures, or spontaneous reinfection.

Etiopathogenesis

    I. Most UTI occur as a consequence of ascending migration of bacteria
through the urethra and/or genital tract to the bladder, ureters, and/or kid-
ney(s).

II. Entrance of bacteria to the urinary tract is not synonymous with infection. Host-defense mechanisms must be transiently or persistently abnormal for bacterial colonization to occur.

III. Factors which may predispose to urinary tract infection are:
   A. Interference with normal micturition
      1. Mechanical obstruction to outflow (e.g., uroliths, neoplasms, urethral strictures)
      2. Incomplete emptying of excretory pathways
         a) Neurogenic micturition disorders (e.g. detrusor areflexia, reflex dyssynergia)
         b) Anatomic defects (e.g. vesicoureteral reflux, diverticulae, especially urachal diverticulae)
   B. Altered urothelium
      1. Trauma (e.g. external trauma, uroliths, catheter or instrumentation-induced
      2. Neoplasia
      3. Drug or chemical-induced (e.g. cyclophosphamide)
   C. Altered urine volume, frequency, or composition
      1. Decreased urine production (e.g. dehydration, oliguric renal failure)
      2. Formation of dilute urine (e.g. polyuric renal failure, Cushing's disease)
      3. Glucosuria
      4. Voluntary or involuntary urine retention
   D. Impaired immunocompetence
      1. Acquired diseases (e.g. Cushing's disease, uremia)
      2. Immunosuppressive drugs (e.g. corticosteroids, cyclophosphamide)
   E. Anatomic defects
      1. Congenital or inherited (e.g. urethral abnormalities, urachal diverticulae, ectopic ureters)
      2. Acquired (e.g. urethrostomies)

Clinical Signs

I. Clinical signs of UTI are related to affected portions of the urinary tract (i.e. urethra-urethritis; bladder-cystitis; kidney(s)-pyelonephritis).
   A. Clinical signs of urethritis may include:
      1. Dysuria
      2. Increased frequency of micturition
      3. Gross hematuria, usually at the beginning of the urine stream
      4. Urethral discharge independent of micturition
   B. Clinical signs of cystitis may include:
      1. Dysuria
      2. Gross hematuria, usually at the end of the urine stream
      3. Cloudy urine
      4. Foul-smelling urine

   5. Absence of systemic signs of illness. Pyrexia and other clinical evidence of systemic disease in animals suspected of having cystitis should prompt a search for disease elsewhere in the body.
   C. Clinical signs of pyelonephritis may include:
      1. Pyrexia
      2. Depression
      3. Anorexia
      4. Vomiting
      5. Pain over the dorsal lumbar region
      6. Polyuria and polydipsia
      7. Absence of clinical signs—most animals with chronic pyelonephritis are clinically asymptomatic.
   D. Dogs and cats may also have asymptomatic bacteriuria or asymptomatic funguria. The incidence and clinical significance of this finding is not clear.

Diagnosis

   I. Bacterial UTI may be suspected on the basis of clinical signs and/or results of urinalysis.
      A. Urinalysis findings suggestive of bacterial UTI include pyuria and visualization of bacteria in unstained urinary sediment. Hematuria and proteinuria may also be observed.
      B. Hematuria, pyuria, and proteinuria suggest inflammatory urinary tract disease, but do not indicate its cause or location within the urinary tract.
      C. Absence of hematuria, pyuria, and proteinuria does not rule out the existence of infection since infection may occur without stimulating a detectable inflammatory response.
  II. Diagnosis of infection should be confirmed by urine culture because detection of inflammation on routine urinalysis is not a reliable index of UTI.
      A. Positive urine culture results indicate that bacterial infection is either a cause of the disease process or a secondary complication of another process such as neoplasia or metabolic stone disease.
      B. The presence of bacteria in urine is not synonymous with UTI because the bacteria may be either contaminants or pathogens.
      C. Significant bacteriuria is a term coined to describe bacteriuria that does represent UTI.
         1. A high bacterial count in a properly collected and cultured urine sample is indicative of UTI.
         2. Small numbers of bacteria obtained from untreated patients usually indicate contamination.
         3. Differentiation between bacterial pathogens and contaminants can usually be made with quantitative urine cultures (Table 12-2).
 III. Diagnosis of candidiasis is based on results of urinalysis and urine culture.

TABLE 12-2. INTERPRETATION OF QUANTITATIVE URINE CULTURES IN DOGS
AND CATS (NUMBER OF BACTERIA/ML URINE)

Collection Method	Significant		Suspicious		Probable Contaminant	
	Dog	Cat	Dog	Cat	Dog	Cat
Cystocentesis	≥ 1000	≥ 1000	100 to 1000	100 to 1000	< 100	< 100
Catheterization	≥ 10,000	≥ 1000	1000 to 10,000	100 to 1000	< 1000	< 100
Voluntary Void	≥ 100,000	≥ 10,000	10,000 to 90,000	1000 to 10,000	< 10,000	< 1000
Manual Compression	≥ 100,000	≥ 10,000	10,000 to 90,000	1000 to 10,000	< 10,000	< 1000

A. *Candida* organisms may be detected by examination of urinary sediment. These organisms may be contaminants, but they should be suspected as pathogens in patients with known predisposition to candiduria
(including diabetes mellitus, long-term antibiotic administration, administration of corticosteroids or immunosuppressive drugs, and/or indwelling urinary catheters), debilitating disease, or bacteriologically
"sterile" pyuria.

B. Definitive diagnosis of candiduria is based on results of urine culture.
1. Unlike bacteriuria, the clinical significance of candiduria cannot be
reliably predicted on the basis of the number of colony-forming-units
per milliliter of urine.
2. The presence of any *Candida* organisms in a properly collected urine
specimen should tentatively be regarded as pathologic.
a) Because true candiduria may occur in low numbers, cystocentesis
is usually required to differentiate true candiduria from contamination.
b) Identification of *Candida* organisms on two properly collected
serial urine specimens should be considered significant.

IV. Urine culture, radiographic studies, and biopsy procedures often provide
information necessary to localize the disease process and to establish its
cause.

V. Bacterial UTI is a common urinary tract disease in dogs but is much less
common in cats.

Treatment

I. An antimicrobial agent should be selected after consideration of the fol-
lowing:
A. Dosage form that is easy for the client to administer
B. Few (if any) undesirable or toxic side effects
C. Inexpensive

D. Produce urinary concentrations that exceed the MIC for the infecting species or strain of bacteria by at least fourfold (Table 12-3).

E. For treatment of lower UTI, select antimicrobial agents that attain high concentrations in urine.

F. For treatment of pyelonephritis, select antimicrobial agents that attain high concentrations in serum and, if possible, in urine.

II. The drug selected should be administered frequently enough to maintain inhibitory concentrations in urine (Table 12-3) and long enough to eliminate the infecting agent from the urinary tract.

A. Data concerning the minimum and optimum duration of antimicrobial therapy for UTI's are not available.

B. It is recommended that acute, uncomplicated UTI be treated for a period of approximately 2 weeks, and that chronic or recurrent UTI be treated for at least 4 to 6 weeks.

C. Some infections involving the kidney(s) and prostate gland may require more prolonged therapy.

III. To ensure adequate concentrations of the drug in the urinary tract overnight, it is recommended that one of the daily doses be administered prior to bedtime (or prior to a period of confinement during which micturition is not permitted) and shortly following micturition.

IV. Avoid use of multiple antibiotics simultaneously. The effect of antibiotic combinations on the infecting bacterial population may be additive, synergistic, antagonistic, or one of indifference. In addition the effect may

TABLE 12-3.   MEAN URINARY CONCENTRATION OF ANTIMICROBIAL DRUGS
USED IN TREATMENT OF CANINE URINARY TRACT INFECTIONS

Antimicrobial Drug	Dose (mg/kg)	Route of Administration	Mean Urine Concentration
Amikacin	2.2 mg/kg q 8 h	S.Q.	100 mcg/ml†
Amoxicillin	11 mg/kg q 8 h	oral	201 mcg/ml
Ampicillin	25 mg/kg q 8 h	oral	309 mcg/ml
Cephalexin	30 mg/kg q 8 h	oral	225 mcg/ml
Chloramphenicol	33 mg/kg q 8 h	oral	123 mcg/ml
Gentamicin	2.2 mg/kg q 8 h	S.Q.	107 mcg/ml
Hetacillin	25 mg/kg q 8 h	oral	300 mcg/ml
Kanamycin	5.5 mg/kg q 12 h	S.Q.	473 mcg/ml
Nitrofurantoin	4.4 mg/kg q 8 h	oral	100 mcg/ml
Penicillin G	36,666 U/kg q 8 h	oral	294 mcg/ml
Penicillin V	25 mg/kg q 8 h	oral	148 mcg/ml
Sulfisoxazole	22 mg/kg q 8 h	oral	1,466 mcg/ml
Tetracycline	18 mg/kg q 8 h	oral	137 mcg/ml
Tobramycin	2.2 mg/kg q 8 h	S.Q.	100 mcg/ml†
TMP-SDZ*	(TMP) 2.2 mg/kg q 12 h	oral	(TMP) 26 mcg/ml
	(SDZ) 11 mg/kg q 12 h		(SDZ) 79 mcg/ml

* TMP-SDZ = Trimethoprim sulfadiazine
† Estimated, Dr. G. V. Ling, personal communication
The above volumes were determined by Dr. G. V. Ling et al in hydrated dogs with normal renal function.

vary unpredictably with the antimicrobials administered, the bacterial species involved, and the site of infection in the body.

V. Use of aminoglycoside antimicrobials (e.g. kanamicin, gentamicin, tobramycin, and amikacin) should be limited to UTI that have persisted in spite of appropriate therapy with other antimicrobials, or in patients concomitantly infected with two or more bacterial species with widely differing antimicrobial susceptibilities.

VI. The efficacy of antimicrobial agents in treatment of bacterial UTI is best predicted by determining the minimum inhibitory concentrations (MIC) of the bacteria isolated from the urinary tract.

    A. The MIC is defined as the least amount of an antimicrobial agent that inhibits growth of a specific species or strain of bacteria in a defined and reproducible set of *in vitro* conditions.

    B. Efficacy of a drug in treatment of bacterial UTI may be estimated by multiplying the determined MIC of the bacteria isolated from the UTI by four. If this product is less than the mean urine concentration for the drug (Table 12-2), the drug has about a 95 percent efficacy.

    C. It is not necessary to routinely perform susceptibility testing on all urinary bacterial isolates.

        1. Data are available that may be used to select an appropriate antimicrobial drug with at least an 80 percent chance of cure for most common bacterial isolates (Table 12-3), provided that the species of the causative agent has been identified.

        2. Susceptibility testing is mandatory:

            a) In cases of UTI caused by multiple organisms

            b) In instances when a drug empirically selected has failed (Table 12-3)

            c) In cases in which the bacteria causing UTI are uncommon or have unpredictable antimicrobial susceptibility

VII. The following protocol is recommended for management of acute, uncomplicated bacterial UTI:

    A. Collect a urine sample for urinalysis and quantitative urine culture, preferably by cystocentesis.

TABLE 12-4. IN VITRO SUSCEPTIBILITY OF COMMON CANINE URINARY TRACT BACTERIAL PATHOGENS TO CERTAIN ORAL ANTIMICROBIAL AGENTS

Organism	Recommended Antimicrobial	Estimated Susceptibility
Staphylococcus spp.	Penicillin	near 100%
Streptococcus spp.	Penicillin	near 100%
Escherichia coli	Trimethoprim/Sulfa	about 80%
Proteus mirabilis	Penicillin	about 80%
Pseudomonas aeruginosa	Tetracycline	about 80%
Klebsiella pneumoniae	Cephalexin	about 80%

Adapted from Ling GV: Treatment of urinary tract infections with antimicrobial agents. *Current Veterinary Therapy* pp. 1051–1055. in Kirk RW: *Current Veterinary Therapy* VIII, Philadelphia, W.B. Saunders Co., 1983

B. Antimicrobial therapy may be initiated either immediately or after identification of the infecting bacteria.

   1. If therapy is initiated immediately, penicillin or ampicillin may be used for gram-positive bacteria, while trimethoprim-sulfa may be used for gram-negative bacteria (based on Gram-stained smear of urinary sediment). Therapy may be modified once results of culture and susceptibility test results are known.

   2. If initiation of therapy is delayed until after identification of the bacteria, the antimicrobial agent may be selected on the basis of known susceptibility of organisms to antimicrobics (Table 12-4), or on the basis of antimicrobial susceptibility tests.

C. Culture a urine sample collected by cystocentesis three to five days following initiation of therapy.

   1. Therapy is considered to be successful only if urine does not contain any pathogenic organisms.

   2. Treatment is ineffective and relapse will occur if the colony count has only been reduced (e.g., from 10^8 to 10^2).

   3. If bacterial growth is detected 3 to 5 days after initiating therapy, treatment has failed and another antimicrobial agent must be selected for use based on results of bacterial culture and susceptibility tests.

D. If urine is sterile after 3 to 5 days, treatment should be continued.

E. Urine may be cultured immediately prior to discontinuation of therapy to insure that the infection has been eradicated.

F. Culture a urine sample obtained by cystocentesis 7 to 10 days after completion of therapy to detect relapses.

G. Reinfection caused by a different organism usually occurs later than a relapse. Therefore urinalysis and culture should be done approximately 4 weeks (and in some instances repeatedly) after cessation of antimicrobial therapy.

VIII. The following protocol is recommended for management of recurrent bacterial urinary tract infections:

A. When reinfection occurs only once or twice each year, each episode may be treated as an acute uncomplicated UTI.

B. Recurrent UTI that does not respond to conventional antimicrobial therapy is an absolute indication to evaluate the patient for a predisposing cause such as uroliths, neoplasms, or diverticula.

C. When reinfection occurs more often than four times in a year and predisposing causes of UTI cannot be identified or eliminated, or their apparent elimination does not prevent recurrence, long-term antimicrobial therapy may be necessary to prevent reinfection.

   1. Long-term preventative therapy is initiated only after effectively treating existing UTI in the patient as outlined for treatment of acute uncomplicated UTI.

   2. Drugs, dosage, and selection criterion for antimicrobial agents used for long-term therapy are summarized in table 12-5.

TABLE 12-5. ANTIMICROBIAL AGENTS USED FOR PREVENTION OF RECURRENT
BACTERIAL URINARY TRACT INFECTIONS

Drug	Indications	Conventional Dose	Prophylactic Dose*
Nitrofurantoin	Gram Negative Infections	4 mg/kg q 8 hr	3–4 mg/kg q 24 hr
Trimethoprim/sulfadiazine	Gram Negative Infections	15 mg/kg q 12 hr	7–8 mg/kg q 24 hr
Ampicillin	Gram Positive	25 mg/kg q 8 hr	25 mg/kg q 24 hr

* Prophylactic medications should be given orally at night after micturition and immediately before bedtime.

3. Antimicrobial drugs are administered nightly after micturition and before bedtime for approximately 6 months.
4. Specimens of urine are collected by cystocentesis for culture approximately once each month.
  a) If urine cultures are negative, therapy is continued.
  b) If bacteria are cultured from urine, the infection is treated as an episode of acute, uncomplicated UTI (see above). If after 2 weeks of such therapy the urine is again sterile, long-term preventative antimicrobial administration is resumed.
5. At the end of six consecutive months of bacteria-free urine, long-term antimicrobial therapy may be terminated.
6. Many patients which remain uninfected for 6 months do not develop additional episodes of infection.
IX. The following protocol is recommended for candiduria.
  A. Because candiduria may be transient and benign, aggressive therapy should probably be reserved for those cases in which clinical evidence suggests that candiduria may be of pathologic significance.
  B. Asymptomatic candiduria should be treated by:
    1. Correcting identifiable predisposing factors, including:
      a) Stop antibiotic, corticosteroid, or immunosuppressive drug therapy (if possible).
      b) Remove indwelling urinary catheters (if possible).
      c) Treat diabetes mellitus.
    2. Alkalinizing the urine by administration of sodium bicarbonate.
      a) The initial recommended dose is 325 mg q 8 h PO.
      b) The dose should be increased until urinary pH remains > 7.5.
  C. A more aggressive therapeutic approach is indicated for patients with symptomatic candiduria and patients that are debilitated, have a grave underlying illness, or whose condition has suddenly deteriorated.
    1. Correct identifiable predisposing conditions (see above).
    2. Alkalinize urine to pH > 7.5 by oral administration of sodium bicarbonate (see above).

3. Initiate therapy with 5-fluorocytosine (5-FC; Ancobon) at a dose of 67 mg/kg q 8 h PO.
    a) Five-FC is excreted in urine in active form.
    b) Rarely encountered toxic side effects include:
        (1) Bone marrow depression
        (2) Hepatic toxicity
        (3) Dermatitis
    c) The dose of 5-FC should be reduced in patients with renal failure.
4. Ketoconazole (Nizoral) may be used instead of 5-FC at a dose of 10 mg/kg q 8 h PO.
    a) The efficacy of ketoconazole as compared to 5-FC in treatment of candiduria is not known. Preliminary trials in our hospital suggest that it may be less effective than 5-FC.
    b) Toxic side-effects of ketoconazole include gastrointestinal upsets and anorexia.
5. Response to treatment should be monitored by urine culture at weekly intervals.
    a) Treatment should be continued until two successive negative urine cultures are obtained.
    b) It has been recommended that cultures of urinary sediment cultures be used to monitor response to treatment because of their greater sensitivity.
    c) As a general rule, patients with renal or systemic candidiasis should be treated for at least four to six weeks.

UROLITHIASIS

Definition

I. Uroliths are polycrystalline concretions that typically contain 95% organic or inorganic crystalloids and less than 5 percent organic matrix.
II. Uroliths recognized in dogs and cats include: magnesium ammonium phosphate, calcium oxalate (2 types), ammonium acid urate, uric acid, calcium phosphate (4 types), matrix calculi, and mixed calculi (mixtures of different minerals in the same calculus).
III. Cystine calculi and silica calculi have been reported in dogs but not yet in cats.

Etiopathogenesis

I. Magnesium ammonium phosphate (struvite) uroliths.
    A. Struvite uroliths are the most common type of urolith found in dogs (about 70 percent) and cats (about 90 percent).

B. Most canine struvite uroliths and some feline struvite uroliths result from UTI due to urease-producing bacteria, primarily *Staphylococcus aureus*. *Proteus* spp. and ureaplasms are also calculogenic microbes. Increased urinary pH and ammonium concentrations resulting from the action of bacterial urease on urea are thought to initiate stone formation.

C. Some canine struvite uroliths and most feline struvite uroliths occur in the absence of bacterial UTI. The mechanisms of sterile struvite urolith formation in these animals are unknown.

D. Struvite uroliths frequently contain calcium phosphate and may contain calcium carbonate.

II. Urate uroliths (ammonium acid urate and uric acid uroliths).

A. Ammonium acid urate uroliths are far more common than uric acid uroliths in dogs. Although Dalmations have a higher incidence of urate uroliths, they have also been detected in many other canine breeds and in cats.

B. Uric acid becomes more soluble as urinary pH becomes more alkaline; ammonium urate becomes less soluble in alkaline urine because of increased ammonium ion concentration.

C. A high prevalence of ammonium acid urate stones has been observed in dogs with portal vascular anomalies. Predisposition of these dogs to urate uroliths probably is associated with concomitant hyperammonemia, hyperammonuria, hyperuricemia and hyperuricosuria.

III. Cystinuria and cystine uroliths.

A. Cystinuria is an inborn error of metabolism characterized by abnormal transport (decreased reabsorption) of cystine and other amino acids by the renal tubules.

B. The exact mechanism of cystine urolith formation is unknown. Since not all cystinuric dogs form uroliths, cystinuria is a predisposing factor rather than the primary cause of cystine urolith formation.

C. Cystine is more soluble in alkaline urine.

D. Many breeds of dogs have been reported to develop cystine uroliths, especially Dachshunds.

E. While cystinuria is observed in both sexes, cystine uroliths occur predominantly in male dogs.

F. Cystinuria has not been documented in domesticated cats.

IV. Calcium oxalate uroliths.

A. Oxalic acid (and its salt, oxalate) is a nonessential endproduct of metabolism produced in the liver and excreted unchanged in urine. Under ordinary circumstances, dietary intake of oxalic acid does not contribute significantly to urinary oxalate.

B. Urinary pH does not appear to alter solubility of calcium oxalate. Factors incriminated in the etiopathogenesis of calcium oxalate urolithiasis include: (1) hypercalciuria, (2) hyperoxaluria, and (3) hyperuricosuria.

V. Silica uroliths.

A. Silica uroliths occur in many breeds, but an apparent predilection exists

for German Shepherd dogs. Silica uroliths occur predominantly, but not exclusively, in male dogs.
  B. Solubility of silica uroliths does not appear to be pH-dependent.
  C. Development of silica uroliths may be related to diet. However, no specific diets or dietary constituents have been incriminated.
  D. Most but not all silica uroliths have a characteristic jack-stone appearance. However, not all jack-stones are composed of silica.
VI. Calcium phosphate (apatite) uroliths.
  A. Formation of calcium phosphate uroliths is influenced by urinary pH, urinary calcium and phosphate concentrations. With the exception of calcium hydrogen phosphate dihydrate (Brushite) calculi, calcium phosphate uroliths are more soluble in acidic urine.
  B. There are four forms of calcium phosphate uroliths: hydroxyl apatite, carbonate apatite, brushite, and whitlockite.
  C. Calcium phosphate uroliths may occur in association with metabolic disorders such as primary hyperparathyroidism, renal tubular acidosis, and excessive dietary calcium and phosphorus intakes.

Clinical Signs

  I. Clinical signs of urolithiasis depend on the location(s) within the urinary tract that are affected.
 II. Clinical signs of uroliths in the urinary bladder and/or urethra include:
  A. Hematuria
  B. Dysuria
  C. Pollakiuria
  D. Inappropriate micturition
  E. Reduced size and force of the urine stream
  F. Spontaneous voiding of uroliths
  G. Abdominal discomfort
  H. Urinary obstruction and its associated clinical signs (postobstructive uremia)
III. Clinical signs of renal and/or ureteral uroliths include:
  A. Hematuria
  B. Abdominal and/or lumbar pain
  C. Vomiting
 IV. Some patients with cystic calculi and many with renal calculi may be asymptomatic.

Diagnosis

  I. Tentative diagnosis of urolithiasis is based on findings obtained by history and physical examination. Diagnosis should be confirmed by urinalysis, urine culture, radiography, and analysis of recovered calculi.
 II. Primary objectives of radiographic evaluation of patients suspected of hav-

ing uroliths are determination of the site(s), number, density, and shape of calculi. Radiographic evaluation is also an important technique to detect predisposing abnormalities and to monitor response to medical or surgical therapy.

III. Determination of the type(s) of urolith(s) found in the patient is essential for planning effective therapeutic and preventive regimens. In patients in which medical dissolution of uroliths is being considered, a tentative diagnosis of the type of urolith may be determined as outlined below:

   A. Radiographic density and physical characteristics of uroliths (Table 12-6)

   B. Urinary pH

      1. Struvite and apatite uroliths—usually alkaline

      2. Ammonium urate uroliths—variable

      3. Cystine uroliths—acid

      4. Calcium oxalate uroliths—variable

      5. Silica uroliths—variable

   C. Identification of crystals in urinary sediment

   D. Type of bacteria, if any, isolated from urine

      1. Urease-producing bacteria, especially staphylococci, commonly are associated with struvite uroliths

      2. Urinary tract infections often are absent in patients with calcium oxalate, cystine, ammonium urate, and silical uroliths

      3. Calcium oxalate, cystine, ammonium urate, and silica uroliths may predispose patients to urinary tract infections; if infections are caused by urease-producing bacteria, struvite may precipitate around them

   E. Serum chemistry evaluation

      1. Hypercalcemia may be associated with calcium-containing uroliths

      2. Hyperuricemia may be associated with urate uroliths

   F. Breed of dog and history of occurrence of uroliths in patient's ancestors or littermates

   G. Analysis of uroliths fortuitously passed and collected during micturition

TABLE 12-6. RADIOGRAPHIC CHARACTERISTICS OF UROLITHS COMMONLY OCCURRING IN DOGS AND CATS

Mineral Type	Degree of Radiopacity	Shape
Cystine	+ to + +	Smooth; usually small; round to oval
Oxalate	+ + + +	Usually rough, often quartz-like, and round to oval
Struvite	+ + to + + + +	Smooth; round or faceted; sometimes assume shape of renal pelvis, ureter, bladder, or urethra; sometimes laminated
Apatite	+ + + +	Smooth; round or faceted
Urate; uric acid	0 to + +	Smooth; round or oval; sometimes jack-stone
Silica	+ + to + + + +	Typically jack-stone

IV. Specific diagnosis of urolith composition should be based on quantitative urolith analysis.* We do not recommend analysis of uroliths by single qualitative chemical analysis because only some of the chemical radicals and ions can be detected by these methods. In addition, one kit (Oxford Stone Analysis Kit) consistently fails to detect calcium.

Dissolution of Struvite Uroliths in Dogs

I. The precise location, size, and number of uroliths present should be determined radiographically. This information is essential to assess response to therapy.

II. If uroliths are available (from previous surgery or spontaneously voided), determine their mineral composition. If unavailable, it may be necessary to make an educated guess about their mineral composition.

III. If UTI is present, institute appropriate therapy to eradicate it. Antimicrobial agents should be administered throughout the course of dissolution therapy and for an appropriate period beyond the time when uroliths are no longer radiographically detectable. Whereas the urine and surface of calculi may be sterilized after appropriate antimicrobial therapy, the original infecting organisms may remain viable below the surface of the urolith. Premature discontinuation of therapy may result in relapse of bacteriuria and infection. Consult the section of this chapter entitled "Urinary Tract Infections" for additional information.

IV. A calculolytic diet** designed for dogs with struvite uroliths should be fed as the *sole* dietary source during therapeutic urolith dissolution. This diet is formulated to contain a reduced quantity of high quality protein and reduced quantities of phosphorus and magnesium. Dietary protein intake is reduced on the basis of the hypothesis that reduced urinary urea concentration (the substrate of urease) would result in reduced urine ammonium concentration. In addition, such diets are supplemented with salt to stimulate thirst and induce compensatory polyuria.

A. Because the calculolytic diet stimulates thirst and promotes diuresis, owners should be informed that dogs with uroliths located in the urinary bladder may have pollakiuria and/or polyuria for a variable time following initiation of dietary therapy. The pollakiuria will usually subside as the infection is controlled and the uroliths decrease in size.

B. The calculolytic diet should be fed throughout the period of urolith dissolution and for an additional 4 weeks beyond the time when uroliths are no longer radiographically detectable.

C. *No other foods or mineral supplements should be fed to the patient*

---

* Urolithiasis Laboratory, P.O. Box 25375, Houston, TX, 77055 and Veterinary Teaching Hospital, School of Veterinary Medicine, University of California, Davis, CA, 95616.

** Prescription Diet s/d, Hills Division, Riviana Foods, Topeka, KS.

during dissolution therapy. Consumption of other foods or dietary supplements may result in therapeutic failure.

V. In the unlikely event that diuresis does not occur while dogs are consuming calculolytic diets, formation of dilute urine may be promoted by administering sodium chloride orally. Dose may range from 0.5 to 10 grams of sodium chloride daily depending on the size of the patient, quantity of urine produced, status of the cardiovascular system, and composition of the diet. Water must be available at all times. A satisfactory increase in volume of urine is indicated by formation of urine with a specific gravity of <1.020.

VI. If antimicrobial drugs and the calculolytic diet do not result in formation of acidic urine, urinary acidifiers may be administered. However, if stones are dissolving, acidifiers may be withheld regardless of urinary pH. Ammonium chloride (200 mg/kg q 8 h P.O.) or DL-methionine (0.2 to 1.0 g/kg q 8 h P.O.) may be used. Dose of urinary acidifiers should be adjusted for each patient on the basis of urinary pH (goal is pH of 6.5 or lower).

    A. Urinary acidifiers may be ineffective in some patients with UTI caused by urease-producing bacteria because therapeutic doses may be insufficient to overcome the continuous production of ammonium by bacterial urease. Combination therapy with appropriate antimicrobial drugs is recommended.

    B. Acidifiers should not be administered to uremic animals since they will aggravate the severity of metabolic acidosis typically associated with renal failure.

VII. Administration of acetohydroxamic acid (AHA, Lithostat), a urease inhibitor, should be considered in patients with persistent urinary tract infections caused by urease-producing bacteria (especially Staphylococci). When given orally at 12.5 mg/kg, every 12 hours, AHA retards alkalinization of urine caused by growth of urease-producing bacteria. It is rapidly and completely absorbed from the gastrointestinal tract of dogs and is excreted and concentrated in urine. Acetohydroxamic acid appears to have a dose-related bacteriostatic effect on gram-positive and gram-negative bacteria and may potentiate the antimicrobial effect of antibiotics. When administered at high doses (50 to 100 mg/kg/day), hemolytic anemia may occur.

VIII. Response to dissolution therapy should be monitored at appropriate intervals.

    A. The size of uroliths should be monitored at periodic intervals by radiography. We recommend monthly re-evaluation for most patients.

    B. Periodic evaluation of urinary sediment for crystalluria may also be considered; struvite crystals should not form if therapy has been effective in promoting urine that is undersaturated with magnesium ammonium phosphate.

C. Urine collected by cystocentesis should be cultured quantitatively during therapy and 5 to 7 days after discontinuation of therapy.

D. If uroliths increase in size during therapy or do not begin to decrease in size after approximately 4 to 8 weeks of appropriate medical therapy, alternative methods of management should be considered. Difficulty in inducing complete dissolution of uroliths by creating urine that is undersaturated with the suspected calculogenic crystalloid should prompt consideration that: (a) the wrong mineral component was identified, (b) the nucleus of the urolith is of different mineral composition than outer portions of the urolith, and (c) the owner or the patient is not complying with therapeutic recommendations.

Prevention of Recurrence of Uroliths

I. Calculi of all types have a tendency to recur after surgical removal or medical dissolution. Unfortunately, the likelihood of recurrence is unpredictable. Recurrence may be related to:
   A. Persistence of the underlying causes of urolithiasis
   B. Failure to remove all uroliths from the urinary tract
   C. Persistence of UTI with urease-producing bacteria
   D. Lack of owner compliance with therapeutic or prophylactic recommendations
II. Increasing volume of urine—Induction of polyuria is recommended for all types of uroliths because it:
   A. Minimizes stagnation of urine by promoting increased urine production and more frequent micturition
   B. Dilutes calculogenic crystalloids which cause uroliths. Consult the section on increasing urine volume under the heading of medical dissolution of struvite uroliths in this chapter for further details.
III. Struvite uroliths
   A. Eradication or control of UTI with urease-producing bacteria is the most important factor in preventing recurrence of infection-induced struvite uroliths in dogs and cats.
      1. Successful eradication or control of UTI *alone* will effectively prevent formation of infection-induced struvite uroliths.
      2. Caution must be used in deciding whether or not to induce prophylactic diuresis in patients with struvite uroliths induced by recurrent UTI. Although formation of dilute urine would tend to minimize supersaturation of urine with calculogenic crystalloids, it may counteract the innate antimicrobial properties of urine and predispose to lower urinary tract infection.
      3. Consult the section of this chapter entitled "Urinary Tract Infections" for additional information.
   B. In light of the effectiveness of diets for dissolution of struvite uroliths,

dietary modification to prevent recurrent of uroliths would appear to be logical and feasible. However, the safety and efficacy of long-term dietary modification remains unproved. We recommend long-term use of the calculolytic diet or low protein diets designed for management of renal failure* especially if patients develop recurrent urolithiasis despite successful eradication or control of infection.

C. Studies to evaluate the effectiveness of acetohydroxamic acid (25 mg/kg/day) in prevention of struvite urolithiasis in dogs with persistent urinary tract infection caused by urease-producing bacteria have been encouraging. Acetohydroxamic acid should be considered for patients with recurrent struvite urolithiasis due to persistent urinary tract infections due to urease-producing bacteria. Consult the section of this chapter on medical dissolution of struvite uroliths for additional information.

D. If urinary pH of patients with previous struvite urolithiasis remains alkaline despite antimicrobial therapy, administration of urinary acidifiers should be considered. Consult the section of this chapter on medical dissolution of struvite uroliths for additional information.

IV. Urate uroliths

A. Adjusting urinary pH is primarily of value in dogs with uroliths composed principally of uric acid. Alkalinizing urine with oral sodium bicarbonate (sodium bicarbonate tablets or baking soda mixed with food) to a pH range of 6.5 to 7.0 significantly enhances the solubility of uric acid. Altering pH has a minimal effect on ammonium urate solubility.

B. Allopurinol (Zyloprim), a synthetic isomer of isoxanthine, inhibits hepatic conversion of hypoxanthine to xanthine and xanthine to uric acid, thereby reducing urinary excretion of uric acid. It should be administered at a dose of 10 mg/kg q 8 h for the first month. The dose may be reduced to 10 mg/kg s.i.d. thereafter. Dose of allopurinol should be reduced in patients with renal failure. In human patients, allopurinol is usually administered only if uric acid stones recur despite fluid and alkaline therapy.

C. Urinary tract infections in dogs with urate urolithiasis are generally considered to be secondary to the urolith. Consult the section of this chapter entitled "Urinary Tract Infections" for information on treatment of UTI.

D. Low-purine (all-vegetable) diets have been advocated as preventive therapy for urate uroliths. The efficacy of such diets remains unproven.

V. Calcium oxalate uroliths

Recommendations concerning prophylaxis of calcium oxalate uroli-

---

* Prescription Diet u/d, Hills Division Riviana Foods, Topeka, KS.

thiasis are extrapolated from studies in human subjects. Recurrence of calcium oxalate uroliths is difficult to prevent.

A. Long-term administration of thiazide diuretics (hydrochlorothiazide 2 mg/kg q 12 h P.O.) should be considered in patients with recurrent calcium oxalate uroliths in association with renal hypercalciuria (hypercalciuria resulting from impaired renal tubular calcium reabsorption). Thiazide diuretics decrease renal calcium excretion by:
   1. Reducing extracellular fluid volume and glomerular filtration rate
   2. Increasing renal tubular reabsorption of calcium
   3. Perhaps contributing a parathormone-like action
   4. Thiazides should not be used in patients with absorptive (intestinal) hypercalcuria because they may cause hypercalcemia.

B. Long-term administration of cellulose phosphate, an intestinal calcium-binding agent, may be considered in patients with recurrent calcium oxalate or calcium phosphate uroliths in association with absorptive hypercalciuria (hypercalciuria that results from primary intestinal hyperabsorption of calcium). Cellulose phosphate is not recommended for patients with renal hypercalciuria because it may induce hypocalcemia. The precise dosage is dependent on urinary calcium excretion, but the approximate recommendation for human beings is 5 grams given 3 times daily after meals. Supplementation with magnesium may be required.

C. Administration of allopurinol may be considered for patients with hyperuricosuric calcium oxalate urolithiasis (i.e. calcium oxalate urolithiasis associated with excessive urinary excretion of uric acid). Consult the section of this chapter on prophylaxis of urate uroliths for additional information on use of allopurinol.

D. Induction of polyuria and/or dietary calcium restriction should be considered for some patients with absorptive hypercalciuria or no metabolic abnormalities.

E. A variety of additional prophylactic therapies have been advocated for human beings, but their efficacy in dogs have not been evaluated. Consult reference material for additional information on these therapies.

VI. Calcium phosphate uroliths

Prevention of recurrent calcium phosphate uroliths includes: control or elimination of underlying causes of hypercalcemia and hypercalciuria (if present), feeding calculolytic diets, eradication or control of UTI, induction of polyuria, and urinary acidification (except for brushite).

A. Feeding of calculolytic diets which are low in calcium and phosphorus content and promotion of polyuria and acid-urine formation should be considered for patients with recurrent calcium phosphate uroliths. While long-term feeding of these diets may be associated with adverse effects such as polyuria, hypoalbuminemia, and mild alteration in hepatic enzymes and morphology, preliminary data indicates that such diets may prevent calcium phosphate urolith formation and growth.

B. Consult the section of this chapter on medical dissolution of struvite uroliths for additional information on induction of polyuria and urinary acidification.

C. Consult the section of this chapter entitled "Urinary Tract Infections" for additional information on treatment of UTI.

VII. Silica uroliths

Since initiating and perpetuating causes of silica urolithiasis are unknown, only nonspecific measures designed to reduce the degree of supersaturation of urine with calculogenic substances can be recommended for prophylaxis.

A. Polyuria should be induced. Consult the section of this chapter on medical dissolution of struvite uroliths for information on inducing polyuria.

B. Although the role of diet in the genesis of canine silica urolithiasis is speculative, it seems reasonable to recommend that the diet of affected patients be changed, especially if the problem is recurrent.

VIII. Cystine uroliths

The relative infrequency with which cystine uroliths occur have precluded extensive clinical evaluation of methods to prevent their recurrence. Recommended methods of prophylaxis which have been extrapolated from human medicine include:

A. Maintaining urinary pH at 7.5 or higher throughout the day by administration of sodium bicarbonate tablets or baking soda mixed with food. Dosage of sodium bicarbonate should be determined by response to therapy (urinary pH).

B. Administering D-penicillamine (dimethyl-cysteine, Cuprimine) orally
   1. Administered at a dose of 15 mg/kg b.i.d., mixed with food or given at mealtime
   2. It is a virtually nonmetabolizable compound which reduces the concentration of relatively insoluble cystine in urine by forming a dimer of cysteine-d-penicillamine disulfide instead of a dimer of cysteine-cysteine.
   3. D-penicillamine is most effective at a neutral to alkaline urinary pH.
   4. Anorexia and vomiting are the major side-effects. If these signs are observed, the dose may be reduced to 10 mg/kg/day and then gradually increased. Antiemetics may also be considered.
   5. Reversible side-effects of D-penicillamine reported in man include: proteinuria, glomerulonephritis, dermatitis, pruritis, pyrexia, neutropenia, arthropathy, and abnormalities of taste and smell. Because of the frequency of adverse reactions, it has been recommended that D-penicillamine therapy only be used when forced

      diuresis and alkalinization of urine are unsuccessful in controlling
      recurrent cystine urolithiasis in man.

  C. Inducing polyuria

  D. Treating urinary tract infections

DISEASES OF THE LOWER URINARY TRACT

DISORDERS OF MICTURITION: INCONTINENCE

Definitions

   I. Urinary incontinence is defined as involuntary loss of urine from the
urinary system. It must be differentiated from inappropriate micturition
which is conscious voiding of urine at inappropriate times or inappropriate locations (see chapter 17).

  II. Urinary incontinence may result from hormonal deficiencies (estrogen
and testosterone responsive incontinence), neurogenic dysfunction (urethral sphincter hypotonus, detrusor hyperreflexia), urinary obstruction
(paradoxical incontinence), and anatomic abnormalities (ectopic ureters,
patent urachus, pseudohermophrodites, and urethrorectal fistulae).

Etiopathogenesis

   I. Estrogen responsive incontinence (ERI)

    A. The etiopathogenesis of ERI has not been determined, but it is believed
that maintenance of adequate vesicourethral sphincter tone, and hence
continence, is dependent upon estrogen activity. Estrogens appear to
exert a permissive effect on alpha adrenergic receptor activity of the
internal urethral sphincter.

    B. Estrogen responsive incontinence is commonly recognized in female
dogs months to years after ovariohysterectomy.

    C. Occurrence of ERI often coincides with onset of polyuria due to any
cause, presumably because the polyuria-induced increase in bladder
volume causes intravesicular pressure to exceed urethral sphincter
tone.

  II. Testosterone responsive incontinence (TRI)

    A. Etiopathogenesis of TRI has not been determined.

    B. TRI apparently occurs in castrated animals and may be related to deficiency of testosterone.

  III. Urethral sphincter hypotonus

    A. Incompetence of the urethral sphincter mechanism may result from
nonneurogenic (diseases of the bladder, urethra, or prostate) or neurogenic causes and may be congenital or acquired in origin.

  B. Incontinence occurs when intravesical pressure exceeds maximum ure-
     thral closing pressure.
     1. The majority of the motor activity of urethral sphincter responsible
        for maintaining continence is mediated by alpha adrenergic recep-
        tors.
     2. Alpha-receptor-stimulating drugs increase tone of the sphincter.
IV. Detrusor hyperreflexia
    Detrusor hyperreflexia results from reduced inhibition of the detrusor
    reflex during the storage phase of micturition and may be caused by partial
    lesions of the long nerve pathways traversing the brainstem or spinal cord
    (C1 to L7) or of the cerebellum.

Clinical Signs

  I. Clinical signs of incontinence in patients with ERI, TRI or urethral sphincter
     hypotonus consist of:
     A. Accumulation of a pool of urine when the patient is lying down
     B. Involuntary dribbling of urine
     C. Accumulation of urine in areas adjacent to the external urethral orifice
     D. The inability to initiate and sustain normal micturition
     E. Normal postvoiding urine volume in the bladder
 II. Clinical signs of detrusor hyperreflexia may include:
     A. Frequent voiding of small quantities of urine, often without warning
     B. Little or no postvoiding residual urine

Diagnosis

  I. Diagnosis of estrogen responsive incontinence is based on:
     A. Recognition of typical clinical signs in spayed female dogs of any age.
     B. Exclusion of other causes of incontinence
     C. Response to estrogen therapy
 II. Diagnosis of testosterone responsive incontinence is based on:
     A. Recognition of typical clinical signs in a castrated male dog
     B. Exclusion of other causes of incontinence
     C. Response to testosterone therapy
III. Diagnosis of urethral sphincter hypotonus is based on:
     A. Recognition of typical clinical signs
     B. Exclusion of other causes of incontinence
     C. Decreased urethral sphincter tone as determined by urethral pressure
        profile
     D. If UPP data is unavailable, tentative diagnosis may be based on re-
        sponse to treatment.
IV. Diagnosis of detrusor hyperreflexia is based on:
     A. Recognition of typical clinical signs

B. Ruling out inflammatory diseases of the bladder
C. Decreased bladder capacity, threshold volume, and threshold pressure as determined by cystometrogram

Treatment

I. Estrogen responsive incontinence
   A. In the past we have empirically recommended oral administration of diethylstilbesterol (DES) at a dose of 0.1 to 1.0 mg/day for 3 to 5 days, followed by a maintenance dose of approximately 1.0 mg per week.
   B. More recently we have observed patients requiring higher doses of estrogens to induce continence. Maximum initial dose of DES is approximately 0.1 to 0.3 mg/kg body weight given daily for 7 days. The same dose may then be given once weekly for maintenance therapy. The maintenance dose should be gradually reduced to the lowest dose that will maintain continence.
   C. Administration of excessive quantities of estrogens may induce signs of estrus and may be toxic to the bone marrow (see chapter 8).
      1. Acute myelotoxicity induced by estrogens in dogs is characterized initially by leukocytosis and thrombocytopenia.
      2. Chronic toxicity with estrogens is characterized by normocytic, normochromic anemia (which may be reversible if detected early), thrombocytopenia, and neutropenia.
      3. Death may result from hemorrhagic diathesis or anemia.
   D. Establishing a safe and effective dose of estrogens (particularly in animals requiring higher doses of estrogens to maintain continence) requires monitoring of packed cell volumes (PCV), white blood cell counts, and platelet counts at monthly intervals. Minimum evaluation should include PCV and examination of a blood smear for leukocyte and thrombocyte numbers.
   E. Various combinations of estrogens and phenylpropanolamine may be used. Unlike estrogens, phenylpropanolamine must be given daily (see the section on urethral sphincter hypotonus).
   F. Older animals and animals with estrogen imbalances of any type may be more susceptible to toxic effects of exogenous estrogens. Phenylpropanolamine may be considered in such patients.
II. Testosterone responsive incontinence
   A. Testosterone propionate given intramuscularly or subcutaneously 3 times per week at a dose of approximately 2 mg/kg body weight has been reported to effectively control TRI in one dog.
   B. Testosterone cypionate (Depotestosterone Cypionate) given intramuscularly at a dose of 200 mg was reported to effectively control incontinence for periods of from 1 to 4 months in a 36 kg dog. No side effects were noted with this drug.

    C. Use of oral testosterone preparations for TRI has not been reported. Oral testosterone therapy may be less effective than parenteral therapy because of hepatic degradation.

III. Urethral sphincter hypotonus

    A. Phenylpropanolamine, an alpha adrenergic stimulating agent which increases urethral outflow resistance, is effective in dogs and cats when given orally at a dose of 12.5 to 50 mg every 8 hours.

       1. Response typically occurs within a few days

       2. Incontinence may recur if even a single treatment is delayed or omitted.

       3. Side effects may include:

         a) Restlessness

         b) Irritability

         c) Hypertension

    B. Alternatively, ephedrine, another alpha adrenergic stimulating agent, may be given orally at a dose of 2 to 4 mg/kg body weight every 8 hours. After efficacy has been demonstrated in the patient, extend the interval between doses to the least frequency which will maintain continence.

       1. Dose-related side effects in dogs include:

         a) Restlessness

         b) Anxiety

         c) Hyperexcitability

         d) Hypertension

       2. In people, tachyphylaxis may develop, and repeated doses may become less effective because of depletion of norepinephrine stores.

       3. Tachyphylaxis has not been reported in dogs and cats.

IV. Detrusor hyperreflexia

    A. Propantheline (Pro-Banthine), an anticholinergic drug, may be administered to dogs at a dose of 0.2 mg/kg given orally every 6 to 8 hours. The dose in cats is approximately 7.5 mg given every third day. Dose may be increased if necessary to the lowest dose which will control hyperreflexia.

    B. The detrusor reflex is mediated by parasympathetic innervation.

       1. Anticholinergic drugs suppress the detrusor reflex.

       2. Signs of drug overdosage include:

         a) Urinary retention

         b) Restlessness

         c) Excitement

         d) Hypotension

         e) Respiratory failure

         f) Paralysis

         g) Coma

    C. Reported side effects (in man) include:

       1. Drying of salivary secretions

       2. Tachycardia

3. Drowsiness
4. Weakness
5. Nausea
6. Vomiting
7. Constipation

DISORDERS OF MICTURITION—URINARY RETENTION

Definitions

I. Detrusor areflexia is defined as the inability of the urinary bladder to initiate and sustain forceful bladder contractions. It may be associated with normal, increased, or decreased urethral sphincter tone.
II. Reflex dyssynergia is defined as loss of coordination between bladder contraction and urethral sphincter relaxation during the voiding phase of micturition. Reflex dyssynergia results in contraction of the bladder without appropriate relaxation of the urethral sphincter.

Etiopathogenesis

I. Detrusor areflexia may result from neurogenic dysfunction or from damage to the detrusor muscle as a result of prolonged overdistension of the urinary bladder.
  A. Lesions of the central nervous system (e.g. neoplasms, intervertebral disc herniations, trauma) from the pontine reticular formation to the L7 spinal cord segments may cause detrusor areflexia with urethral sphincter hypertonus.
  B. Lesions of the brain stem or spinal cord, or trauma to the pelvic plexus which does not injure the pudendal nerve may cause detrusor areflexia with normal urethral sphincter tone.
  C. Prolonged bladder overdistension of any origin may cause detrusor areflexia by interfering with excitation-contraction coupling in the detrusor muscle. Excitation-contraction coupling is prevented by physical separation of the tight junctions between smooth muscle fibers of the bladder which occurs as a result of prolonged stretching of the bladder wall.
  D. Lesions of the sacral spinal cord or the nerve roots may cause detrusor areflexia with urethral sphincter areflexia (hypotonus).
II. The etiopathogenesis of reflex dyssynergia is not known for certain but is thought to result from a partial upper motor neuron lesion cranial to the sacral spinal cord.

Clinical Signs

I. Detrusor areflexia with urethral sphincter hypertonus is characterized by:
  A. Inability to void

    B. Marked distension of the urinary bladder
    C. Difficulty in manually expressing the urinary bladder
    D. Normal or hyperactive perineal reflexes
  II. Detrusor areflexia with normal urethral sphincter tone is characterized by:
    A. Inability to void
    B. Marked distension of the urinary bladder
    C. Ability to manually express the urinary bladder
    D. Intact perineal reflexes
 III. Detrusor areflexia resulting from overdistension of the urinary bladder is
     characterized by:
    A. A history of bladder overdistension
    B. Normal urethral sphincter tone
    D. Partial voiding of urine by abdominal compression
    D. Increased postvoiding residual urine volume
    E. Attempts by the patient to void (sensory pathways of the bladder are
      intact)
    F. Normal perineal reflexes
  IV. Detrusor areflexia with urethral sphincter areflexia is characterized by:
    A. Inability to void
    B. Normal or somewhat increased bladder size
    C. Relative ease in manually expressing the bladder
    D. Intermittent or continuous urine leakage from the bladder (incontinence)
    E. Diminished or absent perineal reflexes
   V. Reflex dyssynergia is characterized by:
    A. Passage of a normal urine stream initially followed by intermittent and
      then complete cessation of urine flow
    B. Straining to urinate after the abrupt cessation of urine flow
    C. Normal or hyperactive perineal reflexes
    D. Overdistension of the urinary bladder may occur

Diagnosis

   I. Diagnosis of detrusor areflexia is based on:
    A. Typical history and clinical signs
    B. Inability to void normally as determined by observation and determination of postvoiding residual urine volume
    C. Reduced or absent bladder tone as determined by palpation of the bladder
    D. Evidence of neurological disease as determined by neurological examination
    E. Absence of detrusor reflex as determined by cystometrogram
    F. Radiographic evaluation of the structural integrity of the urinary system
  II. Patients with detrusor atony should be further classified into those with
    normal, increased, or decreased urethral sphincter tone based on the ease

with which the bladder may be expressed and responses of perineal reflexes.
III. Detrusor areflexia resulting from overdistension of the urinary bladder may be differentiated from other causes of detrusor areflexia on the basis of clinical signs, history or presence of urinary obstruction, and absence of neurologic deficits.
IV. Diagnosis of reflex dyssynergia may be difficult to establish but may be based on:
   A. Clinical signs
   B. Ruling out structural urinary outflow obstruction by radiography
   C. Demonstrating a normal to hyperactive detrusor reflex by cystometrogram
   D. Demonstrating urethral sphincter contraction during the detrusor reflex by simultaneous bladder and urethral pressure measurements or cystometrogram and urethral electromyographic recordings
   E. Response to treatment

Treatment

I. Treatment of detrusor areflexia not resulting from bladder overdistension involves:
   A. If possible, appropriate medical and/or surgical treatment of the neurological disease responsible for urinary retention
   B. .Evacuation of the bladder at *least* three times daily
      1. Except when precluded by urethral sphincter hypertonus, manual compression of the bladder is the preferred method of evacuating the bladder because of lower incidence of iatrogenic UTI.
      2. When urethral sphincter hypertonus is present, manual compression of the bladder should be avoided because it is ineffective and may result in bladder trauma, bladder rupture or vesicoureteral reflux.
      3. When manual compression of the bladder is not effective, intermittent catheterization is preferred over indwelling urinary catheterization because (if properly performed) it is associated with a lower incidence of UTI.
   C. Antibiotic therapy should be considered for prevention of UTI.
      1. Urinalysis should be performed weekly or any time the urine appears to be abnormal.
      2. If results of urinalysis indicate inflammatory disease, urine culture should be evaluated.
      3. If UTI is confirmed, it should be treated as described in the section of this chapter on urinary tract infection.
   D. When urethral smooth muscle sphincter hypertonus is present, administration of phenoxybenzamine (Dibenzyline), an alpha-adrenergic blocking agent, may be of value in reducing internal urethral sphincter tone.

1. The recommended initial dose for dogs is 10 mg given orally once daily. If no response is observed after 4 days, the dose may be increased to 10 mg given every 12 hours, If no response is seen after 4 more days, the dose may be increased to 10 mg given every 8 hours.
2. The recommended initial dose in cats is 0.25 mg/kg given orally every 8 hours. This dose may be gradually increased to 0.5 mg/kg given orally every 8 hours if necessary.
3. Potential side effects of phenoxybenzamine include:
   a) Hypotension
   b) Weakness
   c) Dizziness
   d) Vomiting

E. When urethral skeletal muscle sphincter hypertonus is present, external urethral sphincter tone may be decreased by administration of diazepam (Valium) or dantrolene (Dantrium).
   1. Diazepam may be given orally at doses of from 2 to 10 mg given every 8 hours.
      a) Diazepam is a centrally-mediated skeletal muscle relaxant.
      b) At higher doses diazepam may produce sedation.
      c) Diazepam has been reported to depress detrusor reflex excitability in human beings
   2. Dantrolene has been recommended at a dose of from 0.5 to 2.0 mg/kg q 12 h PO for cats and 1.0 to 5.0 mg/kg q 8 h PO for dogs.
      a) Generalized muscle weakness indicates overdosage.
      b) Dantrolene has caused hepatic enzyme elevations in human patients

F. When urethral sphincter hypertonus is present and neither smooth muscle nor skeletal muscle relaxants alone are effective, combinations of these agents may be tried.

G. If a detrusor reflex is present but insufficient to induce adequate voiding, bethanechol (Urecholine), a cholinergic agent, may be used to stimulate bladder contraction.
   1. Bethanechol enhances but does not initiate a detrusor reflex. It is ineffective if the bladder is areflexic.
   2. Bethanechol may be given to dogs at a dose of 2.5 to 10 mg q 8 h SQ, or 5 to 25 mg q 8 h PO.
   3. Bethanechol may be given to cats at a dose of 2.5 to 5.0 mg q 8 to 12 h PO.
   4. Bethanechol should not be used when urethral resistance is increased except in combination with drugs which effectively reduce urethral outflow pressure.
   5. Potential side effects of bethanechol include:
      a) Vomiting

   b) Diarrhea
   c) Salivation
   d) Anorexia
II. Treatment of detrusor areflexia resulting from prolonged overdistension
   of the bladder involves:
   A. Early relief of bladder overdistension if irreversible damage is to be
      avoided
   B. Complete evacuation of the bladder for one to two weeks.
      1. Because continuous, complete emptying is necessary, a closed in-
         dwelling urinary catheter system may be indicated initially
      2. Manual expression of the bladder is not recommended because it
         will increase intraluminal pressure which in turn adversely affects
         the overdistended bladder wall.
      3. Intermittent catheterization four or more times daily may be used
         initially or after removal of an indwelling catheter.
   C. Antibiotic administration throughout the period of urinary catheteri-
      zation.
      1. Routine urinalysis and urine cultures should be performed weekly
         or more often if indicated during the period of active urine drainage.
      2. If UTI develops, it should be treated (see the section of this chapter
         on treatment of UTI).
   D. Bethanechol may be effective once partial detrusor contraction returns.
      Consult the section of this chapter on treatment of detrusor areflexia
      not resulting from bladder overdistension for additional information on
      use of this drug.
III. Treatment of reflex dyssynergia involves attempting to relax the urethra
   without inhibiting the detrusor reflex.
   A. Therapy directed at urethral smooth muscle, skeletal muscle, or both
      may be required.
   B. For smooth muscle dyssynergia, phenoxybenzamine (an alpha-adre-
      nergic blocking agent) is used. Consult the section of this chapter on
      bladder areflexia for information on usage of phenoxybenzamine.
   C. For striated muscle dyssynergia, diazepam or dantrolene may be used.
      Consult the section of this chapter on bladder areflexia for information
      on use of these drugs.
   D. Detrusor areflexia may result from prolonged bladder overdistension
      associated with reflex dyssynergia.
      1. Overdistension of the bladder during treatment should be prevented.
         a) The patient should be catheterized at least three times daily if
            voiding is ineffective.
         b) The patient should be given the opportunity to void prior to cath-
            eterization to assess response to treatment.
      2. Consult the section of this chapter on detrusor areflexia for rec-
         ommendations on treatment.

CANINE BACTERIAL PROSTATITIS

Definition

I. Bacterial prostatitis is defined as inflammatory disease of the prostate gland which results from microbial invasion of the gland.

II. Benign prostatic hyperplasia, prostatic neoplasia, and cystic disease of the prostate gland are excluded from the definition of bacterial prostatitis except when bacterial infection occurs in association with these diseases.

Etiopathogenesis and Clinical Signs

I. Although the pathogenesis of bacterial prostatitis is poorly understood, it is presumed to be dependent upon a balance between infectious agents and host resistance.

   A. Organisms commonly cultured from dogs with bacterial prostatitis are commensal organisms that normally inhabit the distal portion of the urethra and genital tract.

   B. Conditions which may alter prostatic defense mechanisms and predispose to bacterial prostatitis include urethral disease, bacterial UTI, or non-infectious prostatic diseases (e.g. cysts, benign hyperplasia, neoplasia, or squamous metaplasia of ductal epithelium).

II. Bacterial UTI frequently accompanies bacterial prostatitis; bacterial prostatitis is a major cause of recurrent UTI in male dogs.

Clinical Signs

I. Clinical signs of acute bacterial prostatitis include:

   A. Urethral discharge independent of micturition
   B. Enlarged, painful prostate gland detected by rectal palpation
   C. Tenesmus
   D. Constipation
   E. Abdominal pain
   F. Stilted gait
   G. Dysuria
   H. Fever
   I. Depression
   J. Leukocytosis

II. Clinical signs of chronic bacterial prostatitis include:

   A. Urethral discharge independent of micturition
   B. Recurrent UTI
   C. Enlarged, sometimes asymmetric, usually nonpainful prostate gland detected by rectal palpation
   D. Constipation
   E. Tenesmus
   F. Absence of clinical signs

Diagnosis

I. Diagnosis of bacterial prostatitis is based on clinical signs and results of prostatic fluid, biopsy, and radiographic evaluation.

II. Bacterial culture and cytologic examination of prostatic fluid or semen are the most useful clinical tools for diagnosis of bacterial prostatitis.

    A. Dogs suspected of having bacterial prostatitis should first be evaluated for UTI.

    B. If UTI is not present, diagnostically valid samples of prostatic fluid may be obtained via ejaculation or prostatic massage.

    C. If UTI is present, prostatic massage samples will not yield useful information and samples for bacterial culture and cytology should be obtained by ejaculation if possible.

    D. If UTI is present and a sample of prostatic fluid cannot be obtained by ejaculation, samples for bacterial culture and cytology should be obtained by prostatic massage after attempting control of UTI using an antimicrobial drug which does not penetrate prostatic fluid (e.g., ampicillin).

    E. Detection of increased numbers of WBC in prostatic fluid indicates inflammatory prostatic disease which may be bacterial or non-bacterial in origin.

    F. Quantitative culture of an appropriate sample of prostatic fluid or semen is the optimal method of diagnosing bacterial prostatitis.

        1. Numbers of organisms obtained in these samples may be lower than those observed in bacterial UTI (i.e., samples containing as few as 10^2 bacteria/ml of urine may be significant).

        2. Comparison of numbers of bacteria cultured from urethral samples with numbers cultured from semen obtained by ejaculation may be useful in differentiating urethral contamination from prostatic infection.

III. Prostatic biopsy techniques are useful in differentiating neoplastic from inflammatory prostatic disease, but are less useful for differentiating bacterial prostatitis from non-infectious, inflammatory prostatic disease. Prostatic biopsy samples may be examined microscopically and cultured for microorganisms.

IV. Radiography may be useful in supporting a diagnosis of prostatic disease in some patients, but does not yield findings specific for bacterial prostatitis. Radiographic findings in dogs with bacterial prostatitis may include:

    A. Prostatic enlargement and displacement

    B. Indistinct cranial prostatic margins

    C. Prostatic mineralization

    D. Altered urethral lumen diameter

    E. Reflux of radiographic contrast material into prostatic stroma

V. Diagnostic ultrasonography may be of value in differentiating prostatic cysts and abscesses from diffuse bacterial prostatitis.

Treatment

I. Antimicrobial drugs are the cornerstone of treatment for canine bacterial prostatitis.
  A. For treatment of acute bacterial prostatitis, antimicrobial drugs should be chosen on the basis of susceptibility of organisms isolated by culture of urine, urethral discharge, ejaculate, or fluid obtained by prostatic massage.
    1. Select an antibiotic that achieves high concentrations in blood, tissue, and urine.
    2. The blood-prostatic barrier is apparently not intact during acute inflammation.
    3. Parenteral administration of antibiotics may be indicated for dogs that are very severely ill or septic.
    4. Antimicrobial drugs should be administered for a minimum of 14 days.
    5. Septic animals may require careful attention to fluid, electrolyte, and nutritional needs in addition to antimicrobial therapy.
    6. Dogs with acute bacterial prostatitis should be re-evaluated immediately prior to discontinuation of therapy and after therapy to determine if the infection has been eradicated.
      a) Failure to eradicate acute infections may result in chronic bacterial prostatitis and recurrent UTI.
      b) Physical examination, routine urinalysis, and urine culture should be performed 3 to 5 days before and after terminating antimicrobial therapy.
      c) Prostatic fluid obtained by ejaculation or prostatic massage may be evaluated cytologically and by culture 3 to 5 days before and after terminating antimicrobial therapy.
        (1) If infection is still present before termination of therapy, a different antimicrobial agent should be used.
        (2) If aseptic inflammation is still present before planned termination of therapy, therapy should not be discontinued.
      d) If infection is present after termination of therapy, chronic bacterial prostatitis is present and should be treated accordingly.
  B. Selection of antimicrobial drugs for treatment of chronic bacterial prostatitis is limited by the fact that prostatic fluid concentration of many antibiotics is below the minimum inhibitory concentration required to eradicate infecting pathogens.
    1. The blood-prostatic fluid barrier is thought to remain intact in patients with chronic prostatitis, limiting diffusion of many antibiotics into prostatic fluid.
      a) Antibiotics potentially useful in treatment of chronic bacterial prostatitis include:
        (1) Trimethoprim given at a dose of 2.2 mg/kg q 12 h P.O. or in combination with sulfadiazine at a combined dosage of 13.2

mg/kg q 12 hr P.O. This drug may induce prostatic concentrations of drug two to ten times that of serum concentrations.
  (2) Chloramphenicol given at a dose of 50 mg/kg q 8 h P.O., I.V., S.Q., or I.M. (prostatic concentrations about one half of serum concentrations).
  (3) Erythromycin given at a dose of 10 mg/kg q 8 h P.O.
  (4) Tetracycline may achieve therapeutic concentrations in prostatic tissue. Dose is 20 mg/kg q 8 h P.O.
  b) The antibiotic chosen should be selected on the basis of susceptibility of the organism cultured as well as the ability of the antibiotic to diffuse into prostatic tissue.
  2. Antibiotic therapy should be continued for a minimum of 3 weeks.
  3. Prostatic fluid should be cultured and examined cytologically several days before and 5 to 7 days after the antibiotic is discontinued.
  a) If infection is still present before termination of therapy, administration of a different antimicrobial agent should be considered.
  b) If aseptic inflammation is still present before planned termination of therapy, therapy should not be discontinued.
  c) If infection is present after termination of therapy, treatment should be reinstituted with the same or a different antibiotic, depending on the antibiotic choices available.
    (1) Prostatic fluid should be cultured and examined cytologically several weeks later while the dog is still receiving antibiotics.
    (2) If infection persists at this time, an alternative antibiotic and/or adjunctive therapy should be considered (see below).
    (3) If infection is under control at this time, antibiotic therapy should be continued for at least four more weeks.
    (4) Prostatic fluid should be cultured again prior to and 5 to 7 days after discontinuing therapy.
  d) Reculturing of prostatic fluid approximately two to four weeks after withdrawal of antibiotic therapy may permit detection of recurrent infection at a subclinical stage.
II. Adjunctive therapy for canine bacterial prostatitis
  A. Castration is effective in decreasing recurrent infections in patients with recurrent bacterial prostatitis by reducing the amount of functional prostatic tissue.
    1. Prostatic size begins to decrease within days of castration. Within several months, functional prostatic tissue is replaced by fibrous connective tissue.
    2. Castration usually should not be performed until after antimicrobial drug therapy has effectively eradicated bacterial infection of the prostate gland.
    3. Bacterial prostatitis is unusual in castrated patients.
  B. Surgical drainage of prostatic abscesses is important because of impaired ability of antibiotics to penetrate the abscess cavity.

C. Because of the variable response of the prostate gland to estrogen, and because of the toxic effect of estrogens on canine bone marrow, its routine use in the treatment of bacterial prostatitis cannot be recommended.
D. Oral administration of zinc sulfate has been recommended for treatment and/or prevention of bacterial prostatitis; however, no data exists to confirm the efficacy of this therapy in canine bacterial prostatitis.

FELINE LOWER URINARY TRACT DISEASE

Definition

I. We define the feline urologic syndrome (FUS) as encompassing all cats with evidence of lower urinary tract disease, regardless of specific underlying disease.
II. We define "FUS" in this manner in order to emphasize our belief that it may result from diverse lower urinary tract diseases rather than as a unique disease entity.

Etiopathogenesis

I. Many etiologic agents may produce lower urinary tract diseases in cats (Table 12-7).

TABLE 12-7.   ETIOLOGIC AGENTS WHICH MAY BE
ASSOCIATED WITH FUS

Infection	Anomalies
Bacterial	Persistent urachus
Mycotic	Urethral structures
Mycoplasmal	Other
Viral	
Parasitic (*Capillaria* spp.)	Inflammatory (non-Infectious)
Urolithiasis	Trauma
Struvite	Bladder
Calcium phosphate	Urethra
Calcium oxalate	Herniated bladder
Ammonium urate	
Uric acid	Neurogenic
Matrix	Reflex dyssynergia
Other	Detrusor areflexia
Neoplasia	Idiopathic
Bladder	
Urethra	Iatrogenic
Prostate	
Extra-urinary—impinging on	
urinary tract	

II. Urethral obstruction may be caused by several mechanisms, including:
   A. Intraluminal obstructions
      1. Urethral plugs (matrix and crystals)
      2. Uroliths
      3. Sloughed tissue
   B. Mural or extramural impingment on the urethral lumen.
      1. Neoplasms
      2. Strictures
      3. Urethral and periurethral inflammation
      4. Anomalies
      5. Reflex dyssynergia
   C. Combinations of the above causes

Clinical Signs

I. Clinical signs of lower urinary tract disease that may be observed in obstructed or nonobstructed male and female cats include:
   A. Dysuria
   B. Pollakiuria
   C. Inappropriate micturition
   D. Hematuria
   E. Reduced size and force of the urine stream
   F. Licking of the penis and prepuce
   G. Crying when using the litter pan
   H. Abdominal discomfort
   I. Spontaneous voiding of small uroliths (sand)
II. Clinical signs of urinary obstruction may include:
   A. Depression
   B. Dehydration
   C. Anorexia
   D. Vomiting
   E. Enlarged urinary bladder (unless it has ruptured)
   F. Repeated attempts to micturate
   G. Dysuria
   H. Sitting or lying in the litter box
   I. Abdominal pain
   J. Cardiac arrhythmias
   K. Hypothermia
   L. Coma
III. Clinical signs are often recurrent and intermittent in nonobstructed male and female cats.
   A. In one study, clinical signs were reported to resolve within 5 days in 70 percent of affected cats.
   B. A small percentage of cats have persistent clinical signs.

Diagnosis

I. Diagnosis of "FUS" is based on clinical signs of lower urinary tract disease.

II. Identification of lower urinary tract disease (FUS) should not be a diagnostic endpoint. The etiologic basis of the condition must be sought in order to facilitate effective treatment and prevention of recurrence.

III. A diagnostic approach to cats with "FUS" should begin with a routine urinalysis.

   A. Cats with active signs of lower urinary tract disease and no abnormalities detected on routine urinalysis should be suspected of having behavioral abnormalities or neuromuscular disorders (consult the sections of this chapter on disorders of micturition).

   B. If significant hematuria, pyuria, bacteriuria, and/or crystalluria are detected by routine urinalysis, a sample of urine should be collected by cystocentesis for urine culture. In addition, radiographic studies of the lower urinary tract should be performed (contrast urethrocystography).

      1. Cats with significant bacteriuria and normal radiographic findings may have uncomplicated UTI (spontaneous or iatrogenic) or UTI secondary to metabolic diseases (e.g., diabetes mellitus, renal failure, etc.).

      2. Cats with significant bacteriuria and radiographic abnormalities may be determined to have UTI associated with urolithiasis, structural abnormalities (e.g. urachal diverticulum), neoplasia, neuromuscular abnormalities, or iatrogenic disorders.

      3. Cats without bacteriuria or radiographic abnormalities may have neuromuscular, traumatic, non-bacterial infectious (viral, mycoplasmal, fungal), or idiopathic disorders.

      4. Cats with sterile urine and radiographic abnormalities may have urolithiasis, neoplasia, structural abnormalities, or neuromuscular disorders.

Treatment

I. Treatment of obstruction in cats involves:

   A. Relief of obstruction by various combinations of:
      1. Urethral massage
      2. Cystocentesis
      3. Urethral flushing
      4. Urethral catheterization

   B. Correction of fluid, electrolyte, acid-base, and metabolic abnormalities as described in the section of this chapter on the acute uremic crisis

   C. Identification of and treatment of the underlying cause(s) of lower urinary tract disease and urinary obstruction

II. Treatment of lower urinary tract disease in nonobstructed cats should be based on accurate diagnosis.

III. Treatment of the following causes of lower urinary tract disease in cats are discussed elsewhere in this chapter:
   A. Urinary tract infection
   B. Urolithiasis
   C. Neurogenic micturition disorders
IV. Surgery, chemotherapy, and/or radiation therapy may be considered for patients with neoplasia involving the lower urinary tract.
V. Surgical correction (diverticulectomy) may be considered in patients with urachal diverticula which do not respond to antimicrobial therapy or develop recurrent UTI.
   A. The clinical significance of urachal diverticulae of the bladder in abacteriuric cats with signs of lower urinary tract disease is unknown.
   B. Owners should be advised that diverticulectomy in abacteriuric cats may not result in amelioration of clinical signs or prevention of recurrent episodes of lower urinary tract disease in abacteriuric cats.
IV. There is no proven, effective treatment for cats with idiopathic lower urinary tract disease.
   A. Owners should be advised that:
      1. With the exception of urinary obstruction, the disease is not life-threatening.
      2. Most cats will improve spontaneously within 5 to 7 days.
      3. A high percentage of cats will experience recurrent episodes of lower urinary tract disease.
   B. Careful consideration should be given to the potential adverse effects of any treatments given to cats with idiopathic lower urinary tract disease.
   C. Antibiotics are not routinely recommended in abacteriuric cats.
   D. Propantheline (Pro-Banthine) may be considered during acute episodes for symptomatic treatment of dysuria in nonobstructed cats with idiopathic lower urinary tract disease.
      1. Propantheline has a rapid onset of action.
      2. Care must be used to avoid inducing urinary retention by administration of excessive quantities.
      3. Suggested dose is 7.5 mg of propantheline given orally approximately every 72 hours.

SUGGESTED READINGS

Barsanti JA, Edwards PD, Losonsky J: Testosterone responsive urinary incontinence in a castrated male dog. J Am Hosp Assoc 17:117, 1981

Barsanti JA, Shotts EB, Prasse K, Crowell W: Evaluation of diagnostic techniques for canine prostatic disease. J Am Vet Med Assoc 117:160, 1983

Chew DJ, Meuten DJ: Disorders of calcium and phosphorus-metabolism. Vet Clin North Am 12:411, 1982

Chew DJ, DiBartolla SP: Feline renal amyloidosis. p. 976. In Kirk RW (ed): Current Veterinary Therapy VIII. W.B. Saunders Co., Philadelphia, 1983

Cowgill LD: Diseases of the kidney. p. 1793. In Ettinger SJ (ed): Textbook of Veterinary Internal Medicine, 3rd Ed., Vol. 2. W.B. Saunders Co., Philadelphia, 1983

Greene CE, Wong PL, Finco DR: Diagnosis and treatment of diabetes insipidus in two dogs using synthetic analogs of antidiuretic hormone. J Am Anim Hosp Assoc 15:371, 1979

Hardy RM: Disorders of water metabolism. Vet Clin North Am 12:353, 1982

Lindner A, Cutler RE, Goodman WG: Synergism of dopamine plus furosemide in preventing acute renal failure in the dog. Kidney Intern 16:158, 1979

Ling GV: Treatment of urinary tract infections with antimicrobial agents. p. 1051. In Kirk RW (ed): Current Veterinary Therapy VIII, W. B. Saunders Co., Philadelphia, 1983

Ling GV, Branam JE, Ruby AL, Johnson DL: Canine prostatic fluid. Techniques of collection, quantitative bacterial culture, and interpretation of results. J Am Vet Med Assoc 183:201, 1983

Ling GV, Conzelman GM, Franti CE, et al: Urine concentrations of 5 penicillins following oral administration to normal adult dogs. Am J Vet Res 41:1123, 1980

Ling GV, Conzelman GM, Franti CE, et al: Urine concentrations of chloramphenicol, tetracycline, and sulfisoxazole after oral administration to healthy adult dogs. Am J Vet Res 41:950, 1980

Ling GV, Conzelman GM, Franti CE, et al: Urine concentrations of gentamicin, tobramycin, amikacin, and kanamycin after subcutaneous administration to healthy adult dogs. Am J Vet Res 42:1792, 1981

Ling GV, Hirsch DC; Antimicrobial susceptibility tests for urinary tract pathogens. p. 1048. In Kirk RW (ed): Current Veterinary Therapy VIII. W.B. Saunders Co., Philadelphia, 1983

Ling GV, Ruby AL: Cephalexin for oral treatment of canine urinary tract infection caused by *Klebsiella pneumonia*. j Am Vet Med Assoc 182:1346, 1983

Low DG, Cowgill L: Emergency management of the acute uremic crisis. p. 981. In Kirk RW (ed): Current Veterinary Therapy VIII. W.B. Saunders Co., Philadelphia, 1983

Moise NS, Flanders JA: Micturition disorders in cats with sacrocaudal vertebral lesions. p. 722. In Kirk RW (ed): Current Veterinary Therapy VIII. W.B. Saunders Co., Philadelphia, 1983

Oliver JE: Dysuria caused by reflex dyssynergia. p. 1088, In Kirk RW (ed): Current Veterinary Therapy VIII. W.B. Saunders Co., Philadelphia, 1983

Oliver JE, Lorenz MD; Handbook of Veterinary Neurologic Diagnosis, W.B. Saunders Co. Philadelphia, 1983

Osborne CA, Klausner JS: Calcium oxalate urolithiasis. p. 1177. In Kirk RW (ed): Current Veterinary Therapy VIII. W.B. Saunders Co., Philadelphia, 1980

Osborne CA, Lees GE: Feline cystitis, urethritis, urethral obstruction syndrome, Part I. Mod Vet Pract 59:173, 1978

Osborne CA, Oliver JE, Polzin DJ: Non-neurogenic urinary incontinence, p. 1128. In Kirk RW (ed): Current Veterinary Therapy VII. W.B. Saunders Co., Philadelphia, 1980

Osborne CA, Polzin DJ: Conservative medical management of feline chronic polyuric renal failure. p. 1008. In Kirk RW (ed): Current Veterinary Therapy VIII. W.B. Saunders Co., Philadelphia, 1983

Owen LN: Cancer chemotherapy and immunotherapy. p. 368. In Ettinger SJ (ed): Textbook of Veterinary Internal Medicine, 2nd Ed., Vol. 1, W.B. Saunders Co., Philadelphia, 1983

Park CYC: Should patients with single renal stone occurrence undergo diagnostic evaluation? J Urol 127:855, 1982

Paul MF, Bender RC, Nohle EG: Renal excretion of nitrofurantoin (Furidantoin). Am J Physiol 197:580, 1959

Peterson ME: Treatment of canine and feline hypoparathyroidism. J Am Vet Med Assoc 181:1434, 1982

Polzin DJ, Klausner JS: Treatment of urniary tract candidiasis. p. 1055. In Kirk RW (ed): Current Veterinary Therapy VIII. W.B. Saunders Co., Philadelphia, 1983

Sigel CW, Ling GV, Bushby SRM, et al: Pharmacokinetics of trimethoprim and sulfadiazine in the dog: Urine concentrations after oral administration. Am J Vet Res 42:996, 1981

Thornhill JA: Continuous ambulatory peritoneal dialysis. p. 1028. In Kirk RW (ed): Current Veterinary Therapy VIII. W.B. Saunders Co., Philadelphia, 1983

Thornhill JA: Control of vomiting in the uremic patient. p. 1022. In Kirk RW (ed): Current Veterinary Therapy VIII. W.B. Saunders Co., Philadelphia, 1983

13

Gastrointestinal Disorders

Brent D. Jones, DVM

THE MOUTH

Diseases of the mouth and associated structures are of common occurrence in dogs and cats. Patients with disorders of the oropharynx may be malnourished because of difficulty with eating.

I. Cheilitis
  A. Etiology
    1. Trauma
    2. Dental tartar
    3. Malpositioned teeth
    4. Dermatitis
    5. Bacterial infection
    6. Autoimmune
  B. Clinical signs
    1. Ptyalism
    2. Pawing or rubbing of mouth and muzzle
    3. Halitosis
    4. Alopecia of surrounding skin
    5. Presence of exudate
  C. Treatment
    1. Surgical repair of traumatic lesions
    2. Clip hair from area
    3. Thoroughly cleanse with detergent and antiseptic solutions
    4. Application of topical anesthetic ointments to reduce irritation
    5. Pemphigus (see Chapter 21)

II. Stomatitis
  Generalized inflammation of the mouth which may include the gums (gingivitis) and the tongue (glossitis)
  A. Etiology
    1. Chemical, thermal, or mechanical injury
    2. Infection
      a) Vincent's stomatitis—*Spirochaeta vincenti*
      b) Mycotic—*Candida albicans*

    c) Viral—feline rhinotracheitis virus and calicivirus, canine oral papilloma virus
3. Secondary to:
    a) Uremia
    b) Canine hepatitis
    c) Canine distemper
    d) Leptospirosis
    e) Niacin deficiency
4. Autoimmune disease—Pemphigus
5. "Gray Collie syndrome"
6. Interference with blood supply to tongue—gangrenous glossitis
7. Periodontal disease
8. Neoplasms

B. Clinical signs
1. Highly variable
2. Ptyalism
3. Anorexia
4. Enlarged regional lymph nodes
5. Halitosis
6. Thirst

C. Treatment
1. Pemphigus (see chapter 21)
2. Under general anesthesia, thoroughly clean oral cavity, scale teeth if necessary, extract loose teeth, irrigate with 3% hydrogen peroxide, 40% zinc peroxide suspension, or 1% zinc sulfate solution
3. Ulcers of the mucosa may be cauterized by touching with a silver nitrate stick or application of 10% silver nitrate solution. The action may be terminated by irrigation with saline solution.
4. Most commonly, bacteria causing infectious stomatitis are gram-positive aerobes and anaerobes. Penicillin G should be administered parenterally.
5. "Trench mouth" is caused by a spirochaete and fusobacterium, both of which are sensitive to penicillin G or metronidazole (see Chapter 3).
6. Oral candidiasis
    a) Nystatin (Mycostatin oral suspension)
    b) Clotrimazole cream (Mycelex)
    c) Miconazole cream (Monistat)
    d) Ketoconazole (Nizoral) 10 mg/kg, PO, SID for 2 to 3 weeks

III. Pharyngitis
A. Etiology
1. Usually an extension of disease processes from the oral cavity, sinuses, or nasal cavity
2. Various bacteria
3. Foreign bodies

4. Tonsillitis is often associated with anal sac disease
5. Megaesophagus
6. Pharyngeal cysts
7. Elongated soft palate
8. Neoplasia
  B. Clinical signs
    1. Gagging
    2. Coughing
    3. Anorexia
    4. Expectoration of foamy phlegm
  C. Treatment
    1. Remove foreign bodies
    2. Surgically correct elongated palate
    3. Treat anal sac disease
    4. Most bacterial infections will respond to penicillin, sulfonamides, or tetracycline.

DISEASES OF THE ESOPHAGUS

GENERAL CONSIDERATIONS

Any condition that interferes with passage of a bolus or the normal synchronous relaxation and contraction of the lower esophageal sphincter could result in retention of material in the esophagus. Esophageal disease causes an inability to swallow, a mechanical interference with passage of the bolus, or an interference with the control mechanism of esophageal and gastroesophageal junction motor function.

 I. Clinical signs
  A. May be very obvious or subtle
  B. Location, chronicity, and presence of secondary problems will determine severity of signs.
  C. Dysphagia
  D. Repeated swallowing movements
  E. Copious salivation and drooling
  F. Regurgitation
    1. May immediately follow eating
    2. Or be delayed for several hours
    3. Retching generally absent
    4. pH is usually near neutrality
    5. Tubular-shaped mass of bile-free undigested food
  G. Vomiting
    1. Retching is present
    2. Partially digested, bile-stained mass
    3. Low pH

   H. Coughing, dyspnea, and mucopurulent nasal discharge occur in the as-
      piration pneumonia that frequently accompanies esophageal disease.
   I. Anorexia, weight loss or voracious appetite may accompany esophageal
      diseases
II. Diagnosis
   A. History should include the following:
      1. Onset and course of the problem
      2. Type of dysphagia and relationship to ingestion of food
      3. Any difference in ability to retain liquids and soft food as opposed
         to solid food
      4. Possibility of exposure to:
         a) Caustic agents
         b) Foreign bodies
      5. Previous
         a) Trauma
         b) Neurological problems
         c) Surgery and/or anesthesia
         d) Pharyngitis or tonsillitis
      6. Acute onset is most commonly associated with a foreign body
      7. Slowly developing, progressive regurgitation is more suggestive of
         esophageal stricture or gastroesophageal reflux.
   B. Special procedures
      1. Plain and contrast radiography
      2. Endoscopic examination
      3. Biopsy
      4. Manometry
      5. Electromyography

Esophageal Disease

   I. Vascular ring anomalies
   A. Congenital malformations of the great vessels which interfere with
      esophageal function
   B. Persistent right aortic arch is most common.
   C. Signs
      1. Due to esophageal entrapment with stenosis and subsequent pre-
         cardial esophageal dilatation
      2. Persistent regurgitation in young dogs at the time of weaning to solid
         food
      3. Most common in Irish Setters, German Shepherds, and English Bull-
         dogs
      4. Puppies are malnourished and weak
      5. The food-filled esophagus may be palpated at the thoracic inlet.
   D. Treatment
      1. Surgical correction

2. Complications are frequent
   a) Most cases are poor anesthetic risks
   b) Permanent esophageal dilatation
   c) Dilatation of esophagus caudal to the vascular ring

II. Esophagitis
   A. Primary disease is rare and usually occurs because of trauma or ingestion of caustics. If only the mucosa is involved, the signs are mild and transient. Damage to the muscular layer can lead to severe ulceration with perforation, fibrotic stenosis, or chronic inflammation. Disordered motor activity is an important sequela.
   B. Reflux esophagitis
      1. Associated with hiatal hernia and periesophageal diseases, such as abscesses or neoplasms occurring near the lower esophageal sphincter.
      2. Gastric acid, pepsin, bile salts, and pancreatic enzymes are potent agents for causing damage to the esophageal mucosa.
      3. Severity of the disease is determined by volume and composition of refluxed materials, residence time in esophagus, and competency of antireflux mechanisms.
   C. Treatment
      1. Provide esophageal rest to permit healing. A pharyngostomy tube may be used for feeding.
      2. Feed small meals of soft bland food.
      3. Administer liquid antacids.
      4. Lidocaine gel will provide symptomatic relief.
      5. Reflux esophagitis
         a) Increase pressure at lower esophageal sphincter with bethanechol (Urecholine) 0.5-1.0 mg/kg, PO, q 8 h or metoclopramide (Reglan) 0.5 mg/kg, PO, q 8 h.
         b) Reduce the amount of gastric acid refluxed into the distal esophagus by administration of liquid antacids 30 ml every hour. As this is usually impractical, cimetidine (Tagamet) 5-10 mg/kg, PO, q 6 h may be employed to suppress acid secretion by the stomach. *Do not administer cimetidine with antacids as the two drugs will interact to obviate absorption of the cimetidine.*

III. Esophageal foreign bodies
   A. Common types are steak, chicken, or pork chop bones, wood, string, fish hooks, needles, and other metal objects.
   B. Most common locations are the cranial esophageal sphincter, the thoracic inlet, the heart base area, and the hiatal region.
   C. Complications include perforation of the esophagus, pleuritis or mediastinitis, pyothorax, lacerations, stricture, diverticulosis, and severe esophagitis.
   D. Clinical signs
      1. Regurgitation following eating

        2. Painful dysphagia
        3. Ptyalism
        4. Persistent gulping
        5. Anorexia
    E. Treatment
        1. Should be considered an emergency situation
        2. Attempt removal through the oral cavity via an endoscope
        3. If unsuccessful, you may be able to advance the foreign body into the stomach.
        4. After removal, the esophagus should be examined carefully for presence of perforation, laceration, or extensive mucosal damage.
        5. Treat esophagitis as described above.
        6. If other treatment modalities fail esophagostomy must be done.
IV. Esophageal diverticula
    A. Rarely documented in the veterinary literature
    B. Likely to occur cranial to thoracic inlet or diaphragm (Epiphrenic)
    C. May be congenital or acquired
    D. Predisposing factors
        1. Esophagitis
        2. Esophageal stenosis
        3. Cricopharyngeal achalasia
        4. Vascular ring anomalies
        5. Megaesophagus
        6. Hiatal hernia
        7. Myasthenia gravis
    E. Clinical signs
        1. Gagging
        2. Postprandial regurgitation
        3. Intermittent anorexia
        4. Fever
        5. Pain on abdominal palpation
        6. Reluctance to move, incoordination, or ataxia after eating
    F. Complications
        1. Impaction of ingested material with partial esophageal obstruction
        2. Chronic esophagitis with ulceration
        3. Peridiverticulitis with painful adhesions
        4. Rupture with resultant mediastinitis or tracheoesophageal fistula
    G. Treatment
        1. Soft bland diet
        2. Feed animal while it is standing on its hind legs.
        3. Provide plenty of fluids.
        4. Symptomatic epiphrenic diverticula require surgical excision and reconstruction of esophageal wall.
V. Esophageal stricture
    Can result from either extraluminal masses impinging on the esophagus, or more commonly from intraluminal lesions.

A. Periesophageal masses
  1. Etiology
    a) Cervical neoplasms (thyroid tumors)
    b) Abscesses in cervical (foreign body) or thoracic (nocardiosis) regions
    c) Lymphosarcoma involving anterior mediastinum
    d) Extreme hilar lymphadenopathy
    e) Heart base tumors
    f) Pulmonary neoplasms
  2. Clinical signs
    a) Dysphagia
    b) Regurgitation
    c) Debility
    d) Dilation of esophagus cranial to obstruction
  3. Treatment is directed toward reducing or eliminating the mass.
B. Intraluminal stricture
  1. Etiologic factors
    a) Sequela to esophageal surgery, foreign bodies, ingestion of caustic substances, external trauma
    b) Iatrogenic esophageal stricture
        Develops following elective surgical procedures such as ovariohysterectomy. Probably caused by reflux of gastric acid into the esophagus during surgery. Factors which might facilitate reflux include occlusion of the airway, increased intra-abdominal pressure, lateral or dorsal recumbency with the head lowered and loss of secondary peristaltic contractions during anesthesia.
  2. Clinical signs
    a) Similar to those described for esophageal foreign bodies
    b) Regurgitation immediately follows eating of solid food.
    c) Liquids are well tolerated.
    d) A previously normal animal develops progressive dysphagia.
  3. Treatment
    a) Bougienage to mechanically dilate the esophagus at stricture site
    b) Prednisolone, 1 mg/kg, PO, SID for 2-3 weeks following bougienage

DISEASES OF THE STOMACH

THE CLINICAL EXAMINATION OF PATIENTS WITH
GASTRIC DISEASE
  I. History
    A. Since most patients with gastric diseases have vomiting as their chief complaint, one must differentiate vomiting from regurgitation.
      1. Question owner about:
        a) Color of material—yellow or green color suggests bile which is indicative of vomitus

      b) Whether dog retches—another sign of vomiting and not regurgitation

      c) Composition of material

      d) Time of vomiting or regurgitation

    2. Regurgitation indicates esophageal disorders.

  B. Patient profile: age, breed, sex, weight, and geographical area

    1. Young dogs have a higher incidence of gastric foreign bodies.

    2. Old dogs have a higher incidence of gastric neoplasia.

    3. Deep chested breeds are predisposed to gastric volvulus

    4. Small, hyperactive breeds of dogs have a higher incidence of pyloric diseases and chronic gastritis.

    5. Dogs in the southeastern United States have a higher incidence of *Spirocerca lupi* parasitism.

  C. It is important to record the time of onset, duration, and frequency of the vomiting.

II. Physical examination

  A. Physical appearance

    1. Acute gastric dilation causes the abdomen to be distended and tense.

    2. A normal sized stomach in its normal position cannot be palpated.

  B. Character and location of other abdominal structures are important to note.

    1. Since the stomach is attached to the spleen by the gastrosplenic ligament, abnormal size or position of the spleen may indicate abnormal size or position of the stomach.

    2. Since vomiting causes aerophagia, bowels are often distended with gas.

  C. Evaluate dehydration and depression, as they correlate with the severity of vomiting.

III. Diagnostic tests

  A. Complete bloodwork, urinalysis, and fecal tests are recommended to rule out other conditions that mimic gastric diseases.

  B. Extended bouts of vomition usually produce hypochloremia, hypokalemia and metabolic alkalosis. (However, it should be noted that some authors believe acidosis is the major consequence of vomiting due to the bicarbonate loss that follows sodium depletion.)

  C. Examination of gastric juice

    1. A normal dog that has been fasted for 12 hours will have clear gastric juice with a varying amount of mucus.

    2. Bile is an abnormal component of gastric juices indicating a state of chronic vomition.

    3. Aspirate of gastric juice is tested for pH, WBC's, bacteria, food, parasites, free HCl and total HCl.

  D. Gastroscopy

    1. Definition—a visual examination of the luminal surface of the stomach with the use of an endoscope.

2. Proven most useful in diagnosis of gastric neoplasia and gastric ulcers.
   E. Radiography
   F. Exploratory celiotomy

VOMITING

I. Definition—The forceful expulsion of the contents of the stomach through the mouth
II. Stage of vomiting
 A. Nausea
  1. Associated with hypersalivation
  2. Gastric tone is reduced
  3. Duodenal and proximal jejunal tone is increased.
  4. Reflux of duodenal contents into the stomach
 B. Retching
  1. Spasmodic and abortive respiratory movements with the glottis closed.
  2. Inspiratory movements of the chest wall and diaphragm are opposed by expiratory contractions of the abdominal musculature.
  3. Pyloric end of the stomach contracts whereas the fundus relaxes.
III. Associated phenomena
 A. Hypersalivation
 B. Defecation
IV. Mediation of vomiting reflex
 A. Afferent pathways
  1. Cerebral cortex
    Psychic vomiting
  2. Limbic system
    Head trauma, cytotoxic drugs
  3. Vestibular apparatus
    Motion sickness, labyrinthitis
  4. Chemoreceptor trigger zone (CTZ)
    Drugs, toxins, uremia
 B. Vomiting center
  1. Located in medulla
  2. Coordinates activity of other structures
  3. Stimulated directly by impulses from afferent pathways described above and directly from visceral afferent pathways from GI tract
V. Metabolic consequences of vomiting
 A. Potassium deficiency
  1. Decreased intake
  2. Loss of K+ in vomitus

      3. Renal loss
        a) Potassium bicarbonate
        b) Increased aldosterone
   B. Alkalosis
      1. Loss of hydrogen in vomitus
      2. Hydrogen migrates into cells
   C. Sodium depletion
      1. Loss of sodium in vomitus
      2. Renal sodium loss
   D. Chloride depletion
      Loss of chloride in vomitus
   E. A pancreatic bicarbonate loss due to sodium depletion can produce an acidosis.
VI. Etiology of vomiting
   A. Non-gastrointestinal causes of vomiting
      1. Uremia
      2. Hepatopathies
      3. Pancreatopathies
      4. Infectious diseases
      5. Neurological disorders
      6. Toxemias
      7. Motion sickness
      8. Head injury
      9. Psychic stimuli
    10. Pain
   B. Gastrointestinal causes of vomiting
      1. Esophageal diseases
      2. Gastric diseases
      3. Intestinal diseases
VII. Prophylaxis and treatment
   A. Motion sickness
      Prevented by administration of certain antihistaminics such as diphenhydramine (Benadryl) 4 mg/kg, PO, q 8 h or dimenhydrinate (Dramamine) 8 mg/kg, PO, q 8 h. If greater sedation is desired promethazine (Phenergan) 2 mg/kg, PO, SID may be given one hour before traveling. Recently, it was demonstrated in a controlled trial that the oral administration of ginger was superior to the antihistaminic drugs in prevention of motion sickness.
   B. Broad-spectrum antiemetic drugs
      1. Depress the CTZ so are generally not effective against motion sickness
      2. Chlorpromazine (Thorazine) 0.5 mg/kg, IM, PO
      3. Prochlorperazine (Compazine, Darbazine) 0.13 mg/kg, q 6 h
      4. Triflupromazine (Vesprin) 0.2 mg/kg IM, PO q 8 h
      5. Trifluoperazine (Stelazine) 0.03 mg/kg IM q 12 h

      6. Mepazine (Pacatal) 1.5 mg/kg
      7. Trimethobenzamide (Tigan) 3 mg/kg, IM, PO q 8 h
      8. Diphenidol (Vontrol) 1 mg/kg, IM, PO, q 8 h
      9. Haloperidol (Haldol) 0.02 mg/kg, IM, PO q 12 h
     10. Metoclopramide (Reglan) 0.1-0.5 mg/kg, IM, PO
  C. Correct water, electrolyte, and acid-base disorders (see chapter 2).

ACUTE GASTRITIS

    I. Incidence is high in small animal practice
   II. History
     A. Sudden onset of vomiting is a common observation of the owner.
     B. Because of its self-limiting nature acute gastritis usually has short
        duration.
  III. Abnormal findings on clinical exam
     A. Vomiting (the most frequent sign)
       1. Leads to dehydration and lethargy
       2. Vomitus should be examined carefully for character, amount of
         mucous, foreign material, blood, and should also be cultured for
         infectious agents.
     B. Dehydration is a common clinical finding.
     C. Metabolic changes are apparent in blood chemistry.
       1. Hypochloremia
       2. Hyponatremia
       3. Hypokalemia
     D. Urinalysis shows a high specific gravity unless renal disease is present.
     E. There is usually no fever with acute gastritis unless it is secondary
       to a systemic disease.
  IV. Pathophysiology
     A. Etiology of acute gastritis
       1. Consumption of garbage, foreign material, spoiled food, grass or
         bones
       2. Drugs such as aspirin, indomethacin, ibuprofen, phenylbutazone,
         and corticosteroids
       3. Ingestion of toxic or caustic agents like arsenic, thallium, lead,
         ethylene glycol, herbicides, fungicides, fertilizers, and some poisonous plants
       4. Since the cat is a more fastidious animal than the dog, it is less
         likely to ingest these materials.
     B. A vicious circle is often created in acute gastritis which results in
       severe fluid and electrolyte loss.
       1. Frequent vomiting results in polydypsia.
       2. Polydypsia leads to *more* frequent vomition.

C. The degree of dehydration is:
   1. Dependent on the duration of the vomiting
   2. Evaluated by physical exam, PCV, and total protein
D. The pathology of acute gastritis is inflammation of the mucosal lining which disrupts the gastric-mucosal barrier.
   1. Normally, the gastric-mucosal barrier functions as a dialysis membrane to maintain the million-to-one hydrogen ion gradient between the plasma (pH 7.4) and the gastric contents (pH 1-2).
   2. Back diffusion, the movement of hydrogen ions from the stomach back across the mucosa, is increased by:
      a) Aspirin
      b) Corticosteroids (which decrease hydrochloric acid)
E. Irritated gastric mucosa initiates the reflex act of vomiting.
V. Diagnosis
   A. Based mainly on clinical findings and history
   B. Gastroscopy findings include hyperemia, edema, patchy areas of mucus, petechial hemorrhage, and occasional mucosal erosions.
   C. Biopsy
      1. Oral route
      2. Celiotomy route
   D. Radiographic examination is not a reliable means for diagnosing acute gastritis.
VI. Treatment
   A. An essential part of treatment is to withhold water for 12 hours and food for 24 hours.
      1. Offering ice cubes to lick relieves thirst of vomiting but doesn't provide enough water to stimulate further vomiting.
      2. Follow the 24-hour fast with small amounts of bland food (i/d).
   B. Antacids are recommended to reduce the amount of acid in the gastric juice to decreace back diffusion.
      1. Types of antacids and their precautions:
         a) Sodium bicarbonate—may produce a sodium overload or systemic alkalosis
         b) Magnesium antacids—may cause diarrhea and are contraindicated in patients with renal disease
         c) Calcium carbonate—also contraindicated in patients with renal disease and can cause hypercalcemia
      2. Doses of antacids should be small and frequent to maintain the buffering action.
   C. In refractory cases, antiemetics such as phenothiazine tranquilizers are indicated, but *beware of hypotension in severely dehydrated patients*.
   D. Fluids containing sodium chloride and potassium are used for treating dehydration.
   E. Ice-water lavage is a good non-invasive step to control bleeding of gastric hemorrhage.

VII. Prognosis of acute gastritis is good because the condition is usually self-limiting and will resolve spontaneously when the cause of the problem is removed.
VIII. Information to emphasize to client
  Even though the causative factor is usually of short duration, if it continues to cause acute gastritis, permanent damage may result.

CHRONIC GASTRITIS

  I. Chronic gastritis is usually associated with repeated attacks of acute gastritis.
 II. History usually consists of an owner's report of poor hair coat, inability to gain weight, weight loss, sporadic vomiting.
III. Findings on physical exam
    A. It is not unusual in this disease to find nothing significant on physical exam besides a possible weight loss and minor dehydration.
    B. Sometimes palpation of a foreign body aids in diagnosis of chronic gastritis.
 IV. Pathophysiology and etiology
    A. Chronic gastritis can result from prolonged exposure to agents causing acute gastritis.
    B. In dogs, diffuse follicular chronic hypertrophic-hyperplastic gastritis is caused by chronic uremia.
    C. As a result of their grooming process cats often develop hair ball-induced chronic gastritis.
  V. Diagnosis
    A. The only way to confirm chronic gastritis is by performing a biopsy of the gastric mucosa. Histologic findings are:
      1. Occlusion of pyloric glands
      2. Tiny retention cysts
      3. Presence of chronic inflammatory cells, i.e., plasma cells, lymphocytes, and eosinophils
    B. Laboratory evaluation of blood and serum is usually futile in confirming a diagnosis of chronic gastritis except for finding:
      1. An absolute monocytosis
      2. Signs of dehydration
    C. Gastroscopy reveals a general or local thickening of the gastric mucosa with occasional erosions and hemorrhage.
 VI. Treatment consists of removing the cause.
    A. In foreign body-induced gastritis the inciting cause may be retrieved by endoscopy or laparotomy.
    B. In hair ball-induced gastritis small amounts of petrolatum are given orally for 3 days.
VII. Prognosis is good when the causative agent is removed.
VIII. Clients should be warned that in the event of continued exposure, gastric ulcers or pyloric stenosis may result.

GASTRIC ULCERS

I. Incidence
    A. Age between $2\frac{1}{2}$ and 12 years
    B. Higher incidence in females
    C. Extremely high occurrence in dogs with mast cell tumors
        1. Of 24 dogs with mastocytomas, 20 had gastrointestinal ulceration.
        2. Breed predilection of mastocytomas is in the Boxer and Boston Terrier.

II. History
    A. Chronic vomiting is the most frequent complaint.
        1. Vomitus often has a coffee-ground appearance due to partially digested blood.
        2. Dehydration is prevalent due to vomition.
    B. Blood loss
        1. Melena is sometimes seen.
        2. Anemia may result.
    C. Polydipsia is due to anemia and dehydration.
    D. A history of recent spinal decompression surgery with postoperative corticosteroids often suggests gastrointestinal ulceration.
    E. Gastric ulcers may be asymptomatic until sudden death occurs due to perforation.

III. Abnormal findings on physical examination
    A. Abdominal pain is the most common finding.
    B. Pale mucous membranes indicate anemia is present.

IV. Pathophysiology
    A. Any cause of acute or chronic gastritis may result in gastric ulcers.
    B. Mastocytomas related to peptic ulcers.
        1. These tumors produce histidine-decarboxylase which converts histidine to histamine, the factor responsible for peptic ulcers.
        2. Heparin, which prevents mucosal ulceration by histamine, is inhibited through an unknown mechanism by the mast cell tumor.
    C. Site and nature of peptic ulcers
        1. Usually in the proximal duodenum and non-acid producing areas of the stomach, i.e., pyloric antrum and lesser curvature.
        2. The specific site of gastric ulcer formation is determined by blood flow, mucosal cell turnover, and mucus production.
        3. Ulcers are usually solitary but vary in size from punctate to 4 cm across.
    D. The role of increased bile in gastric ulcers.
        1. Bile causes gastritis by breaking down the gastric mucosal barrier.
        2. Bile also causes increased gastrin levels which cause increased parietal cell density subsequently causing increased acid secretion.
    E. An obstruction or pyloric stenosis can result in gastric ulceration via the pathway just mentioned due to increased gastrin secretion.
    F. Self-protective mechanisms from gastric ulcers:

1. Gastric epithelial cells, with their short four-day life span, offer a continual renewal of the stomach's surface.
2. Mucus of gastric epithelial cells serves to neutralize excess acid.
3. Anti-inflammatory drugs such as aspirin, cortisone, and indomethacin decrease mucous secretion which may lead to gastric ulceration.

V. Diagnostic procedures
  A. Laboratory evaluation of blood and serum reveals:
    1. Regenerative anemia
    2. Liver disease
      In a study of 22 dogs with peptic ulcers, 16 had fatty and degenerative changes of their liver.
    3. Evidence of lead poisoning has been related to gastric ulcer.
  B. Endoscopy reveals two types of ulcers.
    1. Acute
      Inflammatory and bleeding ulcers
    2. Chronic
      Little inflammation with a fibrin-filled crater
  C. Barium contrast radiography demonstrates chronic deep ulcerations but is nearly useless in mucosal erosions.
  D. Abdominal laparotomy offers the best opportunity to diagnose gastric ulcers.

VI. Treatment: medical, surgical, or both
  A. Medical management
    1. Antacids
    2. Antiemetics (promazine tranquilizers) useful except with anemia or dehydration.
    3. Intragastric lavage with ice water for acute gastric hemorrhage.
    4. Norepinephrine at a rate of 8 mg/500 ml may be added to the ice water aid control of acute gastric hemorrhage.
    5. Cimetidine, a new specific H_2-antagonist drug, acts at the final step of acid secretion, involving histamine.
  B. Surgical treatment
    Partial gastrectomy, pyloromyotomy, vagotomy

VII. Prognosis
  Unknown for dogs and cats

VIII. Client education
  Dietary management is the same as for acute gastritis.

GASTRIC FOREIGN BODIES

I. Incidence
  A. A common problem seen especially in younger animals
  B. Two types of foreign bodies are seen:
    1. A swallowed object

2. A bezoar which is a concretion in the stomach or intestines
    a) Trichobezoar (hair ball)
    b) Phytobezoar (composed of fruit and vegetable fibers)
II. History
    A. Most common of the owner's complaints is periodic episodes of vom-
       iting.
    B. Palpation may cause discomfort but rarely detects a foreign body.
III. Abnormal findings
    Unless there is abdominal pain, fluid, or pyrexia associated with sec-
    ondary peritonitis, one cannot usually diagnose gastric foreign body by
    physical examination.
IV. Pathophysiology
    A. Foreign bodies may be responsible for hematemesis.
    B. Perforation of gut by a foreign body often leads to peritonitis.
V. Diagnostic methods
    A. Radiography usually confirms diagnosis.
    B. Endoscopy
    C. A complete clinical history
VI. Treatment
    A. Watchful waiting
       1. Gastric foreign bodies often pass spontaneously (even pins and
          needles) within 72 hours.
       2. Perform consecutive serial radiographs.
       3. If object remains stationary for 24 hours, surgery is indicated.
    B. Endoscopic or surgical retrieval
    C. Vaseline is useful for trichobezoars.
VII. Prognosis is good after removal of foreign body. Gastric erosions will heal
    spontaneously.

Food Allergy

I. Incidence
    A. Occurs early in life
    B. There is no seasonal association as with allergic dermatitis.
II. May be manifested in three forms—all of which may be relieved by
    dietary changes.
    A. Gastric form can be acute or chronic.
       1. Profuse watery diarrhea with or without blood.
       2. Vomition immediately after eating
    B. Skin reaction
       1. Varies in appearance: dry skin, coarse hair, urticaria, angioedema,
          and excoriation with squamous crusts
       2. Intense pruritis of eyelids, nose, jowls, and lips often eliciting self-
          induced trauma

C. Concomitant digestive and dermal signs are occasionally seen.
III. Abnormal findings on physical examination
    A. Thickened intestinal walls can be detected on abdominal palpation.
    B. Signs of dehydration, weight loss, and unthriftiness should be looked for during physical examination.
IV. Pathophysiology
    A. The etiology of eosinophilic gastroenteritis, a sequela to chronic food allergy, is unknown. Possible causes include: low grade bacterial and viral infections, ingestion of toxins, antigen-antibody reactions, or *toxocara canis* infection.
    B. There are four proposed ways for the gastrointestinal tract to participate in an allergic reaction:
        1. An immediate or delayed allergic response at the site of antigen-antibody reaction
        2. A serum sickness-type reaction from IgG and circulating complexes of antigen
        3. Antigens which are absorbed react in distant organs with tissue-fixed antibody (IgE).
        4. An autoimmune response with gastrointestinal tissue mistaken for an antigen.
V. Diagnostic techniques
    A. Diet testing is effective and can be approached in different ways:
        1. First, put animal on a bland diet of mutton and rice. Observe for relief of signs on returning home to eliminate the possibility of environmental factors being the cause of the problem. Then reintroduce foods and check for appearance of signs until the offending agent is identified.
        2. Fast animal for three days, then put it on a bland diet for 10-14 days. Additional foods are added at five-day intervals. Three positive responses, two weeks apart, confirm an offending agent.
    B. Gastric biopsies before and after food challenges
        Look for an increase in plasma cells, eosinophils, macrophages, and neutrophils in the lamina propria.
    C. Hemogram shows absolute eosinophilia.
VI. Treatment
    A. Identification and removal of food
        1. Is the ideal treatment
        2. May lead to dietary deficiency
    B. Of dermal lesions (see chapter 21)
        1. Antihistaminics
            Drug of choice
        2. Corticosteroids
            Parentally and topically
    C. Of eosinophilic gastroenteritis (see chapter 6)
        Corticosteroids

VII. Prognosis is poor.

VIII. Warn clients to be observant of developing signs during changes in diet.

ACUTE GASTRIC DILATATION

    I. Incidence

        A. All breeds at any age are susceptible, but more commonly seen in deep-chested breeds of dogs.

        B. There are two forms of acute gastric dilatation:

            1. Young dogs—overengorgement

            2. Older dogs—gas and fluid accumulation

        C. It is very important to differentiate acute gastric dilatation from gastric volvulus.

   II. History

        A. Complained of distended and painful abdomen

        B. Often results in non-productive retching and excessive salivation

        C. Many times, dogs are greedy eaters which belch and pass flatus postprandially.

  III. Physical examination

        A. Percussion of cranial abdomen reveals a resonant tympanic sound due to air or a dull sound due to large amounts of fluids or food in the stomach.

        B. Succussion reveals a gas and fluid-filled stomach.

        C. Polypnea and tachycardia

        D. Observe for signs of hypovolemic shock.

  IV. Pathophysiology

        A. Two conditions are needed for gastric dilatation.

            1. Presence of gas, fluid, or food

            2. An obstruction that prevents relief of distention such as twisting of fundus

        B. Blocked venous drainage → hypoxia → acidosis

        C. Effects on respiration

            Gastric enlargement → encroachment on the thoracic space → decreased respiratory volume → increased respiratory rate → decreased pulmonary compliance → abnormal ventilation-perfusion ratio → shock lung → hypovolemic shock

        D. Etiology

            1. Acute gastric dilatation in young dog

                Overeating → excessive secretion → even more enlarged stomach → pain

            2. Acute gastric dilatation in older dog

                Many factors possible: emesis, parturition, trauma, gastric neoplasm, overeating, pica, abdominal surgery, and aerophagia

   V. Diagnostic techniques

        A. Radiography is best to confirm acute gastric dilatation and differentiate from gastric volvulus.

B. Passage of stomach tube does *not* always distinguish gastric volvulus from gastric dilatation.
VI. Treatment must be prompt and aggressive.
    A. Early decompression via:
        1. Stomach tube
        2. Trocharization
        3. Gastrotomy
        4. Beware of shock from the rapid release of hypoxemic acidotic fluid.
    B. Fluid therapy with lactated Ringer's solution
    C. Corticosteroid therapy (see chapter 9)
        1. May protect from septic shock
        2. Prevents microvascular damage
    D. Gastric lavage with warm saline or Ringer's solution
VII. Prognosis is good if diagnosed and reduced early.
VIII. Client education
    For the first 3-4 days after recovery from gastric dilatation close observation for vomition, shock, and recurring gastric dilatation is mandatory.

GASTRIC VOLVULUS

I. Incidence
    A. Increased incidence in large deep-chested dogs
    B. Age predilection—older animals
    C. Sex predilection—male
II. History
    A. Postprandial development of unproductive retching with severe abdominal pain
    B. Sometimes a chronic form of gastric volvulus presents as chronic postprandial vomiting often with a history of gastric dilatation.
    C. Dogs are described as "ravenous" eaters which belch and are flatulent after eating.
III. Abnormal findings on physical exam
    A. Abdominal distention with tympany
    B. Polypnea and tachycardia are seen as compensatory attempts against encroachment of thoracic cavity and impeded venous return.
    C. Scleral congestion is usually most pronounced in the dog with significant signs of shock.
    D. On palpation spleen is enlarged and intestines are filled with gas.
IV. Treatment
    A. Relieve distention as above
    B. Surgical repositioning of stomach and spleen and pyloromyotomy
        1. Tube gastrotomy
        2. Gastropexy
        3. Gastrocolopexy
    C. Control shock, cardiac dysrhythmias, and hypokalemia

THE SMALL INTESTINE

DIARRHEA

Diarrhea is the most common sign in intestinal disease. Diarrhea is defined as an increase in the frequency of bowel evacuation and water content of the stool. It nearly always represents an increase in the patient's normal bowel habits.

Pathophysiology of diarrhea

There are four major mechanisms of diarrhea and each enteric disease that causes diarrhea can usually be explained by one or more of the four mechanisms.

I. Osmotic diarrhea

Osmotic diarrhea results from poorly-absorbed solutes in the gut. The solutes may result from:

A. Ingestion (laxatives)

B. Maldigestion or malabsorption

C. Failure to transport a dietary nonelectrolyte

The presence of a non-absorbable solute in the intestine retards water absorption and by its osmotic effect tends to cause net water movement from plasma to the gut lumen. Clinically osmotic diarrhea is distinguished by the fact that diarrhea stops soon after the patient fasts.

II. Secretory diarrhea

The most important mechanism proposed as the cause of increased intestinal secretion is stimulation of active ion secretion by the mucosal cells. Although there probably are a large number of toxins that mediate a secretory diarrhea (e.g., clostridial, escherichial, etc.) knowledge in this area has advanced rapidly, primarily due to the studies with cholera toxin.

The mediator of intestinal secretion in cholera appears to be an elevated intracellular concentration of cyclic AMP(C-AMP) secondary to stimulation of adenyl cyclase by the cholera toxin. Cyclic AMP and agents which raise C-AMP, such as theophylline and prostaglandins, mimic the action of cholera toxin on the small bowel. The response to cholera toxin is not associated with any inflammation to the small bowel mucosa. Active intestinal glucose and amino acid absorption remain normal, because the secretion orginates in the crypts whereas absorptive processes are mainly a villus function.

The major clinical features of pure secretory diarrhea is that the diarrhea persists even when the patient fasts and that stool volumes may be, and often are, very large.

Therapeutically, salicylates (aspirin, Pepto Bismol) may be beneficial in secretory diarrheas caused by enterotoxin. Salicylates inhibit prostaglandin secretion which may in turn decrease intestinal secretion by reducing the intracellular concentration of C-AMP.

III. Increased permeability

There is a continuous flux of water and electrolytes across the intestinal border. In the normal animal absorption exceeds secretion, resulting in net absorption. The bulk of this flux in both directions occurs by passive diffusion through pores in the junctions between epithelial cells. Changes in surface area or specific abnormalities in mucosal cell membranes may increase "pore size" in the mucous membranes causing an increased flow from the blood to the intestinal lumen. If the amount of material exuded exceeds the absorptive capacity of the intestines diarrhea results.

The size of the particles that leak through the mucosa will depend on the magnitude of the increase in pore size. Small increases permit increased diffusion of small molecules such as creatinine and mannitol. Transudation of large amounts of these molecules in solution could result in diarrhea. Large increases in pore size can permit exudation of plasma proteins into the lumen. These diseases are characterized as "protein losing enteropathies." The increase in size of existing pores can be due to: an increase in hydraulic pressure in the mucosa because of obstructed lymph flow or the action of chemical mediators of an inflammatory process acting directly to increase pore size. The channels or pores for protein movement from plasma to the intestinal lumen are ultrastructurally recognizable separations of the functional complexes between epithelial and endothelial cells.

IV. Motility disorders

In the normal animal there are two main types of intestinal motility: rhythmic segmentation and peristalsis. Rhythmic segmentation performs two functions: it mixes the food with digestive enzymes and brings the nutrients into contact with the mucosal absorptive surfaces and it decreases the flow of ingesta down the gastrointestinal tract. In general, animals with diarrhea have a decrease in segmentation thus offering little resistance to the flow of contents through it (e.g., "openpipe"). Peristalsis serves to move ingesta along the intestinal tract. These movements occur in both directions. Forward peristalsis is the most common movement throughout the GI tract. However, reverse peristalsis is important and occurs commonly in the colon. Reverse peristaltic movements have been shown to occur in the horse, cat, and man. Increased reverse peristaltic movements in the colon have been associated with constipation, whereas diarrhea may be associated with decreased colonic peristalsis. Thus diarrhea may be induced by a decrease in segmentation, a decrease in reverse peristalsis, or increase in forward peristalsis.

Therapeutically, drugs such as anticholinergics that decrease intestinal segmentation, reverse peristalsis and sphincter tone are generally contraindicated. Narcotic analgesics (e.g., morphine, meperidine, paregoric [Parepectolin] diphenoxylate hydrochloride [Lomotil], loperamide [Imodium]) are usually more useful because they stimulate segementation and

TABLE 13-1.   PATHOPHYSIOLOGY OF DIARRHEA

I.   Osmotic
   A.   Maldigestion
      1.   Pancreatic enzyme deficiency
      2.   Bile deficiency
      3.   Loss of brush border enzymes
   B.   Malabsorption
      1.   Loss of mucosal absorptive area
      2.   Loss of absorptive mechanisms
      3.   Diseases of the lamina propria
      4.   Circulatory diseases
II.   Secretory
   A.   Bacterial endotoxins
   B.   Drugs
III.   Increased permeability
   A.   Protein losing gastroenteropathies
      1.   Disordered metabolism or turnover of epithelial cell
         a)   Rugal hypertrophy (Menetrier's)
         b)   Allergic gastroenteropathy
         c)   Bacterial enteritis
         d)   Parasitic enteritis
         e)   Histoplasmosis
      2.   Mucosal ulceration
         a)   Carcinoma
         b)   Lymphosarcoma
         c)   Gastric ulcers
         d)   Foreign body (chronic)
         e)   Intussusception
         f)   Parasitic enteritis
      3.   Lymphatic abnormalities
         a)   Lymphangiectasia
         b)   Lymphosarcoma
         c)   Congestive heart failure
IV.   Motility disorders
      German Shepherd diarrhea

sphincter tone to increase resistance to the flow of ingesta, while decreasing forward peristalsis.

Table 13-1 lists the major mechanisms of diarrhea and the major gastrointestinal diseases. Table 13-2 lists the common narcotic analgesics used to treat diarrhea.

TABLE 13-2.   NARCOTIC ANALGESICS

Generic Name	Proprietary Name	Canine Dose
Morphine	—	0.25 mg/kg
Meperidine	Demerol	10 mg/kg
Paregoric	Parepectolin	2–15 ml
Diphenoxylate	Lomotil	0.063 mg/kg

Metabolic consequences of diarrhea

I. Dehydration
   A. The degree of dehydration will depend on the severity and duration of the fluid loss in the stool.
      1. In acute severe diarrhea the major fluid loss is extracellular fluid.
      2. In chronic diarrhea there may be a decrease in all of the fluid compartments.
   B. If the blood volume is considerably decreased, peripheral vasoconstriction will occur. This will cause a lack of oxygen to these tissues and will increase lactic acid production which may contribute to the acidosis.

II. Acidosis
   A. Intestinal bicarbonate loss
   B. Lactic acidosis due to dehydration
   C. Decreased renal H^+ excretion

III. Potassium depletion
   A. Plasma potassium may be increased, normal, or decreased.
      1. Acidosis causes K^+ to move out of the cell. Therefore the intracellular potassium concentration is decreased.
      2. At the same time, potassium is lost in the diarrheal feces. Depending on the relative rates of these potassium losses from the cell and body, the plasma concentration may be increased, normal, or decreased.
   B. Total body potassium is decreased.
   C. Paradoxically potassium toxicity may occur.
      1. Intracellular potassium levels are decreased.
      2. This decreases the intracellular to extracellular potassium ratio (K_i/K_e). If the extracellular potassium increased, this concentration would further decrease the ratio.
      3. If the ratio is decreased sufficiently the result is potassium toxicity even though the total body potassium may be decreased.
      4. Potassium toxicity is illustrated clinically by muscle weakness and cardiac dysfunction (bradycardia and arrhythmias). Electrocardiographic abnormalities are increased amplitude and spiking of the T wave and decreased amplitude of the P wave (see chapter 2).
      5. Therapeutically, the important point to remember is that even though a potassium deficiency exists in patients with diarrhea one should not supplement the fluids given to patients with potassium until the plasma potassium value and/or blood gas status of the patient has been determined.

Clinical evaluation of diarrhea

I. History
II. Physical examination
III. Clinical pathology

A. Fecal examination
   1. Flotation (MgSO₄, saturated sugar solution)
   2. Direct smear
   3. Occult blood (Hematest tablets)
   4. Fecal trypsin activity
      a) X-ray film digestion
         (1) Add feces to 9 ml of 5% sodium bicarbonate to make 10 cc.
         (2) Place film (exposed or unexposed) in the solution.
         (3) Let stand for 2½ hours at room temperature or 1 hour at 37°C.
         (4) Rinse the film with tap water.
         (5) If the film is cleared then trypsin is present.
      b) Gelatin tube test
         (1) Dilute feces 1:10 with water.
         (2) Heat 2 gelatin tubes to 37°C.
         (3) Add 1 ml of 5% sodium bicarbonate and 1 ml feces.
         (4) Add 1 ml of 5% sodium bicarbonate and 1 ml of water to a second tube (control).
         (5) Agitate both tubes.
         (6) Heat to 37°C for one hour or 2½ hours at room temperature.
         (7) Refrigerate (5°C for 20 minutes).
         (8) If the gelatin solidifies digestion did not occur. If no digestion of the gelatin occurs, trypsin is not present in that stool sample or it was destroyed by fecal bacteria. Because of this, at least three negative (no digestion) samples must be obtained to be considered valid results.
   5. Fecal starch (Lugol's iodine stain)
      a) Procedure
         (1) Mix a small aliquot of stool suspension with 1-2 drops of Lugol's iodine stain and coverslip.
         (2) Examine microscopically.
      b) Interpretation
         (1) Bluish-black stained particles are starch granules.
         (2) Talcum powder may mimic dietary starch if sample is contaminated.
         (3) Large numbers of starch granules indicate amylase deficiency.
   6. Qualitative fecal fat
      a) Procedure
         (1) A small aliquot of stool suspension is placed on a slide and mixed with 2 drops of 95% ethanol, followed by 2 drops of saturated ethanolic solution of Sudan III. This is then mixed and coverslipped. Occasionally it helps to slightly heat the microscope slide by placing it on the palm of a hand for 1-3 minutes of placing it over a match flame for 2-3 seconds.
         (2) Examine microscopically.
      b) Interpretation
         (1) Neutral fats appear as large red or orange droplets.

(2) Mineral oil or castor oil may mimic neutral fat.

(3) The normal dog on a commercial dog food (e.g., normal fat content) may not have any fat drops per low power field. At the most there should be no more than 2 drops per low power field.

(4) Because of the low fat content of commercial dog food a patient with maldigestion/malabsorption of fat may not have any fat drops per low power field if it is on a regular dog food. The author likes to have the patients on a moderate fat diet (e.g., c/d) for 24 hours prior to doing this test if he/she does not have fat drops in the stool while on a regular commercial dog food.

(5) The normal dog on c/d (e.g., high fat content) should have no more than 2-3 drops per low power field.

7. Quantitative fecal fat

The total fecal lipid can be quantitated. The total amount of fat in daily fecal samples is measured and expressed as a percent of the dietary intake.

a) Procedure

(1) Feed a known quantity of fat for 3 days (72 hours). Canned c/d is frequently used as it contains 8.4% fat (dry weight).

(2) Collect all of the feces for the last 48 hours and weigh.

(3) Send a fecal sample to a laboratory for fecal fat determination.

(4) Determine fat excreted from laboratory analysis and quantity of feces excreted. Convert to percent of dietary intake.

b) Interpretation

(1) The normal patient will excrete less than 5-8% of the dietary intake.

(2) Greater than normal amounts of fat indicate lipase deficiency, bile insufficiency, and/or intestinal malabsorption.

B. Blood profile
  1. Hemogram (CBC)
  2. Serum chemistries
C. Urinalysis
D. Absorption tests
  1. Xylose absorption test

Xylose is a five carbon sugar that is absorbed by the same mechanism as the hexoses, glucose, and galactose. Assimilation of this sugar does not require the intraluminal pancreatic stage of digestion. An abnormal xylose test then usually indicates a small intestinal disease.

a) Procedure

(1) Fast the patient for 12-24 hours.

(2) Give 0.5 g/kg of 5% xylose solution orally.

(3) Collect plasma samples at 0, 30, 60, 90, 120, and 180 minutes for xylose assay.

    b) Interpretation

        (1) Normal—a net rise of plasma xylose of at least 45 mg/dl by 60-90 minutes.

        (2) Low—malabsorption of carbohydrates, delayed gastric emptying time, or a technical error.

  2. Oral glucose tolerance test.

    Since many factors affect blood glucose levels, this test is not as accurate as the xylose absorption test.

    a) Procedure

        (1) Fast the patient for 12-24 hours.

        (2) Administer 2 g/kg of 25% Dextrose solution orally.

        (3) Collect blood at 0, 15, 30, 60, 120, and 180 minutes.

    b) Interpretation

        (1) Normal—peak greater than 140 mg/dl between 60-90 minutes

        (2) Low—malabsorption of carbohydrates, increased metabolism of glucose, or a technical error

        (3) High—diabetic or pre-diabetic

  3. Fat absorption test

    a) Procedure

        (1) Obtain a plasma sample.

        (2) If plasma sample is clear, give the patient a fatty meal (6 ml/kg Lipomul, or 3 ml/kg corn oil) orally.

        (3) Two hours later collect a plasma sample and check for turbidity.

    b) Interpretation

        (1) If plasma is clear, the patient has maldigestion or malabsorption.

        (2) To rule in pancreatic insufficiency repeat steps a, b, and c except add pancreatic enzymes (Viokase—one teaspoon per 10 kg of body weight) to the fatty meal. If the maldigestion—malabsorption is due to a pancreatic insufficiency the plasma will be lipemic.

  4. BT-PABA absorption test

    N-benzoyl-L-tyrosyl-p-aminobenzoic acid (BT-PABA), a synthetic substrate for pancreatic chymotrypsin, releases PABA in the presence of this enzyme. The amount of PABA in the blood or urine after BT-PKABA administration then serves as an index of pancreatic function. Limited studies indicate that PABA is absorbed normally in most intestinal malabsorptive conditions.

    a) Procedure

        (1) Fast the patient for 12 hours.

        (2) Give 50 mg/kg or 150 mg/kg of 3% solution orally.

        (3) Collect blood samples at 0, 30, 60, 90, 120, and 150 minutes.

    b) Interpretation

        (1) Normal—More than 10 ug/ml in 60-90 minutes at the 50 mg/

kg dose—More than 30 ug/ml in 60-90 minutes at the 150 mg/ kg dose
    (2) Low—Chymotrypsin deficiency due to exocrine pancreatic insufficiency.
E. Bacteriology
F. Virology
G. Serology
H. Miscellaneous tests
    1. Radiography
      Survey and upper G.I. barium studies are often indicated when obstructive intestinal disease is suspected. However, they are less valuable in the study of inflammatory bowel disorders.
    2. Colonic scrapes
    3. Intestinal biopsy
    4. Endoscopy

NON-SPECIFIC ACUTE DIARRHEA

This is one of the most common problems that small animal veterinarians treat.

Etiology

  I. Unknown—In the majority of these cases the veterinarian will never determine the etiology.
 II. Bacteria
III. Viral—See section on Viral Enteritis
IV. Parasitic
 V. Fungal

History

  I. Acute onset
 II. Duration is usually 24 to 48 hours prior to presentation.
III. Usually it is a watery diarrhea and may contain blood.
IV. The frequency of diarrhea is variable.
 V. Borborygmus may be present.

Physical examination

I. The findings are extremely variable depending on the severity and the etiology of the diarrhea.
   A. Dehydration is the most common finding.
   B. Evidence of a generalized disease may be found (e.g., distemper, uremia, etc.).

Clinical pathology

I. All patients with acute diarrhea should have a direct fecal smear and fecal flotation performed to rule in parasitic disease. Numerous fecal examinations are needed to rule out parasitic disease.

II. Depending on the severity of the case, other clinical pathology data may or may not be obtained.

III. To identify complications and to more accurately direct management, additional data may be obtained. The additional data that are *most frequently* obtained at the University of Missouri are the following: CBC, total protein, serum electrolytes, BUN, blood gases, and Wright's stain of a direct fecal smear.

Diagnosis

Based on the history and physical examination findings.

Treatment

The treatment will vary depending on the severity of the case. Most patients with diarrhea will probably recover without any therapy. Listed below are various therapeutic considerations.

I. Dietary management

A. The patient should be kept NPO for the first 12 to 24 hours and should receive no food for the first 24 to 48 hours. When given food it should initially be given in small amounts. It should be a bland diet and consist mainly of carbohydrates and protein.

B. Reasons for not feeding the patient:

1. When inflammation is present in the G.I. tract the loss of mucosal cells is accelerated. Food in the intestine acts as an abrasive and increases the loss of the mucosal cells.

2. Minimizes the chance of colonization of the G.I. tract by foreign bacteria. When the normal flora is upset, as in diarrheal states, transients can enter the G.I. tract and colonize it. Bacteria are present in food and therefore by withholding food one will decrease the number of transients entering the G.I. tract.

3. The small intestinal mucosa loses its brush border enzymes during diarrhea and therefore it loses its ability to digest disaccharides (lactose, sucrose). The inability to digest food may cause an osmotic diarrhea to develop and compound the existing diarrhea.

II. Intestinal protectants

Kaolin and pectin-type drugs are of doubtful value in severe diarrhea. They have not been shown to alter fluid and electrolyte losses. It appears that they are neither beneficial nor detrimental.

III. Drug therapy
   A. Motility modifiers
      1. Decrease the driving force for moving intestinal contents aborally (peristalsis)
      2. Increase resistance to their flow (rhythmic segmentation). Anticholinergics decrease intestinal segmentation, reverse peristalsis and sphincter tone. *They should not be used to treat diarrhea.* Narcotic analgesics (e.g., Lomotil) are the only effective drugs that increase resistance to flow by stimulating rhythmic segmentation. Their major action is on the intestinal smooth muscle producing tonic and phasic contractions of the circular muscle of the bowel. Narcotic analgesics will have either no effect or will cause relaxation of the longitudinal intestinal muscle in the dog. Their net effect is to inhibit the flow of ingesta through the G.I. tract.
   B. Salicylates
      They may be beneficial in secretory diarrheal diseases. Salicylates inhibit prostaglandins which may decrease enterotoxin-induced intestinal secretion.
   C. Corticosteroids, antihistaminics
      These drugs are of dubious value in the treatment of diarrhea.
   D. Antibiotics
      Antibacterial agents may or may not be beneficial. If they only succeed in inhibiting the normal flora they are detrimental. In patients with acute diarrhea it seems logical to use antibiotics when there is evidence that bacteria have induced an inflammatory reaction in the gastrointestinal tract (numerous bacteria and inflammatory cells on fecal smear), invaded intestinal mucosa (blood in the feces), or caused a generalized inflammatory reaction in the body (fever, leukocytosis, etc.). Controlled studies need to be done to determine when antibiotic therapy is needed in dogs and cats with diarrhea. Antibiotics should not be used to treat every case of acute diarrhea. If antibiotics are given in conjunction with intestinal protectants, most are bound to the protectant and are thus ineffective.
IV. Fluid therapy
      In a severe case, proper fluid therapy is extremely important. Proper fluid therapy is based on the state of hydration, serum electrolyte studies, and acid-base studies. If serum electrolyte and blood gas studies are not done it is best to use a balanced electrolyte solution (see chapter 2).

VIRAL DIARRHEA

Etiology

   I. Adenovirus
   II. Astrovirus
   III. Picornavirus

    IV. Paramyxovirus
     V. Rotavirus
    VI. Coronavirus
   VII. Parvovirus
  VIII. From this list it can be seen that a large number of viruses can cause diarrhea. The most important clinically are coronavirus and parvovirus.

Coronavirus enteritis

Coronaviruses affect a large number of animal species including mice, chickens, turkeys, rats, cattle, and swine. The canine pathogenic virus may possibly be related to the transmissible gastroenteritis virus of swine, as both viruses produce gastrointestinal infections in the dog. Coronaviral infections often occur concurrently with other viruses, parasites, and bacterial pathogens, and dogs with complicated infections may develop a more severe syndrome.

    I. History

       One to 3 days postexposure (ingestion of infected feces), the patient may develop signs of the disease. Diarrhea is the main presenting sign. It is usually foul smelling, loose to mucoid, with an orange color, and may contain blood. The patient may also be vomiting, the frequency of which decreases after the first day of diarrhea.

   II. Physical examination

       The patient may show lethargy, depression, anorexia, and slight dehydration. Usually dogs are afebrile or hypothermic. No other specific findings are noted.

  III. Clinical pathology

       Nothing specific

   IV. Diagnosis

       A definitive diagnosis is usually not made.

    V. Treatment

       The therapy will vary depending on the severity of the case. The same considerations should be made as those listed under Treatment of Acute Diarrhea. Generally speaking, most cases will recover in 7 to 10 days.

   VI. Pathological lesions

       The lesions seen microscopically consist of atrophy and fusion of the small intestinal villi, along with lengthening of the crypts.

  VII. Prognosis

       Most will recover with symptomatic treatment.

Parvovirus enteritis

Parvoviruses affect a large number of animals including swine, cattle, cats, and dogs. A parvovirus causes "feline panleukopenia." The canine parvovirus causes an enteritis-leukopenia syndrome, but a myocarditis may also be noted.

I. History
    A. Enteric form
        Initially the patient shows depression, anorexia, and lethargy followed by an acute onset of vomiting and/or diarrhea. The diarrhea is usually seen within the next 24 hours. Usually the diarrhea is bloody and has a characteristic odor. Sometimes it does not contain blood.
    B. Cardiac form
        Myocarditis generally affects puppies 3-8 weeks old due to the virus' affinity for rapidly dividing cardiac muscle fibers. Owners may report the sudden death of a puppy, crying and depression, and/or signs of respiratory distress due to cardiac failure. This form of the viral infection may be the only evidence, or it may follow a viral enteritis 3 to 6 weeks after apparent recovery. Sometimes infection is not apparent and puppies that survive the acute myocarditis may die months later of congestive heart failure due to myocardial fibrosis.

II. Physical examination
    A. The patient with the enteric form is usually afebrile. Anorexia, depression, and dehydration are frequently seen. Many dogs do not have diarrhea until 24 hours after presentation for the chief complaint of anorexia and depression.
    B. The myocarditis patient may show signs of the enteric form in addition to signs of cardiac congestive failure. Yet, previously healthy puppies may present with dyspnea, tachycardia, pale mucous membranes, and froth in the mouth and nostrils without any signs of intestinal disease.

III. Clinical pathology
    Leukopenia is a fairly consistent finding in the enteric form. The total WBC count is usually between 500-2000/mm^3. Frequently, the leukopenia does not occur until 24-72 hours after the development of clinical signs. Creatinine phosphokinase (CPK) may be elevated with the myocardial form in its acute stages.

IV. Diagnosis
    A. History
    B. Physical examination
    C. ECG
    D. Electron microscopy
        Identification of virus particles in intestinal tissue or feces
    E. Serology
        Hemagglutination inhibition tests
    F. Virus isolation

V. Pathological lesions
    In the acute stages of disease there is necrosis of the crypt epithelium and necrosis or depletion of lymphoid tissue (thymus, lymph nodes, spleen). In the myocardial form there is myofiber necrosis with mono-

nuclear cell infiltrate. Occasionally, one may see eosinophilic intra-nuclear inclusions in the intact crypt epithelial and myocardial cells.

VI. Treatment

The therapy depends upon the severity of the case, using those considerations as listed under Treatment of Acute Diarrhea. The goals of therapy should be directed at:

A. Correcting the fluid deficits, acid-base abnormalities, and electrolyte abnormalities

B. Decreasing the loss of fluids and electrolytes from the G.I. tract by controlling the vomiting and diarrhea.

C. Initial studies at the University of Missouri indicate that clostridial overgrowths occur frequently. Therefore, penicillin or penicillin like antibiotics may be indicated.

VII. Prognosis

This is extremely variable. Studies at the Veterinary Teaching Hospital at the University of Missouri have indicated that there is no relationship between the white blood cell counts and prognosis. Mortality is higher among younger patients.

VIII. Prevention

A. Vaccination

The vaccines currently available are of canine cell-line origin. They are either inactivated or attenuated. The killed vaccines offer shorter immunity but are safe to use in pregnant animals. The MLV strains give a longer immunity, greater than one year, but virus particles, while not virulent, may be shed in the feces. Both vaccines are available in combination with other vaccines.

B. Proper hygiene

The virus can survive in the environment for years and can be carried by dog owners from one dog to another. Proper cleaning and disinfection of kennels is extremely important. One part Clorox in 30 parts water is an effective disinfectant.

HEMORRHAGIC GASTROENTERITIS (HGE)

A specific syndrome characterized by a peracute onset of diarrhea and vomiting that becomes hemorrhagic.

Etiology

Not known. Possible theory is abnormal immune response

History

I. The patient was healthy until 4 or 5 hours ago when it started to vomit and/or have diarrhea.

II. Now the vomitus and/or diarrhea is hemorrhagic; patient distressed.

III. Any breed. Schnauzers and Poodles seem to be predisposed.

IV. There does not appear to be any age or sex predilection.

Physical examination

I. The patient is depressed.

II. There is hemorrhagic diarrhea and/or blood flakes on the rectal thermometer.

III. The diarrhea has a characteristic odor.

IV. The rectal temperature is usually normal. If the patient is in shock it may be low.

V. Clinically (skin turgidity, etc.) the patient does not appear to be dehydrated.

VI. Some patients will be in hypovolemic shock.

Clinical pathology

The abnormalities noted will vary with the severity of the case. Most of the abnormalities are secondary to the fluid loss due to the diarrhea. Unlike parvovirus enteritis, the WBC counts are usually normal throughout the course of the disease.

I. Increased packed cell volume

This is a *very* consistent finding and is due to extracellular dehydration. The total protein concentration may be increased from fluid loss or it may be normal because the patients most likely have a protein loss from the GI tract.

II. Azotemia

This is a consistent finding and is mostly due to pre-renal causes. it may also be due to the blood in the G.I. tract.

III. Electrolyte disturbances

See the outline under metabolic consequences of diarrhea.

IV. Acidosis

Treatment

I. Fluid therapy

A. This is the most important aspect of therapy.

B. Even though many of the patients do not exhibit a clinical dehydration they do have an extracellular dehydration as evidenced by the elevated PCV and total proteins.

C. Intravenous fluid therapy should be given in the majority of these cases and should be initiated soon after hospitalization.

D. The choice, volume, and rate of fluid therapy will vary depending on each individual case. As a rule these patients will be acidotic so fluids like lactated Ringer's solution or fluid with bicarbonate are preferred.

II. Dietary management

Same as treatment of other acute diarrheas

III. Antibiotic therapy
  A. At the University of Missouri we observe a pure and heavy growth of *Clostridium* sp. in over 90% of our cases. The significance of this finding is unknown.
  B. Because of the *Clostridial* overgrowth and because there appear to be mucosal alterations (blood in stool) antibiotics are given to these patients.
  C. A penicillin antibiotic appears to be the oral antibiotic of choice because it is effective against anaerobic bacteria and has minimal effects on the normal flora.
IV. Intestinal protectants
  A. These appear to have little, if any, benefit.
  B. Pepto Bismol may have some positive effects because of its salicylate activity.
 V. Motility modifiers
    Usually they are not needed since the diarrhea usually stops shortly after admission. In cases in which this does not occur, motility modifiers may be quite valuable.
VI. Salicylates
    May be of benefit if this is proven to be a secretory type of diarrhea.

Hospital course

   Usually the patient responds nicely in 24 to 48 hours and can go home in 48 to 72 hours after initial hospitalization.

Prognosis

   Most patients will do well with proper therapy, however, some will not survive even with prompt and vigorous treatment.

PARASITIC DIARRHEAS (see chapter 4)

  I. Small intestinal parasitism has long been a notable cause of diarrhea in animal species. A variety of nematodes, cestodes, and protozoal species lead to acute and/or chronic intestinal upset especially if sanitation is poor, nutrition improper, or if animals are overcrowded. Often the problem can be resolved by simple fecal flotation and proper anthelmintic therapy. But special attention must be made to identify certain uncommon parasites. *Giardia canis* is one that may be easily overlooked.
 II. Giardiasis
   A Etiology
      Giardia canis.
   B. Pathogeneis
      1. *Giardia* sp. inhabit the upper small intestine in the normal animal.

They rarely invade tissue, living in the intervillous spaces and on the villous epithelial cells.

2. Originally thought to create a malabsorptive syndrome by forming a physical barrier, they are now thought to cause diarrhea by damaging villous epithelial cells and preventing or interfering with various enzyme systems and cell maturation. This can cause a carbohydrate malabsorption. In addition, their effect on intestinal pH may lead to bile salt deconjugation and fat maldigestion.

C. History
  1. Usually it is a young dog with watery, light colored stools. Diarrhea is often greasy due to fat malabsorption and steatorrhea.
  2. Occasionally older dogs will be affected. They will usually have "cow-pie" stools.

D. Physical examination
  1. Nothing specific will be noted.
  2. Patient may have a secondary fat-soluble vitamin deficiency.

E. Diagnosis
  1. Demonstrate the organism
    a) Direct smears
      Are used to demonstrate the trophozoite. It is very important to use a fresh smear. It is beneficial to initially put a drop of warm saline on the slide. Many times trophozoites are difficult to demonstrate even when a patient has Giardiasis. The most logical explanation for this is that they become damaged and are destroyed as they pass through the intestines from the duodenum where the majority of them reside.
    b) Flotation
      Many times the cyst stage can be seen best by doing a Zinc Sulfate Flotation and staining them with Lugol's solution. Listed below are the steps to be taken:
      (1) Feces in centrifuge tube
      (2) Five drops of Lugol's solution
      (3) Mixed
      (4) Filled halfway with Zinc Sulfate
      (5) Mixed
      (6) Zinc sulfate added until meniscus bulges slightly
      (7) Coverslipped
      (8) Centrifuge (3 to 5 minutes)
    c) Duodenal biopsy or aspiration via flexiable fiberoptic endoscope to demonstrate the trophozoite
  2. Empirical treatment
    If the diarrhea is due to Giardiasis it will resolve within 5 days with proper treatment.

F. Treatment
  1. Metronidazole (Flagyl)

a) 50 mg/kg/day for 5 days
b) This is very effective.
c) Low toxicity
2. Quinacrine hydrochloride (Atabrine; Winthrop)
a) 50-100 mg BID for 5 days
b) For cats: 10 mg/kg/day for up to 12 days
c) Causes remission but does not eliminate infection
3. Glycobiarsol (Milibis-V).
a) 50-100 mg/kg BID for 5 days
b) This drug is not used frequently to treat Giardiasis.

ENDOCRINE DIARRHEAS

Many metabolic and endocrine disorders affect the small intestine indirectly and cause a diarrhea. Diseases such as hypoadrenocorticism (Addison's) and diabetes mellitus are well documented as being causes of intestinal upset. Several others have recently been determined to be part of a diarrhea syndrome.

Feline hyperthyroidism

I. Etiology
   A. Thyroid adenomatous goiter
   B. Thyroid adenocarcinoma
II. Pathogenesis
   A. Unknown
   B. Literature reports human patients with thyroid medullary carcinomas and diarrhea as having high calcitonin levels.
III. History
   Cats are frequently restless, hyperactive, and voracious eaters while weight loss is marked. Polydypsia and polyuria are often observed as is frequent defecation with bulky to diarrheic stools.
IV. Physical examination
   Temperature and heart rate may be elevated. Thyroid gland may be palpated as grossly enlarged.
V. Clinical pathology
   Radioimmunoassays of T_3 and T_4 will show marked elevation.
VI. Diagnosis
   A. History
   B. Physical examination
   C. T_3 and T_4 levels
VII. Pathological lesions
   Multinodular adenomatous hyperplasia (benign adenomatous goiter) is usually the cause of gross enlargement. Adenocarcinoma has been seen in a few cases.

VIII. Treatment

Treatment consists of surgical removal of affected glands being careful to avoid parathyroid tissue. Because of cardiac instabilities, it is best to refer these cases to a referral center for surgical therapy. If both lobes must be removed, replacement treatment with L-thyroxine must be provided daily at 0.05 to 0.1 mg/day. If parathyroid function has been altered one may need to provide a bonemeal-vitamin D_2 supplement.

IX. Prognosis

Prognosis is variable depending upon the type of tumor, size, duration, ease of removal, and ability of owner to supplement.

Zollinger-Ellison syndrome

First recognized in man, this rare syndrome is characterized by recurrent ulcers, hypersecretion of gastric acid and non-β-islet cell pancreatic tumors.

I. Etiology

Non-β-islet cell tumors of the pancreas.

II. Pathogenesis

Gastrin-producing neoplastic cells induce hypersecretion of gastric HCl. The low intestinal pH causes mucosal ulceration, inactivation of lipases and precipitation of bile salts leading to fat malabsorption-maldigestion and protein loss into the gut lumen.

III. History

Owners report vomiting, diarrhea, poor appetite, and weight loss in their dogs. Previous treatment, if any, has been unsuccessful.

IV. Physical examination

Nothing specific. Dogs are lethargic and show weight loss.

V. Clinical pathology
A. Routine hemogram and serum chemistries nonspecific
B. Serum albumin may be low
C. Feces may contain fat.
D. Serum gastrin levels will be elevated.

VI. Diagnosis
A. History
B. Physical examination
C. Clinical pathology
D. Radiology
E. Laparoscopy/laparotomy
F. Histopathology

VII. Treatment

Treatment consists of surgical excision of the pancreatic tumors. Cimetidine therapy will reduce gastric acid secretion.

VIII. Pathological lesions

Lesions consist of non-β-islet cell pancreatic tumors with or without metastasis to regional lymph nodes and liver. The entire gastrointestinal tract may show ulceration due to gastrin secretion and elevated gastric acid production. The thyroid gland may also show C-cell hyperplasia due to the effect of gastrin on calcitonin release.

IX. Prognosis

Poor to grave

Hypersensitivities and Diarrhea

Eosinophilic gastroenteritis

I. Etiology
   A. It is currently believed to be an allergic response to ingesta.
   B. Visceral larval migrans (VLM), an allergic granulomatous syndrome caused by migrating *Toxocara* larvae, may produce a similar disease.

II. Pathogenesis
   A. Ingested antigens evoke a local allergic reaction with subsequent lymphocytic and eosinophilic infiltration of the intestinal wall.
   B. In VLM, migrating larvae are perceived as foreign antigen and incite an immune response with eosinophilic infiltration and granuloma formation.

III. History

Both cats and dogs may be affected. Most have histories of vomiting, diarrhea, anorexia, and sometimes weight loss. Frequently the G.I. signs are cyclic. It is common for these patients to initially have borborygmus followed by diarrhea or vomiting. The G.I. signs usually last two to three days and then resolve until the next cyclic episode. The cycles are usually very regular but can vary from six days to one month for each case.

IV. Physical examination

Not remarkable. Bowel loops might feel thickened on abdominal palpation. Mesenteric lymph nodes may be enlarged.

V. Clinical pathology
   A. Hemogram may show a marked eosinophilia.
   B. Fecal examination may reveal parasite ova or fecal fat with Sudan III stain. Absorption tests usually are within normal limits.

VI. Diagnosis
   A. History
   B. Physical examination
   C. Clinical pathology
      1. Hemogram
      2. Fecal examination
   D. Radiography
   E. Endoscopy
   F. Histopathology

VII. Pathological lesions

Microscopic examination of gastric or intestinal biopsies reveals marked thickening of all layers due to infiltration by eosinophils, plasma cells, and lymphocytes. When VLM is involved, submucosal granulomas may be found surrounding nematode larvae. Local lymph nodes may be hyperplastic and/or contain parasitic granulomas.

VIII. Treatment

A. Treatment consists of oral prednisolone given at 2.2 mg/kg/day and gradually tapered over a 2 to 3 week period. Another treatment plan would be alternate-day therapy.

B. If VLM is suspected anthelmintic therapy might be used in conjunction with steroids. Larvacidal doses of fenbendazole (25–30 mg/kg) may be efficacious.

IX. Prognosis

Most dogs respond well to steroid therapy if VLM is not involved. Cats respond poorly to therapy.

Intestinal mast cell tumors

I. Etiology

Mast cell neoplasms, while common on the skin of dogs, are rare in the gastrointestinal tract. One reported case with involvement of the ileocecal area was implicated as the cause of chronic diarrhea.

II. Pathogenesis

The diarrhea is attributed to the release of mast cell granules which contain heparin, histamine, serotonin, polysaccharides, and hyaluronic acid.

III. History

Chief complaints consist of chronic diarrhea and weight loss.

IV. Physical examination

Nothing specific. An abdominal mass may be palpable depending upon tumor size. Lymph nodes may be enlarged.

V. Clinical pathology

Not significant

VI. Diagnosis

A. History

B. Physical examination

C. Clinical pathology

D. Radiography

1. Survey films
2. Barium upper GI series
3. Exploratory laparatomy

E. Histopathology

VII. Pathological lesions

Macroscopically, the mass may be found to invade the entire intestinal wall. Intussusception may occur secondarily. Microscopic examination reveals malignant mast cells replacing the normal mucosa and submucosa. Cytoplasmic granules may be demonstrated with Giemsa stain. Metastasis to other organs may be seen.

VIII. Treatment

Treatment consists of surgical intervention with intestinal resection when necessary and/or possible. Metastatic tumors should also be excised where possible.

IX. Prognosis

Poor to grave depending upon tumor duration and metastasis.

MALDIGESTION AND MALABSORPTION

Osmotic diarrhea can result from maldigestion or malabsorption. Maldigestion occurs intraluminally when there are deficiences of digestive enzymes or bile acids. This can be due to an absolute deficiency or secondary deficiency when conditions for their action are not optimum. Malabsorption is caused by defective transport of nutrients from bowel lumen into the blood stream.

Etiology

I. Maldigestion
 A. Pancreatic enzyme deficiency (see chapter 15)
  1. Juvenile pancreatic atrophy
  2. Chronic recurrent pancreatitis
  3. Duodenal mucosal disease
  4. Increased degradation of pancreatic enzymes
 B. Bile acid deficiency
 C. Disaccharidase insufficiency
II. Malabsorption
 A. Loss of mucosal absorptive area
 B. Loss of absorptive mechanisms
 C. Disease of the lamina propria
 D. Circulatory disease

History

I. Weight loss is the most common clinical sign. The stool changes are variable. Some patients will have fairly normal stools with just an increase in fecal volume. Others will have a profuse diarrhea. In pancreatic insufficiency it is not uncommon to see undigested food and fat in the stool. The stools may also be foul-smelling.
II. There are no breed or sex predilections for the causes of malabsorption/ maldigestion other than juvenile pancreatic atrophy. The latter is most common in young (18 to 24 months) German Shepherd dogs.

Physical examination

Usually unremarkable except for signs of nutritional deficiency (dry hair coat, thin, etc.).

Clinical pathology

From a practical point of view the veterinarian must restrict the use of laboratory tests to those that establish the presence of impaired assimilation of food or define the defect to a particular stage of the overall process. A rational approach to the sequence of testing is important to accomplish this goal. Figure 13-1 diagrams the sequential use of various laboratory tools currently used at the University of Missouri to evaluate a patient suspected of having maldigestion-malabsorption syndrome.

Histopathology

Many times a definitive diagnosis can only be made after histological examination of the intestine. This is especially true for infiltrative bowel wall disease. Ideally, a small bowel biopsy is best for a diagnosis but, since the only current method of obtaining it is via laparotomy, it may be very risky for the patient. This is especially true if the patient also has a concurrent protein-losing enteropathy (PLE). In order to reduce the risk to the patient, the author frequently obtains a colonic biopsy via colonoscopy or proctoscopy. Many times with infiltrative bowel wall disease (i.e., histoplasmosis, lymphosarcoma, etc.) a definitive diagnosis can be obtained with minimal risk to the patient.

Diagnosis

I. Pancreatic exocrine insufficiency.
   A. Excess fecal fat when the patient is fed Prescription Diet c/d
   B. Lack of trypsin activity in the stools
   C. Normal xylose absorption test
   D. Normal glucose absorption test
   E. Abnormal fat absorption test that becomes normal after the addition of pancreatic enzymes (Viokase)
   F. Abnormal BT-PABA absorption test
   G. Biopsies of the small intestine are normal.
II. Lymphangiectasia.
   A. Excess fecal fat when the patient is on Prescription Diet c/d
   B. There is trypsin activity in the stools.
   C. Normal xylose absorption test
   D. Normal oral glucose absorption test
   E. Abnormal fat absorption test without and with pancreatic enzymes (Viokase)
   F. BT-PABA test is normal.

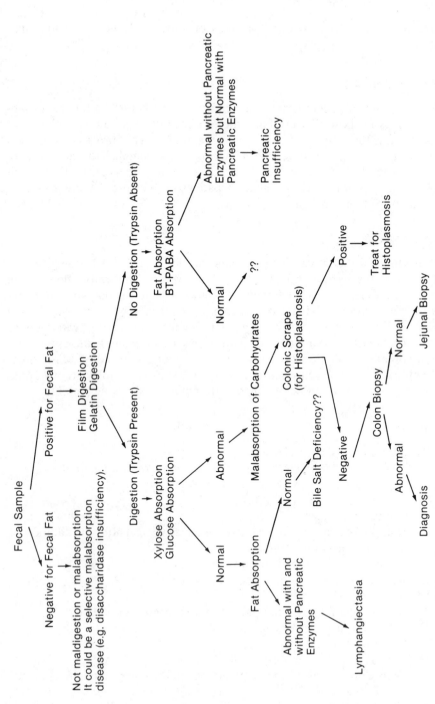

Fig. 13-1. Diagram of the way in which specific tests can be sequentially chosen to evaluate a patient with suspected maldigestion-malabsorption.

G. A small bowel biopsy will document the disease, however, since most of these patients will have a protein-losing enteropathy and a subsequent low serum albumin, the author considers this a very risky diagnostic technique since there is a high incidence of dehiscence when the serum albumin is low.

III. Infiltrative bowel wall diseases (lymphosarcoma, histoplasmosis, etc.)
   A. There is usually excess fecal fat when the patient is fed Prescription Diet c/d.
   B. There is trypsin activity in the stools.
   C. The xylose absorption test is usually not normal. Many times it peaks at greater than 45 mg% but is late to peak (longer than 90 minutes).
   D. Usually the oral glucose absorption test is abnormal.
   E. Abnormal fat absorption with and without pancreatic enzymes (Viokase).
   F. There are not enough data to know if the BT-PABA absorption test has any validity in infiltrative bowel wall disease.
   G. Usually a biopsy of the small intestine is necessary to obtain a definitive diagnosis.

Management

I. Pancreatic insufficiency (see chapter 15)
II. Lymphangiectasia
   A. The most common treatment is the use of a low fat diet (e.g., Prescription Diet r/d) and supplementing it with medium chain triglycerides. (MCT; Mead-Johnson, Portagen; Mead-Johnson). The medium chain triglycerides are absorbed directly into the blood stream and bypass the diseased lymphatics.
   B. Tables 13-3 and 13-4 give other balanced diets for a patient with lymphagiectasia.

TABLE 13-3. A BALANCED LOW FAT DIET FOR A
PATIENT WITH LYMPHANGIECTASIA

This diet supplies 550 calories:

One (1) cup boiled rice (dry)

One (1) pound uncreamed cottage cheese

Two teaspoons of dicalcium phosphate

Balanced vitamin and mineral supplement

300 cc of MCT

(From Gerald Johnson, D.V.M.; Unpublished data.)

TABLE 13-4.   A BALANCED LOW FAT DIET FOR A PATIENT WITH
LYMPHANGIECTASIA.

	Protein (gm)	Fat (gm)	kCal
Two (2) cups of Portagen	16	17	480
Twelve (12) ounces uncreamed cottage cheese	45	—	240
Four (4) medium baked potatoes	8	—	400
Two cups rice (dry)	6	—	360
Two ounces MCT	—	60	500
Vitamin/Mineral supplement	—	—	—
Total	$\overline{75}$	$\overline{77}$	$\overline{1980}$

(From Gerald Johnson, D.V.M.; Unpublished data.)

PROTEIN-LOSING GASTROENTEROPATHY

Leakage of plasma proteins into the gastrointestinal tract is a major cause of hypoproteinemia in many diseases and may play a role in the normal degradation of plasma proteins. Protein-losing gastroenteropathy is a disease syndrome characterized by excessive protein loss through the gastrointestinal tract. The gastrointestinal signs are extremely variable. The protein loss can be so severe as to cause a hypoproteinemia and the clinical signs associated with it.

Etiology

I. Disordered metabolism or turnover of epithelial cells
   A. Rugal hypertrophy (Menetrier's)
   B. Allergic gastroenteropathy
   C. Bacterial enteritis
   D. Parasitic enteritis
   E. Histoplasmosis
II. Mucosal ulceration
   A. Carcinoma
   B. Lymphosarcoma
   C. Peptic ulcers
   D. Foreign body (chronic)
   E. Intussusception
   F. Parasitic enteritis
III. Lymphatic abnormalities
   A. Lymphangiectasia
   B. Lymphosarcoma
   C. Congestive heart failure

History

I. Usually it is a semi-chronic to chronic course.

II. Gastrointestinal signs may or may not be present. Generally speaking most of the diseases that cause a protein-losing gastroenteropathy will have vomiting and/or diarrhea. Lymphangiectasia, however, frequently exhibits no gastrointestinal signs.

III. Usually weight loss is present.

IV. The patients may present because of clinical signs associated with hypoproteinemia (e.g., ascites, edema, etc.).

Physical Examination

I. Many times no specific abnormalities will be found.

II. Weight loss may be evident.

III. The patient could have ascites and/or edema.

Diagnostic Techniques

I. Figure 13-2 diagrams the sequential use of diagnostic techniques that can be used in a practice setting to work up a case of hypoproteinemia.

II. Clinical pathology

A. Total protein

In the majority of cases both albumin and globulin will be decreased since all components are lost at an equal rate. This is different from a glomerulopathy where the majority of the protein that is lost is albumin. In chronic liver disease one will see a hypoalbuminemia due to a decreased production of a albumin. Therefore of the three major causes of hypoproteinemia (proteinuria, chronic liver disease, and protein-losing gastroenteropathy) a protein-losing gastroenteropathy is the only one that will cause a panhypoproteinemia. However, there are cases of protein-losing gastroenteropathies in which albumin was the only protein that was decreased. The reason for this, in these cases, might be due to an increased production of immunoglobulins.

It is therefore important to measure both the albumin and globulin concentrations to determine which fraction is causing the serum protein abnormality.

B. Urinalysis

This should be performed on each patient that has a hypoproteinemia (hypoalbuminemia) to rule out renal losses.

C. Liver function tests (LFT's)

These are needed to rule out chronic liver disease.

D. Fecal examination

1. Parasitic examination

2. Cytology

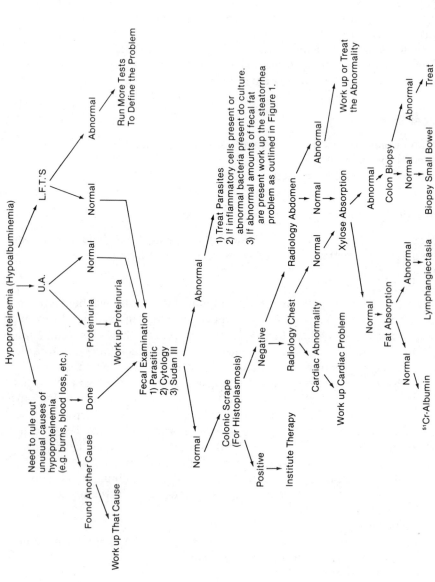

Fig. 13-2. Diagram of the way in which specific tests can be sequentially chosen to evaluate a patient with hypoalbuminemia.

    If an inflammatory reaction is present or if abnormal bacteria are present one should perform a stool culture.

  3. Sudan III

    Many diseases (histoplasmosis, lymphosarcoma) that cause a protein-losing gastroenteropathy will also cause malabsorption of fats and perhaps other foods as well. If the Sudan III stain is positive one will need to work up the problem of steatorrhea as outlined in Figure 13-1.

E. Xylose absorption test

    An abnormal xylose absorption test would indicate that the patient is unable to absorb carbohydrates. In patients with a protein-losing gastroenteropathy it usually indicates an infiltrative bowel wall disease (e.g., lymphosarcoma, histoplasmosis, etc.). For a definitive diagnosis a biopsy is necessary.

F. Fat absorption test

    If the xylose absorption test is normal and the patient does not absorb fats (without and with pancreatic enzymes) the most likely cause would be intestinal lymphangiectasia. Fat malabsorption is common with lymphangiectasia since the transport of chylomicrons through lymphatics is impaired. The only way to make a definitive diagnosis of lymphangiectasia is to obtain a small intestinal biopsy.

III. Cytology

A. Colonic scrape

B. In Missouri, histoplasmosis is a common GI disease. The purpose of this procedure is to diagnose GI histoplasmosis with a noninvasive technique. The colonic mucosa is scraped with a platinum spoon or a small wood tongue depressor. It is then smeared on a microscope slide and stained. If present the Histoplasma organisms will be found in the macrophages. If they are not found it *does not* rule out histoplasmosis as a diagnosis.

IV. Radiology

A. Thoracic radiographs

    These are taken to rule out cardiac disease as the cause of the protein-losing gastroenteropathy. If cardiac disease is the cause it is usually right-sided cardiac disease.

B. Abdominal radiographs

    Survey radiographs are usually helpful to rule out intestinal obstructive diseases (e.g., foreign bodies, carcinomas, etc.). They are not useful in ruling in or out mucosal diseases.

C. Upper G.I. barium study

    An upper GI barium study is useful in ruling out occult intestinal obstructive diseases that were not evident on the survey radiographs. It is also useful in ruling in mass lesions of the stomach. It may have limited usefulness in ruling in infiltrative bowel wall disease (e.g., intestinal lymphosarcoma, etc.). Generally speaking a G.I. series is not useful in diagnosing mucosal diseases. It is the author's opinion that for the cost of doing an upper GI barium study, it is a low yield diagnostic technique when evaluating inflammatory bowel disease.

V. Endoscopy

    A. Endoscopy is a new and emerging diagnostic and therapeutic tool in veterinary medicine. In addition to visualizing the lesions, one is also able to obtain tissue (biopsy, brush cytology, aspirate cytology) from the lesions for a specific diagnosis.

    B. With gastrointestinal endoscopy one would be able to diagnose any intraluminal or mucosal gastric disease as well as any colonic disease that would cause a protein-losing gastroenteropathy.

VI. Histopathology.

    For patients that have an abnormal xylose absorption test, a small intestinal biopsy is necessary for a definitive diagnosis. Because of the increased incidence of dehiscence a small intestinal biopsy can be a dangerous procedure in a patient that has hypoalbuminemia. Because of this, the author currently biopsies the colon or stomach first via endoscopy. This is a noninvasive technique and many times a definitive diagnosis can be made because the same disease entity that involves the small intestine also involves the colon or stomach. If the gastric and/or colonic biopsies are normal then one has no choice but to obtain a small intestinal biopsy by celiotomy if a definitive diagnosis is to be obtained.

Diagnosis

The diagnosis is based on the results obtained from the history, physical examination, and laboratory data.

Treatment

The treatment will depend on the diagnosis.

THE COLON

GENERAL CONSIDERATIONS

    I. Major physiologic function of the colon

        A. Absorption of water and electrolytes

            Primarily in ascending, transverse and proximal part of descending colon

        B. Storage with periodic expulsion of fecal material from distal descending colon and rectum

        C. No nutritional function from microbial digestion

        D. High volatile fatty acids may facilitate sodium absorption.

    II. Absorption of water and electrolytes reduced if colon is inflamed.

    III. Inflammation reduces motility.

    IV. Some 50% of chronic diarrhea cases attributed to colonic dysfunction.

V. Colonic disease is uncommon in the cat.
   A. Whipworm infection very rare in cat (common in dog).
   B. Cats are more fastidious eaters (unlike the dog).
      1. Fewer toxins
      2. Less trauma from dietary indiscretion
   C. Cats lead a quieter and less stressful life.

SIGNS OF COLONIC DISEASE

Diarrhea

   I. Results when there is:
      A. Increase in the rate of delivery of intestinal contents from the small
         intestine sufficient enough to overwhelm the reserve capacity of the
         colon
      B. The reserve capacity of the colon is impaired.
   II. Pathogenesis of colonic diarrhea
      A. Abnormal mucosal permeability occurs when there is inflammatory dis-
         ease of the colon.
      B. Abnormal motility
         1. A poorly understood entity in the dog
         2. May be similar to irritable bowl syndrome in man
         3. Probably increased in inflammatory and infiltrative diseases of the
            colon
         4. Probably increased when the colon is exposed to fatty acids and bile
            salts
      C. Abnormalities of secretion
         1. Mediated via cyclic AMP
         2. Occurs in enterotoxin-induced diarrhea
      D. Abnormal microbial digestion
            Most commonly associated with malabsorption and maldigestion dis-
         eases
   III. Character
         Listed below are the "classical" descriptions of colonic diarrhea. The
      author feels that this description has been overemphasized in the past. This
      type of diarrhea is very compatible with colonic disease but a patient may
      still have colonic disease and not have this type of diarrhea.
      A. Small volume, frequently mucoid and bloody
      B. Defecation frequent, often with tenesmus and a sense of urgency
      C. Alternate diarrhea and normal stool

Constipation—Pathogenesis

   I. Dietary and environmental
      A. Bones, hair, foreign material, etc.
      B. Change in the environment

II. Painful conditions prevent defecation or positioning.
   A. Anal saculitis
   B. Anal abscesses
   C. Rectal strictures
   D. Perianal fistulae
   E. Fractured pelvis, etc.
III. Obstruction preventing fecal flow
   A. Extraluminal
     1. Perianal hernia
     2. Pelvic fracture
     3. Pelvic tumors
   B. Intraluminal
     Colonic or rectal tumors
IV. Neurogenic
   A. Unable to assume position to defecate
   B. Disturbance to smooth muscle of colon
 V. Metabolic and endocrine
   A. Dehydration
   B. Muscle weakness
   C. Electrolyte imbalances which alter smooth muscle function

Tenesmus—ineffectual effort to defecate

  I. Associated with many organ systems
 II. Associated with inflammatory diseases of rectum or anus
III. With constipation it occurs before defecation.
IV. In diarrheal diseases it occurs after defecation and results from an inflamed mucosa.
 V. Continuous tenesmus is rare and is often associated with a rectal foreign body or tumor.

Vomiting

 I. Absorbed toxins stimulate the chemoreceptor trigger zone.
II. Common in severe colitis or prolonged cases of constipation

Dyschezia—painful or difficult defecation

 I. Associated with lesions in or near the anus
   A. Pseudocoprostasis
   B. Perianal fistula
   C. Anal spasm
   D. Perianal hernia
II. Animal may cry out as it defecates.

Hematochezia—fresh blood in the
feces

I. Bloody diarrhea
   A. Uncommon
   B. Associated with severe colonic inflammatory disease
II. Normal feces with streaks of blood
   A. Indicative of a solitary bleeding lesion such as a polyp or bleeding ulcer

DIARRHEAL DISEASES

Inflammatory

I. Acute nonspecific colitis
   A. Most cases the cause is unknown
      1. Garbage or foreign material ingestion
      2. Parasites
      3. Allergic colitis—food-induced
   B. History
      1. Sudden onset
      2. Severe, watery, occasionally bloody, mucoid diarrhea
      3. Vomiting may be present or absent.
      4. Usually presented within 48 hours of onset of signs
      5. No age, sex, or breed predisposition
   C. Physical examination
      1. Depends on severity and nature of insult and the amount of fluid
         loss
      2. Fever or afebrile
      3. Pain may or may not be elicited on abdominal palpation.
      4. Foreign material on rectal palpation
   D. Diagnostics
      1. Hemogram and blood chemistries are not diagnostic.
      2. Fecal exam mandatory (direct and flotation)
   E. Treatment
      1. The treatment will vary depending on the severity of the clinical
         signs. Usually the treatment is supportive and symptomatic and
         will consist of the following:
         a) Fluid and acid/base restoration
         b) Broad spectrum antibiotics indicated if the patient is febrile, has
            leukocytosis or an inflammatory bowel disease (WBC's on fecal
            smear, etc.).
         c) Non-absorbable antibiotics (Neomycin) are not indicated
         d) Liquid antidiarrheals—Pepto Bismol
         e) Motility modifiers

        (1) Diphenoxylate hydrochloride—Dose (canine—0.063 mg/kg Q4–6H)

           (one tablet/20 lbs).

        (2) Propantheline bromide

      f) Appropriate anthelminthic drugs

      g) Dietary manipulations

        (1) Fast for a minimum of 24 hours

        (2) Free access to water

        (3) Resume feeding on 2nd or 3rd day with a bland diet that consists mainly of carbohydrate and protein such as cottage cheese, chicken, or broiled hamburger and rice.

        (4) Appropriate doses of bran or psyllium hydrophilic mucilloid (Metamucil) (see chapter 1)

  F. Prognosis

     Usually good although a few may develop chronic colitis

II. Chronic colitis

  A. Exact cause unknown

    1. After a bout of nonspecific gastroenteritis

    2. May follow whipworm or hookworm infection

    3. Possibly psychogenic, genetic, immunological factors are involved

  B. History

    1. All ages and breeds susceptible (6 months to 4 years seem particularly susceptible)

    2. Chronic diarrhea that is unresponsive or temporarily responsive to treatment

    3. Semiformed to liquid feces, hematochezia may be present

    4. Increased defecation frequency (2 to 3x normal)

    5. Sensé of urgency to defecate

    6. Tenemus after defecation plus mucus in stool are very common historical findings.

    7. Vomiting may be present.

  C. Physical examination

    1. Most dogs are physically normal.

    2. Underweight or dehydrated if severe

    3. Feces on perianal hair if it is a long haired breed, along with painful moist dermatitis of the perineum.

    4. Tenesmus may be present upon rectal palpation if distal bowel is involved.

  D. Diagnostics

    1. No characteristic hematological changes

    2. Repeated fecal examination for parasites is mandatory.

    3. Contrast studies

      a) Diagnostic changes in some 50% of cases

      b) Mucosal irregularities, filling defects

4. Endoscope—flexible fiberoptic or rigid (human sigmoidoscope).
   a) Submucosal vessels disappear.
   b) Granular appearing mucosa, nonglistening
   c) Thick tenacious mucus adheres to the mucosa and free in the lumen.
   d) Ulceration is variable.
5. Biopsy
   a) Can be obtained with the following instruments.
      (1) Quinton multipurposed suction biopsy capsule
      (2) Uterine biopsy forceps
      (3) Welch-Allyn biopsy forceps
      (4) Through the flexible endoscopes
   b) Appearance
      (1) Acute and chronic changes are both present.
      (2) Acute changes are characterized by edema of the lamina propria and infiltration with acute inflammatory cells and a decrease of goblet cells.
      (3) Chronic changes are characterized by fibrosis of the lamina propria and a depletion of colonic glands.
6. Cytology of direct fecal, rectal, or colonic smears
   a) Loeffler's Methylene Blue or Harleco Diff-Quick stain
   b) Appearance
      Erythrocytes and inflammatory cells are present.
E. Differential diagnosis
   1. Small intestinal disease
   2. Colitis
   3. Noninflammatory colonic diarrhea diseases
   4. Parasitic colitis
F. Treatment
   1. Supportive care in the severely sick animal
   2. Antibacterials
      a) Sulfasalazine drug of choice
         Combination of sulfapyridine and 5-aminosalicyate. It is reduced in the colon. Dog: 50 mg/kg/day in 3–4 equal doses. Dosage not determined in the cat but probably lower due to sensitivity to salicylates.
      b) Treat 3 to 4 weeks usually
      c) Side effects: allergic dermatitis, nausea, vomiting, cholestatic jaundice, keratoconjunctivitis sicca
   3. Antispasmotics
      a) Anticholinergics contraindicated since colonic motility is already decreased.
      b) Narcotic analgesics (diphenoxylate [Lomotil], Loperamide [Imodium], morphine) reduce propulsive peristalsis by acting directly on intestinal smooth muscle.

4. Nutritional
   a) Nutritionally balanced and palatable diet
   b) High bulk diets may decrease overall colonic motility. This can be obtained by feeding Prime or Top Choice or by adding 2 tablespoons of unprocessed bran per 400 gms (one can) or one teaspoon of Metamucil per 20 pounds of body weight.
5. Corticosteroids
   a) Some dogs reportedly deteriorate when treated.
   b) May be warranted on a trial basis (inflammatory disease of unknown etiology) if unresponsive to other therapy
   c) Prednisolone 1–2 mg/kg/day, PO

G. Prognosis guarded
1. Some recover completely with no recurrence.
2. Chronicity for a year may result in fibrosis that decreases colonic surface area and impairs absorptive function—poor prognosis.
3. Client should be warned of possible long-term therapy and cost of therapy.

III. Whipworm-induced colitis
A. Signs (primary diarrhea) depend on number of parasites and individual response of the host.
B. Signs similar to chronic colitis
C. Parasites induce mucosal and goblet cell hyperplasia which can cause increased mucus in the stool.
D. History
   1. Mucoid diarrhea
   2. Rare tenesmus
   3. Signs of typhlitis are unusual
      a) Biting at flank
      b) Irritability
   4. Exposure to contaminated environment (dirt run, local park, etc.)
   5. Light infections may have weight loss with increased appetite and no diarrhea
E. Physical examination
   1. Body weight and hydration vary with severity.
   2. Rectal examination is normal.
F. Diagnosis
   1. Fecal exam
      a) Shedding of eggs by adult is not continuous.
      b) A minimum of four negative exams over a four-day period is necessary to rule out infection.
      c) May even have infection when repeated exams are negative for Trichuris eggs
   2. Colonoscopy
      a) Mucosa hyperemic with excessive mucus
      b) Focal hemorrhagic areas occasionally present

      c) May see white adult worms (5–10 mm long) embedded in the mucosa

   3. Histology

      a) Mucosal hyperplasia with parasites surrounded by an intense cellular reaction

      b) Goblet cell proliferation

      c) Plasma cell and lymphocyte accumulations in the mucosa and submucosa

      d) Increased mononuclear cellularity in the lamina propria

   4. Eosinophilia not consistent (must consider other causes)

   5. Occasionally see a gas-filled cecum on plain film radiographs

  G. Differential diagnosis

     Must consider noninflammatory chronic diarrheal disease if diarrhea continues after anthelminthic therapy.

  H. Treatment

   1. Whipworms require rigorous treatment.

      a) Two doses given 3 weeks apart

      b) More than one course of therapy often necessary

   2. Must eliminate possibility of reinfection from the environment

   3. Mebendazole (Telmin), butamisole (Styquin), and fenbendazole (Penacar) are probably the most effective agents

   4. Sulfasalazine may be beneficial in severe cases.

IV. Hookworm-induced colitis

  A. Generally a small intestinal parasite

  B. May be found in large numbers in the colon

  C. Mucoid diarrhea, occasionally bloody, with increased frequency of defecation

  D. Suspect with chronic weight loss, diarrhea, and hookworm eggs in the feces

  E. May have eosinophilia

  F. Small ulcers may be seen on colonoscopy.

  G. Treatment

   1. Two doses given 3 weeks apart

      a) Disophenol (DNP)

      b) Dichlorvos (Task)

      c) Mebendazole (Telmin)

      d) Butamisole (Styquin)

   2. Improve husbandry or environment to reduce reinfection.

   3. Signs may persist past parasite elimination and should then be treated for chronic colitis.

V. Entamoeba infection

  A. Southern U.S., India, China, Indochina, Egypt, Panama

  B. Signs dependent on parasite numbers and host susceptibility

   1. Mild gelatinous, occasionally mucoid diarrhea

   2. Can have acute fulminating dysentery

    C. Diagnosed by identifying trophozoites in feces
       1. Feces suspended in physiologic saline
       2. Staining with iodine or iron hematoxylin
       3. Colonic mucosal biopsy
    D. Differential diagnosis
       1. Chronic colitis
       2. Hemorrhagic gastroenteritis
       3. Parvovirus
    E. Treatment
       1. Supportive therapy
       2. Metronidazole (30 mg/kg/day for 7–10 days)

  VI. *Giardia canis* infection
    A. One reported case of giardiasis in a dog presented for chronic ulcer-ative colitis
    B. Signs similar to chronic colitis
    C. Diagnosed by detecting *giardia canis* cysts or trophozoites in the feces
    D. Uncommon in the cat (primarily a small intestinal disease)
       One case reported with a rectal prolapse associated with severe diarrhea.
    E. Treatment
       1. Specific chronic colitis therapy
       2. Quinicrine hydrochloride or metronidazole is effective.

  VII. *Balantidium coli*
    A. Protozoal organism that normally resides in the mucous lining of the colonic mucosa.
    B. Disease associated with concomitant *Trichuris* infection
       1. *Trichuris* causes mucosal damage that allows the protozoal organism to penetrate.
       2. Proteolytic enzymes from *B. coli* produce necrosis and ulceration of the mucosa.
    C. Diagnose on a fresh fecal smear
    D. Treatment
       1. Elimination of whipworms may be sufficient.
       2. Metronidazole reportedly effective

 VIII. Salmonella infection
    A. Generalized entero-colitis
    B. Fairly uncommon

  IX. Protothecal infection
    A. Extremely rare cause of colitis
    B. May also be systemic and CNS involvement
    C. Prothotheca is a pathogenic alga.
       1. Colonize the laminae propria and submucosa of the intestinal tract (predilection for the colon)
       2. Produces an inflammatory response
         a) Severe transmural colitis

        b) Secondary lymphadenitis

        c) Occasionally lymphangiectasia

    D. Thickened, corrugated, friable mucosal folds with variable ulceration

    E. Diagnosis

       1. Organism in the feces

       2. Biopsy

    F. No reported treatment

  X. *Histoplasma capsulatum* infection

    A. May directly infect the intestinal tract

    B. Organism colonizes the lamina propria and submucosa of intestinal tract

       1. Elicits a prominent macrophage response

       2. Macrophages filled with *Histoplasma* organisms distend the mucosa and submucosa.

         a) Distortion and corrugation of mucosa

         b) Lumen narrowed from thickened wall

         c) Results in decreased water and electrolyte absorption and a change in motility (diarrhea)

    C. History.

       1. Diarrhea (frequently profuse and watery when small intestine is involved)

       2. Chronic weight loss

       3. Cough, abdominal distension, and depression when the colon is involved secondarily

    D. Physical examination

       1. Compatible with chronic debilitating fungal disease

       2. Abdominal palpation may reveal thickened intestines, hepatomegaly, or ascites

       3. Rectal exam: thickened mucosa and narrowed lumen, enlarged iliac lymph nodes

    E. Diagnosis

       1. Colonoscopy

         a) Mucosa corrugated, ulcerated

         b) Colon does not distend readily when insufflated with air

       2. Biopsy or mucosal smears reveal organism

 XI. Granulomatous colitis (regional enteritis of the colon).

    A. Analagous to Crohn's disease in man

    B. Affects both the small and large intestine

    C. Uncommon disease

    D. Unknown etiology

    E. Severe patchy inflammation with extensive intestinal scar formation

    F. Most affected dogs are under 4 years of age

    G. History

       1. Chronic bloody, occasionally mucoid, diarrhea

       2. Listlessness

   3. Anorexia
   4. Weight loss
   5. Tenesmus if distal colon and rectum are involved
   6. Constipation if constriction of rectum or anus occurs
   7. Vomiting may or may not be reported.
  H. Physical examination
   1. Depends on duration, location, and severity of disease.
   2. Animal appears severely sick and malnourished.
   3. Dehydration.
   4. Fever or afebrile
   5. Rectal exam: thickened mucosa and maybe strictures
  I. Diagnosis
   1. Hemogram
      a) Mild anemia
      b) Leukocytosis with left shift
   2. Hypoalbuminemia
   3. Colonoscopy
      a) Severe granulomatous mucosal proliferation
      b) Narrowed lumen
      c) Failure to dilate with air insufflation
      d) Mucosa corrugated and hyperemic
      e) Lesions interspersed between relatively normal areas
   4. Contrast radiography.
      a) Segmental constrictions of the lumen
      b) Mucosal serrations and ulcerations
   5. Only biopsy is diagnostic
      a) Ulceration of the mucosa and submucosa
      b) Infiltration with mononuclear cells, eosinophils, and poly-
         morphs
  J. Treatment
   1. Surgical excision if lesions are sparse (may recur).
   2. Corticosteroids along with tylosin or sulfasalazine are reported to
      help
   3. Prognosis is grave.
XII. Histiocytic ulcerative colitis
  A. Very uncommon
  B. Once only reported in purebred Boxer but now has been reported in
     a French Bulldog (probable genetic predisposition)
  C. Characterized by infiltrates of large periodic-acid Schiff (PAS) pos-
     itive macrophages and progressive superficial ulceration
  D. History
   1. Young Boxers (less than 2 years) of either sex
   2. Bloody mucoid diarrhea
   3. Good overall body maintenance with a good appetite
   4. Tenesmus (often involves distal colon)

    E. Physical exam unrewarding

    F. Diagnosis

       1. Hemogram: some dogs may have a mild anemia and a leukocytosis.

       2. Rectal mucosal or fecal smear reveals numerous erythrocytes and neutrophils if stained with new methylene blue.

       3. Colonoscopy

          a) Mucosa hyperemic and edematous

          b) Can have strictures and deep bleeding ulcers

       4. Biopsy

          a) Thickening of the lamina propria and submucosa by histiocytes, plasma cells, and lymphocytes

          b) Most histiocytes are PAS positive

    G. Treatment

       1. Symptomatic and life long

       2. Some respond to chloramphenicol and tylosin combined

       3. Sulfasalazine has been used with some success by the author.

       4. Steroids are of little benefit.

    H. Prognosis is guarded.

XIII. Feline histiocytic colitis (one case)

    A. Histiocytic granulomatous inflammation having macrophages laden with bacteria and phagolysosomes

    B. Mucosa more friable, bleeds easily when rubbed

    C. Barium studies

       1. Some diameter reduction of the distal colon

       2. Papular projections suggestive of ulceration

       3. Length, diameter, and pliability were good

    D. Biopsy

       1. Lamina propria distended with large eosinophilic (pale) macrophages.

       2. Intracytoplasmic bacilli found in the macrophages (stained faintly with PAS)

       3. Epithelium thin and contained no bacteria

    E. Treatment

       Chloramphenicol continued for 7 months past signs.

XIV. Eosinophilic colitis.

    A. Uncommon, more frequently seen in association with eosinophilic gastroenteritis.

    B. The etiology is unknown.

    C. Regarded as allergic in origin

       1. Elimination diet trials generally unrewarding

       2. Other causes of allergic reactions are rare.

    D. Diagnosis

       1. Circulating eosinophilia (consider other causes)

       2. Eosinophils in rectal smear

       3. Eosinophilic infiltration of colonic mucosa on biopsy

     E. Treatment.
       1. Prednisolone (1–2 mg/kg) initially
       2. Taper dosage to a maintenance dose over 3 to 4 weeks.
       3. Lowest dose should then be tapered off after a 6-week course.
       4. Symptomatic therapy
XV. Other causes of colitis
     A. Mycotic colitis
     B. Traumatic colitis
     C. Antibiotic—associated pseudomembranous colitis
     D. Self-limited proctitis
     E. Lymphocytic mucosal colitis
     F. Colitis cystica profunda
     G. Colitis secondary to chronic pancreatitis
       1. Hematochezia, diarrhea, and mucoid feces often seen
       2. Transverse colon adjacent to the pancreas
       3. Diagnosis
         a) Fiberoptic endoscopy
         b) Biopsy
         c) Contrast radiography
       4. Treatment
         a) Sulfsalazine
         b) Pancreatitis therapy (see chapter 15)
         c) *Corticosteroids are contraindicated.*

Non-inflammatory colonic diarrheal disease

  I. Ten to 15% of chronic diarrheas
 II. Assumed to be a primary colonic motility defect
     A. Unknown cause
     B. No evidence for colonic motor dysfunction
     C. Possibly an abnormal myoelectrical activity producing the dysfunction
     D. May be similar to irritable bowel syndrome in people
III. History.
     A. Similar to chronic colitis
       1. Mucoid diarrhea that may be intermittent.
       2. Not the same urgency to defecate as in colitis
       3. May have normal stool and diarrhea in the same defecation
     B. Failure to respond to treatment including sulfasalazine
     C. Predilection for larger breeds and may have an unusually high incidence in working breeds such as seeing eye, guard, and police dogs
     D. Those affected are usually hyperexcitable although others may not be.
IV. Diagnosis
     A. Afflicted dogs clinically normal
     B. Made by exclusion of organic colonic disease and other functional diarrheas

      1. Colonoscopy

      2. Biopsy

V. Treatment

  A. No present treatment is curative and disease may be lifelong.

  B. Should attempt to alleviate environmental causes

  C. Sedation (especially before periods of stress)

      1. Phenobarbital

      2. Chloropromazine

  D. Increase dietary fiber.

      1. Frequently this is all that is needed.

      2. Psyllium hydrophilic mucilloid is beneficial in many cases.

      3. Feeding Prime or Top Choice many times is of benefit.

VI. Prognosis is guarded.

    Clients more apt to accept the situation if it is explained fully to them.

CONSTIPATION/DYSCHEZIA DISEASES

Colonic impaction

    I. Commonly a mixture of feces and ingested hair and foreign material (bones most commonly)

   II. These hard masses are difficult to eliminate.

  III. More frequent with age, low residue diets, painful rectal or anal disease and with narrowing of the pelvic canal (secondary to fractures)

  IV. More common in the cat

  A. Defecates less frequently

  B. Hair ingestion when grooming

   V. Many lead to secondary megacolon

  VI. History

  A. A failure to defecate for days to weeks

  B. Animal makes frequent unsuccessful attempts to defecate

  C. Some may pass liquid feces containing blood or mucus after a lot of straining

  D. Unobserved animals may be dull, listless, anorectic, and vomit intermittently.

 VII. Diagnosis

  A. Physical examination

      1. Animal depressed, dehydrated

      2. Unkempt appearance

      3. Crouching, hunched attitude (abdominal discomfort)

      4. Palpation reveals a hard fecal mass.

      5. Rectal exam

         a) Identify location of fecal mass.

         b) Identify underlying causes: rectal foreign bodies, prostatic hypertrophy, narrowed pelvic canal, rectal sacculation.

  B. Radiographs

VIII. Treatment
    A. Gentle removal of fecal concretions
        1. Feces softened
           a) Softening agents
           b) Mineral oil for lubrication
           c) Docusate (DSS)
               (1) Wetting agent and colonic irritant
               (2) Patient should be well hydrated since DSS stimulates colonic secretion
        2. Enemas
        3. Manual removal under general anesthesia
        4. Some patients are dehydrated and sick so supportive therapy (fluids, etc.) should be instituted before removal of the impaction
    B. Remove inciting cause if possible
    C. Prevent recurrence
        1. No bones in diet
        2. Regular grooming
        3. Provide opportunity for regular defecation
        4. Fecal softeners to the diet
           a) Methylcellulose
           b) Psyllium hydrophilic mucilloid (Metamucil). This is probably the best treatment.
           c) Docusate (DSS)
           d) Bran to the diet

Idiopathic megacolon

    I. More common in the cat than dog
   II. An unusual cause of constipation
  III. Possibly related to degeneration or relative absence of myenteric ganglion cells in the colonic wall (erroneously called Hirschsprung's disease)
  IV. History
    A. Cats greater than or equal to 6 years (dogs earlier age)
    b. Signs similar to colonic impaction
    C. Insidious onset and progressive
   V. Diagnosis—Physical
    A. Depressed, unkempt appearance
    B. Rectum empty and dilated on digital exam
    C. Hard mass of feces in pelvic inlet
    D. Abdominal palpation reveals large colonic concretions.
  VI. Treatment
    A. Same as colonic impaction
    B. Preventive measures to guard against future impactions
    C. Surgical resection of the atonic colon *only* as last resort

Cecal inversion

I. Infrequent
II. Associated with a weak ileo-ceco-colic ligament
III. Parasites and garbage ingestion predispose an animal
IV. History
    A. Chronic sometimes bloody diarrhea
    B. Weight loss
    C. Dehydration
V. Diagnosis
    A. Contrast radiography
    B. Fiberoptic colonoscopy
VI. Treatment is by surgical removal of cecum (typhlectomy).

COLONIC PERFORATION FOLLOWING NEUROSURGICAL PROCEDURES AND CORTICOSTEROID THERAPY

I. Etiology/pathogenesis (Figure 13-3)
    A. Spinal injury and surgical stress
        1. Increased sympathetic activity causing decreased colonic motility
        2. Increased transit time, fecal retention, and colonic distension resulting in physicochemical trauma
    B. Steroids.
        1. Decreased mucus production allowing the mucosal cells to be less resistant to trauma
        2. Decreased mucosal cell renewal
        3. Decreased immune response
        4. Decreased fibroblast proliferation
        5. Decreased inflammatory response
        6. Increased collagen breakdown
    C. The above factors allow intestinal wall damage to occur and progress.
    D. Dexamethasone seems to be a major cause (no deaths in neurological patients not receiving it).
II. Low incidence: Approximately 2% will die from gastrointestinal complications.
III. Higher doses of dexamethasone did not result in higher prevalance of hemorrhage.
IV. Early diagnosis of colonic perforation is difficult in the corticosteroid-treated patient. The signs of a perforated viscus are modified by the effects of the steroid drugs.
    A. Anti-inflammatory effects
    B. Lysosomal stabilization
    C. Reduced polymorphonuclear leukocytic migration

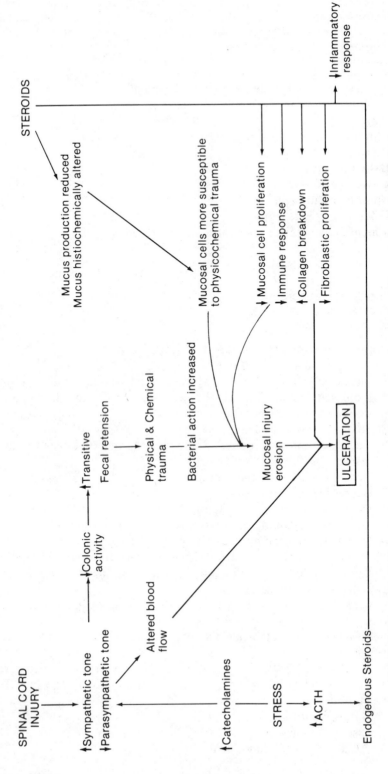

Fig. 13-3. Schematic of the events leading to colonic ulceration due to steroid administration and neurological injury.

   D. Kallikrein release prevented
   E. Antipyrogenic effect (hypothalamic)
V. To minimize complications
   A. Corticosteroid administration for as short a time as possible
   B. Intestinal protectants

SUGGESTED READINGS

Anderson NV (ed): Veterinary Gastroenterology. Lea & Febiger, Philadelphia, 1980

Burrows CF: The treatment of diarrhea. p. 784. In Kirk RW (ed): Current Veterinary Therapy VIII. WB Saunders, Philadelphia, 1983

Burrows CF: Metoclopramide. J Am Vet Med Assoc 183:1341, 1983

Bywater RJ, Newsome PM: Diarrhea. J Am Vet Med Assoc 181:718, 1982

Davis LE: Pharmacologic control of vomiting. J Am Vet Med Assoc 176:214, 1980

Ettinger SJ (ed): Textbook of Veterinary Internal Medicine. p. 1126–1371. 2nd Ed. WB Saunders, Philadelphia, 1983

Hirsch DC, Enos LR: The use of antimicrobial drugs in the treatment of diseases of the gastrointestinal tract. p. 794. In Kirk RW (ed): Current Veterinary Therapy VIII. WB Saunders, Philadelphia, 1983

Ridgway MD: Management of chronic colitis in the dog. J Am Vet Med Assoc 185:804, 1984

Strombeck DR: Small Animal Gastroenterology. Stonegate Publishing, Davis, CA, 1979

Twedt DC: Gastric ulcers. p. 765. In Kirk RW (ed): Current Veterinary Therapy VIII. WB Saunders, Philadelphia, 1983

Willard MD: Newer concepts in treating secretory diarrheas. J Am Vet Med Assoc 186:86, 1985

Willard MD: Some newer approaches to the treatment of vomiting. J Am Vet Med Assoc 184:590, 1984

14

Hepatic Diseases
Robert M. Hardy, D.V.M.

Major therapeutic objectives for patients with hepatic diseases include elimination of causative agents, if known, suppression or elimination of mechanisms that potentiate the illness, provision of optimal conditions for hepatic regeneration, and controlling manifestations of complications that develop. Little in the way of specific therapy exists. Etiologic diagnoses are infrequently made for hepatic diseases and even if established, therapy often remains supportive and symptomatic. No controlled clinical trials have been reported for treating spontaneous hepatobiliary disorders in dogs and cats.

INFLAMMATORY HEPATIC DISEASES

The majority of hepatic disorders in small animals are characterized biochemically by necrosis or inflammation. Inflammation is implied by significant increases in the serum concentration of alanine aminotransferase, (S-ALT), aspartate aminotransferase (S-AST), or arginase. Such diseases may be infectious or, more commonly, noninfectious in nature. Hepatic biopsy should be considered in all functionally impaired inflammatory hepatic disease. Biochemistry serves a localizing function, while biopsy aids in etiologic, prognostic, and therapeutic considerations.

INFECTIOUS INFLAMMATORY DISEASES

Viruses

I. Infectious canine hepatitis virus and canine herpesvirus are the only known important hepatotropic canine viruses.
II. Treatment is supportive and symptomatic.

Bacteria

I. Even though the liver harbors a normal population of anaerobic bacteria, they rarely assume clinical importance.

II. Hepatic anaerobes become important whenever hepatic arterial oxygenation is reduced.

III. Penicillin, or its newer derivatives, are usually effective in controlling these organisms.

IV. Bacterial cholangitis occurs in both dogs and cats, but is uncommon.
   A. Signs are often low-grade and chronic.
   B. Diagnosis is made on a combination of laboratory findings and biopsy.
   C. Associated lesions include pancreatitis and cholelithiasis.
   D. Treatment involves appropriate antibiotics based on antibiotic sensitivity testing and corrective surgery, if indicated (cholecystostomy, cholecystectomy, or cholecystoduodenostomy).

Parasites

I. Trematode infestations are uncommon. The gallbladder and bile ducts are primary sites for these organisms.

II. Specific proven therapy for these infestations has not been established.

Mycotic Infections

Systemic mycoses, particularly histoplasmosis, may cause considerable hepatic injury. Therapy utilizing amphotericin B or ketoconazole can be curative (see chapter 3).

Non-Infectious Inflammatory Diseases

I. Most common hepatic diseases seen in clinical practice.

II. May be secondary to diseases in other organ systems, i.e., acute pancreatitis, chronic colitis, or trauma, or may be related to primary liver diseases, i.e., chronic hepatitis/chronic active hepatitis (CAH), toxic and drug-induced hepatitis, chronic copper toxicity of Bedlington terriers, and cirrhosis.

III. Chronic hepatitis/chronic active hepatitis
   A. Chronic inflammatory hepatic disease is a common problem in dogs. Numerous recent articles have appeared describing a canine syndrome similar to CAH in human patients.
   B. Chronic active hepatitis in people is a well-defined clinical entity.
      1. A definitive diagnosis requires precise clinical, biochemical, immunologic, and most importantly, histologic confirmation.
      2. Increases in serum ALT (5–10 times normal) for over 12 weeks, hypergammaglobulinemia, and circulating antibodies to hepatocyte-associated antigens are consistent clinical findings.
      3. Histopathology is characterized by periportal and portal inflam-

mation. Lymphocytes and plasma cells predominate in the reaction. Both bridging and piecemeal necrosis occur, and if unchecked, progress to cirrhosis.
4. The etiology of CAH is often unknown. Certain drugs, and viruses (hepatitis B) are known to induce typical lesions.
C. Therapy in human patients involves glucocorticoids singly or combined with other immunosuppressive drugs.
  1. Glucocorticoids are only used in cases that are non-drug-, nonviral-induced, and only if evidence for severe disease exists.
  2. Nearly 50% of nonviral CAH patients improve spontaneously.
  3. Prednisone or prednisolone are primary drug choices in human therapy. Even though prednisone must be converted by the liver to prednisolone for activity, either drug works equally well.
  4. Prednisone dose used in human patients is 60 mg daily, tapered slowly (over 6 weeks) to a maintenance dose of 20 mg daily.
  5. An alterative therapeutic regimen, with fewer steroid side effects employs 30 mg/day of prednisone initially, plus 50 mg azathioprine daily. Daily prednisone doses are reduced over 6 weeks to maintenance levels of 10 mg with 50 mg azathioprine.
  6. Clinical and biochemical remissions should occur in 3 months.
  7. Duration of maintenance therapy in people is for a minimum of 2 years.
  8. Therapy is discontinued only if clinical, biochemical, and repeated biopsy findings indicated the disease is in remission.
  9. The "cure" rate in human CAH is between 11 and 17%. Relapses occur in 50% of patients in remission when therapy is stopped.
D. Immunosuppressive drug recommendations for dogs remain speculative. No controlled clinical trials utilizing steroids in this syndrome have been performed. Serious doubts exist as to the similarities of this disease to human CAH.
  1. Dose recommended for the dog is 1–2 mg/kg daily until clinical remission is evident. The dose is then reduced to maintenance levels of 0.4 mg/kg daily or less.
  2. Optimal duration of therapy in dogs is unknown.
  3. Because of the unique susceptibility of the canine liver to glucocorticoid-induced enzyme changes, it will be difficult on a biochemical basis to assess therapeutic efficacy.
E. D-Penicillamine (Cuprimine) has had limited clinical trials as an antifibrotic drug in human CAH. Preliminary evidence indicates it may be more effective than steroids in reversing or delaying hepatic fibrosis in CAH. Recommended dose in dogs is 10–15 mg/kg twice daily. Vomition and anorexia are frequent side effects of this drug.
F. Polyunsaturated phosphatidyl choline (PPC, lecithin) has been tried as adjunctive therapy in a controlled clinical trial of human patients with CAH.

1. This essential phospholipid is hypothesized to block or modify cytotoxic effects of antibodies reacting with liver cell membranes.
2. Polyunsaturated phosphatidyl choline therapy (3 g/day) significantly reduced histologic severity and no relapses were encountered.
3. It has been recommended that PPC be used for patients inadequately controlled by conventional therapy (prednisone + azathioprine).

G. Supportive and symptomatic care will be discussed below.

IV. Toxic hepatitis
A. The liver is subject to damage by a wide variety of chemical compounds by virtue of its central role in metabolism and detoxification.
B. Therapy for most toxicoses is supportive and symptomatic. If a definitive toxin can be identified and an antidote exists, such therapy is obviously indicated.
C. Acute fulminant hepatitis, toxic or otherwise, will be discussed below.

V. Drug-induced hepatitis
A. A wide variety of therapeutic agents have been incriminated as causing hepatic injury in dogs and cats. This list includes arsenicals, phenytoin, primidone, glucocorticoids, methoxyflurane, mebendazole, tolbutamide, phenazopyridine, and acetaminophen.
B. The incidence of toxic hepatic injury associated with drugs is currently unknown.
C. Therapy involves withdrawing the drug and providing supportive care. Steroids have not been shown to be beneficial in toxic hepatitis.

VI. Copper-associated hepatitis in Bedlington terriers
A. Bedlington terriers have a unique, genetically predisposed liver disease caused by the excessive accumulation of copper within hepatocytes.
B. Definitive diagnosis requires hepatic biopsy and special stains for copper (rubeanic acid, rhodanine, Timm's) coupled with quantitative hepatic copper assay.
C. Hepatic copper concentrations should be less than 350 μg/g on a dry weight basis.
D. Therapy is both specific and symptomatic. Specific therapy involves utilizing the copper-chelating drug D-penicillamine.
1. Data supporting efficacy of D-penicillamine are limited. However, extensive use in human patients for copper storage diseases supports its clinical use in dogs.
2. Dosage—250 mg once daily, 30 minutes prior to eating. If vomition occurs, may be given as 125-mg dose A.M. and P.M. Product available as 125- or 250-mg capsules (Merck, Sharpe and Dohme) or 250-mg scored tablets (Wallace Laboratories)
3. No other toxic side effects noted except vomition in long-term use
4. Therapy is lifelong once instituted.

5. Criteria for selecting patients to receive D-penicillamine have not been conclusively established.
   a) Clinically evident signs of hepatic failure warrant therapy.
   b) Patients with persistent elevations in serum alanine aminotransferase (ALT) of 300–400 IU/L should be considered candidates for therapy.
   c) Patients receiving long-term D-penicillamine therapy should be monitored biochemically and histologically to determine if the expected therapeutic benefits are occurring. Weeks to months may pass prior to noting biochemical or histopathologic improvement.
   d) Many affected Bedlingtons live normal lives without treatment even though they have significant hepatic lesions.
6. Oral zinc sulfate therapy has been used in people as an alternative to D-penicillamine to reduce hepatic copper concentrations. Oral zinc sulfate binds intestinal copper, impairing its absorption.
   a) Dose recommended in man is 200 mg three times daily.
   b) No data are available for dogs to support clinical efficacy of this drug, nor are dosage recommendations available.

VII. Chronic lymphocytic cholangitis of cats is a rare clinical syndrome associated with increased alkaline phosphatase, serum ALT and hepatomegaly.
   A. Lesions resemble primary biliary cirrhosis in people.
   B. The etiology and pathogenesis of this disease of cats are unknown, but immune-mediated processes are likely.
   C. Therapy utilizing prednisolone at 1–2 mg/kg for varying time intervals was reported to result in clinical remissions.

VIII. Cirrhosis
   A. Cirrhosis is an end-stage to many inflammatory liver diseases (CAH, toxic, copper-associated hepatitis, and so forth).
   B. Histologically, cirrhotic livers are characterized by increases in connective tissue, areas of necrosis, and unsuccessful attempts at regeneration.
   C. Many cirrhotic patients develop clinical signs of advanced hepatic failure, i.e., portal hypertension and ascites, depression, anorexia, weight loss, and hepatic encephalopathy.
   D. Because of the advanced nature of this disease, the majority of therapeutic efforts remain supportive and symptomatic (see sections below).

NONINFLAMMATORY HEPATIC DISEASES

A number of important noninflammatory hepatic diseases occur in dogs and cats. The most common include portal vascular anomalies, congenital urea cycle enzyme deficiencies, steroid hepatopathy, lipidosis, amyloidosis, and glycogenosis.

PORTAL VASCULAR ANOMALIES

 I. An important congenital disease of dogs and occasional cats
 II. Characterized clinically by stunting, depression, anorexia, seizures, and other signs of hepatic encephalopathy
III. Therapy may be medical and/or surgical
    A. Medical therapy combines all the techniques used to modify the signs of hepatic encephalopathy. (see section on Supportive and Symptomatic Care, pg 470).
    B. Although a few affected animals will do well for long periods (years) using medical therapy alone, most animals will likely develop progressive hepatic atrophy and ultimately, hepatic failure if surgical correction is not attempted.
    C. Surgery to completely or partially ligate anomalous portal vessels is associated with complete reversal of clinical and biochemical evidence of hepatic failure.
        1. Since both intrahepatic (patent ductus venosus) and extrahepatic portal-systemic shunts exist, it is critical to perform portal angiography to determine the nature and location of the shunting vessels.
        2. Ligation of shunts that develop secondary to portal vein atresia or cirrhosis will result in death of the patient.
        3. Patients with extrahepatic portal-caval or portal-azygous shunts are technically easiest to correct.
        4. It is important to measure portal vein pressures following shunt vessel attenuation. Pressures postligation should not exceed 20–25 cm water or severe portal hypertension and death will ensue.

UREA CYCLE ENZYME DEFICIENCIES

 I. Rare instances of congenital urea cycle enzyme deficiencies have been reported in dogs.
 II. Signs are similar to those for dogs with portal vascular anomalies.
III. Therapy utilizing dietary modifications to reduce intestinal ammonia production controlled the clinical signs of the disease. (See Complications of Hepatic Failure, below.)

STEROID HEPATOPATHY

 I. Administering glucocorticoids or production by the adrenal gland of excessive cortisol (hyperadrenocorticism) leads to dramatic increases in

serum alkaline phosphatase, and mild to moderate increases in serum ALT and hepatomegaly in most dogs.
II. Clinical signs of illness are rarely present except for steroid-induced polydipsia/polyuria.
III. Therapy for this disorder is directed at withdrawing the steroids, if possible, or recognizing that hyperadrenocorticism may exist.

LIPIDOSIS

The accumulation of excessive quantities of fat within the liver is a complex process which may be induced by a multitude of factors. The most common causes for fatty liver in the dog and cat are starvation, obesity, diabetes mellitus, drugs and toxic states. In many patients, the exact etiology goes undefined. Generally, lipidosis is not associated with severe signs of hepatic decompensation. Exceptions are advanced diabetes mellitus in the dog and feline idiopathic lipidosis.
I. Therapeutic efforts are directed at removing the cause, if known.
II. Lipotropic drugs, those containing methionine, choline, betaine, casein, or raw pancreas, are only useful in situations where dietary deficiencies of these substances exist and should be reserved for those cases.
   A. Methionine, in particular, may be harmful to patients with hepatic failure as its metabolites can induce hepatic coma in marginally compensated animals.
   B. Very few clinical hepatic diseases are benefited by the use of lipotropic drugs.
III. Oral antibiotics may be useful in some cases of "toxic" lipidosis. Bacterial endotoxins absorbed from the large bowel can induce a fatty liver. Antibiotics suppressing bacterial toxin production lead to improvement in hepatic function.
IV. Fatty liver syndrome in cats is a much more serious entity than its canine counterparts. The majority of cats with this lesion have died.
   A. The etiology is unknown, although most cases have been in obese cats that had recent, dramatic weight losses.
   B. Lesions are compatible with severe starvation-induced lipidosis.
   C. Therapeutic recommendations include vigorous nutritional rehabilitation. Usually this requires force feeding manually or via a pharyngostomy tube.
   D. Dietary modifications should provide a high-carbohydrate, moderate-protein combination to allow for mobilization and catabolism of stored hepatic lipid.

AMYLOIDOSIS

No specific therapy exists for treating the rarely encountered case of hepatic amyloidosis. Attempting to define and eliminate the cause (usually nonhepatic inflammatory or neoplastic processes) elsewhere in the body is the therapy of choice.

Glycogen Storage Diseases

Familial glycogen storage diseases associated with deficiencies of glycogenolytic enzymes have no specific therapy. Supportive and symptomatic therapy may be palliative for a time.

Hepatic Neoplasia

Therapeutic efforts in primary hepatic neoplasia are usually unrewarding due to the extensive involvement of the liver at the time of diagnosis. Occasional hepatocellular carcinomas may be surgically correctable. For metastatic hepatic disease, efforts directed at controlling the primary cancer with chemotherapy may have short-term benefits (see Chapter 7).

SUPPORTIVE AND SYMPTOMATIC CARE

Regardless of the cause for hepatic failure in dogs and cats, most patients will receive supportive and symptomatic therapy in addition to any specific drugs that may be given. Such care is designed to reduce the severity of clinical signs and provide optimal conditions for hepatic regeneration. Even though a cure may be unlikely in most patients with advanced hepatic disease, improvement in the patient's quality of life and functioning may be attained.

Rest and Confinement

I. Facilitates hepatic regeneration by increasing hepatic blood flow and reducing unnecessary metabolic work
II. Reduces pain associated with distention and stretching of the liver capsule
III. In people, subjective signs of illness are reduced (anorexia, nausea) if activity is curtailed.
IV. Exercise restriction is unnecessary once biochemical recovery is noted.

Dietary Modifications

I. Dietary therapy is probably the single most important means of modifying the course of most spontaneous liver diseases.
II. Dietary modifications are most effective in chronic liver diseases because these patients will often consume adequate quantities of nutrients and calories.

III. Goals of dietary therapy
  A. Reduce signs of hepatic failure.
  B. Provide optimal conditions for repair and regeneration.
IV. Intake of nutrients is adjusted to match the patient's ability to metabolize them in a failing liver.
 V. The type and quantity of protein are the most important considerations when formulating a diet for patients with hepatic failure.
  A. Appropriate protein adjustments will lead to reductions in blood ammonia concentrations and return abnormal ratios of circulating amino acids toward normal.
  B. Cottage cheese can serve as a beneficial single protein source for dogs with hepatic failure.
    1. Has high biologic value, is easily digested, contains no additives, and has a desirable ratio of branched-chain to aromatic amino acids
    2. Beneficial effects of cottage cheese over other protein sources are related to
      a) Reduced putrefaction and ammonia production by gut bacteria
      b) Reduction of urease-positive bacteria in the colon
      c) A high bacterial population of favorable organisms (lactobaccilli) which may aid in partial repopulation of the colon
      d) Lack of additives is beneficial as colonic bacteria metabolize some food additives to potent hepatotoxic compounds
      e) High digestibility reduces residues available for colonic bacterial degradation
        (1) Reduces bacterial numbers
        (2) Reduces toxic bacterial metabolites of protein degradation
        (3) Reduced residue decreases intestinal desquamation and loss of protein from lymphatics
  C. Protein provisions for dogs with hepatic failure should initially be 2 g/kg body weight/day of high biologic value protein. Normal adult maintenance requirements for protein are 4.8 g/kg/day.
    1. If hypoalbuminemia is present, such restriction may not allow for adequate protein synthesis.
    2. If clinical signs improve, but hypoalbuminemia persists or worsens, increase protein content slowly (by 0.5 g/kg/day) until clinical signs worsen or protein anabolism is evident.
  D. A commercial, balanced, low-protein diet that has worked well in many dogs with signs of hepatic failure is k/d.*
    1. When dogs will eat their recommended caloric allowance, this diet will deliver approximately 2 g/kg body weight per day of high-biologic-value protein.
    2. If protein malnutrition is evident, in spite of adequate caloric intake, this diet may be supplemented with cottage cheese.

---

* Prescription diet—k/d, Hills Division, Riviana Foods, Topeka, Kansas.

    VI. Carbohydrates should form the bulk of the diet for patients with hepatic failure.
       A. Carbohydrate sources should be easily digested so that minimal residues reach the colon where bacteria may convert them to volatile fatty acids.
       B. An inexpensive and useful carbohydrate source is boiled white rice.
    VII. Fats should be given so that they comprise 6% of the diet on a dry weight basis, which is equivalent to supplying 1.32 g/kg/day.
       A. Fats are necessary to supply essential fatty acids, fat-soluble vitamins, and to improve palatability.
       B. Excessive fat intake may worsen clinical signs.
         1. Certain fatty acids induce or aggravate signs of encephalopathy.
         2. Cholestatic liver diseases may have reduced bile salt secretion, leading to impaired fat assimilation and steatorrhea.
    VIII. Vitamin and mineral supplementation is necessary if home-formulated diets are used. Hypovitaminosis is common in liver failure.
       A. Vitamins most often deficient in human patients with hepatic failure are folic acid, vitamin B_6, vitamin B_{12}, thiamine, vitamin A, vitamin E, riboflavin, nicotinic acid, and pantothenic acid.
       B. Most frequently deficient minerals are zinc and cobalt.
       C. B-Complex requirements should be doubled for patients with hepatic failure.
       D. For patients on home-formulated diets, a good quality, high-potency vitamin-mineral supplement should be added to their daily ration (e.g., Centrum, Lederle Laboratories).
    IX. Lipotropic drugs containing methionine should be avoided in animals with hepatic failure.
       A. Oral methionine will consistently induce hepatic coma in experimental dogs with stable hepatic failure.
       B. Metabolites of methionine act synergistically with short-chain fatty acids and ammonia to induce encephalopathy.
       C. Lipotropic drugs are only of value where proven deficiencies of methionine or choline exist.

DRUGS IN HEPATIC FAILURE

The liver is quantitatively the most important organ involved in drug metabolism. Duration of action for many drugs may be prolonged in hepatic failure. However, most commonly used drugs can be safely administered to dogs and cats with hepatic failure, if patients are observed conscientiously for signs of overdosage.

Antibiotics

Normal hepatic function does not seem to be a critical factor in handling of most antibiotics.

I. Of primary value for treating specific bacterial hepatic diseases (hepatitis, cholecystitis, cholangitis)
II. Very beneficial for suppressing intestinal flora when signs of hepatic encephalopathy exist (See Section Therapy for Complications of Hepatic Failure, below.)
III. Selection of antibiotics for treating nonhepatic infections in patients with hepatic failure should be made with caution. If possible, avoid antibiotics requiring hepatic inactivation or excretion in such patients.
IV. Tetracyclines are concentrated in the liver and excreted in bile. Biliary concentrations reach 5–32 times those of plasma.
   A. High doses of IV tetracycline may be toxic to small animals, as they are in people, and should be used with caution.
   B. Chlortetracycline can induce a reversible toxic lipidosis in dogs.
   C. Tetracycline may be useful in bacterial cholangitis due to the high drug concentrations attained.
   D. Penicillins are minimally dependent on hepatic function for elimination from the body.
      1. Pencillins have a low order of toxicity in dogs and cats.
      2. Significant hepatic tissue concentrations develop.
      3. Useful and safe in patients with hepatic failure where indications for antibiotics exist
   E. Chloramphenicol
      1. Should *not* be used in patients with hepatic failure unless no other choices exist
      2. Requires hepatic conjugation prior to renal excretion
      3. Plasma half-life increased in cirrhosis
      4. Profoundly depresses hepatic microsomal enzymes and results in inhibition of many important hepatic metabolic activities
   F. Lincomycin
      1. Primarily metabolized by liver and excreted
      2. Serum half-life may double in hepatic failure
      3. Toxicity possible

Sedatives

I. Avoid in patients with hepatic failure as they can induce hepatic coma.
II. Phenobarbital is safest hypnotic as it is excreted by the kidneys
   A. Phenobarbital is a potent enzyme inducer and can improve the ability of the liver to perform many metabolic functions.
   B. Low doses of phenobarbital can augment hepatic albumin synthesis in hypoalbuminemic human patients.
   C. Drug of choice for seizure control in dogs and cats with hepatic failure
      1. For short-term anticonvulsive therapy, diazepam (Valium) or chlordiazepoxide may be given at reduced dosage.
      2. Avoid the use of primidone or phenytoin, if possible, in patients with

known hepatic disease as these drugs have been associated with the development of cirrhosis in dogs.

Anesthetics

I. The inhalant anesthetic, halothane, has been incriminated in the etiology of fulminant hepatic failure in people.
II. Repeated exposures are most often associated with this syndrome.
III. Little support exists for a similar problem in animals unless halothane anesthesia is administered to hypoxic, acidotic dogs.
IV. If an alternative inhalant anesthestic is available, i.e., methoxyflurane, it has a theoretical advantage over halothane in patients with underlying hepatic disease.

Anabolic Agents

I. Anabolic steroids have been reported to have therapeutic benefits in treating chronic liver diseases in people.
II. Mesterolone has been evaluated in cirrhotic human patients and was shown to improve both clinical and biochemical status of these patients. Mesterolone was administered at a dose of 25 mg three times daily for several weeks.
III. Testosterone propionate has also been suggested to have a positive therapeutic effect in some human cirrhotic patients. No published data are available supporting such beneficial effects in dogs or cats.
IV. For anabolic steroids to be effective, patients must consume sufficient nonprotein calories to meet their metabolic needs or no anabolic effects will be seen.
V. Methyltestosterone has been shown to have a mild toxic effect in the dog and should be avoided.

Glucocorticoids

I. Glucocorticoid use in hepatic disease is controversial.
II. The only condition where glucocorticoids have been shown to be of benefit is severe CAH (in human patients).
III. Positive effects of glucocorticoids include
   A. Increased appetite
   B. Decreased serum bilirubin
   C. Decreased serum transaminase activity
   D. Decreased sulfobromophthalein (BSP) retention
   E. Increased serum albumin concentration

IV. Negative aspects
  A. Failure to prevent progression of most acute diseases to chronic diseases
  B. Increased chances for intercurrent infection
  C. Usually do not change life expectancy
  D. Failure to alter histologic pattern in most diseases
  E. May aggravate management of ascites
 V. Patients most likely to benefit are those with severe anorexia and weight loss, in which steroids may improve appetite and thus favor nutritional rehabilitation.
VI. Doses of prednisone or prednisolone used in people are generally small, after an initial loading period. Five to 10 mg/day may be a reasonable maintenance dose for dogs.
  A. Even though prednisone is not efficiently converted to prednisolone (its active form) in patients with hepatic failure, clinically they are equally effective.
  B. Since the elimination of glucocorticoids requires hepatic activity, the half-life of most glucocorticoids is prolonged in severe hepatic failure.
  C. Initial dose may have to be reduced if excessive side effects are noted.

Antifibrotic Drugs

  I. One of the most significant pathologic changes in chronic liver diseases is the development of fibrosis.
 II. In cirrhosis, the normal rate of collagen synthesis is greatly accelerated.
III. A number of drugs has been tried experimentally to reduce fibrosis in patients with chronic liver diseases.
  A. Colchicine has been advocated for use in inhibiting and reversing hepatic fibrosis in people.
    1. Colchicine inhibits intracellular collagen assembly and extracellular transport while accelerating collagen degradation.
    2. Significant reductions in hepatic fibrosis in human cirrhosis have been observed when using this drug.
    3. Dosage in humans was 1 mg/day, 5 days/week.
    4. Therapeutic dosage for dogs has not been established. Dogs given 4 mg daily for 14 days have developed significant toxicities.
    5. A recent single case study recommended a dose of 0.03 mg/kg, SID.
    6. Clinical use of this drug in patients should be undertaken only with the full understanding by the owner of its experimental nature.
  B. D-Penicillamine has been shown to decrease hepatic fibrosis in experimental animals (rats).
    1. Dose recommended in antifibrotic therapy was 300 mg/kg/day.
    2. Usual recommended dose for D-pencillamine in the dog is 10–15 mg/kg twice daily.

THERAPY FOR COMPLICATIONS OF HEPATIC FAILURE

Multiple serious complications may develop in patients with hepatic failure. These complications frequently result in death of the patient or produce such severe clinical signs that euthanasia is requested.

HEPATIC COMA

  I. Hepatic coma is a serious complication of hepatic failure. Clinical signs of encephalopathy are recognized more frequently in congenital hepatic disorders than in acquired acute or chronic diseases.
  II. Most clinical signs result from a failure of the liver to remove from portal blood toxic metabolites absorbed from the gastrointestinal (GI) tract.
 III. Several factors are important in the pathogenesis of hepatic encephalopathy.
    A. Hyperammonemia is important in the production of clinical signs of encephalopathy.
      1. Major source of blood ammonia is colonic production by urea-splitting bacteria.
      2. Excess dietary protein is also an important source of blood ammonia.
    B. Methionine degradation products (mercaptans) can induce coma and act synergistically with other coma inducers.
    C. Altered amino acid metabolism in hepatic failure predisposes to encephalopathy.
      1. Increases in aromatic amino acids (phenylalanine, tyrosine, tryptophan) and decreases in branched-chain amino acids (valine, leucine, isoleucine) occur.
      2. Increased entry of aromatic amino acids into brain is proposed to lead to increases in false neurotransmitters and inhibitory neurotransmitters within the brain.
      3. Intestinal (colonic) bacteria are also capable of synthesizing false neurotransmitters from aromatic amino acids.
    D. Short-chain fatty acids (octanoic, butyric, valeric) can induce signs of hepatic encephalopathy in dogs. Sources include ingested medium-chain triglycerides and synthesis by intestinal bacteria.
    E. Multiple precipitating factors may induce hepatic coma in susceptible animals.
      1. Increased dietary protein
         Source of ammonia, short-chain fatty acids, false neurotransmitters
      2. GI hemorrhage
        a) Substrate for ammonia production
        b) May cause hypovolemia, decreased cerebral perfusion, prerenal uremia

    3. Diuretics
       a) Cause hypokalemic, alkalosis
       b) Increase renal ammonia production
       c) Enhance ammonia entry into brain
       d) May cause dehydration, prerenal uremia
    4. Sedatives and anesthetics may have direct depressive effect on cerebral function.
    5. Uremia results in increased quantities of urea entering the gut, and urea-splitting bacteria cause ammonia production to be increased.
    6. Infection causes increased tissue catabolism and increased urea production, and causes increased ammonia to be produced.
    7. Constipation allows increased production and absorption of ammonia and other nitrogenous breakdown products.
IV. The mainstays of therapy for hepatic encephalopathy include reduction of protein intake, gut "sterilization," and catharsis.
  A. All oral intake of food should cease in cases of acute hepatic encephalopathy until central nervous system signs abate. Cessation of protein intake eliminates exogenous sources of ammonia, aromatic amino acids, short-chain fatty acids, and toxic amines.
  B. Complete catharsis of the colon should be done as soon as possible after signs of encephalopathy develop.
    1. Catharsis flushes out colonic bacteria and any potentially toxic products contained within the colon.
    2. Enemas using acidifying agents such as vinegar and water (1:10 ratio) or lactulose (Merrell-Dow Pharmaceuticals, Cincinnati, Ohio) are much more effective than warm water in reducing blood ammonia concentrations and improving clinical signs.
       a) Lactulose is diluted with warm water (30% lactulose:70% water) and given as a retention enema.
       b) A volume of 20–30 ml/kg is infused and retained for 20–30 minutes before allowing the patient to evacuate.
       c) Experimental data in man suggest the pH of the evacuated colon contents should be <5.0.
       d) If the colonic pH is >5.0, a second dilute lactulose enema should be given.
       e) By acidifying the colon to a pH of 5.0 or less, lactulose effectively traps ammonia within the colon, preventing its absorption.
       f) Improvement in neurologic status can occur within two hours in human patients.
       g) Lactulose enemas may also be useful for controlling blood ammonia in cases where oral liquids are not tolerated.
    3. Reducing intestinal ammonia production with nonabsorbable oral antibiotics and/or lactulose is also an important means of reversing the signs of encephalopathy.

a) Neomycin is used most often, but kanamycin, vancomycin, or paromomycin may be used interchangeably.

b) Neomycin is administered at a dose of 20 mg/kg every 6 hours.

c) Patients unable to tolerate oral drugs in acute encephalopathy may be given neomycin liquid rectally.

d) Rare, but important, complications of neomycin therapy are oto- and nephrotoxicity, severe diarrhea, and malabsorption.

e) Lactulose may be given orally in acute or chronic encephalopathy.

    (1) Lactulose is the drug of choice if renal or hearing problems exist.

    (2) Lactulose is the drug of choice for long-term control of hepatic encephalopathy in human patients.

    (3) Lactulose is given at a dose of 5–15 ml three times daily. The drug should induce two to three soft stools per day. If diarrhea develops, the dose is reduced.

    (4) The combination of lactulose with neomycin may be superior to either drug alone in some cases.

    (5) Adding viable lactobacillus acidophilus organisms to the therapy may augment lactulose fermentation and improve its effects.

V. Additional supportive measures are often required in patients with hepatic coma.

  A. Fluids with 5% dextrose added may be beneficial. The ideal fluid for use in such patients is controversial.

    1. Although respiratory alkalosis is common, and considered to worsen clinical signs, lactated Ringer's solution has been shown to be beneficial.

    2. We currently add sufficient dextrose to lactated Ringer's solution to make a 5% dextrose solution (50 g/L).

  B. Specially formulated IV amino acid preparations can be useful in acute hepatic encephalopathy.

    1. These solutions contain a high ratio of branched-chain amino acids to aromatic amino acids and when given IV, reverse the deranged amino acid ratios seen in encephalopathy.

    2. Such a preparation is commercially available as Hepatamine (American-McGaw Laboratories, Irvine, California). Such preparations are very expensive ($65.00/500 cc) and require strict asepsis for IV catheter placement and maintenance.

    3. Recent evidence indicates they do little to improve human patients with low-grade *chronic* encephalopathy.

    4. Do not use commercial amino acid hydrolysates designed for partial nutritional support in veterinary medicine. They contain very high ammonia concentrations, 1,500–1,900 mg/dl.

    5. Stored blood also contains very significant ammonia concentrations.

Only fresh blood should be used for transfusions in patients with hepatic encephalopathy.

C. L-Dopa (Larodopa, Roche Laboratories) has been used with some success in human patients with acute hepatic coma.
1. L-Dopa is a precursor to norepinephrine and dopamine.
2. Given orally, L-dopa raises cerebral dopamine concentrations.
3. L-Dopa has been given to human patients at 2–4 g/po initially, followed by 0.5–1 g q6h.
4. Patients usually respond by regaining full consciousness in 6–12 hours. Responses may be transient, with patients relapsing into coma even though drug therapy is continued.
5. A canine dose has not been established.

ASCITES AND EDEMA

I. Ascites is a relatively common late-stage development in dogs with progressive hepatic disease.
II. Edema is an uncommon event.
III. Ascites develops secondary to varying degrees of hypoalbuminemia, portal hypertension, and renal salt and water retention.
IV. Unless ascites is severe and causing respiratory distress, medical means are preferred over mechanical drainage.
V. Medical control of ascites is accomplished by two means.
  A. Low-sodium diets
  B. Diuretics
VI. Low-sodium diets should be tried in all ascitic patients.
  A. Moderately restricted sodium intake can be provided by diets such as k/d (prescription diet K/d, see footnote, above). Since this diet is also restricted in protein, it meets two dietary needs of patients in hepatic failure fairly well.
  B. If moderate salt restriction does not control or eliminate fluid formation, severe salt restriction may be necessary.
    1. Specially formulated very-low-salt diets, h/d, may be useful in this regard.
    2. Specially home-formulated diets may also be used (See chapter 9).
    3. Ultralow sodium intake is on the order of 15 mg/kg/day in dogs.
VII. Diuretics should be used if low-sodium diets are ineffective in controlling ascites.
  A. Furosemide may be tried initially at 0.12–0.25 mg/kg q12h. This dose may be doubled if no effective diuresis is noted in 2–3 days.
  B. Furosemide is often ineffective in mobilizing ascites in human cirrhotic patients.
  C. Spironolactone, an aldosterone antagonist is usually much more effective.

1. Spironolactone is administered at 1–2 mg/kg twice daily.
2. If no response is noted in 4–5 days, this dose is doubled for an additional 4–5 days.
3. One additional doubling, i.e., 4–8 mg/kg twice daily should be tried if no response is noted to initial increases.

D. Do not allow patients to become dehydrated by excessive diuretic use.
   1. Maximal volumes of ascites mobilization in human patients per day are 700–900 ml.
   2. Patients should be weighed daily and should not lose more than 0.25–0.5 kg/day.

E. The most common adverse reactions associated with diuretic use in cirrhosis are volume and electrolyte depletion. Periodic electrolyte panels should be performed on dogs given continuous diuretic therapy.

F. Diuretics should be stopped once ascites has been controlled, i.e., is no longer clinically evident.

G. If the serum albumin concentration can be raised via nutritional rehabilitation, diuretics usually can be withdrawn.

VIII. Mechanical removal of ascites may be accomplished by several means.

A. Paracentesis should be avoided unless dyspnea or patient discomfort are noted and the ascites has not responsed to medical therapy.
   1. Small quantities may be removed for diagnostic purposes.
   2. Complications of ascites removal include albumin depletion, peritonitis, hypovolemia, hepatic coma, and oliguria.

B. Two surgical procedures for long-term control of ascites can be considered in medically nonresponsive ascites.
   1. A one-way, pressure-activated valve, the La Veen shunt, may be used to reduce chronic ascites in dogs.
      a) The valve is inserted into the peritoneal cavity and connected by SQ tubing to the jugular vein.
      b) Such valves allow for continuous, endogenous reinfusion of ascitic fluid back into the systemic circulation.
   2. Surgically created portal-systemic venous shunts may be used to reduce ascites formation.
      a) Creating a large communication between the portal venous system and the vena cava reduces portal hypertension, slowing the rate of the ascites formation.
      b) Major drawbacks include high surgical risk and a tendency for hepatic coma to develop postoperatively.

INTERCURRENT INFECTION

I. Intercurrent infections are common complications of chronic liver diseases.

II. Gram-negative sepsis, presumably arising from the GI tract is frequent in human patients.
III. Prophylactic, systemic antibiotic therapy may be useful in the early medical management of dogs and cats in hepatic failure.

MALABSORPTION

I. Clinically important malabsorption is uncommon in dogs and cats with hepatobiliary disorders.
II. Steatorrhea due to reduced bile salt excretion probably occurs in many cholestatic liver diseases. Its magnitude has not been documented.
III. Oral bile salt preparations may increase fat emulsification and subsequent digestion and absorption. Diarrhea is a frequent side effect of these drugs.
IV. Adding water-soluble medium-chain triglycerides (Portagen, Meade Johnson) will increase caloric intake. These fats do not require pancreatic lipase or bile salts for absorption. Some medium-chain triglycerides can aggravate signs of hepatic encephalopathy.

HEMORRHAGE AND ANEMIA

Coagulopathies associated with hepatic disease are common, but overt bleeding is rare except in patients with very advanced stages of disease. Prothrombin deficiencies are frequent.

I. Decreased hepatocellular mass impairs synthesis of prothrombin from dietary precursors.
II. Chronic cholestatic diseases and prolonged bile duct obstruction can induce vitamin K-responsive coagulopathies.
III. Therapy of acute bleeding is managed by *fresh* whole blood transfusions.
IV. Vitamin K_3 (Menadione) injections may reverse prolonged prothrombin times in cases of obstructive jaundice within 24–48 hours.
V. Vitamin K is of no use in correcting coagulopathies secondary to decreased hepatocellular mass.

ACUTE FULMINANT HEPATIC FAILURE

I. Acute fulminant hepatic failure is a major therapeutic challenge. The clinical syndrome is associated with massive necrosis of hepatocytes and acute onset of severe functional failure of the liver. No specific drugs are available to treat acute hepatic failure.
II. The primary therapeutic goals are to preserve life until sufficient regeneration occurs to allow recovery and to manage complications. Supportive measures include the following
   A. Frequent monitoring of vital signs and repeated physical examinations; particular notice of neurologic status should be made.

B. Discontinuation of all drugs not absolutely indicated
C. Prevention of hypoglycemia
D. Careful monitoring of acid-base, fluid, and electrolyte balance
E. Control of hyperammonemia
F. Prompt recognition and control of infections and bleeding episodes
G. Glucocorticoids have never been proven to be of benefit in acute hepatic
    failure and could be harmful.

SUGGESTED READING

Barsanti JA, Jones BD, Spano JS, Taylor HW: Prolonged anorexia associated with hepatic lipidosis in three cats. Feline Pract 7:52, 1977

Bishop L, Strandberg JD, Adams RJ, et al: Chronic active hepatitis associated with leptospires. Am J Vet Res 40:839, 1979

Breznock EM: Surgical manipulations of portosystemic shunts in dogs. JAMA 174:819, 1979

Breznock EM, Berger B, Pendroy D, et al: Surgical manipulations of intrahepatic portal caval shunts in dogs. J Am Vet Med Assoc, 182:798, 1983

Bunch SE, Castleman WL, Hornbuckle WE, Tennant BC: Hepatic cirrhosis associated with long-term anticonvulsant drug therapy in dogs. J Am Vet Med Assoc 181:357, 1982

Campra JL, Reynolds TB: Effectiveness of high-dose spironolactone therapy in patients with chronic liver disease and relatively regractory ascites. Am J Dig Dis 23:1025, 1978

Chen TS, Zaki GF, Leevy CM: Studies of nucleic acid and collagen synthesis: current status in assessing liver repair. Med Clin N Am 63:583, 1979

Ericksson LS, Persson A, Wahren J: Branched chain amino acids in the treatment of chronic hepatic encephalopathy. Gut 23:801, 1982

Fenton JCB, Knight EJ, Humperson PL: Milk and cheese diet in portal systemic encephalopathy. Lancet 1:164, 1966

Figueroa RB: Mesterolone in steatosis and cirrhosis of the liver. Acta Hepato-Gastroenterol 20:282, 1973

Freund H, Yoshimura N, Fischer J: Chronic hepatic encephalopathy. Long-term therapy with a branched-chain amino acid enriched diet. JAMA 24:347, 1979

Hardy RM: Hepatic diseases. p. 1372. In Ettinger SJ (ed): Textbook of Veterinary Internal Medicine. 2nd Ed. WB Saunders, Philadelphia, 1983

Hardy RM, Stevens JB, Stowe L: Chronic progressive hepatitis in Bedlington terriers associated with elevated liver copper concentrations. Minn Vet 15:13, 1975

Heywood R, Chesterman H, Ball SA, Wadsworth PF: Toxicity of methyltestosterone in the beagle dog. Toxicology 7:357, 1977

Hoenig V: Management of acute liver damage in man. p. 269. In Popper H, Schaffner F (eds): Progress in Liver Diseases. Vol. 3. Grune & Stratton, New York, 1970

James IM, Sashat S, Sampson D, et al: Effect of induced metabolic alkalosis on hepatic encephalopathy. Lancet 2:1106, 1969

Jenkins PJ, Portmann ALW, Eddleston F, William R: Use of polyunsaturated phosphatidylcholine in HB_sAg negative chronic active hepatitis: results of prospective double-blind controlled trial. Liver 2:77, 1982

Kershenobich D, Uribe M, Suares GI, et al: Treatment of cirrhosis with colchicine: a double-blind, randomized trial. Gastroenterology 77:532, 1979

Levy M, Wexler MJ, McCaffrey C: Sodium retention in dogs with experimental cirrhosis following removal of ascites by continuous peritoneovenous shunting. J Lab Clin Med 94:933, 1979

Maddrey WC, Weber FL: Chronic hepatic encephalopathy. Med Clin N Am 59:937, 1975

Martin AJ: Portal systemic encephalopathy: should lactulose and neomycin be used together? Br J Clin Pract 35:323, 1981

McGhee A, Henderson JM, Millikan WJ: Comparison of the effects of Hepatic-Aid and a casein modular diet on encephalopathy, plasma amino acids and nitrogen balance in cirrhotic patients. Ann Surg 197:288, 1983

Millikan WJ, Henderson JM, Warren WD: Total parenteral nutrition with FO80 in cirrhotics with subclinical encephalopathy. Ann Surg 197:294, 1983

Muting D, Winter G, Fischer R, et al: Is chronic active hepatitis curable? Lancet 1:905, 1982

Naranjo CA, Pontiga E, Valdenegro C, et al: Furosemide-induced adverse reactions in cirrhosis of the liver. Clin Pharmacol Ther 25:151, 1979

Olsson R: Oral zinc treatment in primary biliary cirrhosis. Acta Med Scand 212:191, 1982

Orlandi F, Freddara U, Condelaresi MT, et al: Comparison between neomycin and lactulose in 173 patients with hepatic encephalopathy: a randomized clinical study. Dig Dis Sci 26:498, 1981

Perez-Ayuso RM, Arroyo V, Planas R, Gaya J: Randomized comparative study of the efficacy of furosemide versus spironolactone in non-azotemic cirrhosis with ascites. Relationship between the diuretic response and the activity of the renin-aldosterone system. Gastroenterology 84:961, 1983

Prasse KW, Mahaffey EA, De Novo R, Cornelius L: Chronic lymphocytic cholangitis in three cats. Vet Pathol 19:99, 1982

Pulliyel MM, Vyas GP, Mehta GS: Testosterone in the management of cirrhosis of the liver—a controlled study. Aust N ZJ Med 7:596, 1977

Rautio A, Sotaniemi EA, Pelkonen RO, Luoma P: Treatment of alcoholic cirrhosis with enzyme inducers. Clin Pharmacol Ther 28:629, 1980

Rojkind M, Kershenobich D: Regulation of collagen synthesis in liver cirrhosis. p.195. In Popper H, Becker K (eds): Collagen Metabolism in the Liver. Stratton Intercontinental Medical Book Corp., New York, 1973

Rosenoer VM, Gualberto G, Jr: Management of patients with chronic obstructive jaundice. Med Clin N Am 56:759, 1972

Rossoff IS: Handbook of Veterinary Drugs. A Compendium for Research and Clinical Use. Springer, New York, 1974

Schalm SW: Treatment of chronic active hepatitis. Liver 2:69, 1982

Smith AR, Rossi-Fanelli F, Freund H, Fischer JE: Sulfur-containing amino acids in experimental hepatic coma in the dog and monkey. Surgery 85:677, 1979

Strombeck DR, Gribble D: Chronic active hepatitis in the dog. J Am Vet Med Assoc 173:380, 1978

Strombeck DR, Meyer DJ, Freedland RA: Hyperammonemia due to a urea cycle enzyme deficiency in two dogs. J Am Vet Med Assoc 166:1109, 1975

Strombeck DR, Schaeffer MC, Rogers QR: Dietary therapy for dogs with chronic hepatic insufficiency. p. 817. In Kirk RW, (ed): Current Veterinary Therapy. Vol. 8. WB Saunders, Philadelphia, 1983

Szczerban J, Rozya J: Treatment of acute and chronic portal encephalopathy with the precursors of dopamine. Acta Med Pol 20:249, 1979

Tanner AR, Powell LW: Corticosterids in liver disease: possible mechanisms of action, pharmacology and rational use. Gut 20:1109, 1979

Thornburg LP, Simpson S, Digilio K: Fatty liver syndrome in cats. J Am Anim Hosp Assoc 18:397, 1982

Van Waes L: Emergency treatment of portal-systemic encephalopathy with lactulose enemas. A controlled study. Acta Clin Belg 34:122, 1979

Whitcomb FF: Chronic active liver disease: definition, diagnosis and management. Med Clin N Am 63:413, 1979

15

Pancreatic Diseases
William D. Schall, D.V.M.

Pancreatic disorders are relatively common in the dog and cat. They may be acute or chronic, inflammatory or functional, and may involve the exocrine and endocrine portions of the organ. Etiologic factors are commonly obscure so therapy often is symptomatic and supportive.

EXOCRINE DISORDERS

Acute Pancreatitis

I. Clinical signs
   A. Lethargy
   B. Anorexia
   C. Vomiting
   D. Diarrhea
   E. Abdominal pain
      1. "Prayer"stance
      2. Elicited by palpation
   F. Fever
   G. Shock in severe cases
   H. Abdominal distension
II. Etiologic factors
   A. More common in the bitch than in the dog
   B. Rare in cats
   C. Obesity
   D. Hyperlipemia
   E. Uremia
   F. Biliary tract disease
   G. Drugs
      1. High doses of corticosteroids
      2. Thiazide diuretics
      3. Chlorthalidone

    4. Sulfasalazine

    5. Azathioprine

    6. Tetracyclines which produce hepatic damage

    7. Estrogen/progestin

  H. Duodenal reflux

   I. Trauma

   J. Immune mechanisms

III. Pathogenesis

  A. Enzymatic autodigestion following some precipitating insult

  B. Systemic effects of enzymes, inflammatory mediators, and myocardial depressant factors

  C. Hepatic lesions and cholecystitis

  D. Nephrosis

  E. Hypocalcemia and hyperglycemia

  F. Cardiomyopathy

  G. Pulmonary edema

  H. Disseminated intravascular coagulopathy

IV. Diagnosis

  A. No clinical sign is pathognomonic.

  B. Abdominal radiographs

  C. Laboratory studies

    1. Hemogram

      a) Leukocytosis

      b) Neutrophilia

      c) Lymphopenia

      d) Monocytosis

    2. Serum amylase and lipase

    3. Lipemic serum

    4. Hypocalcemia

    5. Hyperglycemia

    6. Elevated hepatic enzyme values

    7. Abnormal lipoprotein electrophoresis

    8. Methemalbuminemia

 V. Treatment

    Therapy of acute pancreatitis is symptomatic. The objectives of therapy are to reduce pancreatic exocrine secretion and to maintain fluid and electrolyte balance.

  A. Suppression of pancreatic secretion

    1. Fasting

      It is generally agreed that pancreatic secretion is reduced primarily by fasting. Permitting nothing by mouth reduces pancreatic secretory activity by eliminating food-caused gastric distension and secretagogues such as fats and amino acids. Complete restriction of oral intake is usually necessary for 3 to 5 days after the onset of acute pancreatitis; feeding should not resume until clinical signs disappear and serum amylase and lipase activity approach normal.

2. Pharmacologic inhibition

   Cimetidine, glucagon, propantheline and other anticholinergics have been used in attempts to inhibit pancreatic secretion. Convincing evidence of the efficacy of these drugs in reducing the morbidity or mortality associated with acute pancreatitis is lacking.

3. Mechanical methods

   Nasogastric suction is routinely used by some physicians. Others reserve it for instances when severe ileus and gastric distension occur. Nasogastric suction has been used little in the therapy of acute pancreatitis in the dog.

B. Fluid and electrolyte balance (see chapter 2)

   1. Type

      A balanced electrolyte solution such as lactated Ringer's solution or isotonic saline with potassium added should be administered intravenously until normal alimentation resumes.

   2. Amount

      The total amount of fluid administered should include quantities to correct dehydration, balance continued losses, and provide maintenance requirements.

   3. Rate

      If the dog is in shock or if there is evidence of marked decrease in circulating volume, fluids should be administered at a rapid rate (40 to 90 ml/kg of body weight) for the first hour. When intensive fluid therapy is used, it is recommended that central venous pressure be monitored. After circulatory volume is restored, the rate of fluid administration should be reduced to rates that restore total body deficits and supply maintenance over 24 hours (2 to 10 ml/kg/hr).

C. Other therapeutic considerations

   1. Antibiotics

      There is no evidence that spontaneous pancreatitis of dogs is caused by bacteria nor is there evidence of bacteria-caused complications. For these reasons, antibiotics are not recommended unless there is clear evidence of sepsis (see chapter 3).

   2. Glucocorticoids

      It is generally agreed that glucocorticoids should be administered to dogs with acute pancreatitis that are in shock. Whether glucocorticoids are otherwise efficacious in reducing mobidity or mortality has not been clearly established (see chapter 9). Because it is known that glucocorticoids in high dose can induce pancreatitis, the question of their usefulness in treating pancreatitis is being reexamined.

   3. Analgesics

      Because of the severity of pain associated with human pancrea-

titis, either meperidine or morphine is routinely used in man regardless of effects on the sphincter of Oddi. Analgesics should be considered for use in dogs that appear to be experiencing excruciating pain (see chapter 1).
   4. Protease inhibitors
      Because released pancreatic proteolytic enzymes are thought to be important in the systemic effects of acute pancreatitis, protease inhibitors such as aprotinin have been used therapeutically. Efficacy has not been established.
   5. Heparin
      The use of heparin has been evaluated in experimental pancreatitis based on potential improvement in pancreatic microcirculation and activation of lipoprotein lipase. Efficacy has not been clearly established.
   6. Miscellaneous drugs
      A variety of other drugs, such as fibrinolysin and vasopressin, have been suggested for treatment of acute pancreatitis. Efficacy has not been established.
   7. Non-medical therapy
      Peritoneal dialysis and surgical intervention have not been critically evaluated.

CHRONIC PANCREATITIS

  I. Usually relapsing with frequent episodes of acute pancreatitis
 II. Dogs
     A. Episodes of abdominal distress, vomiting, and diarrhea
     B. Abnormal laboratory values during bouts of illness
     C. Clinically normal between episodes
     D. May proceed to pancreatic insufficiency or diabetes mellitus or both
     E. Treatment is same as for acute pancreatitis
III. Cats
     A. A persistent, inflammatory disease with vague clinical signs
     B. More common in the tom
     C. Anorexia, cachexia, depression, and polydipsia are common.
     D. Cats are not in pain and laboratory values are commonly normal.
     E. Often accompanied by interstitial nephritis and/or cholangitis
     F. Effective therapeutic regimens have not been defined.

PANCREATIC EXOCRINE INSUFFICIENCY

  A syndrome characterized by impaired acinar cell function, maldigestion, and malnutrition. Occurs in chronic pancreatitis, following recovery from acute hemorrhagic pancreatitis, in idiopathic pancreatic acinar atrophy and secondary to protein-calorie malnutrition.

I. Clinical signs
   A. Do not appear until over 90% of the acinar cells are nonfunctional
   B. Steatorrhea with voluminous, malodorous stools
   C. Weight loss
   D. Polyphagia and pica
   E. Signs of diabetes mellitus, if insufficiency is secondary to pancreatitis
II. Diagnosis (see chapter 13)
   A. Clinical signs
   B. Fecal smear stained with Sudan III
   C. X-ray film digestion test
   D. Gelatin-digestion test
   E. Plasma turbidity test
   F. Peptide-paraaminobenzoic acid (BT-PABA) test
   G. D-xylose absorption
   H. 72-hour fecal fat assay
   I. Fecal trypsin analysis
III. Treatment
   Therapy of pancreatic exocrine insufficiency is directed at enzyme replacement.
   A. Pancreatic enzyme replacement
      1. Many formulations are available
         a) Powder
         b) Tablets
         c) Enteric-coated tablets
         d) Tablets which include bile salts
      2. Most veterinarians prefer powder products.
         a) Although definitive data are not available, most veterinarians believe powder, especially when pre-incubated with moistened food for 15 to 20 minutes, is superior to tableted products.
         b) Pancreatic enzymes in tablet form are generally considered to be less efficacious than powder, and considerable objective data support this notion.
         c) Enteric-coated tablets, designed to diminish gastric acid hydrolytic inactivation, are less efficacious in objective studies.
         d) Tablets which include bile salts are less efficacious than the same product without added bile salts.
   B. Methods to limit acid hydrolysis of administered enzymes
      1. Because much of orally administered enzymes is destroyed by gastric acid, attempts have been made to limit inactivation.
         a) Pre-incubation
         b) Neutralization of gastric acid
         c) Inhibition of gastric acid secretion
         d) Enteric coating
      2. Methods attempted either are not efficacious or are not cost effective.

a) Pre-incubation of enzymes in powder form has not been adequately studied. Many veterinarians are convinced of the efficacy. One experimental study failed to provide convincing data.

b) Sodium bicarbonate and aluminum-magnesium hydroxide gels have been documented to lack efficacy in limiting acid hydrolysis.

c) The administration of the H-2 antagonist, cimetidine (10 mg/kg, PO), in most studies has documented enzyme-sparing properties but is not cost-effective.

d) Enteric coating of enzyme tablets is not efficacious based on most *in vivo* studies.

C. Clinical application
  1. The manufacturer's recommendations should be followed initially.
  2. The dose recommended may prove to be inadequate and may have to be exceeded to alleviate clinical signs.

ENDOCRINE DISORDERS

Non-Insulin-Dependent (Type II) Diabetes Mellitus

I. Infrequently diagnosed in animals because the hyperglycemia is of insufficient magnitude to cause an obligatory diuresis.

II. Without solute diuresis, the usual signs of diabetes (polyuria, polydipsia, and weight loss) are absent.

III. If an insulin response to glucose challenge can be documented by insulin assay, then therapy with oral hypoglycemic drugs is warranted in canine patients.
  A. Glipizide (Glibenese, Pfizer)—Dose: 0.25 to 0.5 mg/kg, q 12 h.
  B. Glibenclamide (Daonil, Hoechst)—Dose: 0.2 mg/kg, SID.
  C. Not to be used in diabetic ketoacidosis

IV. Hypoglycemic drugs have not been evaluated in treatment of feline diabetes.

Uncomplicated Insulin-Dependent (Type I) Diabetes Mellitus

I. Characteristics of patient
  A. Has appetite
  B. Not vomiting
  C. Not dehydrated
  D. Appears to be feeling well
  E. May have moderate ketonemia or ketonuria

II. Therapeutic decisions
  A. Insulin
    1. Type
    2. Dose
    3. Frequency
  B. Diet
    1. Food type
    2. Caloric requirements
    3. Frequency and timing of feedings
  C. General approaches
    1. Insulin therapy is best initiated in the home environment.
    2. If the owner cannot observe the pet throughout the day, initiate therapy in the hospital.
    3. Provide written instructions to the client.
    4. Plan to counsel the average client by telephone every morning for the first week of home insulin administration.
III. Assessing the home environment
  A. Before recommending an insulin administration and feeding protocol, the veterinarian should determine the current and past characteristics of the home environment so that a therapeutic plan can be formulated that is compatible with the demands of the household. In many cases, sub-optimal control of diabetes may be the only alternative to a request for euthanasia. Specifically, the veterinarian should determine:
  B. Will the diabetic cat or dog have constant supervision?
    1. Whether or not the pet owner(s) work and will be unavailable to observe the diabetic pet during the day
    2. The presence of strong detractors to close observation in spite of a non-working pet owner, including:
      a) Infant children
      b) Invalids in household
      c) Other pets
  C. What has been the eating pattern of the cat or dog in the past? This information is important because:
    1. It may be impossible to change an *ad libitum* fed cat to scheduled feedings.
    2. Dogs accustomed to scheduled snacks may not thrive if snacks are eliminated.
  D. What have been the urinary habits of the diabetic cat? Important because it may prove impossible to monitor urinary glucose of:
    1. Cats which void outdoors
    2. Cats which void indoors but are private in their voiding habits
  E. Does the diabetic dog owner wish to achieve the best possible control of diabetes?
    1. Although definitive data are lacking, the common complication of cataract formation in dogs may be minimized by "tight" control.

    2. The best possible (tight) control requires a commitment by the veterinarian and pet owner that is substantially greater than that required for the usual degree of diabetic control.

IV. Selecting an insulin preparation

  A. Much of what has been published about insulin preparations and administration to cats and dogs was extrapolated from information that relates to man. It has now been established that much extrapolated and published information is erroneous. For this reason, a brief review of current knowledge of commercially available insulin preparations and their usefulness in cats and dogs follows. In all, 46 different insulin preparations are now available; only those most useful to veterinarians will be reviewed.

  B. Origin

    1. Beef-pork

      Insulin used in cats and dogs is usually derived from pancreata of cattle and hogs obtained at slaughter. A combination preparation is the least expensive and most commonly used by veterinarians.

    2. Pork

      Insulin derived from pork pancreata is available as single peak insulin (99% pure) and as single component (99.8% pure). Single component insulin is expensive and rarely has been used by veterinarians. Pork insulin is theoretically useful in the dog because the insulin amino acid sequence is the same for the two species and acquired anti-insulin antibodies are less likely to develop if purified pork insulin is administered to dogs. In actual practice, the development of clinically important anti-insulin antibodies following the administration of beef-pork insulin is a rare occurrence. When anti-insulin antibodies do develop, it is usually after four months of exogenous insulin administration. No theoretical advantage exists for the cat because feline insulin amino acid sequence is unknown.

    3. Synthetic and semi-synthetic purified human insulin

      Human insulin, made by substituting one amino acid on the pork insulin molecule or by means of recombinant DNA technology, is expensive and of no theoretical or practical use in the dog or cat.

  C. Types of insulin preparations

    1. Background

      Many textbooks of veterinary medicine and therapeutics list insulin preparations and expected peak effect and duration of effect of each. For the most part, such listings were derived from information regarding insulin administration in man. It is now clear that peak effect and duration of effect of insulin preparations when administered to cats and dogs is different than when administered to human beings. In general, the peak action is earlier and the duration shorter in cats and dogs when compared to man. Wide variation exists, however, between individual animals, and the veterinarian must be alert for unexpected responses.

  a) Regular or crystalline insulin

   Regular insulin is used for the treatment of diabetic ketoacidosis and, when used for this purpose, is administered either intravenously or intramuscularly. Regular insulin is occasionally used in conjunction with intermediate-acting insulins for the maintenance of diabetic cats and dogs. When so used, it is usually administered at meal time by the subcutaneous route.

  b) The duration of action of regular insulin is dependent on the route of administration. When used for the treatment of diabetic ketoacidosis and administered intramuscularly or as an intravenous bolus, its duration of action is only about two or three hours. Its action is continuous when it is infused intravenously at a low dose for the treatment of diabetic ketoacidosis but ceases almost immediately when the infusion is stopped. When regular insulin is administered by the subcutaneous route in conjunction with intermediate-acting insulins for the maintenance of diabetic cats and dogs, the duration of action is about four to six hours.

3. Neutral protamine Hagedorn (NPH) insulin

  a) NPH insulin has been widely used by veterinarians based on the contention that the duration of action is 24 hours when administered to cats and dogs. It is now clear, however, that NPH insulin is effective for about 12 rather than 24 hours in most dogs; the duration of action is slightly less than 12 hours in most cats. Because the duration of action is generally shorter than previously thought, most dogs and cats require two rather than one daily injection of NPH insulin for adequate glycemic control.

  b) In addition to a shorter duration of action than previously thought, the peak action of NPH insulin is quite variable but, in general, much earlier in cats and dogs than in man.

  c) Because great variation exists in the duration of action and peak action of NPH insulin between different animals, there is no reliable time at which the veterinarian can assume that the nadir in blood glucose concentration has been reached. The time of nadir in blood glucose concentration can be established for the individual cat or dog only by performing multiple blood glucose determinations.

  d) Once the time of low blood glucose concentration for the individual animal is established, the clinician usually can rely on its timing after each dose of insulin.

4. Lente insulin

   Lente insulin has not been used in cats and dogs to the extent that NPH insulin has been used. It is similar to NPH insulin and usually can be interchanged with like response.

5. Protamine zinc insulin (PZI)
   a) The use of PZI is currently on the increase. Although it was once thought that the duration of action is 36 or more hours, it is now apparent that the duration of action of PZI when administered to a cat or dog is usually about 24 hours.
   b) The peak action of PZI, although variable, tends to occur six to ten hours after administration. The time of peak action in an individual animal can be determined with greater precision by performing serial blood glucose determinations.
   c) Because most diabetic dogs and cats can be adequately maintained with a single daily injection of PZI, many veterinarians and pet owners find it to be the most satisfactory insulin for routine use.
6. Ultralente insulin
   Ultralente insulin seldom has been used by veterinarians. Its action is similar to that of PZI.

D. Concentration of insulin
   1. Most insulin types are available in concentrations designated U-40 and U-100, the designation referring to the number of units per ml. The more concentrated preparation of U-500 is of little use in diabetic cats and dogs. Insulin preparations which are U-100 are preferred because the simplicity of the metric system makes errors less likely.
   2. Insulin syringes which correspond to the concentration of insulin should be used. For U-100 insulin, low-dose U-100 syringes should be used in most cases. Low-dose U-100 syringes have capacity for a total of 50 units of insulin. With their use, the pet owner can approximate the insulin dose to the nearest one-half unit and is unlikely to err in determining insulin dose. Tuberculin syringes and insulin syringes that are not designed for the concentration of insulin in use should not be used.
   3. If necessary, insulin can be diluted with pH-adjusted diluents obtained from the manufacturer.

E. Dose of insulin
   1. Dog
      The starting dose of PZI in the dog is approximately 1.0 unit per kg of body weight (0.5 unit per pound) administered once daily, usually in the morning. If NPH insulin is used, it may be administered once daily at the same dose as PZI, but the clinician should be alert to the probability that the duration of action will be substantially less than 24 hours and that adequate glycemic control will be achieved only by twice daily NPH insulin injections.
   2. Cat
      Because cats are more insulin-sensitive than dogs, the initial dose of PZI should not exceed 0.5 unit per kg of body weight (0.25 unit per pound). A single daily dose of PZI is adequate for the regulation

of most insulin-dependent cats. If NPH insulin is used, most cats will require twice daily insulin administration.

F. Establishing a protocol

1. Objectives

a) The veterinarian should make reasonable efforts to determine how much time the pet owner can devote to regulation of the diabetic pet and attempt to formulate a therapeutic plan and protocol for monitoring that will best fit with the family routine.

b) In general, the objective should be to control glycemia within reason but allow hyperglycemia sufficient to produce mild transitory glycosuria within each 24-hour period. The detection of small amounts of urinary glucose provides a means, in most instances, of insuring reasonable confidence in the unlikelihood of hypoglycemia.

2. Standard protocol

a) For most owners of insulin-dependent pets, the most convenient protocol is morning monitoring of urinary glucose followed by feeding and insulin administration. An afternoon or evening feeding concludes the day. For most cats and dogs, PZI is the most satisfactory insulin for this sort of protocol. In some dogs and a few cats, the duration of action of NPH insulin is sufficiently long that this same protocol can be adopted even if NPH insulin is used.

b) Monitoring

Initially, the pet owner should monitor urinary glucose every morning, and if after two consecutive mornings there is deviation from the desired 100 mg/dl to 250 mg/dl urinary glucose estimation, they should either increase or decrease the dose of insulin by 5 to 10% of the administered dose to correct the lack of glycosuria or the excessive glycosuria.

c) Feeding

The pet should then be fed approximately one-half of its caloric requirements. If the appetite is good, insulin should then be administered. The remainder of the daily food should be offered in the late afternoon or evening. If the pet refuses food in the morning, approximately one-half of the usual insulin dose should be administered.

d) Adjusting insulin dose

The dose of insulin should be adjusted based on the urinary glucose concentration. If after reasonable stabilization no urinary glucose is detected on two consecutive mornings, the dose of insulin should be decreased by 5 to 10%. If urinary glucose concentration exceeds 250 mg/dl on two consecutive mornings, the dose of insulin should be increased by 5 to 10%.

3. Alternative protocol using twice daily NPH insulin

a) In many dogs and most cats, the duration of action of NPH insulin is sufficiently short that twice daily NPH insulin injections are required for adequate glycemic control. Twice daily administration of NPH or Lente insulin is more likely to result in "tighter" control and may minimize or delay cataract formation for those dog owners willing to commit the extra time necessary for optimal control of diabetes.

b) Monitoring

When twice daily NPH insulin administration is used for the regulation of an insulin-dependent cat or dog, the urinary glucose concentration may be monitored twice daily. Urinary glucose concentration in the morning is a reflection of the effect of the insulin administered the previous evening whereas urinary concentration in the evening is a reflection of the effect of the insulin administered the previous morning. Deviations from the desired 100 to 250 mg/dl urinary glucose concentration should prompt changes in the dose of insulin that is administered 12 hours prior to urine collection.

c) Feeding

In most cases, feeding immediately after insulin administration is adequate for cats and dogs receiving twice daily NPH insulin. In some cases, additional feedings are necessary four to eight hours after insulin administration.

d) Insulin

The dose of insulin should be adjusted based on the urinary glucose concentration that corresponds to insulin administered 12 hours earlier. Negative urinary glucose determination, if present for two consecutive days, should prompt a decrease in insulin dose of 5 to 10%.

G. Additional considerations regarding monitoring

1. Urine

Inherent in the use of urinary glucose estimations for the regulation of insulin-dependent cats and dogs are disadvantages and advantages. For glucose to be present in urine, the blood glucose concentration must have exceeded the renal threshold at some point during the formation of the tested urine. Inasmuch as blood glucose concentration of 180 to 200 mg/dl is necessary to exceed renal threshold, constant euglycemia is impossible if the pet owner is to adjust insulin dose so as to intermittently detect glycosuria. The detection of intermittent glycosuria, however, does offer some assurance that impending hypoglycemia is unlikely.

2. Urine methods

Several products are available for estimation of urinary glucose concentration. Those that detect urinary ketones as well as glucose are generally most useful.

3. Blood

Blood (serum or plasma) glucose determinations have limitations in terms of simple interpretation because the anticipated time of peak insulin action is often incorrect. In general, urinary glucose determinations are more useful in the regulation of the diabetic pet unless the peak action of administered insulin is determined by serial blood glucose determinations over 24 hours. Once the peak action is determined from blood samples obtained at two to three-hour intervals over 24 hours, meaningful interpretation is possible because the lowest blood glucose concentration in response to peak insulin action tends to occur at the same time following insulin administration. Such determinations, however, are time consuming, fairly expensive, and only necessary for diabetic pets that are difficult to regulate.

4. Blood methods

Blood glucose concentration can be determined by several methods. Substantial improvement in glucose oxidase color-developing strips have made blood glucose monitoring more simple, practical, and inexpensive. In addition, reflectance meters are now available that provide digital read-out of blood glucose concentration derived from the strips.

5. Glycosylated hemoglobin

The determination of the glycosylated hemoglobin concentration can be used to assess glycemic control. Glycosylation of hemoglobin occurs non-enzymatically, and the concentration is a reflection of the average blood glucose concentration during the preceding four to six weeks. It is particularly useful in monitoring dogs that are "tightly" controlled inasmuch as urinary glucose is likely to be absent and blood glucose determinations do not provide an indication of the average blood glucose concentration.

6. The "Somogyi" effect

The "Somogyi" effect is most likely to occur when urinary glucose is used to monitor control of diabetes. The effect occurs when the animal responds to over insulinization and subsequent hypoglycemia by the release of catecholamines, and to a lesser extent glucagon, which causes rebound hyperglycemia. Resultant hyperglycemia usually occurs in the evening and, in turn, causes morning glucosuria which prompts the pet owner to increase the dose of insulin. Increase in insulin dose aggravates the situation. Eventually overt signs of hypoglycemia are evident during the day. The phenomenon can be documented by performing serial blood glucose determinations and is remedied by slight reduction in insulin dose.

THERAPY OF DIABETIC KETOACIDOSIS

For the purpose of therapeutic segregation, the ketoacidotic diabetic pet is defined as one that is obviously ill and anorectic as well as ketoacidotic. Animals that are not dehydrated or anorectic are treated as uncomplicated diabetics even if they have modest ketosis and metabolic acidosis. The therapeutic plans that follow entail substantial effort and are recommended for the ano-rectic, weak, depressed, and dehydrated ketoacidotic diabetic patient. In ad-dition to decisions regarding insulin therapy, the veterinarian must restore fluid, electrolyte, and acid-base balance in the patient.

I. Fluids
   A. Dogs and cats with diabetic ketoacidosis (DKA) are often dehydrated to the equivalent of 10 to 15% of the body weight.
   B. Because of the magnitude of dehydration, fluids should be administered intravenously. A jugular venous catheter is preferred because central venous pressure can be monitored.
   C. Although the total water deficit can be corrected over 24 to 48 hours, circulating blood volume initially should be restored by the rapid in-fusion of fluid for the first one to two hours.
   D. Although some free water loss is characteristic of DKA, an isotonic fluid such as lactated Ringer's solution or 0.9% NaCl is preferred. Spe-cific additional electrolytes such as potassium may need to be added later.

II. Electrolytes
   A. Although serum potassium concentration may be normal or increased, total body potassium deficit is often profound. This apparent paradox is caused by the flow of potassium ions from the intracellular com-partment into the extracellular compartment. Dehydration accompan-ied by free water loss further masks the extent of total body potassium deficit. The objectives of potassium replacement therapy are to main-tain extracellular potassium on an acute basis and to more gradually replace the total body deficit. An acute decrease in extracellular po-tassium concentration is most likely to occur as insulin is administered. As blood glucose concentration decreases in response to insulin ad-ministration, serum potassium concentration often drops dramatically. Although hypokalemia is best documented by serum potassium deter-minations, its occurrence should be suspected if the patient becomes weaker at a time that blood glucose concentration is decreasing as a result of insulin administration but is still greater than 200 mg/dl. If hypokalemia is documented or suspected, potassium should be added to the rehydrating fluid at the rate of 30 to 40 mEq/L of fluid. The rate of fluid administration should then be adjusted so that the rate of po-tassium administration does not exceed 0.5 mEq/kg/hr. The intravenous administration of potassium is a therapeutic maneuver to maintain serum (and extracellular) potassium concentration within the normal range. Correction of the total body deficit of potassium is accomplished over days as normal alimentation returns.
   B. Inasmuch as hypophosphatemia often accompanies hypokalemia, po-tassium may be added to intravenous fluids in the form of potassium phosphate rather than potassium chloride.
   C. Other electrolyte derangements are usually corrected once insulin and balanced electrolyte therapies are initiated.

III. Acidosis
   A. In the past, it has been recommended that metabolic acidosis associated with diabetes should be treated with alkalizing agents such as bicarbonate and lactate.
   B. Although critical studies comparing therapy of metabolic acidosis of diabetic cats or dogs have not been done, such studies of human diabetics have been done. In Type I (IDDM) human patients, there is no significant difference in correction of acidosis, reversal of ketosis or return of blood glucose to normal in those patients treated with alkalizing agents compared to those treated with insulin and fluids alone.
   C. Because of the lack of proven superiority and because of potential deleterious side effects such as aggravation of hypokalemia, leftward shift of the oxyhemoglobin dissociation curve, and the induction of paradoxical CSF acidosis, the administration of alkalizing agents to ketoacidotic dogs and cats, remains controversial.

IV. Insulin
   A. Regular or crystalline insulin should be used to treat diabetic ketoacidosis. The relatively high-dose intravenous-bolus method is no longer recommended because it is complicated, not physiologic, and frequently associated with complications.
   B. Low dose intravenous infusion
      1. The low dose intravenous infusion method provides the patient with physiologic doses of insulin without wide fluctuations in concentration, is simple, and can be instantaneously stopped.
      2. 1.0 unit of regular insulin is added to each 100 ml of fluid, and the fluid is administered at a rate such that the animal receives between 0.5 and 1.0 units per hour or 0.025 to 0.05 units per kg of body weight per hour. The lowest dose should be used for cats and very small dogs.
      3. To adequately regulate the rate of administration, either a pediatric-drip set or volumetric infusion pump should be used. In some instances, a separate intravenous line may be necessary for hydrating purposes, but the second line can often be avoided if circulating volume is restored in an hour preceding insulin administration.
   C. Low dose intramuscular
      1. The low dose intramuscular method is nearly as physiologic as the intravenous infusion method but cannot be controlled as precisely.
      2. The initial dose should be 2 units of regular insulin for dogs under 10 kg and 0.25 unit per kg for dogs over 10 kg of body weight.
      3. Thereafter, the hourly intramuscular dose is 1 unit for dogs under 10 kg and 0.1 unit per kg for dogs over 10 kg of body weight.
   D. Monitoring
      1. Regardless of which method is used, blood glucose concentration should be determined hourly and insulin administration at the above dose schedules stopped when blood glucose concentration is be-

tween 200 and 250 mg/dl. This usually occurs about four hours after starting insulin.

2. Therapy

At this time, the clinician can either treat to promote peripheral ketone utilization by infusing glucose and insulin, or the clinician can treat with subcutaneous insulin as for the uncomplicated diabetic.

E. Promoting ketone utilization

1. After blood glucose has returned to normal, as a result of initial insulin administration, ketones often persist. Although it is not clear whether survivability is increased, some internists prefer to promote peripheral ketone utilization.

2. This can be done by infusing glucose (2 to 3 mg/kg/min) and insulin (about 0.035 U/kg/hr) until the animal is eating and not vomiting. The added intensive step of glucose-insulin infusion is omitted by many internists who treat with subcutaneous insulin once the blood glucose reaches the 200 to 250 mg/dl range after low dose intramuscular or intravenous infusion insulin administration.

F. Converting to conventional insulin therapy

1. After the glucose concentration is between 200 to 250 mg/dl or after ketonemia is reversed as outlined above, the animal must be converted to subcutaneous insulin administration as for uncomplicated diabetes.

2. If the time for conversion occurs in the morning, the clinician can proceed. If, however, the blood glucose returns to the 200 to 250 mg/dl range at a time other than morning, a plan is needed to maintain blood glucose in that range until it is convenient to start subcutaneous insulin therapy.

3. One such means is to infuse glucose and insulin as outlined above. A less labor intensive alternative is to administer regular insulin every four to six hours subcutaneously at a dose one-fourth of that total dose which was required to decrease blood glucose to the 200 to 250 mg/dl range.

V. Complications

A. Pancreatitis

1. The most common complication of diabetic ketoacidosis in the dog but is extremely rare in the cat.

2. The effectiveness of medications used for treating pancreatitis remains unsubstantiated, and for this reason they are not recommended.

3. The diabetic ketoacidotic animal with pancreatitis should receive nothing by mouth until vomiting has ceased and serum amylase and lipase activity approach normal.

B. Hyperosmolality

1. This is a rather rare occurrence in cats and dogs and is usually present in the absence of ketoacidosis.

2. Hyperosmolality usually results from the combination of profound hyperglycemia and marked hypernatremia.
3. Clinical signs include depression and stupor which can progress to coma.
4. Serum osmolality can be measured directly or estimated from the formula:

$$\text{Osmolality} = 2(\text{Na} + \text{K}) \times \frac{\text{blood glucose}}{18}$$

when sodium and potassium are expressed in mEq/L and blood glucose in mg/dl. Normal osmolality is about 300 mOsm/L. The clinician should be concerned if serum osmolality exceeds 350 mOsm/L although clinical signs may not be obvious until serum osmolality exceeds 370 mOsm/L.
5. Isotonic fluids or fluids no less hypotonic than 0.45% saline should be used to treat hyperosmolality. If hypotonic fluids are used, a substantial osmotic gradient may be created between ECF and brain and fatal cerebral edema may result.

THERAPY OF SECONDARY DIABETES

Diabetes mellitus can occur secondary to several diabetogenic factors most of which are hormone excesses. Some of the more common factors are obesity, glucocorticoids, progestogens, estrogens, catecholamines, glucagon, growth hormone, and thyroxine. Therapy of two syndromes of secondary or complicated diabetes will be discussed.

I. Diabetes secondary to progestogens
   A. Diabetes in both cats and dogs can result from the chronic administration of progestogens (usually megestrol acetate in the USA) or from chronic endogenous production in the intact bitch in which corpora lutea produce progesterone regardless of conception.
   B. The progestogens, whether of exogenous or endogenous origin, stimulate excess growth hormone production which causes peripheral insulin resistance. Peripheral insulin resistance is followed by ineffective hyperinsulinemia and hyperglycemia.
   C. At this stage, if exogenous progestogen is stopped or, in the case of the elderly, intact bitch, if the ovarian source of endogenous progestogens is removed, the diabetes disappears. If the progestogen influence is not eliminated, however, the pancreatic beta cells may continue to maximally produce insulin and eventually lose their insulin-producing capability. At this stage, the diabetes is permanent and insulin-requiring.
   D. If the association between progestogens and diabetes is made early by the clinician, the results of treatment are dramatic. When exogenous progestogen administration is stopped, exogenous insulin requirements usually diminish to nil within weeks. When the elderly bitch is spayed, the decrease in exogenous insulin requirements, which is often dramatic

in its own right (up to 8 U/kg/day), is profound. For example, a bitch that required 240 U of insulin per day to control ketoacidosis in preparation for ovariohysterectomy may lose all exogenous insulin requirements within four days after surgery.

E. Because of the sharp drop in insulin requirements, close postsurgical monitoring is important. In contrast, if the diagnosis of diabetes secondary to endogenous progestogens is not made early, exogenous insulin requirements may gradually diminish over a period of weeks but never reach zero.

II. Diabetes with hyperadrenocorticism
   A. Although many dogs with insulin-requiring diabetes will, when tested for adrenal function, yield results suggestive of hyperadrenocorticism, their adrenal function studies sharply contrast with those dogs that actually have diabetes and hyperadrenocorticism. Dogs with both diseases yield adrenal function test results that are dramatically indicative of hyperadrenocorticism and often have clinical signs indicative of hyperadrenocorticism.
   B. The breeds of dogs most often afflicted with both conditions are Miniature Poodles, Dachshunds, and Schnauzers.
   C. Although some dogs will have signs of both diseases, the clinician should suspect the occurrence of hyperadrenocorticism if polyuria persists after adequate control of diabetes.
   D. When it is established that a dog has both conditions, diabetes should be adequately controlled first and hyperadrenocorticism treated next.

HYPERINSULINISM

   I. A rare condition of dogs and cats caused by a functional tumor of the beta cells of the islets of Langerhans. It is most commonly observed in Boxers, Standard Poodles, and Fox Terriers.
  II. Clinical Signs
   A. Generalized seizures
   B. Ataxia
   C. Weakness
   D. Muscle fasciculation
   E. Syncope
   F. Polyphagia
   G. Hysteria
   H. Nervousness
    I. Tachycardia
    J. Provoked by fasting, exercise, or excitement.
 III. Diagnosis
   A. Blood glucose determination.
   B. Simultaneous plasma immunoreactive insulin concentrations
   C. Insulin:glucose ratio or glucose:insulin ratio

D. Amended insulin:glucose ratio is of no increased diagnostic value
E. Glucagon tolerance test.
IV. Treatment
  A. Hypoglycemic crisis
    1. Intravenous administration of 50% dextrose solution to effect.
    2. Xylazine, 1.1 mg/kg, IM.
       May be useful along with dextrose solution IV. Suppresses insulin release from normal beta cells. Has not been evaluated in treatment of insulinoma.
  B. Surgical laparotomy, exploration, and removal of tumor.
  C. Medical management of metastatic disease.
    1. Prednisone, 0.25 mg/kg, q 12 h, PO.
       Efficacy not established
    2. Diazoxide, 10 mg/kg, q 12 h.
       May be used up to a dose of 20 mg/kg q 12 h. Inhibits release of insulin. Effectiveness may decrease over a period of months
    3. Streptozotocin, 500 mg/m^2
      a) Approx. 14.5 mg/kg
      b) Infused IV over a period of 1 hr, on two to three consecutive days each month
      c) May induce renal tubular acidosis

SUGGESTED READINGS

Allen TA: Canine hypoglycemia. p. 845. In Kirk RW (ed): Current Veterinary Therapy VIII. WB Saunders, Philadelphia, 1983

Chastain CB, Nicholas CE: Low-Dose intramuscular insulin therapy for diabetic ketoacidosis in dogs. J Am Vet Med Assoc 178(6):561–564, 1981

Church DB: Diabetes mellitus. p. 838. In Kirk RW (ed): Current Veterinary Therapy VIII WB Saunders, Philadelphia, 1983

Church DB: A comparison of intravenous and oral glucose tolerance tests in the dog. Res Vet Sci 29:353–359, 1980

Eigenmann JE: Diabetes mellitus in elderly female dogs: recent findings on pathogenesis and clinical implications. J Am Animal Hosp 17:805–812, 1981

Feldman EC, Nelson RW: Insulin-induced hyperglycemia in diabetic dogs. J Am Vet Med Assoc 180(12):1432–1437, 1982

Giulian BB, Mitsuoka H, Mansfield AO, et al: Treatment of Pancreatic Exocrine Insufficiency: II. Effects on Fat Absorption of Pancreatic Lipase and Fifteen Commercial Pancreatic Supplements as Measured by I^{131} Tagged Triolein in the Dog. Ann of Surg 165(4):571–579, 1967

Kaneko JJ, Mattheeuws D, Rottiers RP, Vermeulen A: Glucose tolerance and insulin response in diabetes mellitus of dogs. J Small Animal Practice 19:85–94, 1978

Knowlen GG, Schall WD: The amended insulin-glucose ratio. Is it really better? J Am Vet Med Assoc 185(4):397–399, 1984

Marmor M, Willeberg P, Glickman LT, et al: Epizootiologic patterns of diabetes mellitus in dogs. Am J Vet Res 43(3):465–470, 1982

National Diabetes Data Group: Classification and Diagnosis of Diabetes Mellitus and Other Categories of Glucose Intolerance. Diabetes 28:1039–1057, 1979

Nelson RW: Use of insulin in small animal medicine. J Am Vet Med Assoc 185:105, 1984

Pairent FW, Howard JM: Pancreatic exocrine insufficiency. IV. The Enzyme Content of Commercial Pancreatic Supplements. Arch Surg 110:739–741, 1975

Pidgeon G, Strombeck DR: Evaluation of treatment for pancreatic exocrine insufficiency in dogs with ligated pancreatic ducts. Am J Vet Res 43(3):461–464, 1982

Regan PT, Malagelada JR, DiMagno EP, et al: Comparative effects of antacids, cimetidine and enteric coating on the therapeutic response to oral enzymes in severe pancreatic insufficiency. N Engl J Med 16:854–858, 1977

Rogers WA: Diseases of the exocrine pancreas. pp. 1435–1455. In Ettinger SJ (ed): Textbook of Veterinary Internal Medicine. 2nd Ed. WB Saunders, Philadelphia, 1983

Rottiers R, Mattheeuws D, Kaneko JJ, Vermeulen A: Glucose uptake and insulin secretory responses to intravenous glucose loads in the dog. Am J Vet Res 42:155–158, 1981

Schall WD, Cornelius LM: Diabetes mellitus. In Feldman EC (ed): Symposium on Endocrinology. Vet Clinics No Amer 7:613, 1977

Strombeck DR, Feldman BF: Acute pancreatitis. p. 810. In Kirk RW (ed) Current Vet Therapy VIII. WB Saunders, Philadelphia, 1983

16

Seizure Disorders

William J. Kay, D.V.M.
David P. Aucoin, D.V.M.

In this chapter the terms *epilepsy, fit, ictus, seizures,* and *convulsions* will be used interchangeably. These are names of the neuronal, cerebral events characterized by abnormal electrical discharges. The following are necessary for the successful treatment of chronic recurring epilepsy.

GENERAL COMMENTS

I. The veterinarian must first establish the nature of all events, i.e., the attack(s), episodes, spells, fits, and/or convulsions.
II. Events that are historically reported or experienced by the veterinarian and his or her staff must be categorized.
III. Classification of events is essential to the development of a therapeutic objective.
IV. The veterinarian must be familiar with the actions of several compounds currently and historically used for the control of epileptic seizures.
V. After establishing the above criteria, the veterinarian must
  A. Rule in or rule out organic lesions
  B. Determine if the lesion is within the brain (intracranial)
  C. Determine if the lesion is outside of the brain (extracranial)
  D. Determine the specific localization if the lesion is intracranial
  E. Determine the symmetrical diffuse nature of the process if it is extracranial
VI. Chronic therapy of epilepsy is successful over an extended period only if nonprogressive lesions are selected for treatment with an appropriate anticonvulsant or anticonvulsants.

OBJECTIVES

I. Confirming that clinical events are epileptic or nonepileptic
II. Classifying epileptic events into specific forms or types of epilepsy
  A. Major motor

    B. Partial

    C. Nonmotor

  III. Choosing or accepting of a therapeutic objective

      1. Total control

      2. Partial control

      3. Shortening seizures

  IV. Understanding the basic pharmacology and actions of each widely used anticonvulsant

   V. Proper dosage

  VI. Determining appropriate response to therapy

 VII. Recognizing side effects (toxicity) and what to do about side effects

VIII. Treating status epilepticus

  IX. Rules of thumb for use in the treatment of epilepsy

   X. Eliminating epileptic animals with severe, progressive intracranial diseases and extracranial diseases

DEFINITIONS

  I. Epilepsy

    A. *Epilepsy* is cerebral dysrhythmia and excessive neuronal energy.

    B. The energy is in cerebral cortical neurons.

    C. It flows through the brain to the spinal cord, peripheral nerves, and muscles.

 II. Epileptic seizures

    A. Epileptic seizures are clinical manifestation of an active, cerebral, bizarre neuronal irritative process involving billions of cortical neurons.

    B. They originate in cortical grey matter.

    C. Epileptic seizures are characterized by loss of consciousness, gross or minor body movements, and incontinence.

COMPONENTS OF AN EPILEPTIC ATTACK

Each epileptic event has components. They should be observed by client and clinician.

  I. Prodrome or aura

    This constitutes signs that precede or herald an epileptic event.

 II. Ictus

    The actual seizure, which lasts seconds to several minutes and may be generalized, partial, or nonmotor

III. Postictus, postictal, or postseizure phase

    The period of confusion, depression, coma, blindness, moving in circles, and so forth that follows the seizure

IV. Interictal phase

This is the period between seizures, which lasts seconds to months, and can be a time of normal or mild to severely abnormal behavior.

V. Status epilepticus

These are seizures that run together and do not have a period of normalcy in between.

CLASSIFICATION OF SEIZURES

Epilepsy in companion pet animals is classified by several methods including nature of the seizure, neuroanatomic location of the origin of the seizure, and etiology of the seizure. For the purpose of this chapter, classification will be based on the overt, viewed, clinical form of the seizure.

I. Major motor seizure

Tonic-clonic, the most common, easiest to recognize, and most overt type of seizure

II. Minor motor seizure

This is a partial, nongeneralized seizure which orginates in one part of the brain and is reflected by the movement of only part of the body.

III. Behavioral seizure

This is a nonmotor seizure, characterized by periodic, paroxysmal events of personality or behavior. The occurrence of behavioral or nonmotor seizures has a wide variety of clinical manifestations including staring, growling, vomiting, retching, fly snapping, and viciousness.

IV. Sensory seizure

This is a hysterical, running seizure. The pet runs aimlessly, as if possessed.

SEIZURE WORKUP

I. The veterinarian must first determine whether or not events or attacks are epileptic seizures.

A. Many animals may exhibit events which resemble epileptic seizures. While there are similarities between the spells exhibited by other organ systems and those of epilepsy, a careful history and complete physical examination usually will eliminate other organ systems and other neural disorders.

B. It may be necessary to rule out other diseases including cardiovascular, hepatic, adrenal, pancreatic, pulmonary, neoplastic, drug-induced, and hematologic disease.

II. A seizure evaluation is composed of four parts

A. A detailed seizure history is designed to accomplish the following

1. Establish the event as epileptic

      2. Characterize its severity

      3. Characterize its length

      4. Characterize its specific parts

      5. Determine response to medication

      6. Evaluate severity and direction

    B. A complete physical examination, including thoracic and abdominal radiography, to determine if extracranial conditions are involved.

    C. A complete neurologic examination to determine if the epilepsy is secondary to a localized, focal, discrete lesion residing in a lateralizing process located within the substance of the brain (organic or structural epilepsy) or is a functional manifestation without a discernible lesion (idiopathic symptomatic epilepsy)

    D. Diagnostic tests including skull radiography, cerebrospinal fluid analysis, and electroencephalography (EEG)

III. The seizure workup is constructed to answer the following questions

    A. Does the patient have a neurologic disease?

    B. Does the neurologic disease originate within the brain?

    C. If it originates within the brain, does it originate within the cerebrum?

    D. If it originates within the cerebrum does it originate from the left cerebral hemisphere or the right cerebral hemisphere (or both?)

    E. Is there evidence that the lesion is enlarging, is staying the same, or is getting smaller?

    F. Is there evidence of multiple lesions or is the process multifocal diffuse and therefore global?

  These questions must be answered, hopefully in the sequence they are asked here, in order to narrow the focus to functional disorders. The functional disorders are easier to treat.

THERAPEUTIC OBJECTIVES

    I. The objective of long-term seizure control is to stop the seizures by removing or treating the cause (i.e., tumor, infection, hemorrhage, and so forth) or to control the seizures, either independently of the cause or in addition to the cause.

   II. By far the most frequent seizure control objective in companion animal practice is the long-term control of functional seizures.

  III. While 100% control is the objective, veterinarians must frequently accept lesser degrees of control; lesser control is defined as the improvement in a seizure disorder without 100% control.

  IV. The goals of therapy are to

    A. Modify the frequency of seizures

    B. Modify and lessen the severity of seizures

    C. Shorten the postseizure period (postictal phase)

    D. Prevent status epilepticus and cluster seizures

V. The accomplishment of these objectives is achieved by the use of phar-
   macologic agents which meet certain criteria including
   A. Absence of side effects considered unacceptable to the client and animal
      (e.g., depression, sleepiness, viciousness)
   B. Affordable cost
   C. Easy administration
   D. Absence of short- or long-term harm to the client and animal
VI. Veterinarian and client must clearly understand
   A. The objectives
   B. The limitations of the objectives
   C. How to achieve the objectives

STATUS EPILEPTICUS

Status is a fixed or enduring state. As applied to epilepsy, status is defined
as seizures, the frequency, duration, and severity of which are so serious and
violent that the patient does not adequately recover between seizures. Alternatively, status may be defined as seizures, the clinical manifestation of which
is constant, repetitive, and persistent. There is no discernible interictal period.
The seizures are continuous, in status epilepticus, over an extended period of
time (minutes, hours, or days). The treatment of status epilepticus is a medical
emergency.

CLINICAL MANAGEMENT

   I. Determine whether or not the observed event is actually cerebral dys-
      rhythmia. Several acute intracranial crises may mimic status epilepticus
      A. Head trauma with coma
      B. Brain herniation
      C. Acute intracranial cerebrovascular accident (CVA)
      D. Severe hepatic encephalopathy (entracranial seizures)
      E. Encephalitis (bacterial, viral)
      F. Severe hypoglycemia (functional)
      G. Secondary to a variety of extracranial etiologies
  II. Collect blood samples for laboratory testing.
 III. Establish and maintain a patent airway.
  IV. Administer anticonvulsant drugs parenterally.
   V. Maintain a patent IV catheter.
  VI. Evaluate the patient for metabolic disturbances including hypokalemia,
      hypercalcemia, acidosis, and so on.
 VII. Evaluate and treat the patient for pulmonary edema.
VIII. Attempt to terminate parenteral IV medication.
  IX. Begin oral anticonvulsant therapy as early as possible.
   X. Maintain overall homeostasis.

CLIENT MANAGEMENT

INFORMING THE CLIENT

The treatment of chronic epilepsy requires excellent rapport with the client. The veterinarian must help the client to

I. Understand the nature of epilepsy as a disease and as a sign of a disease.

II. Recognize the futility of tests in many patients—test results routinely are normal.

III. Recognize the absence of a permanent cure—seizures as a functional phenomenon occur without overt seizure.

IV. Accept partial seizure control as a legitimate objective compatible with the client's well-being and that of the pet.

V. Develop the willingness to medicate an animal chronically for years; the medications are usually given two to three times daily.

VI. Learn that epileptic seizures are not directly indicative of the seriousness of disease and are not a reflection of the ultimate outcome.

QUESTIONS TO ASK THE CLIENT

It is crucial that the veterinarian spend enough time with the client early in the course of symptomatic treatment of a chronic disease often fraught with upset, recurrences, crises, and misunderstandings. Ictus means, literally, "fear of the unknown." Seizures are spontaneous, sudden, intermittent, and often unpredictable. It is very important for the client to react but not to overreact! This is especially true with large dogs. Clients should be asked if they will

I. Bring the pet to a veterinarian under certain circumstances.

II. Give medication daily.

III. Have tests performed intermittently for toxicities brought on by the chronic use of certain anticonvulsants.

IV. Have the animal boarded or closely observed during the client's vacation.

V. Learn to recognize signs of drug toxicity.

THE MEDICAL RECORD

The keeping of a log, list, or chart will help both client and veterinarian. The direction, increase, or decrease in severity, frequency, characteristics, and length of postictal phase of seizures are all-important. Without adequate records the worsening or improvement of a seizure disorder is often difficult to determine, as well as the efficacy or lack thereof of certain medications. The chart should include

I. Medication regimen

II. Date of seizure

III. Length of seizure

IV. Postictal phase—signs, severity, length
 V. Response to medication
VI. Timing of medication, details of administration (route, dose, frequency)
VII. Testing frequency for concentrations of anticonvulsants and toxicity (see chapter 22)

CLINICAL MANAGEMENT OF SEIZURES

CLINICAL CHARACTERISTICS

I. The patient's history, even when taken with great care, changes each time it is taken and changes according to who is taking the history.

II. To classify an animal as having symptoms of periodicity as a sign is not always easy. Some examples of periodicity are subtle because the periods are long (hours to days).

III. Periods change. They become shorter or longer.

IV. A period or episode or event or convulsion can have a wide range of presentations, from a subtle twitch to a violent seizure and from complete collapse to transient staggering of a few seconds duration.

V. Making a distinction between the period or episode or event or convulsion and the context in which they (it) occur is an objective of a detailed history.

VI. The grounding of a case, i.e., separating the event from the nonevent.

VII. The more events noted or reported the more likely the event is an epileptic seizure.

VIII. The more paroxysmal the event the more likely the event is an epileptic seizure.

IX. The longer the duration (in terms of months or years) the more likely the event is an epileptic attack.

X. Fainting or collapsing, or falling without movement is routinely a feature of cardiovascular disease, syncope, narcolepsy, or cataplexy.

XI. Narcolepsy or cataplexy—short periods of collapse (cataplexy) or collapse and sleeping (narcolepsy) can occur hundreds of times without serious consequences.

XII. Therapeutic diagnostics are necessary to determine the nature of many events.

XIII. The loss of consciousness associated with many events and spells is often subjective. It can be assessed historically.

XIV. The dementia and depression associated with many events and spells are subjective. They, too, can be assessed historically.

XV. Spells and periods of a cardiovascular nature including congestive heart failure, arrhythmias, and heart block generally are associated with discernible disease of the cardiovascular system.

XVI. A good way to determine the cause of spells and periods and events is the assessment of intracranial signs (brain) or appendicular signs (extremities) using reflexes, state of consciousness, cranial nerves, cerebral status, and so forth.

XVII. The period, spell, event, and so forth is not always seen in many of the diseases in which it is a routine feature.

XVIII. Nearly all systemic diseases have waxing and waning features. This does not make them episodic diseases.

XIX. The periodicity of a disease is a useful prognostic tool.

XX. Some pharmacologic agents produce intermittent signs. Many of these signs are not recognized adverse effects.

XXI. Epileptic seizures are the most common of the epileptic events.

XXII. Animals seldom die from epileptic seizures, unless status epilepticus occurs.

XXIII. Epileptic seizures will usually worsen if not controlled.

XXIV. In almost every epileptic seizure disorder, relapses occur.

XXV. Discontinuation of medication (anticonvulsants) will precipitate recurrence of seizures.

XXVI. Younger animals (early-onset seizures) are less likely to have progressive diseases than older animals (late-onset seizures).

XXVII. The exacerbation of a seizure disorder after successful management is a common sign and may require increased doses of medication.

XVIII. Exacerbation of a seizure disorder does not imply a serious etiology—exacerbations are routine.

XXIX. The most common causes of failure in epileptic seizure management are
A. Poor client education
B. Inadequate medication levels
C. Failure to administer medication properly or in a timely fashion
D. Incomplete neural diagnostics, i.e., failure to rule out progressive disease

XXX. Clients must be made aware of the individual nature of seizure medications. They need to know about trial and error techniques. Raising and lowering dose levels.

XXXI. Oral medication takes several days to be effective. Seizures will, therefore, occur after medication is instituted.

XXXII. The prognosis of severe epilepsy, even status epilepticus is not grave unless accompanied by a severe structural disease.

XXXIII. Evaluating an epileptic animal shortly following a seizure is difficult. The neurologic examination cannot be adequately performed.

XXXIV. There is no correlation between severity of a seizure disorder and the underlying disease. Severe seizure disorders can be idiopathic and a progressive structural lesion can be associated with very mild seizures.

XXXV. Changing seizure patterns are routine and are unrelated to the etiology of the seizure.

XXXVI. In some seizures the postictal phase is more disturbing than the actual seizure.

XXXVII. Most seizures have a prodrome and aura. It should be observed and noted.

XXXVIII. Therapeutic diagnostic techniques are often requested to determine the nature of events.

PHARMACOLOGY OF ANTICONVULSANT DRUGS

I. General comments
  A. There is a wide variety of causes for seizures but the pathologic mechanism appears to be the same for all. Normal neural discharge is asynchronous. A seizure is precipitated when a focal area of neural tissue starts to fire homogeneously, which can activate synchronous firing in adjacent tissue, leading to the spread of the seizure focus.
  B. There are two general mechanisms of anticonvulsant action
    1. The capacity of the focal area for synchronous repetitive firing can be abolished by raising the threshold for firing.
    2. Stopping the propagation of the discharge into contiguous neural tissue. Each of the drugs discussed in this chapter operates by one of the two mechanisms. The exact biochemical pathways of these mechanisms are still under investigation.

II. Phenytoin (Dilantin)
  A. Also known as diphenylhydantoin, this drug acts by stopping the propagation and spread of a focal neural discharge.
  B. It is one of the most widely used anticonvulsants in human medicine because of its efficacy and need for treatment only once or twice daily. However, in dogs controversy exists regarding its usefulness as a sole agent in the treatment of epilepsy.
  C. Phenytoin has a very rapid metabolism in dogs with a half-life of only 2–4 hours, and at least three treatments daily are required. No well-documented studies have correlated serum concentrations with clinical efficacy but it appears that signs of toxicity occur at serum concentrations of greater than 20 μg/ml which is similar to that in humans.
  D. If we use values for therapeutic serum concentrations of 10–20 μg/ml, the recommended dosage to achieve those concentrations in the dog is from 20 to 35 mg/kg TID. There is a great deal of variability in serum concentrations because of erratic absorption, making predictable serum concentrations difficult. The drug has a long half-life in cats and should be administered less frequently.

    E. Toxic side effects are vomition, ataxia, and delirium. Hepatotoxicity has been reported with chronic use.

III. Primidone

    A. This drug is metabolized by the liver into two active metabolites. The one that is probably most contributory to anticonvulsant effect is phenobarbital. The other metabolite, phenylethylmalonamide (PEMA) has some anticonvulsant properties but has been estimated to contribute less than 15% to the total effect. The effects of unmetabolized primidone are probably unimportant inasmuch as the serum concentrations in the dog are extremely low.

    B. The mechanism of action for primidone is the same as that of its most active metabolite, phenobarbital. The threshold for repetitive firing for neurons is raised, thus blocking the initiating synchronous focal firing of the epileptogenic site.

    C. The recommended dose for primidone has been correlated recently with clinical efficacy and phenobarbital serum concentrations. The dosage range is 11–22 mg/kg TID.

    D. Phenobarbital concentrations of 25–40 μg/ml appear to be therapeutic, but some dogs require much less. Concentrations greater than 40 μg/ml usually result in excessive sedation.

    E. Side effects are polyuria, polydipsia, and polyphagia. During the first few weeks of treatment or when the dose is increased, sedation and ataxia may occur but these signs resolve with continued treatment. It has been recommended to start the dose at 3–5 mg/kg and raise the dose over 2 weeks to prevent sedation. Until the dose is high enough, seizures may occur and the owner should be forewarned.

    F. Hepatotoxicity has been reported. It is suggested that liver function and enzyme tests be performed periodically, and monitoring of plasma concentrations of phenobarbital may be useful (see Chapter 22).

    G. Contrary to information provided in package inserts, primidone is not exceptionally toxic to cats.

IV. Phenobarbital

    A. This drug is slowly metabolized by the liver and has a serum half-life of 22–42 hours. Therefore, 7–10 days of treatment are required before steady-state concentrations of the drug are achieved.

    B. The mechanism of action has been discussed in the section on Primidone, above.

    C. The dose varies, depending on whether or not the dog has been on previous anticonvulsant medication. This can greatly speed up the metabolism of phenobarbital in which case a higher dosage is required. The initial dose is 1–2 mg/kg BID to TID. Tolerance develops to barbiturates with chronic use and even with higher dosages anticonvulsant activity may not be maintained without overt sedation.

    D. It is frequently added to other anticonvulsants (phenytoin, primidone) for added efficacy with less chance of toxicity.

E. The effective plasma concentrations appear to be 20–40 μg/ml.

F. Side effects are the same as those listed for primidone. This drug is the safest anticonvulsant.

G. Interactions—both primidone and phenobarbital are potent inducers of hepatic microsomal enzymes. This will increase the rate of biotransformation of other drugs.

V. Valproic acid

A. Rapid metabolism of this drug occurs in the liver, and two metabolites have some anticonvulsant activity. The serum half-life of valproic acid in dogs is much shorter (3 hours) than that in humans (9–22 hours).

B. The mechanism of action remains speculative at this time. It is currently used in treating different forms of epilepsy in humans, however, its Food and Drug Administration (FDA) approval is for petit mal or other absence seizures and not for grand mal or generalized motor seizures.

C. In one clinical trial the dose was 30–45 mg/kg/day in divided doses. The response to treatment was equivocal. Reported therapeutic serum concentrations in human patients are 40–100 μg/ml; however, massive doses (220 mg/kg TID) are required to obtain these concentrations in the dog. A suggested initial dose is 170–185 mg/kg/day divided BID to TID.

D. In people this drug is reported to potentiate the sedative properties of the other anticonvulsants.

E. A side effect is gastrointestinal upset. Hepatotoxicity has been reported in human patients.

F. This drug is expensive, has little advantage over the previously discussed anticonvulsants, and is not highly recommended for treatment of epilepsy in the dog. ·

VI. Alternative anticonvulsants

A. Carbamazepine (Tegretol)

1. Structurally this drug is related to the tricyclic antidepressants and has been used commonly in Europe for grand mal seizures.

2. Its mechanism is the same as that for phenytoin.

3. The drug is metabolized 25 times faster in the dog than in people.

4. With continued treatment metabolism is induced even further, making this drug a poor choice for use in this species.

B. Diazepam (Valium)

1. A benzodiazepine, this is the drug of choice for treatment of status epilepticus.

2. The dose necessary to achieve the desired effect is seldom more than 10 mg per dog IV.

3. The half-life is 6–8 hours (including its metabolites).

4. More than two or three doses of this drug should not be given since tolerance can develop and its sedative property is additive with that of the barbiturates.

    5. The drug should NOT be given by IM injection since poor absorption occurs.

    6. The drug has not been evaluated as an oral anticonvulsant in the dog.

    7. Diazepam injections should not be stored in plastic containers as this drug adsorbs to the plastic, removing it from the solution.

VII. Summary of useful anticonvulsant drugs in veterinary practice

    A. Phenobarbital is the safest and most efficacious anticonvulsant for therapy in the dog.

    B. Primidone is an effective anticonvulsant, with phenobarbital contributing an estimated 85% of its anticonvulsant properties. Hepatotoxicity is a potential problem.

    C. Phenytoin can not be recommended as sole treatment because of its rapid metabolism and erratic absorption. In combination with phenobarbital it is effective. However, clinical trials in dogs have shown it not to be more effective than phenobarbital alone.

    D. Monitoring phenobarbital serum concentrations is an effective way of determining whether or not the drug is being given as directed and will also help the clinician decide if treatment failure is the result of inappropriate dosing or drug failure or if a change in a dog's mental status is related to drug overdose or progression of the disease.

SUMMARY OF PRINCIPLES

I. To be successful in the treatment of chronic seizures, it is important to

    A. Establish the event, episode, spell, or period as an actual epileptic event.

    B. Categorize the event, after it has been classified as epileptic, as functional epilepsy or symptomatic epilepsy.

    C. Classify the event as having an intracranial or extracranial origin (remove the etiology if possible, especially if extracranial).

    D. Rank the possible etiologies.

    E. Establish a treatment regimen if the etiology is functional or idiopathic.

    F. Educate and advise clients on all aspects of epilepsy.

    G. Monitor medication based on clinical signs, side effects, and possibly measurement of drug concentrations in plasma.

    H. Evaluate the animal periodically for side effects and toxicity.

    I. Evaluate medication and dosage if there are any breakdowns, setbacks, flare-ups, or occurrences of status epilepticus.

II. The rational treatment of chronic epilepsy is based on

    A. Selecting the right case

    B. Giving the right medication

    C. Selecting the right dosage regimen

    D. Administering the medication at the right time

III. Prognosis
   A. Even with everything in order, seizures will recur.
   B. This is especially true with large breed dogs and cats.
   C. Our experience suggests that large breed dogs respond poorly and that small breed dogs respond well.
   D. Few large breed dogs are completely or even adequately cured.

SUGGESTED READINGS

Chrisman C: Problems in Small Animal Neurology. Lea and Febiger, Philadelphia, 1982

Holliday T: Seizures. Proc. Am. An. Hosp. Assn, 1982

Kay WJ: Epilepsy. In Kirk RW (ed.): Current Veterinary Therapy V, W.B. Saunders Co., Philadelphia, 1974, p. 686–699

Kay WJ, Fenner WR: In Sattler F, Knowles R, Willick W (eds): Emergency Management of the Epileptic Animal. Veterinary Critical Care. Lea & Febiger, Philadelphia, 1981

Kelly MJ: Periodic Weakness. Proc. Am. An. Hosp. Assn. 1980, p. 181

Russo ME: The pathophysiology of epilepsy. Cornell Vet 71:221 1981

17

Behavioral Disorders
Victoria L. Voith, D.V.M.

GENERAL COMMENTS

I. The behavior of a companion dog or cat is as important to the owner as its physical well-being. The veterinarian is usually the first person to whom owners turn regarding advice about the behavior of their pet, and therefore whether the practitioner decides to treat the problem or refer it to a specialist, he or she is in the position of having to make the initial differential diagnoses.

II. A behavioral problem may be a normal behavior (species-typical or learned behavior) or an abnormal behavior (a pathophysiologic disorder or a deleterious learned behavior). A good differential diagnosis, prognosis, and treatment plan necessitates knowledge about principles of learning, developmental processes, physiologic states, and the pervasive effects of early experience. The short space available in this book can not be devoted to detailed descriptions and explanations of these factors. The reader is therefore referred to the material listed in the Suggested Readings at the end of this chapter.

DEFINITION

I. *Behavior* is essentially what an animal does. Behavior can be affected by many factors, both internal and external. Because behavior can be influenced by numerous variables, behavioral problems can be influenced in a variety of ways.

II. Behavioral problems may be influenced by
   A. Altering the environment
   B. Physiologic manipulation via pharmacologic or surgical intervention
   C. Behavior modification techniques utilizing learning principles
   D. Depending upon the problem, the constraints of the owner, and the

physical dictates of the patient, one or all of the above therapeutic avenues could be utilized.

III. Classification of behavioral problems
- A. Normal behavior
  1. Species-typical behaviors, i.e., innate or unlearned behavior patterns
  2. Learned behavior patterns that are somewhat adaptive to the animal
- B. Abnormal behaviors
  1. Acquired or genetic pathophysiologic disorders.
  2. Experiential factors
     a) Early experience of the animal
     b) Phobic developments
     c) Psychosomatic disorders
- C. Descriptive

  This is exactly what the name implies, a precise behavioral description [aggression, elimination (urination, defecation, spraying), vocalization, and so forth] derived from observation or history.
- D. Functional or motivational

  The circumstances, context, and physiologic status of the animal allow the clinician to classify the behavior functionally.

BEHAVIOR MODIFICATION TECHNIQUES

I. Ways of reducing the occurrence of learned behaviors are by extinction, counterconditioning (reinforcement of alternative behaviors), systematic desensitization, punishment, and flooding or response prevention. Application of these methods requires a clear understanding of the concepts of shaping (successive approximation), reinforcement (reward), punishment, schedules of reinforcement, and time contingencies.

II. Definitions
- A. Positive reinforcement
  1. A *positive reinforcement* is an event or state of affairs that following a response tends to increase the probability that the response will recur. The reward is most effective when it occurs 0.5 seconds after the response. In essence, the animal should be rewarded as soon as possible.
  2. Behaviors acquired or enhanced as the result of reinforcements will extinguish, or reduce in frequency, if reinforcements cease.
  3. The frequency and intervals at which the rewards are administered influence acquisition of a response and its rate of extinction.
  4. For acquisition of a response, immediate, continuous reinforcement is best. This means that every response is immediately followed by a reinforcement.
  5. For perpetuation of the response intermittent reinforcement is su-

perior to continuous reinforcement. Intermittent reinforcement means that not every response is followed by a reinforcement.

6. Although delay of reward retards acquisition of a response, varied delays of reward increase resistance to extinction of an acquired response.

B. Punishment

1. *Punishment* is the application of an aversive event that stops or prevents a behavior from occurring.

2. Punishment can have side effects.

a) Anxiety

b) Aggression

3. Punishment is contraindicated in the treatment of fear-related behaviors.

C. Shaping

1. *Shaping* (successive approximation) is a technique used in training an animal to perform a precise behavior by, initially, reinforcing an approximation of the ultimately desired response.

2. Finally only the precise behavior is reinforced.

D. Counterconditioning

1. *Counterconditioning* is training or conditioning an animal to acquire a response to a stimulus which is incompatible with a response previously evoked by the stimulus.

2. Classically, counterconditioning has been used to reduce anxieties by conditioning the animal to respond to the anxiety-producing stimulus in a way that is physiologically incompatible with the undesired response.

3. Pleasant stimuli are paired with the anxiety-producing stimuli.

4. Frequently the pleasant stimuli are also used as an operant reinforcement for the new behavior.

E. Systematic desensitization

1. *Systematic desensitization* is a technique of gradually exposing an animal to increasing intensities of a stimulus without evoking an undesirable response.

2. It is usually used to break down anxiety and fear response habits in a piecemeal fashion by repeatedly exposing a subject to a weak fear-eliciting stimulus during a physiologic state that is inhibitory of fear or anxiety.

F. Flooding

1. *Flooding* or response prevention is a technique used to treat fear responses.

2. The patient is forced to experience the intense anxiety of a phobic situation, but is prevented from leaving the situation until the anxiety has been markedly reduced or ceases.

3. This technique has not been used often to treat extreme phobic responses of animals in clinical situations.

BEHAVIORAL PROBLEMS IN CATS

ELIMINATION BEHAVIOR PROBLEMS

General Comments

I. A cat presented for an elimination problem may be either urinating, defecating, or urine-marking. The cat assumes a squatting position for urinating and defecating, and generally scratches before and afterward. Urination and defecation problems are usually treated by manipulating the environment. Most squatting urination behavior problems occur because cats have developed a new location or surface preference regarding elimination and are *not a urine-marking problem.*

II. Urine-marking can occur in a spraying or squatting posture. The cat generally does not engage in scratching or covering-up behavior when it urine-marks. Urine-marking in a squatting posture usually occurs in the same locations or contexts where spraying is likely to occur.

Urine-marking

I. Diagnosis
A. Spraying
1. Occurs in a standing posture with the tail erect and quivering. Frequently the hind limbs step alternately.
2. The urine is sprayed or squirted backward onto vertical objects.
3. The cat may expel small or large amounts of urine and may pick one or several locations in the house.
4. Frequently occurs near doors and windows and after an encounter (auditory or visual) with another cat
5. Directly proportional to the number of cats in the household
B. Urine-marking in a squatting posture
1. Usually involves smaller amounts of urine than the cat normally voids when eliminating
2. Occurs in the same locations and contexts as does spraying
II. Treatment techniques
Any one of the following techniques may be effective.
A. Environmental manipulation
1. Reduce the number of cats in the household.
2. Restrict accessibility of outside, visiting cats to the windows and doors of the housed, spraying cat.
3. Increase or decrease amount of time the spraying cat spends outdoors.
4. Prevent accessibility to stimuli that elicit spraying (i.e., novel objects, garden equipment, firewood sprayed by visiting cats, and so forth).
5. If the cat is spraying only in a few locations, either changing the significance of the location by placing food or toys in these areas or

making the location aversive with mothballs or a commercial product that contains methyl-nonyl-ketone may repel the cat and stop the problem. If the latter is used in a large area, the odor dissipates and the cat will habituate to the odor, rendering the repellent useless.

B. Physiologic intervention
  1. Surgical
    a) Castration has a 90% probability of stopping spraying behavior in male cats, regardless of their age or duration of the spraying problem.
    b) Spaying is unlikely to affect spraying behavior in the female cat unless the spraying is related to her estrous cycle.
    c) Olfactory tractotomy
       This procedure is reported to reduce or stop spraying in 50% of cats refractory to castration and drug therapy.
  2. Drug therapy
    a) No drugs are marketed for treatment of behavioral problems in cats and owners should be advised of this.
    b) Drug therapy should be gradually stopped every 1–2 months to assess whether the cat is still motivated to spray.
    c) There appears to be a wide range of minimum therapeutic doses and the clinician should determine the lowest possible dose required by a particular animal.
    d) Diazepam
       1–2 mg per cat PO BID will suppress spraying in some cats.
    e) Progestin therapy
      (1) Potential side effects to progesterone therapy
        i) Elevated serum glucose levels, diabetes, and mammary gland hyperplasia are the most likely side effects to occur.
        ii) In dogs, the probability of developing diabetes is age-related—the older the animal the more likely it is to develop a problem.
        iii) Prolonged, elevated progesterone levels may lead to pyometra/endometritis complex and consequently prolonged administration of progesterone in the intact bitch or queen is contraindicated.
        iv) Libido and spermatogenesis should return when progestin therapy ceases.
        v) Adenocarcinomas have been reported in the cat following prolonged, repeated use of repository medroxyprogesterone.
      (2) When using progestins
        i) Obtain a baseline glucose level prior to treatment and thereafter periodically monitor the cat.
        ii) Instruct owners how to palpate the mammary glands of their cats and to watch for mammary gland hyperplasia or lactation.

   iii) Oral progesterone can be withdrawn if side effects develop.
   iv) The oral form of megestrol acetate is more effective than
       the injectable repository medroxyprogesterone acetate.
       There may be an occasional cat that will respond to one
       form of the synthetic progesterone over another.
    v) Dosage varies considerably. This author has used *either* 5–
       10 mg per cat PO megestrol acetate for 7–10 days, decrease
       the dose to 5 mg once a week for 1 month, then reduce the
       dose to 2.5 mg once a week for a second month, and then
       stop therapy *or* 10–20 mg/kg IM or SQ of repository me-
       droxyprogesterone acetate repeated as necessary and ac-
       companied by monitoring for side effects. These are not the
       author's drugs of choice.
  3. Behavior modification
     Reward and/or punishment are not effective in treating urine-mark-
     ing problems, although some cats will inhibit themselves from urine-
     marking in the presence of the owner.
  4. Treating pathophysiologic processes
     It is undetermined at this time if cystitis, urethral blockage, or ir-
     ritation are inciting causes of urine marking, particularly spraying.
     The possibility of disease processes should be explored utilizing ap-
     propriate history taking techniques and physical examination.

Urinating and/or Defecating Problems

   Both males and females, intact or neutered, declawed or not, can develop
a preference for urinating and/or defecating somewhere in the house other than
in the litterbox. Usually the cat has acquired a new location and/or substrate
preference. Drug therapy is unlikely to have any effect on this behavior. Any
one or a combination of the following treatments may work.
   I. Treat pathophysiologic disorder, if one exists.
  II. Increase the attractiveness of the litterbox.
      A. Change litter frequently.
      B. Avoid using specific cleaning compounds or specific commercial kitty
         litters, e.g., some cats avoid use of litter with perfumed pellets.
      C. Increase number of litterboxes in multicat households.
      D. Place litterboxes in convenient locations.
      E. Try other loose substrates such as sand, sawdust, wood chips, dirt,
         shredded newspaper; if the cat is eliminating on smooth surfaces such
         as tile, linoleum, or bathtub give it access to an empty litter box.
      F. Put litterbox in a location the cat prefers; then if cats resumes use,
         gradually move the litterbox to a location convenient for both owner
         and cat.
 III. Decrease the attractiveness of location cat has chosen to eliminate.
      A. Change significance of location by making area a feeding or play station.

B. Make entire area aversive by using repellent.
C. Alter substrate surface where cat has chosen to eliminate.
   Cover with plastic, aluminum foil, newspaper, water (tubs or sinks); or if cat prefers smooth surfaces, cover with newspaper or blanket. Gradually remove covering over a period of several months.
D. Clean area well with cleaning compounds that do not contain ammonia.

AGGRESSION TOWARDS PEOPLE

Play Aggression

I. Diagnosis
   A. Either male or female cats that are usually under 3 years of age (often less that 1 year of age).
   B. Usually in households without other cats
   C. May scratch and bite (inhibited but not completely) one or more persons in the household.
   D. Situations that often elicit the attacks are walking up and down stairs, entering a room, stepping out of the shower, and so forth.
   E. Often associated with stalking, pouncing, hopping sideways, and appearing as a "Halloween cat"
   F. The injury inflicted is usually not severe unless the person is a child or elderly.
   G. If not stopped, the intensity of the aggression may escalate
II. Treatment
   A. A combined approach of redirecting the active play to appropriate objects and immediately and consistently punishing the cat when it attacks a person
   B. If an attack can be predicted, the owner might redirect play prior to onset of an incident—by throwing a ball down the steps, and so forth
   C. Throughout the day, other activities should be initiated that encourage active play.
   D. If punishment is immediately and consistently administered, it need only be used two or three times. Loud sounds such as a foghorn or siren are usually effective.

Redirected Aggression

I. Diagnosis
   Redirected aggression can be exhibited by cats of either sex and is not age-related. It involves biting or scratching a person who has interfered or interrupted the cat in an aggressive mood, e.g., when the cat is threatening or fighting another cat.

II. Treatment

A. Treatment involves avoiding disturbance of the cat when it is in aggressive state.

B. The owner should wait before touching or picking up a cat that is or has recently demonstrated agitation until the cat exhibits a neutral or unaggressive behavior such as grooming or eating.

C. Identify and treat the cause of the primary aggressive behavior.

Idiopathic, Serious, and Repeated Aggressive Attacks

I. Such aggressive attacks are rare, may be exhibited by males or females, and are not age-related. There does not appear to be any eliciting stimulus and the behavior is not accompanied by signals of play, and the like. The behavior usually involves severe, *repeated* scratching, growling, and biting of a person; sometimes even chasing the person.

II. Some of these episodes may be psychomotor seizures, and might respond to antiepileptic medication. However, to date, psychomotor epilepsy has not been definitely confirmed as the etiology of these serious attacks. The author is not aware of any successful treatment of this type of aggression and considers it dangerous to keep cats with this problem.

AGGRESSION TOWARD CATS

Intermale Aggression

I. Diagnosis

A. Yelling, yowling, scratching, hissing, and attacking other male cats usually accompanied by ritualized threat displays.

B. Usually develops sometime after sexual maturity, at 2 or 3 years of age.

II. Treatment

A. Castration has a 90% probability of stopping or reducing this behavior regardless of the age of the cat or duration of the problem.

B. Progestin therapy may also suppress this behavior at the same dosage used to treat spraying behavior. A change in this behavior is usually drug-dependent and will resume when drug is withdrawn.

Territorial Aggression

I. Diagnosis

A. Threats, scratching, and biting directed towards a new cat being introduced, a former cat being reintroduced into a home, or when one cat in a household reaches behavioral maturity (2 or 3 years of age)

B. May be exhibited by males or females

C. Generally involves one cat seeking out and harassing the other cat

D. If it involves cats that have previously lived together amicably, the onset is usually slow; one cat taking the role of the offensive aggressor and the other cat simply trying to avoid the aggressive cat.
II. Treatment
A. Not easily treated
B. Tedious counterconditioning and habituation techniques may be effective
C. Drug therapies are not usually effective.
D. These cats are often friendly toward people and can make excellent pets in households where they are the only cat.

Fear or Defensive Aggression

I. Diagnosis
A. Usually of sudden onset toward another cat in the household
B. May be exhibited by males or females and is not age-related
C. The cats do not seek each other out as do territorially aggressive cats but rather assume a defensive aggressive attitude (ears back, body hunched, piloerection) whenever they accidentally run into each other.
D. The initiating causes are not always known but frequently involve an initial misinterpretation of the other cat's intentions.
II. Treatment
A. Desensitization and/or counterconditioning are usually effective.
B. Until the problem is resolved, the cats should be isolated from each other except during treatment sessions.

INGESTIVE BEHAVIOR PROBLEMS

Grass or Plant Eating

I. Grass and plant eating appear to be normal behaviors of cats. The behavior is not sex or age-related.
II. Providing the cat with its own plants or grass may decrease its grazing behavior on the owner's greenery.
III. Immediate and consistent punishment with a loud noise or splashing with water may help, however, the most effective solution is to prohibit the cat's access to forbidden plants. Toxic plants should always be kept out of reach.

Pica

I. Chewing and ingesting nonfood items, particularly wool and cloth, is not uncommon in Siamese and Siamese-crosses. It can be exhibited by males and females and is not known to be age-related.
II. Treatment techniques that *might* work are immediate punishment and sab-

otaging the items with aversive-tasting substances, but generally these techniques are not highly effective. Prohibiting the cat's access to all tempting materials is the only sure way to prevent consumption.

Play

The most common reason cats are presented for overactive behavior is simply the result of exuberant play.

I. Diagnosis
  A. Can be exhibited by males or females usually less than 3 years of age.
  B. Often occurs in households where
    1. The owner does not actively initiate play.
    2. The cat is frequently confined for long periods of time.
    3. It is the only cat in the household.
  C. Involves running, knocking things over, dashing to and from the owner, and so forth.
II. Treatment
  A. Provide ample and appropriate opportunity for sufficient activity and play.
  B. Perhaps take the cat outside to play.
  C. Initiate play with movable toys.
  D. Acquire another friendly, playful cat as a companion for the problem cat.

Hyperthyroidism

I. Diagnosis
   Physical signs are often excessive nervousness, dyspnea, weight loss, ravenous appetite, easily palpable enlarged thyroid gland, cardiac abnormalities, and other signs of a disease disorder. Occurs in both male and female cats and usually in older cats.
II. Treatment
   See Chapter 19.

Attention-Seeking Behaviors

I. Diagnosis
  A. Male or female cats
  B. Not age-related
  C. Meowing or otherwise pestering the owner until he or she gets up or moves
  D. Usually occurs early in the morning before the owner arises
  E. May be play behavior and/or a food-seeking behavior

II. Treatment

Treatment involves one or more of the following

A. Punishment and/or ignoring the behavior

B. Shift feeding schedule to another time of day so the cat is not immediately rewarded for disturbing the owner.

EXCESSIVE GROOMING BEHAVIORS

Disease or Dermatologic Condition.
See Chapter 21.

Displacement Activity

I. General Comments

The most common form of displacement activity exhibited by animals, when they are in a conflict situation, is grooming. A cat may excessively lick or pull out its hair.

II. Diagnosis

A. Not sex or age-related

B. The history should support the existence of a conflict situation.

III. Treatment

A. The preferred method of treatment is to
1. Identify the anxiety-eliciting stimulus.
2. Desensitize or countercondition the cat to the stimulus.
3. Alter the environment such that the animal is not kept in an anxiety-producing situation.

B. Antianxiety drugs, such as amitriptyline HCl (5–10 mg per cat per day PO) or progestins (dosage as for spraying cats) may also be helpful. Clinicians should be familiar with potential side effects and contraindications.

"Claw sharpening"

I. Diagnosis.

"Claw sharpening" is not sex- or age-related. It is usually directed toward furniture, carpets, draperies, owner's clothing, and so forth. Scratching serves a function of removing old sheaths from claws and perhaps as a visual marking behavior.

II. Treatment

A. Provide the cat with its own scratching post or scratching materials. It may be necessary to encourage the cat to use the provided scratching post.

B. Punish if discovered scratching on inappropriate items—sounds such as foghorns or water are sufficient aversive stimuli. Punishment techniques may only work when the owner is present.

C. Declaw the cat. The author is not aware of any evidence that indicates declawing is psychologically harmful to cats. Cats continue to engage in "claw sharpening" and other behaviors after declawing that they engaged in prior to declawing. While engaging in such behaviors the cats do not appear to be "distressed" or "frustrated."

BEHAVIOR PROBLEMS IN DOGS

ELIMINATION

General Comments

I. When a dog is urinating and/or defecating in the home, the possibility of disease processes should be explored by using the appropriate laboratory tests, history interviews, and physical examinations. If a dog is both urinating and defecating in the house, disease processes are usually not the etiology of the problem.

II. A dog may eliminate in the home because it is not housebroken, is marking, exhibiting a submissive gesture, or as a consequence of excitement, fear, or separation anxiety. A correct differential diagnosis is necessary prior to initiating appropriate treatment techniques. On the whole, punishment does not work well in treating elimination behavior problems. Only if the animal is caught in the act of eliminating would it be appropriate to punish the dog, and then only if the problem was unrelated to fear or submissive responses. The observation that dogs "only look guilty when they have done something wrong" can be explained more parsimoniously; the dog assumes a submissive or fearful expression only when two stimuli are simultaneously present (feces or urine and owner) because it has learned to anticipate punishment in such a context.

Urinating

I. Disease process

II. Urine-marking

A. Diagnosis

This involves leg-lifting behavior in the home by male dogs after they have reached sexual maturity. It is usually unrelated to the presence or absence of the owner, although it may be initiated by specific stimuli such as entrance of the owner into the home or entrance of a visitor; it usually involves small amounts of urine.

B. Treatment

1. Castration has a 50% probability of decreasing this behavior in male dogs regardless of the age of dog or duration of the problem.

2. Progestins may also suppress urine-marking. The recommended in-

itial dose is 1.0–2.2 mg/kg for 1 week followed by a decrease of the dose to the smallest amount necessary to control the problem. The clinician should be familiar with the side effects of progestin therapy, take appropriate monitoring precautions and periodically cease drug therapy. (See section on Potential Side Effects of Progestin Therapy in general section Behavioral Problems in Cats, above.)

3. Consistently and immediately punishing the dog *when it begins to urine-mark* may prevent the dog from urine-marking in the presence of the owner. If the dog only urine marks in a few locations, teaching it to avoid or prohibit access to these areas may prevent urine-marking.

4. Behavior modification

    If specific stimuli that elicit urine marking can be identified, the dog could be counterconditioned to engage in alternative behaviors during those circumstances.

III. Submissive urination

A. Diagnosis

   This behavior is frequently exhibited by puppies although it can also extend into young adulthood. Both males and females may engage in this behavior. It usually occurs during a greeting situation or when a person reaches toward the animal. The urinating is generally accompanied by submissive postures of lowered head, ears back, tail down, and even rolling over on the side.

B. Treatment

1. Ignore the behavior—either reward or punishment may facilitate the behavior.

2. Avoid the eliciting stimulus, i.e., do not reach for the dog or greet it immediately upon entry.

3. Redirect the dog's greeting behavior to play. For example, as the owner enters, he or she can throw a ball and switch the animal from a greeting mode to a play mode.

4. Construct a desensitization or counterconditioning program during which the dog is conditioned to assume a standing and nonurinating posture in situations that elicited the behavior.

5. Punishment is contraindicated.

IV. Excitement urination

A. Diagnosis

   Some dogs, either males or females of any age, urinate when they become excited. The dog may still be in a standing position. The behavior often occurs in a greeting or playing context.

B. Treatment

1. Avoid the eliciting stimuli if possible.

2. Desensitize or countercondition the animal's response to the eliciting stimuli.

3. Do not associate punishment or reinforcements with this behavior.

V. Housebreaking

Housebreaking problems generally involve both urination and defecation. Diagnosis and treatment procedures are described in the section Urination and Defecation in the Home, below.

VI. Separation anxiety

Separation anxiety is often accompanied by urination and/or defecation. Diagnosis and treatment is discussed in the section Urination and Defecation in the Home, below.

VII. Fear-induced elimination behavior

Animals frequently urinate and/or defecate in response to a fear-eliciting stimulus. Treatment is desensitization and counterconditioning. Antianxiety drugs may temporarily alleviate or reduce the fear response.

Defecation

I. Disease

II. Marking

Dogs rarely mark with feces, although this behavior is occasionally seen in outdoor situations. Feces-marking is usually performed by male dogs and the feces are deposited on an obvious landmark or object such as against a tree or on the tops of bushes or fenceposts. No treatment techniques have been developed for treating defecation-marking behaviors in the dog.

III. Fear-induced elimination

A. Diagnosis

Defecation as part of a fear response may be exhibited by males or females of any age. It is accompanied by other manifestations or expressions of fear—e.g., ears down, head down, pacing, salivating, hyperventilation, expression of anal sacs, and so forth. The behavior is frequently elicited by stimuli such as punishment, loud noises (particularly thunderstorms), strangers, and the like.

B. Treatment

Treatment involves identifying the eliciting stimuli and then desensitization and counterconditioning. Punishment is contraindicated.

IV. Housebreaking—see section Urination and Defecation in the Home, below.

V. Separation anxiety—see section Urination and Defecation in the Home, below.

Urination and Defecation in the Home

I. Disease—rarely the cause for both problems

II. Fear-induced behavior. See section on Fear-Induced Elimination, above.

III. Housebreaking

A. Diagnosis

1. Housebreaking problems are generally manifested by both urination

and defecation and can be exhibited by either males or females at any age.

2. These dogs often have a history of eliminating in the house since puppyhood.
3. The behavior is usually unrelated to the presence or absence of the owner.
4. The behavior is related to the length of time since the dog last had access to an appropriate place to eliminate.
5. The urine and/or feces may be found in one or more locations in the house.
6. Large amounts, as opposed to small spots, of urine are voided at a time.

B. Treatment

Treatment involves a combination of one or more of the following housebreaking techniques:

1. Supervising the dog when it is unrestricted in the home in order to detect when it appears to need to eliminate and then immediately taking it to an appropriate place.
2. Frequently taking the dog outside so it can develop a preference for eliminating outdoors.
3. When the dog cannot be supervised, restrict the dog's access to large amounts of space, particularly if the dog has not recently been outdoors or had an opportunity to eliminate in an appropriate location.
4. If the dog is observed eliminating in the house, immediate punishment in the form of scolding, yelling, or a loud noise, is appropriate. Punishment after the dog has eliminated is counterproductive.
5. Rewarding the dog with praise or tidbits when it eliminates in an appropriate place may help.
6. If the behavior is very location-specific, preventing access to or repelling the dog from that area may solve the problem.

IV. Separation anxiety
A. Diagnosis
1. Urination and/or defecation occurs when the dog is prevented access to its owner. This can occur when the owner departs for work or simply is separated from the dog at home by a door or barrier.
2. Both males and females exhibit this behavior and it can occur at any age.
3. The behavior may occur within minutes of separation—usually within 30 minutes.
4. These dogs may be very well housebroken. The manifestation of this problem is unrelated to the length of time since the last elimination. The dog will eliminate regardless of whether it has recently eliminated outside prior to the owner's departure.
5. These dogs usually show signs of distress as the owner prepares to depart. They follow the owner closely, pant, pace, salivate, and sometimes even tremble.

    6. The dog usually does not eat anything while the owner is away.

    7. When the owner returns, the dog often exhibits an exceedingly exuberant and prolonged greeting.

    8. While the owner is home, the dog often follows him or her from room to room, leaning against and staying as close as possible to the person.

    9. Histories of these dogs often reveal that they were rarely left alone as they grew up, have recently spent several weeks or months in constant contact with owner, were acquired as adults after having been in a kennel or a shelter for abandoned animals, or had been found as strays.

  B. Treatment

    Treatment involves gradually getting the dog used to being alone without being distressed.

    1. Gradual exposure or desensitization and counterconditioning techniques that modify the dog's response to specific stimuli related to departure—rattling of car keys, and the like and length of time the owner departs

    2. Antianxiety medication is often helpful, either alone or in combination with behavior modification techniques. Drugs that have been found helpful are amitriptyline HCl at 1.1–2.2 mg/kg PO and megestrol acetate at 1.1–2.2 mg/kg PO. Medication should be given an hour prior to departure. If there is a positive response the dog should be medicated at the initial dosage for 1–2 weeks and then the drug is gradually withdrawn over a period of 4–6 weeks. The clinician should be familiar with the side effects and contraindications to the use of these drugs. It is advisable for owners to first try the medication when they will be home for the entire day, in order to observe potential side effects.

EXCESSIVE VOCALIZATION

Separation Anxiety

  I. Separation anxiety may be manifested by howling, whining, or barking at the time of the owner's departure or shortly thereafter. Occasionally dogs with separation anxiety vocalize several hours later, but this is rare.

  II. The diagnosis and treatment of separation anxiety are outlined in the section on Elimination, above.

Reaction to Specific Eliciting Stimuli

  I. Diagnosis

    A. Some dogs bark excessively to certain stimuli such as mailmen, airplanes, persons passing by, and so on. This may be an arousal response or a combination of some protective or fearful behaviors.

    B. The behavior may be self-reinforcing.

    C. Occasionally, excessive vocalization is facilitated by the barking or howling of other dogs.

II. Treatment

    A. Treatment is to identify the stimuli that elicit the excessive vocalizations and then countercondition the animal's response.

    B. If fear is not part of the response, punishment might be effective. Common forms of punishment are water administered via a hose, an electric shock collar activated by barking, or simply scolding or startling the animal whenever it barks. For punishment to be effective, if should be administered immediately at the onset every time the animal engages in the behavior. If bark-activated electric shock collars are used, the owners should be certain nothing else in the vicinity will trigger the shock, that the collar works appropriately, and that there is not a negative feedback loop of bark, shock, yelp, shock, yelp, and so forth.

    C. Punishment is not an effective way to treat any type of barking that is related to anxiety or fear.

    D. Debarking is another procedure to be considered, particularly if eliciting stimuli cannot be identified or controlled and/or the dog cannot otherwise be treated.

Play Behavior

    I. Vocalization is often part of play behavior

  II. Play behavior can occur at any age, but is generally exhibited by younger animals.

 III. Play vocalizations are usually accompanied by play postures such as the "play bow," "happy face," and so forth.

 IV. Circumstances which elicit play should be identified and the animal counterconditioned or trained to terminate play behavior at the owner's request.

  V. The owner should not continue to unwittingly reward the animal for vocalizations by giving in and paying attention to it.

Fearful Behavior

    I. Vocalization elicited by fear can be identified by the facial and body expressions of the animal while it is vocalizing.

  II. Treatment involves identifying the eliciting stimuli and then desensitization and counterconditioning.

Aggression

Some forms of aggression are accompanied by excessive barking. The type of aggression must be identified by the facial and body expressions of the animal and the context in which the aggression occurs. Depending on the type of aggression (see section on Aggressive Behavior, below) treatment may be instituted.

Reinforcement

I. Many dogs bark because it gets attention, gives them access to indoors, brings the owner at a run, and the like.
II. If barking is being reinforced, treatment involves extinction or counter-conditioning. If fear is not part of the problem, extinction combined with punishment may be appropriate.

DESTRUCTIVE BEHAVIOR—CHEWING AND DIGGING

Separation Anxiety

I. Diagnosis
   A. One of the most common reasons an animal engages in destructive chewing and digging is separation anxiety.
   B. Destruction is often directed at items in the direction of the owner's departure, such as doors and windows.
   C. The diagnostic histories are described in the section on Elimination, above. The treatment would be the same as for separation anxiety expressed in excessive vocalization or elimination. Crating the dog is usually contraindicated because these dogs often injure themselves if so confined.

Fearful Behavior

I. Diagnosis
   A. Males and females of any age may manifest destructive behavior as a part of a phobic response.
   B. The behavior is diagnosed by the facial and body expressions of the animal which are usually paired with a specific class of stimuli. The destructive behavior is often exaggerated when the owner is not there.
II. Treatment
   A. The stimuli that elicit the phobic response must be identified and the animal must then be desensitized and counterconditioned.
   B. High levels of antianxiety drugs, such as diazepam at 1.1–2.2 mg/kg often suppress but do not completely eliminate phobic responses of dogs.

Play

I. Diagnosis
   A. Destruction or digging may be part of play behavior.
   B. This behavior is exhibited by both sexes and usually by dogs less than 2 years old.
   C. The destruction is often directed to objects that are easy to pull apart or shred and objects that permit shaking.

D. It may occur in the presence or absence of the owner, and often occurs when the dog does have access to the owner but is not being attended to.

II. Treatment

A. Ensure an adequate amount of exercise

B. Appropriate play items should be available and the dog encouraged to play with them.

C. In addition to redirecting the play, punishment might also be incorporated in the treatment program. Inappropriate objects can be "booby trapped," or if the animal is caught in the act of chewing or digging, it can be disciplined. Punishment by itself usually does not correct a play behavior problem but it may facilitate correction of it.

D. Puppies may need to be restricted to areas where they do not have access to forbidden objects until they grow older. As they demonstrate their ability to leave inappropriate objects alone, they can be allowed access to larger and more complex areas.

OVERACTIVITY

Play Behavior

I. Diagnosis

By far the most common reason dogs are overactive is because of play and/or reinforcement from the owner. Play behavior can be exhibited by males and females and generally is manifested by dogs under 2 years of age. Common histories include lack of exercise, confinement to small areas, and reinforcement by the owner of the exuberant behavior.

II. Treatment

A. Avoid reinforcing the behavior.

B. Allow ample opportunity for active exercise.

C. Countercondition the animal to assume quiet behaviors in circumstances in which it exhibits overactivity.

D. Drugs are not an appropriate method of treating this behavior.

Hyperkinesis

I. Diagnosis

Hyperkinesis is a physiologic disorder characterized by overactivity, intolerance of restraint, inability to learn to sit and stay, and lack of response to tranquilizers such as the phenothiazines and meprobamate. Physiologic signs include elevated heart and respiratory rates, and increased oxygen consumption. Hyperkinesis is not a common finding in dogs.

II. Treatment
  A. Methylphenidate: 2–4 mg/kg PO
  B. Dextroamphetamine: 0.2–1.3 mg/kg PO
  C. Levoamphetamine: 1.0–4.0 mg/kg PO
  D. The dogs generally resume a hyperactive state in the absence of the drug therapy.
  E. Hyperkinetic dogs can be overdosed with amphetamines. Excessive dosage of amphetamines to either normal or hyperkinetic dogs results in an increase of activity, stereotypic behaviors (nonsensical, repetitive behaviors such as circling or running backwards), anorexia, hyperthermia, and convulsions. Amphetamine poisoning has been reported to be treatable with 0.1–1.0 mg/kg of acetylpromazine maleate IM, immersion in cold water, and if necessary, barbiturate anesthesia.

Hyperthyroidism

I. Diagnosis
  Hyperthyroidism in the dog is often accompanied by clinical signs of polydypsia, loss of body weight, and polyphagia as well as other signs in proportion to the severity and duration of the hyperthyroid condition. These may include cardiac abnormalities. Increased activity level is not always associated with hyperthyroidism; in fact, such dogs are often weak and lethargic. See Chapter 19.
II. Treatment
  See Chapter 19.

Breed Predisposition for High Activity Levels

I. Diagnosis
  A high and prolonged activity level has been selected for in various hunting breeds such as pointers and setters. This level of activity is not related to hyperkinesis or hyperthyroidism, nor is it directly related to excessive play or reinforcement.
II. Treatment
  A. Sufficient exercise.
  B. Training the animal to inhibit itself on command.
  C. Sometimes confining the dog in circumstances when it is likely to be active but cannot be supervised.

Separation Anxiety

I. Diagnosis
  A. Sometimes the presenting complaint by owners of dogs with separation anxiety is that of overactivity. These dogs engage in prolonged and ex-

treme activity at the time of the owner's return—running and dashing through the house, excessively pestering the owner and so forth.
  B. Diagnosis is made from the history and/or observation of dog at time of departure and ways the dog relates to the person throughout the day while at home. See section on Diagnosis of Separation Anxiety, above.
II. Treatment
  A. Redirecting the behavior or counterconditioning the dog at the time of owner's return.
  B. If necessary, treating it as other separation anxiety cases.

EXCESSIVE GROOMING AND SELF-LICKING

Disease/Pathophysiology

  I. Dermatologic conditions
 II. Phantom pain—referred or residual effect of an injury.

Displacement Activity

  I. Grooming is a common form of displacement activity exhibited by animals when they are in a conflict or anxiety-producing situation.
 II. Separation anxiety
      Some dogs with separation anxiety will excessively lick or nibble on their legs when left alone. Diagnostic features and treatment of separation anxiety are delineated in the section on Separation Anxiety, above.
III. Other stressors
  A. Identify stressors (e.g., other animals or people in the household, and so forth) that may be producing anxiety.
  B. Either eliminate stressors that are producing anxiety or desensitize and countercondition the dog's response to these stimuli.
  C. Antianxiety drugs such as amitriptyline, progestins, benzodiazepines, or phenobarbital may reduce anxiety and consequently also alleviate the excessive licking.

Flank-Sucking

  I. This behavior is almost exclusively demonstrated by Doberman pinschers. It is not sex- or age-related.
 II. The dog grabs its flank with its mouth. It may remain that way for a few seconds to several hours.
III. The behavior is often brought on by an exciting stimulus, such as a person entering the room.
IV. Rarely do these dogs inflict any injury to themselves.
  V. There is no known treatment.

FEARS AND PHOBIAS

General Comments

I. A *phobia* is an excessive fear response that is out of proportion to the real threat of the stimulus. The behaviors the dog engages in are often detrimental; excessive vocalization, pacing, panting, hyperventilation, digging, escape behaviors (including jumping through windows, digging through doors or ceilings), shivering, and sometimes collapsing into flaccid paralysis.

II. The method of treatment of any fear is for the animal to experience the fear-eliciting stimulus without being afraid. This can be accomplished via gradual desensitization, counterconditioning, or flooding. Antianxiety medication may also help an animal to experience a phobic situation without being afraid; however, generalization to the nondrug state does not always occur.

Fear of Noises

I. Diagnosis

Noise phobias are not sex or age-related; they generally get progressively worse and generalize to other similar stimuli. Dogs are often afraid of thunderstorms, firecrackers, or similar noises.

II. Treatment
   A. Identify the eliciting stimuli.
   B. Be able to replicate the stimulus in order to use in treatment sessions.
   C. Desensitization and counterconditioning
   D. Flooding
   E. Drug therapy—0.5–1.0 mg/kg PO of diazepam frequently suppresses phobic responses to thunderstorms.

Fear of People

I. Diagnosis

This behavior can occur in either males or females of any breed and at any age. It is diagnosed by observing facial and body expressions indicative of fear. In addition to fearful body expressions, the dog might also manifest aggression or submissive urination.

II. Treatment
   A. Identify the eliciting stimulus
   B. Present the stimulus to the dog on a gradient and desensitize and countercondition the dog's response.
   C. Flooding
   D. Avoid reinforcing the fearful behavior with petting and praise.
   E. If at all possible, the fearful stimulus should be avoided between treatment sessions until the dog has demonstrated it can tolerate that level

of stimulus intensity. The prognosis is usually good following treatment of this behavior disorder.

AGGRESSIVE BEHAVIOR

General Comments

I. Aggression can be manifested by biting, snapping, nipping, growling, baring the teeth, and barking. Aggression is not a unitary phenomenon; there are many reasons and different physiologic states that predispose to aggression. To maximize the probability of successful treatment of aggression, a functional classification is essential.

II. Owners should always be advised that there is never a guarantee that treatment will completely eliminate the dog's aggressive behavior. Appropriate treatment generally reduces the frequency and intensity of the aggression, but not always to zero. The owner must assess whether or not the benefit is worth the potential risk. The reader is referred to other textbooks that discuss aggression in greater detail (see Suggested Readings).

Intermale Aggression

I. Diagnosis
   A. This involves aggression directed by one male dog to another.
   B. Onset is usually between 1 and 3 years of age.
   C. The aggression may occur regardless of the distance between dogs, or only when one dog approaches within a critical distance of the other.
   D. Generally, the body and facial expressions are indicative of dominance but there may be a superimposition of fear. Many of these dogs are ambivalent.

II. Treatment
   A. Castration
      1. Castration has a 62% probability of reducing aggressive behavior between male dogs.
      2. It is more likely to be effective if both males involved are castrated.
   B. Progestin therapy
      1. Synthetic progestins can also suppress intermale aggression at doses of 1.0–2.0 mg/kg of megestrol acetate or 10.0 mg/kg/IM or SQ of repository medroxyprogesterone acetate.
      2. Unless the dog is counterconditioned to assume an unaggressive behavior in the presence of other male dogs, the aggressive behavior will gradually return as the drugs are withdrawn.
      3. Clinicians should be familiar with the potential side effects and contraindications of progestin therapy. Elevated serum glucose levels, diabetes, and mammary gland hyperplasia are the most likely side effects to occur. The probability of developing diabetes is age-re-

lated—the older the animal the more likely it is to develop a problem. Progestins will also suppress spermatogenesis although libido and spermatogenesis should return when progestin therapy ceases. It is advisable to obtain a baseline glucose value prior to treatment and thereafter monitor the patient periodically. (See section on Progestin Therapy in general section Behavioral Problems in Cats, above.)

C. Counterconditioning. The dog can be trained to assume a nonaggressive or immobile stance when encountering other male dogs.

D. Prohibit access to other male dogs when not under supervision.

E. Finding a new, separate home for one of the aggressive dogs is always an alternative. A dog aggressive toward other dogs can make a perfectly fine pet in a household without other dogs. These dogs do not necessarily manifest aggression toward people.

Interfemale Aggression

I. Diagnosis
  A. This is aggressive behavior directed by one female dog toward another.
  B. It may involve dominant gestures or dominant/fearful postures.
  C. Onset of the behavior is usually between 1 and 3 years of age.
II. Treatment
  A. Spaying is not likely to affect this behavior unless the aggression is related to the estrous cycle of the dog.
  B. Countercondition the dog to assume a nonaggressive attitude in circumstances known to precipitate aggression.
  C. Maintain the dogs separately.
  D. Find one of the dogs a new home. This aggression is not directed to people.
  E. Progestin therapy is unlikely to suppress interfemale aggression.

Parental Aggression

I. Diagnosis
  Parental aggression may be exhibited by the mother of a litter of puppies or by other adult dogs in the household when a lactating bitch and her puppies are approached by other dogs or people.
II. Treatment
  A. Avoid eliciting the aggressive encounters.
  B. Countercondition the animal to assume a nonaggressive attitude in situations likely to elicit aggression.

Aggression Related to Pseudocyesis

I. General comments
  A bitch in false pregnancy, or *pseudocyesis*, may suddenly begin exhibiting protective behavior of nesting areas, surrogate puppies, or small alien

animals. She may or may not show physical signs of false pregnancy such as distended abdomen, engorged uterus, development of mammary glands, and/or lactation. Interestingly, other dogs in the household may also protect a bitch in pseudocyesis from people or other dogs.

II. Diagnosis

Diagnosis is based on sudden onset of signs 6–8 weeks postestrus, behaviors associated with false pregnancy, and physical signs of false pregnancy.

III. Treatment

A. Avoid eliciting the aggressive behavior.

B. Countercondition.

C. To prevent recurrence of the problem, spay the dog after cessation of false pregnancy.

D. Drug therapy

1. Megestrol acetate at 2 mg/kg PO for 5–7 days administered immediately after the onset of false pregnancy is reported to be effective 80% of the time in shortening or terminating the false pregnancy cycle.

2. Androgens are currently recommended in the treatment of pseudocyesis (see chapter 20).

3. Bromocriptine, a dopamine agonist, is used to treat hypergalactia in human patients and may be an effective treatment for false pregnancy. Emesis is a side effect of bromocriptine administration.

4. Drugs that inhibit or antagonize dopamine (dopamine is a prolactin-inhibiting factor) are likely to enhance the pseudocyesis phenomenon. Such drugs include the phenothiazines and butyrophenones.

Pain-Induced Aggression

I. Diagnosis

This aggressive behavior is not sex- or age-related. The aggression is usually directed toward a person who attempts to groom, medicate, touch, manipulate, or even approach a painful area. The onset may be sudden or gradual and is related to a disease process or injury.

II. Treatment

A. Treat the etiology of the painful disorder.

B. Avoid eliciting pain.

C. Countercondition the animal to exhibit nonaggressive behaviors when approached.

D. Painful punishment is contraindicated.

Redirected Aggression

I. Diagnosis

This type of aggression may be directed toward people or other animals. It occurs in situations where the dog is motivated to manifest aggression toward a target but is inhibited or prevented from attacking it. Instead, the dog, either male or female and of any age, may turn and attack a person or other animal nearby. When aggression is directed toward a person, it is often an indication that the dog is also dominant toward that individual. If so, the possibility of dominance aggression should always be explored.

II. Treatment.
    A. Avoid directly interfering in aggressive situations.
    B. Treat the cause of the initial aggression.
    C. If relevant, increase the dominant status of the person in the household relative to the dog.

Predatory Aggression

I. General comments
    This aggressive behavior is often accompanied by a chase, predatory stalking, and behaviors associated with hunting. The aggression may be directed toward animals or people and is frequently elicited by quick-moving stimuli. It can be exhibited by males or females and is not age-related; although there are histories of bitches who instigated predation of livestock when their puppies reached 3–4 months of age. Occasionally an attack of a person may be initiated because of territorial or protective aggression; however, once the attack ensues, it can lead to predatory aggression, killing, and actual consumption of flesh of the person.

II. Treatment
    A. *Confinement.* This is the most reliable prevention of predatory aggression.
    B. Punishment such as shock delivered by remote control might be effective if the predatory chase is not pack-facilitated.
    C. "Garcia effect" (inducing nausea after consumption of prey) is unlikely to inhibit the predatory chase and kill.
    D. Counterconditioning (training the dog to inhibit itself when it sees a predatory prey stimulus) is usually only effective if the owner is present.

Fear-Induced Aggression

I. Diagnosis.
    This aggressive behavior can be directed toward dogs or people, is equally exhibited by males and females, and is not age-related. It is diagnosed by concurrent fearful body and facial expression. Some dogs with fear-induced aggression are inhibited when people face them but will bite when the person passes or turns away.

II. Treatment (Also see section on Fears and Phobias, above.)
    A. Identify the fear-eliciting stimuli.
    B. Desensitize and countercondition.
    C. Flooding
    D. Avoid punishment.

Protective and Territorial Aggression

I. Diagnosis

Such aggressive behavior is often accompanied by piloerection. It is often manifested toward people or other animals when they approach another person, animal, or area that the dog is motivated to defend. It can be exhibited by males or females and usually develops after 9 months of age.

II. Treatment
   A. Castration or spaying is unlikely to affect this behavior.
   B. Prohibiting access to the vulnerable target is the most effective means of preventing injury.
   C. Countercondition (train the animal to assume a nonaggressive stance). However, since the presence of the owner is part of the training process, the dog is still likely to manifest its aggressive behavior when the owner is absent.
   D. Punishment might help suppress this behavior, however, it should be used in conjunction with counterconditioning.
   E. Some breeds are more predisposed than others to exhibiting this behavior.
   F. Protective and territorial dogs are often ambivalent and may also show signs of fear.

Aggression Over Food

I. Diagnosis

This aggressive behavior is directed toward animals or people when either approaches the dog in possession of food. It may be exhibited by males or females and is not age-related. It is not necessarily related to dominance; however, it is often one of the circumstances in which a dominant dog exhibits aggression.

II. Treatment
   A. The most effective treatment is to countercondition the dog to assume a nonaggressive stance as it is approached.
   B. Punishment, in the form of scolding or grabbing the dog by the muzzle and neck, might be effective if applied when the animal first begins exhibiting the behaviors.
   C. Painful punishment often exacerbates the problem and instigates fear-induced aggression.

Dominance Aggression

I. Diagnosis
   A. This is one of the most common forms of aggression presented to the behavioral therapist.
   B. It is generally exhibited by intact, purebred male dogs, and occurs at 2–2.5 years of age.

C. The behavior is usually described as sudden, unprovoked, aggressive attacks; however, a detailed history usually reveals that the aggression had a gradual onset and that the dog is aggressive in a number of circumstances.

D. Circumstances in which dominant dogs frequently manifest aggression are
1. If disturbed while resting: either being awakened or while being physically displaced and/or ordered from a resting place
2. When a person approaches food, an estrous bitch, a "favorite person," or the dog's resting area, (even if the dog is not in it)
3. While being petted, restrained, being pushed against, being pushed into a down position, being rolled over, having collars or leashes put on or taken off, having the muzzle or back or neck held, being stared at, disciplined, or threatened, and/or meeting at a passageway
4. During grooming, toweling, or having its nails trimmed
5. When scolded, threatened, or physically disciplined

E. The dog often assumes dominant postures such as placing its feet on the owner, pressing its chin down on the shoulder or lap of the owner, staring at the owner, assuming a "stand-over" posture when the owner is in a recumbent position.

F. The dog may not be aggressive to all members of the family.

G. The dog often shows no aggression toward strangers.

II. Treatment
A. Primary goals of treatment are to avoid having a person injured and to get the dog to assume submissive and nonaggressive behaviors in circumstances that previously elicited aggression.

B. All stimuli or situations known to elicit the behavior should be identified and avoided in order to prevent the dog from reinforcing its dominance stance as well as to prevent injury. Gradually the dog should be put into these situations while it exhibits nonaggressive behavior.

C. The dog should be slowly habituated or counterconditioned to assume nonaggressive behaviors while the owner engages in dominant gestures such as touching, pushing, pulling on the dog, approaching the dog, holding its muzzle, and so forth.

D. Progestin therapy frequently suppresses dominance aggression exhibited by both male and female dogs. Clinicians should be familiar with contraindications to use of progestin therapy. (See section on Progestin Therapy in general section Behavioral Problems in Cats, above.) Megestrol acetate at 1.0–2.0 mg/kg PO or medroxyprogesterone acetate at 10 mg/kg IM or SQ appear to reduce the dog's motivation to be aggressive and allows behavior modification techniques to be implemented. In the author's experience, unless concurrent behavioral techniques are implemented, the aggression returns as the drug therapy is reduced.

E. Castration may be effective in reducing dominance aggression in some male dogs.

F. Physical punishment usually should be avoided in cases of long-standing aggression because it often escalates the aggression. If used at all, punishment should not be instigated until the frequency and intensity of aggression has been reduced. Immediate and consistent punishment (grabbing the muzzle, pushing the dog onto its side, or even hitting the dog) might be effective if used the first time the dog manifests aggressive dominance.

G. The use of remote control electric shock collars by specialists utilizing "safety training" methods is reportedly a highly effective mechanism of reversing dominance aggression; however, once the collar is removed there may be a regression of the problem.

H. Behavior modification procedures and drug therapy will usually reduce the frequency and intensity of dominance aggression but rarely eliminate the behavior completely. Therefore, the prognosis is guarded. Persons with small children in the household should be carefully advised of the risk in keeping such a dog.

I. Electroconvulsive therapy (ECT) may reduce or eliminate dominance aggression for a few months to several years. The effectiveness of ECT may be based on memory loss and the dog subsequently being subjugated to a lower social status. Subsequent behavioral procedures, such as described above, may help reduce the incidence of recurrence.

J. This behavior appears to have a genetic predisposition and may be passed on to subsequent generations. Dominance aggression appears more frequently in some families of purebred dogs than in others.

Aggression Toward Infants

I. Aggression is rarely directed toward small infants, but when it is it can be fatal. Aggression toward babies (1–90 days) is generally manifested by dogs that have not seen the child before or have had little contact with the child. The attack usually occurs in an unsupervised situation. The aggression is unlikely to be dominance-related, but is rather a predatory response.

II. Dogs should be gradually exposed to infants in controlled situations and allowed considerable contact with them under supervision.

Aggression Toward Small Children

I. Aggression toward small children (1.5–5 years of age) generally stems from fear or pain-elicited aggression and responds to desensitization and counterconditioning. The child should be restricted in his or her unsupervised access to the dog and should be taught to approach, touch, and pet the dog in an acceptable manner.

II. If a dog has shown no previous signs of aggression to adults, treatment of aggression toward small children that is related to fear is usually successful. Parents should of course be advised that they are responsible for the dog's behavior, and so forth.

III. Treatment should involve multiple visits to behavioral therapists, and the participation of conscientious and intelligent parents.

Aggression Related to Pathophysiologic Disorders

  I. Aggression related to disease processes usually does not fit the description of a normal species-typical behavior or an adaptive, learned behavior. The animal should show some evidence of concurrent neurologic or pathophysiologic signs.

 II. Epileptogenic drugs such as phenothiazines are likely to elicit the aggressive behavior.

III. Antiepileptic medication might suppress the behavior (see chapter 16.)

IV. There have been several reports of dogs that, when presented with food, growl, snap, and attack the air about them as well as anything else that may get in their way. This may be a psychomotor seizure elicited by food and sometimes other exciting stimuli. Occasionally this behavior will stop when the dogs are treated with antiepileptic drugs.

SUGGESTED READINGS

Rimm DC, Masters JC: Behavioral Therapy. Academic Press, New York, 1975

Voith VL: Behavioral problems. pp. 499–537. In Chandler EA, Sutton JB, Thompson DJ (eds): Canine Medicine and Therapeutics. Blackwell Scientific Publications, Oxford, 1984

Voith VL: Behavioral disorders. pp. 208–227. In Ettinger SJ (ed): Textbook of Veterinary Internal Medicine: Diseases of the Dog and Cat. Vol. 1. WB Saunders Co., Philadelphia, 1983

Voith VL, Burchelt PL (eds): Veterinary Clinics of North America. Small Animal Practice Vol. 1, No. 4. Symposium on Animal Behavior. WB Saunders Co., Philadelphia, 1982

18

Ophthalmic Diseases
William A. Vestre, D.V.M.

ORBIT

ORBITAL CELLULITIS AND RETROBULBAR
ABSCESS

I. General comments
   A. Orbital cellulitis is diffuse inflammation originating from within the orbit or it may be an extension from adjacent tissues.
   B. True abscessation is localized.
II. Clinical signs
   A. Abnormal position of eyeball
   B. Decreased ocular motility
   C. Chemosis and injection of conjunctiva
   D. Elevated membrana nictitans
   E. Blepharedema
   F. Periorbital pain
   G. Exposure keratitis
   H. Pain on opening the mouth
   I. Rapid onset of signs with severe pain and pyrexia are generally associated with a retrobulbar abscess.
III. Treatment
   A. Orbital cellulitis and abscess are treated similarly and often the distinction cannot be made until after the response to therapy has been evaluated.
   B. Establish ventral drainage.
      1. General anesthesia
      2. Incise oral mucosa 0.5–1 cm posterior to the last upper molar.
      3. Insert closed hemostat dorsally through the pterygoid muscle and open when the tip is positioned behind the globe.
      4. Avoid excessive trauma but establish adequate drainage.
      5. Flush with a solution containing a wide-spectrum antibiotic such as gentamicin or ampicillin.

   C. General therapy
      1. Administer ampicillin, gentamicin, or chloramphenicol systemically for 5–7 days.
      2. Apply hot packs to the orbital area three times daily for 3 days or until the swelling subsides.
      3. Protect the cornea and conjunctiva
         a) Ophthalmic antibiotic ointment several times a day
         b) Temporary tarrsoraphy
      4. If clinical signs do not resolve in 2 days, supplemental therapy with prednisolone (0.5 mg/kg SID) for 1 week is indicated.
   IV. Further diagnostic tests are indicated if signs recur within a few weeks.
      A. Radiography
      B. Cytology of aspirated material

TRAUMATIC PROPTOSIS OF THE GLOBE

   I. General comments
      A. Proptosis of the globe is dependent somewhat on conformational predisposition, e.g., brachycephalics, but in all cases indicates severe trauma necessitating rapid and thorough evaluation and treatment.
      B. Chemosis develops quickly and the eyelids are often turned in, thus trapping the globe outside the orbit.
   II. Evaluation
      A. The prognosis for vision is based on the presence of consensual and direct pupillary light reflexes and a normal-appearing retina and optic disk.
      B. A poor prognosis is given to animals with rupture of one or more extrinsic muscles, marked hyphema, scleral or corneal laceration, or retinal detachment.
      C. Absolute pupil size and the direct light response are not accurate prognostic indicators.
   III. Treatment
      A. Objectives
         1. Globe replacement
         2. Prevention and treatment of optic neuritis
         3. Protection of the ocular surface
         4. All proptosed globes without corneoscleral rupture should be repositioned
         5. Even if vision is lost the eye will be cosmetic and pain free.
      B. The anesthesia required will vary with the animal from only topical and local infiltration to general.
      C. Systemically atropinize the animal well before replacing the globe to prevent the oculocardiac reflex and severe bradycardia.
      D. Surgical procedures
         1. A lateral canthotomy is performed and the eyelids freed from the globe with a blunt muscle hook.

2. Preplace three horizontal mattress sutures of 3-0 or 4-0 silk in the eyelids 1–2 mm from the eyelid margin.
3. Replace the eye by pulling the eyelids forward with the sutures while applying gentle pressure on the globe.
4. Tuck the globe under the eyelids and tie sutures.
5. The lateral canthotomy is closed in two layers.
6. Keep the eyelids closed until swelling subsides (7–10 days).

E. Follow-up care
1. Hot packs are applied to the eye three times per day.
2. Systemic wide-spectrum antibiotics such as ampicillin are administered for 10 days.
3. Topical antibiotic and 1% atropine ophthalmic ointments are applied three times per day between the tarsorrhaphy sutures.
4. If corneal damage is minimal, topical corticosteroids may be used.
5. Systemic corticosteroids (0.5–1.0 mg/kg prednisone SID) are administered for 7 days to help control the traumatic optic neuritis.
6. If the cornea appears damaged when the eyelid sutures are removed or if lagophthalmos causes the cornea to remain dry, suture the membrana nictitans over the cornea for another 7–10 days.
7. If lagophthalmos is severe or persistent, perform a permanent lateral tarsorrhaphy to shorten the palpebral fissure.

EYELIDS

ANKYLOBLEPHARON

I. General comments
A. Ankyloblepharon or adhesion of the eyelid edges to each other is physiologic in dogs and cats up to 10–15 days of age.
B. If there is an associated infection (conjunctivitis neonatorum), excess swelling and a purulent discharge at the medial or lateral canthus will be noted. The infection is usually caused by *Staphylococci* sp. or *Escherichia coli* in puppies and by *Chlamydia* sp. or herpesvirus in kittens.

II. Treatment
A. The goal is to minimize corneal damage by opening the eyelids and cleansing the exudate from the conjunctival sac.
B. Usually the edges will separate with gentle traction or the use of a blunt instrument, e.g., muscle hook.
C. Incising with corneal scissors may be required in a few cases.
D. Culture and antibiotic sensitivity testing should be performed. Topical broad-spectrum antibiotic ointments are applied every 4 hours and systemic antibiotics such as ampicillin added in severe cases.
E. Warm to hot compresses and repeated drainage and irrigation of discharge from the conjunctival sac are recommended.

EYELASH DISEASES

I. Distichiasis
    A. General comments
        1. This is the most common form of eyelash disease with most cilia arising from the meibomian gland openings of both upper and lower lids.
        2. These cases must be evaluated carefully as only those causing a problem need be corrected. Often cocker spaniels and poodles have a few fine soft lashes which are not causing a problem.
        3. The main clinical signs are epiphora and blepharospasm.
        4. Secondary corneal damage may ensue necessitating therapy for the ulceration.
    B. Treatments
        1. The abnormal lashes must be removed.
        2. Several methods are available depending on the degree of distichiasis.
            a) Epilation
            b) Electrolysis
            c) Eyelid splitting
                (1) This is used when an entire row of cilia is present.
                (2) This procedure is not advised for small dogs with thin eyelids as entropion may result and further damage the cornea.
                (3) Alternatives are to remove only the base of the meibomian glands by two parallel conjunctival incisions or remove the middle portion of the lid containing the glands.

II. Ectopic cilia
    A. General comments
        1. A hair or bundle of hairs may be found growing through the conjunctival surface of the upper lid at about the base of the meibomian gland usually near the center of the lid and 3–4 mm from the eyelid margin.
        2. Clinical signs are blepharospasm and lacrimation and occasionally a keratitis often nonresponsive to standard medical therapy.
    B. Treatment
        The abnormal cilia are destroyed by electroepilation, cryosurgery, or a wedge resection of the affected eyelid.

ENTROPION

I. General comments
    A. The rolling in of the eyelids may be congenital (primary) e.g., in chows, bulldogs, St. Bernards, golden retrievers, or acquired (secondary) such as spastic entropion due to corneal pain, or cicatricial due to prior eyelid damage.
    B. Entropion is most common in dogs but does occur occasionally in cats (primarily Persians).

II. Treatment
  A. The amount of correction must be estimated prior to anesthesia.
  B. Surgical correction in mild cases in young animals is often postponed until the adult conformation is attained.
  C. Routine surgical correction involves removing a fold of skin and a small strip of orbicularis oculi muscle parallel to the lid margin.
  D. Closure is with interrupted 5-0 or 6-0 nonabsorbable sutures.
  E. The major error with this method is for the incision to be placed too far from the lid margin. The incision should be only 1–2 mm from the margin.

ECTROPION

  I. General comments
  A. Rolling out of the eyelid may be congenital, e.g., in St. Bernards, spaniels, and hounds, cicatricial following injury, or paralytic following facial nerve damage.
  B. Correction should be undertaken only if it is causing corneal disease or excessive ocular discharge.
  II. Treatment
  A. A V-to-Y correction is used for cicatricial ectropion. This frees the skin overlying the scar tissue and allows the lid margin to retract to a more normal position.
  B. For congenital or conformational ectropion, various sliding skin graft techniques have been developed.

BLEPHARITIS

  I. General comments
  A. Inflammation of the eyelids, especially the eyelid margins, is common but may be overlooked if it is part of a more generalized dermatitis.
  B. There are numerous etiologies, including bacterial (*Staphyloccus aureus*); parasitic (*Demodex* or *Sarcoptes* mites); metabolic, e.g., blepharitis associated with generalized seborrhea; actinic; fungal, e.g., dermatomycoses; and traumatic.
  C. The relative severity of the different signs will vary somewhat with the underlying etiology.
  II. Clinical signs
  A. Pruritis
  B. Epiphora
  C. Blepharospasm
  D. Hyperemia
  E. Edema
  F. Alopecia
  G. Ulceration

    H. Serous to purulent exudate

    I. Scaling

    J. Encrustations

    K. Conjunctivitis or keratoconjunctivitis

III. Treatment

    A. Gently express the meibomian glands using a flat surface, e.g., Bard Parker handle on the inner lid with digital pressure on the outer eyelid. Examine and culture the expressed material.

    B. Bacterial blepharitis will often respond to topical antibiotic/steroid ophthalmic ointment three times a day for 1–2 weeks. In most cases also use systemic antibiotics, e.g., ampicillin and hot packs three times a day for 2 weeks.

    C. For parasitic blepharitis apply physostigmine ophthalmic ointment $\frac{1}{4}\%$ or demecarium bromide (Humersol) drops $\frac{1}{8}\%$ or $\frac{1}{4}\%$ into the fornices with gentle massage.

    D. For blepharodermatomycosis treat the eyelids with miconazole nitrate topically and oral griseofulvin for 6 weeks.

    E. Allergic blepharitis requires topical and systemic corticosteroids to control the inflammation. In extreme cases a hyposensitization regimen may be employed.

CHALAZION

I. General comments

    A. This is a nodular mass formed by a granulomatous reaction to the oily meibomian secretion which has escaped into surrounding tissue.

    B. The mass is usually painless, visible through the conjunctiva, and located near the lid margin.

II. Treatment

    A. Surgical excision using a Desmerres chalazion clamp and a conjunctival incision is required.

    B. The skin is not excised.

    C. Aftercare consists of topical antibiotic and corticosteroid drops for 5–7 days.

    D. Always submit the tissue for histopathology as the differential diagnosis is sebaceous adenocarcinoma.

MEMBRANA NICTITANS

PROLAPSED GLAND OF THE MEMBRANA NICTITANS

I. General comments

    A. This is primarily a disease of young dogs (less than 2 years old), most commonly beagles, cocker spaniels, Pekingese, and bulldogs.

    B. The gland protrudes above the free border of third eyelid, becoming inflamed and enlarged.

    C. The onset is sudden and is usually accompanied by epiphora, mucoid discharge, and a variable amount of conjunctival inflammation.

    D. Histologically, there is plasma cell and lymphocyte infiltration and glandular hyperplasia.

    E. The cause is felt to be a defective formation of the normal fibrous attachments to the base of the gland.

II. Treatment

    A. Surgical excision at the base of the gland is by using topical anesthesia, topical 1/1,000 epinephrine, and a crushing technique with a mosquito hemostat across the base prior to cutting. The third eyelid itself should not be removed. Clinical signs of keratoconjunctivitis sicca should be discussed so that therapy can be initiated quickly if necessary as removal of the gland predisposes the animal to keratoconjunctivitis sicca later in life.

    B. An alternative technique which preserves the gland uses an elliptical incision through the conjunctiva over the gland. The deep (epibulbar) connective tissue is exposed by blunt dissection. 6-0 absorbable suture material is placed subconjunctivally in the epibulbar tissue and near the margin of the third eyelid near the gland. A second suture is placed similarly on the opposite side of the gland. As the sutures are tied the prolapsed tissue is inverted and the conjunctival margins apposed.

EVERTED CARTILAGE

I. General comments

    A. This is clinically significant only in the dog and is usually spontaneous, occurring most frequently in young dogs of the large breeds, primarily Great Danes.

    B. It can be acquired following injury or improper third eyelid suturing.

    C. The cartilage curls outward forming a scroll.

    D. There is usually an associated ocular discharge and conjunctivitis.

II. Treatment

    A. Surgical excision of the deformed piece of cartilage is required.

    B. A saline or saline/epinephrine solution injected into the third eyelid will separate the surfaces and prevent "buttonholing" of the bulbar conjunctival surface.

    C. The conjunctiva on the bulbar surface is incised and the deformed cartilage isolated by blunt dissection and removed.

    D. The conjunctival incision is closed with 6-0 gut in a continuous pattern with buried knots to avoid corneal irritation.

PROTRUSION OF THE MEMBRANA NICTITANS

I. General comments

This is a common complaint in small animal practice and has numerous etiologies the therapy of which will vary.

II. Etiologies

    A. Decreased orbital mass—dehydration and emaciation lead to loss of orbital fat, thus, the eyes become enophthalmic and the membrana nictitans protrudes bilaterally. Usually, there will be other associated clinical signs.

    B. Decreased ocular mass—microphthalmia or phthisis bulbi will lead to elevation but usually no associated systemic signs.

    C. Increased orbital mass or pressure—neoplasia or inflammation behind the globe will cause unilateral protrusion.

    D. Denervation (Horner's syndrome)—symptomatic relief is provided by topical epinephrine but usually this is not treated.

    E. Ocular pain—globe retraction will be self-limiting once the cause of the pain is treated.

    F. Encephalitis and meningitis, e.g., tetanus, rabies, distemper

    G. Conjunctivitis—cats primarily, usually due to herpes or chlamydial infection.

    H. Idiopathic—in cats, protrusion may be associated with gastrointestinal problems. Therapy is dependent on the specific cause. Many dolicocephalic dogs with deep orbits may have chronic protrusion. In these cases surgical resection of the third eyelid may be required.

PLASMOCYTIC INFILTRATION

I. General comments

    A. This presents as a white-grey bilateral thickening near the margin of the third eyelid, most commonly in adult German shepherds.

    B. There may be an associated keratitis (chronic superficial keratitis).

II. Clinical signs

    A. Hyperemia

    B. Nodular thickening and depigmentation along the free edge of the membrane

    C. Mucoid discharge

III. Treatment

    A. Topical corticosteroids three to six times a day are used for two to three weeks to get the disease in remission; then one to two times a day for control.

    B. Subconjunctival repositol steroids are used on initial presentation or during exacerbations to induce remission.

C. The lowest dose of topical corticosteroids that will maintain remission is recommended.

D. Frequent exacerbations are to be expected.

CONJUNCTIVA

CONJUNCTIVITIS

I. General comments
   A. Inflammation of the conjunctiva is the most common eye disease of animals.
   B. Classification is based on cause and duration of the inflammation and the type of discharge.
II. Clinical signs
   A. Will vary with duration and severity of the process
      1. Hyperemia
      2. Chemosis
      3. Follicles
      4. Ocular discharge—beginning as serous but progressing to mucoid then to mucopurulent
      5. Pain
      6. Pruritis
III. Etiologies
   A. Infectious
      1. Bacterial conjunctivitis is usually purulent and usually has an underlying initiating cause, e.g., foreign body or eyelid disease.
      2. Viral conjunctivitis is usually bilateral and usually part of a systemic disease, e.g., canine adenovirus I or feline herpesvirus.
      3. Chlamydia causes chemosis which is more severe than with other etiologies and follicle development usually is evident after several days.
      4. Mycoplasma causes mucopurulent discharge. Pseudomembrane formation on the palpebral conjunctiva is considered a classic sign.
      5. Mycotic conjunctivitis usually is associated with a concurrent mycotic keratitis.
   B. Parasitic—e.g., *Thelazia californiensis*
   C. Allergic conjunctivitis may be associated with generalized allergic manifestations (atopy) or can be a localized reaction to a wide variety of antigens including many topical drugs, e.g., pilocarpine and neomycin.
   D. Physical irritation
   E. Decreased tear production
IV. Differential diagnosis
   A. Various causes and types of conjunctivitis may merge, depending on

the lack of response to treatment or in some cases, such as allergy, because of treatment.

B. Serous to mucoid discharge of acute onset is suggestive of irritants, allergy, or virus.

C. If the discharge is mucopurulent to purulent, a bacterial cause or complication is implied.

D. Diagnostic techniques used to determine an etiology for conjunctivitis include cultures, conjunctival scrapings, conjunctival stains, and Schirmer tear test.

V. Treatment

A. Eliminate any physical cause and treat any systemic disease present.

B. Clean the eye thoroughly as often as required to keep the animal comfortable and free of accumulated discharge.

C. Antibacterials are often chosen empirically, but specific sensitivity tests may indicate a change in the drug being used. Usually ocular penetration is not important. Use drugs not generally administered systemically, thus not sensitizing the patient to drugs which may be required in the future and also minimizing the development of resistant strains. The first recommended therapy is a neomycin–polymyxin B–bacitracin mixture. Ointments are generally recommended due to longer contact time than liquid medications. Other recommended antibacterials are chloramphenicol, gentamicin, and sulfacetamide.

D. Corticosteroids are used in combination with antibiotics to reduce the inflammatory response. Always evaluate corneal integrity before dispensing steroids for ocular use. Irritant and allergic conjunctivitis respond very well to steroid medication.

E. Nonspecific decongestants, such as 10% phenylephrine (Neo-Synephrine) can be incorporated into the treatment regimen in nonspecific conjunctival inflammation.

FOLLICULAR CONJUNCTIVITIS

I. General comments

A. This is a very common disease in dogs in which any prolonged ocular irritation or immunologic stimulus causes follicle development primarily on the bulbar but occasionally on the palpebral surface of the third eyelid.

B. Often the follicles will persist even after the initial stimulus is removed.

II. Clinical signs

A. Persistent mucoid discharge

B. Hyperplastic follicles leading to a raised, roughened, or "cobblestone" appearance.

III. Treatment

A. Mild cases will respond to a topical antibiotic or steroid ointment, but discharge often returns when the medication is withdrawn.

B. Removal of the follicles by debridement with the curved end of a Bard-Parker handle, gauze sponges, or a Kimura spatula followed by a steroid and antibiotic ophthalmic ointment for 5–7 days, is usually curative.

LACRIMAL SYSTEM

DACRYOCYSTITIS (CANALICULITIS)

I. General comments
  A. This is typically a recurrent, chronic problem.
  B. There will be a mucoid to purulent discharge which can usually be flushed out of the puncta or nasolacrimal opening.
  C. In acute cases, there may be a swollen area medial and ventral to the lower lid margin.
II. Treatment
  A. Flush the ducts and use topical antibiotic therapy, e.g., gentamicin three times a day.
  B. In many cases daily flushing may be required.
  C. In chronically recurring cases, placement of an indwelling catheter of 2-0 monofilament suture material or PE 90 tubing in the nasolacrimal system for 2–3 weeks is used to dilate a stenotic duct and assure that antibiotic therapy traverses the entire system. Long-term (3 to 4 week) antibiotic therapy is often required in these patients.

EPIPHORA

I. General comments
  A. Epiphora is a common complaint in small animal practice and has numerous etiologies.
  B. A thorough ocular examination is required as such differing etiologies as distichiasis, entropion, trichiasis, nasal folds, atresia of the puncta, and posteriorly placed puncta may present as excess tearing.
II. Treatment
  A. If no underlying cause can be found, oral tetracycline (50 mg/day) may alleviate the staining problems although this will not affect tear production.
  B. Naphazoline hydrochloride topically once or twice a day will decrease the tearing in some cases and should be used on a trial basis before surgical correction of any form is attempted.
  C. As a last resort the gland of the membrana nictitans may be removed. This should not be done unless tear production is well above normal as it may predispose an animal to keratoconjunctivitis sicca.

D. A dacryocystoconjunctivorhinostomy may be performed in problem patients to provide permanent drainage to the nasal sinus.

KERATOCONJUNCTIVITIS SICCA

I. General comments
   A. Keratoconjunctivitis sicca (KCS) is due to a failure of formation of the aqueous portion of the precorneal tear film by the lacrimal and membrana nictitans glands.
   B. The majority are idiopathic although systemic diseases, e.g., distemper, trauma, and drug reactions, e.g., sulfonamides have been shown as causes.
   C. Clinical signs are proportional to the degree of hyposecretion and duration of the disease.
II. Clinical signs
   A. Chronic mucopurulent discharge
   B. Pain initially, but more of a discomfort or irritation
   C. An inflamed, thickened conjunctiva
   D. Corneal neovascularization, melanosis, keratinization, and occasionally ulceration
III. Diagnosis
   The disease is confirmed and monitored by the Schirmer tear test with 5.0 mm/min diagnostic, 5–15 mm/min questionable, and above 15 mm/min considered normal.
IV. Treatment·
   A. Supplementation of the tear film by artificial tears as often as possible but at least four times a day
   B. Ointments are used at night or if frequent application of tears is not possible.
   C. Stimulation of lacrimation by oral pilocarpine one to four drops of 1–2% solution added to the food (roughly one drop/5 lb). The dose is increased to the maximum the animal will tolerate. Always warn the owners of side effects of salivation, vomition, or diarrhea.
   D. Topical pilocarpine $\frac{1}{4}$% may stimulate glandular activity. Do not exceed 1% pilocarpine topically.
   E. Control infection by the use of broad-spectrum antibiotic solution or ointment.
   F. Keep the eye and eyelids clean and comfortable by gentle, frequent cleansing.
   G. Use 5% acetylcysteine in artificial tears to liquify excess mucus if present.
   H. Topical and subconjunctival steroids are used if the corneal epithelium is intact and vascularization excessive.
   I. Bromhexidine systemically is safe and effective in human patients and may be available for animals in the future.

J. Usually this treatment regimen is used for 1–2 months. If there is some response it is continued for another month.

K. The goal of medical management is to control corneal changes and ocular discomfort with the minimal amount of medication required. Often the disease is progressive and may eventually become refractory even to intensive medical therapy.

L. If there is no response to medical management or the condition becomes refractory over time, a parotid duct transposition is recommended. Saliva will keep a cornea healthy but often two to three times a day therapy (artificial tears and/or corticosteroids) may still be required. Potential complications include torsion and failure of the transposition, excess mineralization along the eyelids, excess epiphora, and calcium deposition in the cornea. The transposition should be successful in 90% of cases operated.

CORNEA

BURNS

I. General comments
   A. Alkali burns penetrate and soften the tissue and the further release of hydroxyl ions causes the injury to progress, whereas acid is neutralized quickly by the tissues and precipitated protein acts as a barrier to further penetration.
   B. The cornea is extremely sensitive to heat and hyperthermic injury will usually be accompanied by delayed healing.

II. Treatment
   A. The most important consideration is immediate copious irrigation, ideally with collyrium but in an emergency situation tap water can be used.
   B. Citric and boric acids are advised for alkali burns, sodium bicarbonate for acid burns if the pH of the offending compound is known.
   C. Burns should be treated with topical antibiotics and atropine until the corneal epithelium is renewed, and then topical steroids may be added to minimize scarring.
   D. Five percent acetylcysteine in artificial tears or in the antibiotic solution may be added to the treatment regimen for alkali burns to help inhibit the collagenase released.

ABRASIONS AND ULCERATION

I. General comments
   A. A corneal abrasion (erosion) indicates loss of epithelium while ulceration indicates stroma involvement as well.

II. Clinical signs
   A. Pain (manifested by blepharospasm)

    B. Serous or purulent discharge

    C. Photophobia due to ciliary spasm

    D. Loss of corneal transparency

    E. Changes in corneal contour

    F. Neovascularization of the cornea which develops 3–6 days after the original insult.

III. Diagnosis

    A. Clinical signs and history and a thorough examination with magnification will usually lead to the diagnosis.

    B. Stain the cornea with fluorescein.

    C. Examine carefully to eliminate mechanical causes, e.g., eyelash diseases or foreign bodies behind the membrana nictitans.

    D. A very deep ulcer (to Descemet's membrane) will not retain stain, thus clearing in the center of a deep ulcer is a very unfavorable sign.

    E. Perform culture and sensitivity tests on any progressing ulcer.

IV. Treatment

    A. Broad-spectrum topical antibiotics to control the infection.

    B. Begin treatment with a broad-spectrum drug at least four times a day initially until culture results are received.

    C. Relieve pain with a cycloplegic drug (atropine topically).

    D. If there is corneal necrosis or liquefaction an anticollagenase drug (5% acetylcysteine) may be added to the topical medication.

    E. Subconjunctival injections of antibiotics, e.g., chloramphenicol or gentamicin are frequently used to insure high levels of drug for rapidly progressing ulcers or for hard-to-treat animals.

    F. If there is a marked uveitis prostaglandin inhibitors e.g., oral aspirin are used for 3–5 days.

    G. Evaluate the ulcer at least daily and continue antibiotics for at least 1 week after the epithelial defect is closed.

    H. If the ulcer is very deep (desmetocoele) or if there is danger of rupture the cornea should be covered with a membrana nictitans or conjunctival flap.

LACERATION

  I. General comments

    If the laceration is full thickness it should be sutured and the anterior chamber re-formed.

 II. Treatment

    A. Careful, accurate apposition with fine suture material is necessary to minimize scarring.

    B. Sutures should be placed to one half to two thirds of the depth of the cornea.

    C. Either absorbable or nonabsorbable sutures can be used and a membrana

nictitans flap, conjunctival flap, or temporary tarsorrhaphy can be used to support the cornea.
D. Treat postoperatively similarly to an ulcer, i.e., antibiotics and cycloplegics.
E. Penetrating wounds should also be treated with systemic antibiotics for several days.
F. If there is no infection, steroids may be added to the treatment regimen to minimize scarring.
G. If there is prolapse of uveal tissue, it can be replaced if viable or an iridectomy may be required.

CHRONIC SUPERFICIAL KERATITIS

I. General comments
   A. Chronic superficial keratitis (CSK, degenerative pannus, Uberreiter's syndrome) is a chronic progressive disease of the canine cornea characterized by an invasion of blood vessels and mononuclear inflammatory cells into the anterior corneal stroma.
   B. It is bilateral but not necessarily symmetrical.
   C. After the initial inflammatory reaction has occurred pigment cells invade the stroma and a grey band is often present in the stroma adjacent to the advancing edge of the lesion.
   D. As the lesion advances pigmentation increases and eventually the entire cornea is affected.
   E. The majority of patients are 3–6 years of age and 83% of patients are German shepherds.
   F. More cases and increased severity of the cases are reported in higher altitudes, the presumed relation being increased exposure to ultraviolet light.
   G. The temporal quadrant is affected in 96% of the patients.
II. Treatment
   A. Objectives
      1. Because the underlying etiology is not known, treatment of CSK is not aimed at curing but at controlling the disease.
      2. Client education is important as they must be instructed that lifelong medication and frequent reevaluation will be required.
   B. Subconjunctival repository steroids, e.g., 10 mg triamcinolone acetonide (Kenalog) are used initially and as required if there are exacerbations.
   C. Topical ophthalmic steroids, e.g., dexamethasone at least three times a day.
   D. On reevaluation examinations the injections are repeated as needed and the frequency of topical applications adjusted.
   E. Eventually, once a day application may be adequate to control the disease.

F. In some areas, e.g., at high altitudes, a superficial keratectomy and possibly β-radiation may be needed to remove the pigmented tissue.

G. Occasionally infections and ulceration may occur and the owner must be counseled to watch for these and discontinue steroids as required.

H. Secondary mycotic infection appears to be relatively rare.

INDOLENT ULCER

I. General comments
   A. Indolent ulcer or corneal erosion syndrome is a reoccurring type of epithelial erosion due to defective attachment of basal epithelial cells to the basal lamina.
   B. It is more prevalent in older boxers but can be present in any breed.
   C. When fluorescein is applied it will readily spread under the loosely adherent lip of epithelium.

II. Treatment
   A. Remove the poorly adherent epithelium with a cotton-tipped applicator.
   B. Iodine cautery (2–5% tincture) of the loose edges is used to enhance adhesion.
   C. Treat as for a fresh corneal ulcer.
   D. The stripping may have to be repeated several times at 1 to 2 week intervals.
   E. In very resistant cases (three or four debridements with no success) a membrana nictitans or preferably a conjunctival flap can be put up to enhance healing.

MYCOTIC KERATITIS

I. General comments
   A. Mycotic keratitis should be suspected in animals with refractory keratitis and a history of chronicity and numerous unsuccessful therapies especially topical corticosteroid usage.
   B. The most common agents are *Aspergillus* sp., *Fusarium*, and *Mucor*.

II. Diagnosis
   A. History
   B. Clinical signs
      1. White plaques in the cornea
      2. Satellite lesions in the cornea
      3. Marked subepithelial neovascularization
   C. Corneal and conjunctival scrapings
   D. Culture results

III. Treatment
   A. Specific antifungal drugs topically every 4 hours for 2 days, then two

times a day, e.g., miconazole. The IV forms can be used topically undiluted.
   B. Pimaracin (Natamycin) is a topical broad-spectrum ophthalmic preparation useful in confirmed cases.
   C. In many cases a superficial keratectomy to decrease the fungal mass is required in addition to medical therapy.
   D. Prolonged medical therapy e.g., 4–6 weeks is often required.

SUPERFICIAL PUNCTATE KERATITIS

 I. General comments
   A. This syndrome in dogs is characterized by very small, superficial ulcers and epithelial and subepithelial infiltrates giving the cornea a stippled appearance.
   B. Clinical signs are variable, from absent to marked epiphora and pain.
II. Treatment
   A. Treat as a fresh corneal ulcer.
   B. Topical corticosteroid therapy is added after the epithelium has healed over the lesions or if the lesions are nonresponsive to ulcer therapy.
   C. Reevaluate the animal every 2–3 days. When improvement is noted the frequency of steroid medication is decreased.
   D. Continued low-dose (one to two times a day) steroid therapy is often required to keep the disease in remission.

FELINE HERPES KERATITIS

 I. Clinical signs
   A. A serous to seromucoid discharge
   B. Blepharospasm
   C. Conjunctival injection
   D. Superficial neovascularization
   E. Mild corneal edema
   F. Superficial ulcers usually in a branching or dendritic pattern.
   G. Clinical diagnosis is based primarily on the finding of superficial linear ulcers.
II. Treatment
   A. Topical antiviral drugs, e.g., idoxuridine, vidarabine, or trifluridine one drop every 4 hours for 1–2 days, then four times a day.
   B. Treatment should be continued for 10–14 days following reepithelialization of the cornea.
   C. If a mucopurulent discharge is present topical broad-spectrum antibiotics are combined with the antiviral medication.
   D. The client should be advised of the high recurrence rate.

ANTERIOR EPISCLERITIS

I. General comments
  A. This can present as either a diffuse or nodular reaction in the episclera, usually of the temporal globe.
  B. It is primarily unilateral and usually nodular.
  C. If the nodule is near the cornea there may be some neovascularization and leukoma formation.
  D. Episcleral vessels will be engorged and the overlying conjunctiva congested.
II. Treatment
  A. Systemic steroids (5 mg/kg prednisone) once a day for 2–3 weeks. Gradually decrease the steroid dose after 3–4 weeks.
  B. Topical steroids e.g., dexamethasone 1%, three times a day, then decreased to once a day as the animal is in remission.
  C. Subconjunctival repositol steroids are used in acute exacerbations.

ANTERIOR CHAMBER

HYPHEMA

  I. General comments
    A. Blood in the anterior chamber can be associated with both local and systemic disease.
    B. There are numerous etiologies including trauma, uveal neoplasia, systemic neoplasia, chronic glaucoma, infections, and retinal detachment.
    C. The significance of hyphema varies with the cause and response to therapy in the first few days of treatment.
  II. Treatment
    A. Topical mydriatics and cycloplegics (atropine and phenylephrine) three or four times a day for 2–3 days, then once a day
    B. Topical steroids, e.g., dexamethasone three times a day
    C. Systemic steroids (1 mg/kg prednisone) can be added if the uveal inflammation associated with the hyphema is intense.
    D. If the hyphema is due to a penetrating wound systemic antibiotics are indicated as well.
    E. Surgical removal of clotted blood is rarely needed.
    F. Keep the animal very quiet for 48 hours then relatively quiet for the next 5 days.
  III. Prognosis
    A. The prognosis varies somewhat with the underlying etiology.
    B. If hemorrhaging stops and the blood clots in the first 1–2 days the prognosis is good.
    C. If bleeding continues, secondary glaucoma may develop and necessitate enucleation or prosthesis implantation.

UVEITIS

I. General comments
    A. Uveitis is a composite of clinical diseases in which the inflammatory response itself is the predominant cause of altered ocular structure and function.
    B. Inflammatory processes of the anterior uveal tract, i.e., anterior uveitis usually have an iris component or iritis and a ciliary body component or a cyclitis, i.e. anterior uveitis is iridocyclitis.
    C. Inflammation of the choroid by itself is a choroiditis, and total uveal inflammation is panuveitis.

II. Clinical signs
    A. Subjective
        1. Pain
        2. Photophobia
        3. Epiphora
        4. Visual loss.
    B. Objective
        1. Congestion of the short, brush-like deep circumcorneal vessels (ciliary injection)
        2. Miosis
        3. Congestion and swelling of the iridic stroma
        4. Aqueous flare due to increased protein concentration of the aqueous humor.
        5. Sedimented and organized exudate in the anterior chamber (hypopyon)
        6. Cellular and proteinaceous precipitates adherent to the corneal endothelium (keratic precipitates)

III. Classification
    A. Uveitis is classified by combinations of description (granulomatous or nongranulomatous), source of inflammation (endogenous versus exogenous), etiology (hypersensitivity, toxic, traumatic), and association with systemic disease or idiopathic.
    B. Most cases of uveitis fall into the endogenous category with an unknown etiology.

IV. Diagnosis
    A. Presenting clinical signs and history
    B. Complete physical examination for signs of systemic diseases
    C. Routine blood counts, chemistries, and urinalysis
    D. Immune profile, e.g., antinuclear antibodies (ANA), Rh factor
    E. Protein electrophoresis, e.g., for feline peritonitis
    F. Centesis of the anterior chamber for fluid and cell analysis

V. Etiologies
    A. Almost any insult to an eye and most systemic diseases can cause uveal inflammation.
    B. Trauma

    C. Bacterial

    D. Viral

    E. Fungal

    F. Parasitic diseases such as ascariasis and filariasis

    G. Hypersensitivity

    H. Autoimmune diseases

    I. Primary and secondary ocular neoplasms

VI. Treatment

    A. Objective

       To quickly and effectively suppress the inflammatory cycle by inhibiting as many of the separate steps as possible, including inhibiting normal immune reactions.

    B. Treatment of active ocular inflammation can be divided into the 4 phases of stimulus control, control of host response, preservation of ocular structures, and control of symptomatology.

    C. When possible, specific therapy is used in eliminating known antigenic stimuli. Despite the low overall incidence of overt microbial infections as a cause of uveitis, blanket antimicrobial therapy, both topical and systemic is frequently instituted.

    D. Control of host response is usually nonspecific and consists of topical and systemic corticosteroids. Systemic steroids are primarily utilized if the uveal inflammation is part of a systemic immunologically mediated disease.

    E. In most cases of uveitis, subconjunctival and topical steroid administration is adequate to control inflammation and prevent structural alteration.

    F. The systemic use of prostaglandin inhibitors such as aspirin is also advocated.

    G. To preserve ocular structure and function, mydriasis and cycloplegia must be established. Usually 1–4% atropine sulfate topically two to three times a day is adequate.

VII. Sequelae

    A. Synechia

    B. Seclusion and occlusion of the pupil

    C. Cataracts

    D. Ciliary body atrophy and hypotony

    E. Cyclitic membranes

    F. Chorioretinal atrophy

    G. Glaucoma

    H. Phthisis bulbi

GLAUCOMA

  I. Clinical signs

    A. The clinical signs can be divided into those of acute versus chronic glaucoma, although the clinician must remember that there can be a great deal of overlap and blending of signs as the disease progresses.

B. Acute glaucoma
1. Pain as evidence by blepharospasm, an elevated membrana nictitians, epiphora, and photophobia
2. Conjunctival inflammation
3. Episcleral vessel congestion if there is a relatively large pressure increase
4. Corneal edema
5. Pupillary dilation and nonresponse to light
6. Decreased visual acuity
7. Decreased retinal vascularity
8. Cupping of the optic disc

C. Chronic glaucoma
1. Long-standing increases in intraocular pressure lead to irreversible damage.
2. A gradual enlargement of the globe or buphthalmos will occur although this can be rapid in young animals. This is rarely reversible even if the pressure is reduced.
3. Episcleral congestion and enlargement of vessels. The veins may remain dilated even after the pressure is controlled.
4. The corneal edema present in acute cases remains, and striae (white endothelial stretch marks) (striate keratopathy) occur as linear ruptures form in Descemet's membrane.
5. Corneal neovascularization and pigmentation
6. Pupillary dilation remains and is often more pronounced than in early glaucoma.
7. The lens often becomes cataractous and may luxate.
8. Retinal and optic nerve atrophy with cupping of the optic disc and retinal vascular attenuation

II. Diagnosis
A. Presenting signs and history, e.g., breed predisposition and previous recurring episodes of "reddened eyes"
B. Measurement of intraocular pressure: Schiotz tonometry or applanation tonometry if available. (Pressures above 30 mmHg with clinical signs are diagnostic of glaucoma.)
C. Gonioscopic evaluation of the iridocorneal angle
D. Fundoscopic examination for evidence of glaucomatous cupping and retinal degeneration
E. Biomicroscopy of the anterior chamber
F. Tonography to determine coefficient of aqueous outflow

III. Classification of glaucoma
A. Glaucomas can be classified by mechanism of action and by stage of disease. Stage of disease is valuable in deciding on most applicable therapy and in offering a prognosis to the owner.

B. Classification by stage of disease
  1. Enlarged blind eye
     a) No therapy will improve the eye.
     b) If the pressure is still elevated and the eye painful or if an exposure keratitis is beginning, the options are cyclocryosurgery, an intraocular prosthesis, or enucleation.
     c) If the pressure is decreased owing to ciliary atrophy and the animal is comfortable it may be best to do nothing.
  2. Blind but not enlarged eye
     The pressure will almost always be elevated and the eye painful, so either cyclocryosurgery, an intraocular prosthesis, or medical therapy should be performed.
  3. Recent attack of congestive glaucoma
     Intense and early medical therapy is required to decrease pressure and save vision.
  4. Very early attack of glaucoma
     a) Emergency medical treatment is required.
     b) Once the cause (mechanism) is established, a long-term medical and/or surgical treatment regimen can be started.
     c) This may include prophylactic medication if the pressure has returned to normal.
IV. Treatment
  A. Medical therapy must be started as soon as the diagnosis of glaucoma is made, as even a few hours of highly elevated pressure can cause irreversible damage.
  B. Medical treatment is directed at opening the drainage angle with miotics and then decreasing production of aqueous humor.
  C. The emergency medical treatment regimen includes combinations of the following drugs.
     1. Mannitol: 1–3 g/kg IV of a 20% or 25% solution is given. Water must be withheld for the first few hours after administration. Mannitol administration can be repeated two to four times in the first 48 hours, but the animal must be monitored for signs of dehydration.
     2. Cholinergic stimulation
        a) Direct cholinergics: pilocarpine 1%, 2%, or 4% is given topically every hour until the pupil constricts and then three times a day. This increases the facility of outflow and decreases the amount of aqueous production slightly.
        b) Indirect cholinergics: these are organophosphates, which cause irreversible blockade of the cholinesterases, and are more powerful and longer acting than the direct-acting drugs. The two commonly used are demecarium bromide (Humorsol) and echothiophate (Phospholine iodide).

3. Carbonic anhydrase inhibitors
   a) These act by decreasing aqueous humor production by creating a local acidosis.
   b) IV acetazolamide is available for management of acute cases (50 mg/kg administered one time).
   c) Acetazolamide 7 mg/kg orally three times a day or dichlorphenamide 2–5 mg/kg orally three times a day is used.
   d) The individual dose may need adjustment to balance the pressure reduction with the side effects of vomition, panting, and weakness.
4. Sympathomimetics
   Epinephrine 1–2% applied topically one to three times daily decreases production and increases the outflow of aqueous humor.
5. Combination drugs
   a) Pilocarpine plus epinephrine (P_2E_1) seems to be very effective in the dog.
   b) The pupillary size remains small to moderate, and the facility of outflow is increased.
6. Autonomic blocking agents
   These include the β-antagonists, e.g., timolol maleate (Timoptic) and atenolol, and the α-antagonists, e.g., thymoxamine, applied two times a day.
D. The owners must be counseled that life-long therapy is required and frequent reevaluation of these animals is necessary.
E. Surgical management
   1. Long-term control of glaucoma is not often achieved medically in animals, so the owner should be counseled that surgical procedures may be necessary. Many owners are unwilling or unable to medicate frequently enough to control the pressure and may desire surgery in the early stages of the disease.
   2. If possible, the pressure should be brought to a normal range by medical management before surgery is attempted.
   3. Cyclocryosurgery
      This is selective destruction of the ciliary body by freezing and is the currently recommended therapy.
   4. Heat cautery is very damaging and results in a large percentage of phthisical eyes and can no longer be recommended.
   5. Cyclodialysis
   6. Iridencleisis
   7. Corneoscleral trephination and iridectomy
   8. Numerous combinations of these methods are available.
   9. For blind painful enlarged eyes and a glaucoma nonresponsive to cyclocryosurgery, e.g., that due to nonseptic uveitis an intraocular prosthesis is recommended.

LENS

CATARACTS

I. General comments
   A. Cataract is any opacity of the lens or its capsule. It is associated with vacuolation and local precipitation of protein.
   B. Cataracts are classified by stage of development, clinical groupings, and location within the lens.
II. Treatment
   A. Medical
      1. Medical treatment for cataracts has included numerous drugs none of which has proved successful.
      2. Medical therapy is indicated if the lens protein is leaking through the capsule, causing a lens-induced uveitis.
      3. Topical cycloplegics (1% atropine) and corticosteroids (dexamethasone 1%) are applied two to three times daily.
      4. Mydriatics may be used alone in cases of hypermature or incipient cataracts to facilitate vision around the focal opacities.
   B. Surgical
      1. Surgical treatment is the only routinely effective therapy available for cataracts at this time.
      2. The various forms available include phacofragmentation, discussion and aspiration, intracapsular and extracapsular removal.
      3. The standard approach in most canine patients remains the extracapsular extraction. An ophthalmic surgical textbook should be consulted for indications, procedures, and potential complications.

LENS LUXATION

I. General comments
   A. Lens displacement may be either a subluxation with the lens still partially in the patellar fossa or complete luxation with loss of all zonular attachments and complete displacement of the lens from the fossa.
   B. The condition may be hereditary, or secondary to trauma or concurrent ocular disease such as glaucoma.
II. Clinical signs
   A. Iridodonesis
   B. Aphakic crescent
   C. Altered depth of the anterior chamber
   D. Corneal edema
   E. Glaucoma
   F. With glaucoma or corneal pain there may be blepharospasm, epiphora, inflammation, and decreased vision.

III. Treatment
  A. If the lens is subluxated posteriorly, long-acting miotics (0.03% echo-thiophate) once or twice a day can occasionally maintain the lens behind the iris.
  B. Total posterior luxation without concurrent inflammation or glaucoma should be reevaluated every 3 months but usually further medical therapy is not indicated.
  C. Anterior luxations or anterior subluxations causing glaucoma should be treated surgically. A standard intracapsular extraction is recommended in sighted eyes while a couching procedure is recommended in blind eyes.

RETINA

FELINE CENTRAL RETINAL DEGENERATION

  I. Feline central retinal degeneration begins in the area centralis as a small, well-defined area of increased granularity then hyperreflectivity and progresses to a band-shaped area dorsal to the optic disc.
 II. The degeneration begins in the outer retinal layers but eventually total retinal degeneration is present.
III. If untreated, the degeneration progresses to total retinal atrophy. Feline central retinal degeneration is due to taurine deficiency and has been reproduced by feeding experimental diets and diets of only low-quality dog food. Changing to a taurine-rich diet (fish, clam juice) will stop progression of the disease but will not correct the area already affected.

RETINITIS

  I. General comments
  A. Inflammation of the retina and choroid is usually referred to as chorioretinitis because these structures are so closely related that inflammation of one will involve the other.
  B. It should be remembered that some conditions will have an effect on one layer primarily, e.g., toxoplasmosis is primarily a retinitis while feline infectious peritonitis is primarily a choroiditis with secondary retinal involvement.
 II. Classification
     The posterior segment inflammation is classified as granulomatous or nongranulomatous primarily on histology but often on ophthalmoscopic appearance as well. The etiologic agent of granulomatous chorioretinitis is more likely to be found on histopathology than with nongranulomatous lesions.

III. Nongranulomatous retinitis/chorioretinitis
   A. Unless both eyes are severely enough involved to cause a noticeable decrease in visual acuity there are no presenting complaints.
   B. When evaluating a systemic disease that can cause retinitis always examine the eye thoroughly.
   C. With active inflammation there is retinal edema as evidence by dull, ill-defined areas, gray or white exudates, congested blood vessels, perivascular cuffing, retinal hemorrhage, or serous retinal detachment.
   D. In inactive lesions there is increased reflectivity due to retinal atrophy, hyperpigmentation over the tapetum due to pigment epithelial reaction, loss of pigmentation in the nontapetal area, decreased vascularity and well defined edges to the lesion.
   E. Healed scars are a common finding in "normal" animals.
   F. The numerous etiologies include viral, bacterial, parasitic, hypersensitivity and toxic reactions.
   G. The retinitis is usually part of a systemic disease.
   H. Treatment
      1. If possible, treat the underlying disease.
      2. Systemic steroids, e.g., prednisone 0.5 mg/kg for 2–3 weeks
      3. Systemic antibiotics for 2–3 weeks
      4. Diuretics are added if there is retinal detachment.
IV. Granulomatous chorioretinitis
   A. This usually will present as part of a systemic disease or as part of a severe uveitis.
   B. There is evidence of exudate, subretinal material, irregular borders to the lesions, and a more marked inflammatory response than with nongranulomatous disease.
   C. The numerous etiologies include fungal infections, e.g., blastomycosis, and feline infectious peritonitis, tuberculosis, and toxoplasmosis.
   D. Treatment
      1. Systemic therapy of the associated disease if identified
      2. Systemic steroids (if infectious disease is not involved) to control the inflammation

RETINAL DETACHMENT

 I. General comments
   A. This often will not present for ocular examination unless bilateral and thus causing blindness.
   B. Early after the detachment the pupillary reflexes will still be normal but will gradually decrease as the retina degenerates.
   C. A total detachment will cause syneresis of the vitreous body.
II. Clinical findings
   A. A white to grey membrane with blood vessels in it can be seen behind the lens with a light and loupe.

B. The retina remains attached at the optic disc giving a cone or funnel appearance.

C. If there is a small partial detachment the lesion may only be detected with indirect ophthalmoscopy.

III. Treatment

A. Systemic corticosteroids at anti-inflammatory levels for up to 6 weeks, e.g., prednisone 1.0 mg/kg daily tapering to 0.5 mg/kg after 2 weeks

B. Furosemide 2–4 mg/kg orally once or twice a day for 2–3 weeks

C. Therapy is empirical and a poor prognosis should always be given. Surgical correction is possible but not often effective in animals.

OPTIC NEURITIS

I. General comments

A. This disease will usually present as a case of sudden blindness with fixed, dilated pupils.

B. Fundoscopic lesions are usually absent but occasionally an inflamed optic disc and exudates and focal retinal detachments are found.

C. The disease was originally thought to be a simple bilateral retrobulbar inflammation of the optic nerves.

D. Canine distemper virus and neoplastic and inflammatory neurologic diseases (e.g., reticulosis) are now considered as etiologies.

II. Patient evaluation

Prior to therapy a thorough evaluation of the patient including cerebro-spinal fluid examination is recommended to determine an etiology. Most patients are idiopathic.

III. Treatment

A. Systemic corticosteroids, e.g., 1–2 mg/kg prednisone daily for up to 3 weeks.

B. If no improvement is noted at 3 weeks, medication is reduced and then discontinued with a very poor prognosis for return of vision.

SUGGESTED READINGS

Ellis PP: Ocular Therapeutics and Pharmacology. 5th Ed. CV Mosby, St. Louis, 1977

Gelatt KN: Veterinary Ophthalmic Pharmacology and Therapeutics. 2nd Ed. VM Publishing, Bonner Springs, Kansas, 1978

Gelatt KN (ed): Textbook of Veterinary Ophthalmology. Lea and Febiger, Philadelphia, 1981

Martin CL (ed): Ophthalmological diseases. p. 530. In Kirk RW (ed): Current Veterinary Therapy. VIII. Small Animal Practice. WB Saunders, Philadelphia, 1983

Slatte DH: Fundamentals of Veterinary Ophthalmology. WB Saunders, Philadelphia, 1981

19

Endocrine Disorders
John A. Mulnix, D.V.M.

ADENOHYPOPHYSIS (ANTERIOR
PITUITARY)

Hormones from the Adenohypophysis

Pars distalis

I. Growth hormone (GH). somatotropic hormone (STH)
   A. Has basic effects of
      1. Increased rate of protein synthesis in all cells of the body
      2. Decreased rate of carbohydrate (CHO) utilization
      3. Increased mobilization of fats and use of fats for energy
   B. By basic actions it promotes growth, conserves CHO, mobilizes fat, and enhances body protein.
   C. For GH to be effective, CHO and insulin must be available.
   D. Growth hormone increases release of fatty acids from adipose tissue and accentuation of ketogenesis in diabetics.
   E. Growth hormone has a diabetogenic effect; it causes decrease in use of CHO for energy—cells become saturated with glycogen—therefore, less glucose uptake by cells and a resulting increase in blood glucose concentration.
   F. Regulation of GH by somatotropic-releasing factor from hypothalamus
II. Thyroid-stimulating hormone (TSH)
   A. Controlled by
      1. Thyrotropin-releasing hormone (TRH)
      2. Direct effect of thyroxine on pituitary gland
   B. Effects
      1. Induces release of fatty acids from fat deposits.
      2. On thyroid gland
         a) Increases blood flow through gland.
         b) Increases rate of breakdown of colloid thyroglobulin, thereby increasing thyroid hormone discharge.

  c) Increases biosynthesis of thyroid hormone, thus increasing iodine
   uptake

III. Adrenocorticotrophin (ACTH)
 A. Control
  1. Corticotropin-releasing factor (CRF)
  2. Glucocorticoid feedback to pituitary
 B. Effects
  1. Three sites of action
   a) Zona fasiculata and zona reticularis of adrenal cortex
   b) Fat deposits with lipolytic effect
   c) Stimulates melanocytes, causing darkening of skin
  2. Effect on adrenal cortex
   a) Decreases ascorbic acid content
   b) Increases secretion of glucocorticoids by converting cholesterol
    to pregnenolone
   c) Increases metabolic activity of cortex
    (1) Increases size
    (2) Increases O_2 consumption

IV. Gonadotrophins
 There are three
 A. Luteotropic hormone (LTH) (prolactin)
 B. Luteinizing hormone (LH). Interstitial cell-stimulating hormone (ICSH)
  is less in the male.
 C. Follicle-stimulating hormone (FSH)

Pituitary Dwarfism

 I. A result of decreased secretion of all hormones of anterior pituitary gland.
  The clinical signs are related to growth hormone deficiency.
 II. Two types in human youth—do not usually recognize difference in canine
  patients.
  A. Larain dwarf
  B. Senile dwarf
 III. Incidence
  A. Relatively rare, predominantly in German shepherd and Cornelian bear
   dog
  B. Probably many cases destroyed by owner
 IV. Etiology
  A. Agenesis or hypoplasia of pituitary
  B. Cystic Rathke's cleft
  C. Cystic malformation of craniopharyngeal duct
  D. Decreased activity of the acidophil with subsequent decreased pro-
   duction of growth hormone
 V. Clinical syndrome
  A. Lethargic and listless

B. Eyes bright and alert
C. Hair coat wooly and fine—puppy coat
D. Bilaterally symmetrical areas of alopecia
   1. Head, neck, top of shoulders
   2. Underline—medial surfaces of legs
E. Denuded areas
   Hyperpigmentation and hyperkeratosis on posterior abdomen and inguinal area
VI. Diagnosis
   A. Clinical signs and history
   B. Blood and urine normal or may reveal findings consistent with hypothyroidism and/or secondary adrenocortical insufficiency.
   C. Determine adrenal cortex and thyroid hormone levels before and after stimulation.
   D. Radiographs
      1. Delayed closure of epiphysis due to decreased osteoblastic activity—usually not closed by 1.5 years
      2. Many radiographic lesions associated with achondroplasia.
   E. Skin biopsy reveals changes typical of dermal endocrinopathy
      Decreased amount and size of dermal elastin fiber very suggestive
   F. Plasma growth hormone levels
      1. Radioimmunoassay method
      2. Stimulation of growth hormone secretion by clonidine. Dose 10–30 mg/kg IV. Sample before and 15 minutes and 30 minutes postinjection.
VII. Treatment
   Bovine or porcine growth hormone has been used. Recommended dosage is 5–10 U SQ every other day for 5–15 injections. Beneficial response may be seen in 1–3 months, and remission may last from 6 months to over 3 years.

CANINE ACROMEGALY

I. Caused by hypersecretion of growth hormone in the mature animal
   In the dog has been reported in association with
   A. Hyperplasia of the anterior pituitary gland
   B. Pituitary adenocarcinoma
   C. Diestrous in the intact cycling bitch
   D. Administration of progestational compounds
II. Clinical signs
   A. Thickened skin
   B. Hypertrichosis
   C. Inspiratory stridor
   D. Abdominal enlargement

    E. Polyuria/polydipsia

    F. Fatigue

III. Diagnosis

    Measurement of plasma growth hormone levels. Values significantly elevated. Elevated levels not suppressible with IV glucose load (1 g glucose/kg).

IV. Treatment

    A. Depends on underlying factors

    B. Pituitary ablation for tumors

    C. Ovariohysterectomy or cessation of progestational hormones

NEUROHYPOPHYSIS

Diabetes Insipidus (DI)

This is the syndrome which results from failure of the neurohypophysial system to produce or release a quantity of antidiuretic hormone (ADH) sufficient to bring about the normal homeostatic renal conservation of free water. Diabetes insipidus (DI) may be complete or partial, permanent or temporary and is *usually* characterized by the production of large volumes of hypotonic urine.

Antidiuretic Hormone

    I. Has the fundamental role in homeostatic regulation of volume and osmolality of body fluids by its action on renal tubule

    II. Is present in all mammals

  III. Specialized hypothalamic nuclei (supraoptic and paraventricular) and the neurohypophysial tract (axons originating in these nuclei) and terminating in the posterior lobe (pars nervosa) comprise the neurohypophysial system.

  IV. Biologically active octapeptides have been identified in lower vertebrates.

    A. Only three have antidiuretic activity

      1. Arginine-vasopressin (AVP)

      2. Lysine-vasopressin (LVP)

      3. Arginine-vasotocin (AVT)

    B. Arginine-vasopressin appears to be present in representative species from most of the major groups of mammals.

    C. Lysine-vasopressin appears only in members of suborder, suina (pigs, peccaries, hippopotami), although these mammals also secrete AVP

    D. Arginine-vasotocin (AVT) is the only neurohypophysial hormone in the bony fishes as well as the teleosts (all nonmammalian vertebrates). Arginine-vasotocin produces both antidiuretic and milk ejection effects when injected into mammals, but is not nearly so potent in this regard as vasopressin. Arginine-vasotocin enhances water transport in the nephrons of birds, reptiles, and amphibians but not in bony fishes, cartilaginous fishes, or cyclostomes; it appears to enhance sodium excretion in these latter vertebrates.

V. Formation and storage
   A. Posterior lobe of pituitary is storage site for ADH and oxytocin formed in nerve cell bodies
      1. Antidiuretic hormone formed primarily in supraoptic nuclei
      2. Oxytocin formed primarily in paraventricular nuclei
   B. Neurophysins are the physiologic "carrier proteins" for the intra-neuronal transport of ADH and oxytocin from their site of synthesis to the neurohypophysis
   C. Neurophysin is *not* confined to the neurohypophysis but is released into the circulation with ADH or oxytocin.
   D. It is probable that all stimuli that enhance release of ADH also enhance its synthesis.

VI. Secretion and release of ADH
   A. The actual release of the hormone is strongly Ca^{2+} ion-dependent
   B. Acute hemorrhagic hypotension is one of the most powerful stimuli for the immediate release of ADH.

VII. Osmotic and nonosmotic stimuli and inhibitors to ADH release
   A. Stimuli
      1. Osmotic—contracted intracellular volume of supraoptical hypophysial nuclei
      2. Nonosmotic—decreased arterial pressure; decrease in tension of left atrial wall and pulmonary veins; emotional stress or pain; increased temperature of blood; drugs (cholinergic, barbiturates, nicotine); low O_2 tension; stimulation of renin-angiotensin system
   B. Inhibitors
      1. Osmotic—expansion of intracellular volume of neurons at supraoptic hypophysial nuclei
      2. Nonosmotic—increased arterial pressure; increased tension of left atrial wall and pulmonary veins; occasionally emotional stress; decreased temperature of blood; drugs (alcohol, atropine, anticholinergic drugs)

VIII. Circulation and metabolism of ADH
   Once secreted into the circulation, AVP has a half-life of only 16–20 minutes.

Incidence

  I. Seen occasionally in the dog
 II. Rare in the cat
III. Has been reported in mice, rats, horses
IV. In human beings and in some dogs, rapid in onset.

Etiology

   I. Idiopathic—majority of cases
  II. Congenital
 III. Surgical
 IV. Traumatic
  V. Ischemia
 VI. Inflammatory
VII. Neoplasia

Clinical signs

   I. Usually the sudden onset of moderate to marked polyuria and secondary polydipsia
  II. Because of severe polyuria, some patients become dehydrated.
 III. Because of secondary polydipsia, some patients vomit due to water overload.
 IV. Other secondary signs
     A. Weight loss
     B. Anorexia
     C. Depression
     D. Weakness

Diagnosis

 DI must be differentiated from the other important polyuric disorders.
   I. In DI blood and urine chemistries are usually normal with the exception of mild to severe plasma hyperosmolality (dehydration is present)
  II. Differential diagnosis
     A. Compulsive water drinker (psychogenic polydipsia)
     B. Renal tubular failure to respond to vasopressin—nephrogenic DI
     C. Chronic renal diseases (pyelonephritis, glomerulonephritis, and so forth)
     D. Diabetes mellitus
     E. Pyometra—endometritis
     F. Hyperadrenocorticism
     G. Hyperthyroidism
     H. Chronic severe liver disease (persistent ductus venosus syndrome)
     I. Pseudohyperparathyroidism
     J. Sodium washout
 III. Diagnosis of DI is assured when it has been demonstrated that one or more of the major stimuli to ADH release (careful water restriction, hypertonic saline, nicotine) do not cause a significant antidiuresis or the production of hypertonic urine, but that the kidney is responsive to exogenous ADH or pitressin.

A. Water restriction in a DI patient should be done with extreme caution while the patient is observed closely.

B. Stop dehydration test when patient has lost 3–5% of body weight

IV. It was formerly thought that DI was an "all or none" disease, and that mild or moderate forms of the disease did not exist.

A. Partial DI clearly established in humans

B. Partial DI now reported in dog

Treatment

I. Some form of ADH is the mainstay of treatment.

II. Pitressin tannate in oil (5 U/ml) is the most common form (Parke-Davis, Morris Plains, New York)

A. Dosage is individualized for each patient.

B. Usually start with 1–2 U SQ or IM every 36 to 72 hours.

C. Adjust dose and frequency for each case.

D. The residual amount in each ampule may be covered with alcohol sponge and stored in the refrigerator. The ampule must be warmed by hand and completely mixed (5 full minutes).

E. Overdosage may lead to water intoxication.

III. Aqueous pitressin

A. Use in emergency situations, 1–2 U is administered SQ every 4–6 hours.

B. Main use is for diagnostic purposes

IV. Desmopressin acetate (DDAVP) Armour Pharmaceutical Co., Tarrytown, New York, intranasal drops are supplied in 2.5-ml vials.

A. Store in refrigerator.

B. Administer one drop intranasally every 8 hours, or in patients that will not tolerate intranasal instillation, use conjunctival sac.

V. Lypressin (Diapid nasal spray) Sandoz Pharmaceuticals, East Hanover, New Jersey

Very short duration of action, not as suitable for treatment of dog or cat.

VI. Nonhormonal forms of therapy

A. Thiazide diuretics—chronic administration of these products to human patients with NDI and DI can cause approximately 50% reduction in 24-hour urinary volume. The reduced urine volume although less hypotonic, is never hypertonic. Must be used with rigid salt restriction. Is the specific form of therapy for NDI (see Chapter 12).

B. Sulfonylurea products (chlorpropamide)—main use is as an oral hypoglycemic agent. Has now been clearly established that this drug (chlorpropamide, Diabenese) has an ADH-like effect and can be used successfully in the treatment of vasopressin-sensitive DI. Has no effect in NDI. Results in production of hypertonic urine. Shown to be effective in treating partial DI in the dog. Fifty to 250 mg q12h orally depending on size. Use for diagnostic purposes only.

THYROID GLAND

HYPOTHYROIDISM

Definition

A state resulting from inadequate quantities of the circulating thyroid hormones, triiodothyronine and thyroxine

Classification

I. Primary hypothyroidism
   A. An absence or destruction of functioning thyroid tissue
   B. May be congenital or acquired
   C. Disease develops insidiously
   D. More in young adult dogs
II. Secondary hypothyroidism
   A. Deficiency of TSH production
   B. May be caused by pituitary tumors

Clinical Signs

   I. The disease usually develops slowly over a course of many months. The owner may not be aware of the development of clinical signs at first.
  II. History usually suggests the diagnosis.
       A. Cold intolerance
       B. Slowing of mental and physical activities
 III. Decrease in metabolic rate
       A. Weight gain—mild to severe
       B. Cold intolerance
       C. Rectal temperature—occasionally 1–2°F lower than normal
       D. Reduced exercise tolerance in some animals
  IV. Skin and hair coat
       A. Changes dependent upon duration of hypothyroidism
       B. Occasional alopecia—especially chest, flanks, and thighs.
       C. Pigmentation in areas of alopecia
       D. Thickening of the dermis
       E. Puffiness of skin of face and forehead
   V. Cardiovascular—pulse rate may be below normal.

VI. Gastrointestinal
   A. Increased appetite in some animals, fair to poor appetite in others
   B. Occasional diarrhea, dry feces
VII. Reproduction
   A. Irregular or abnormal estral cycles in some females. Occasionally complete anestrus.
   B. Hypogonadism in males
   C. Lack libido
   D. See chapter 20

Diagnosis

I. Clinical signs
II. Laboratory evaluation
   A. Normal or reduced hematocrit (packed cell volume)
   B. Cholesterol levels elevated in majority of cases, may occasionally be in normal range.
III. Measurement of serum triiodothyronine (T3) and serum thyroxine (T4) levels by radioimmunoassay.
   A. Use laboratory that has assays standardized for use in dogs and cats.
   B. Interpret values based on the normal ranges established by the laboratory performing assays.
   C. Factors that may alter (decrease) serum T3 and T4 values: Certain drugs—glucocorticoids, exogenous or endogenous; phenylbutazone; mitotane; phenobarbital
   D. Thyroid-stimulating hormone response test: evaluate only response of T4 as T3 quite variable; administer 5–10 U bovine TSH IM; take blood sample before and 8 hours after TSH administration; euthyroid animals show two- to threefold rise in serum T4 levels; hypothyroid animals show minimal or no elevation in T4 levels.

Treatment

I. Thyroid hormone replacement is for life of the patient.
II. Several preparations available
   A. l-thyroxine, T4 (levothyroxine)
      1. Twenty to 32 μg/kg/24 hr
      2. Administer once daily during morning hours.
      3. Drug of choice in the dog
   B. Triiodothyronine, T3 (liothyronine)
      4.4 μg/kg given every 8 hours
   C. Dessicated thyroid, thyroglobulin
      15–20 mg/kg once daily

THYROID TUMORS

Since the work of Rijnberk (1971) on iodine metabolism and thyroid disease in the dog, recognition of the significance of thyroid tumors, especially toxic thyroid tumors (hyperthyroidism), has become more apparent.

Euthyroidism and thyroid tumors

I. The majority of thyroid tumors are nontoxic (i.e., do not result in clinical signs of hormone excess).
II. Average age affected is 9 years (range 4–13 years).
III. Boxer most commonly affected breed
IV. Clinical manifestations
   A. Reason for presentation usually an enlargement in the neck region.
   B. Frequency of clinical signs in 45 dogs (Table 19-1)
V. Laboratory findings
   Erythrocyte sedimentation rate (ESR) was greater than 5 mm/hr in 13 of 45 dogs; in only 4 was anemia observed, and Ca and P levels were normal in all cases.

Hyperthyroidism

I. Thyrotoxicosis—a group of clinical and metabolic abnormalities that arises when there is an excess of circulating thyroid hormone.
   A. Two forms of hyperthyroidism in people.
      1. Graves's disease—diffuse hyperplasia of thyroid and sometimes exophthalmos
      2. Plummer's disease—solitary autonomous hypersecreting adenoma without exophthalmos
   B. Canine hyperthyroidism so far only reported to be similar to Plummer's disease.
II. Incidence of clinical signs in 13 dogs (Table 19-2)

TABLE 19-1. FREQUENCY OF CLINICAL SIGNS IN 45 DOGS WITH THYROID TUMORS

Unilateral goiter	39	Tracheal deviation	12
Bilateral goiter	6	Palpable regional LN	6
Consistency soft	4	Dysphagia	6
Consistency firm	26	Local pain	4
Consistency hard	15	Respiratory distress	3
Irregular shape	13	Weight loss	3

Data from Rijnberk, 1971.

TABLE 19-2. INCIDENCE OF CLINICAL SIGNS IN 13 DOGS
WITH HYPERTHYROIDISM

Goiter	13
Polydipsia	13
Weight loss	10
Polyphagia	8
Weakness and fatigue	8
Intolerance to hot environment	7
Nervousness	6
Hyperdefecation	3
Tremor	3
Absence of estrus (eight bitches)	2

Data from Rijnberk, 1971.

PARATHYROID GLANDS

PRIMARY HYPERPARATHYROIDISM

   I. Rarely seen
  II. Usually associated with neoplasms (adenoma)
 III. Clinical signs related to increased Ca levels
    A. Anorexia, vomiting, constipation
    B. Muscle weakness
    C. Lameness—pathologic fracture, arthritis—due to Ca deposits in joints
    D. Loose teeth
    E. Polyuria/polydipsia due to Ca nephropathy
    F. Cardiac arrhythmia
 IV. Radiographic findings
    A. Decreased bone density, subperiosteal cortical resorption, loss of lamina-dura around teeth, bone cysts, general decrease of bone density, multiple fractures (advanced)
    B. Ca deposits in soft tissue
  V. Laboratory values
    Elevated Ca values
    A. Over 11.0 mg/dl—reports as high as 27 mg/dl
    B. Low phosphorus—below 4 mg/dl
    C. Increased alkaline phosphatase
    D. Increased urinary excretion of Ca and P—may predispose the animal to development of nephrocalcinosis and urolithiasis.

VI. Differential diagnosis of hypercalcemia
   A. Physiologic—young growing dog
   B. Neoplasia
      1. Lymphosarcoma
      2. Anal sac adenocarcinoma
      3. Other tumors with or without bone involvement
   C. Hypoadrenocorticism
   D. Renal disease
   E. Hypervitaminosis D
   F. Primary hyperparathyroidism
   G. Other—i.e., laboratory error, hemoconcentration and the like
VII. Diagnosis
   A. Rule out all other causes by systematic evaluation of patient.
   B. Measure immunoreactive parathormone (IPTH) levels.
      1. Test difficult to perform—special handling
      2. Expensive
      3. Elevated levels are diagnostic.
VIII. Treatment of hypercalcemia
   A. Marked hypercalcemia and acute symptoms—treat first, then diagnose.
   B. Definite but not greatly elevated Ca levels—need diagnostic work
   C. Marginal Ca elevations (probably will tend to ignore)
      1. At present we measure bound Ca whereas ionic Ca (Ca^{2+}) is the cause of most problems.
      2. Serum protein reduction (albumin) changes the level of Ca (as albumin decreases measured Ca levels decrease).
      3. It is possible to measure ionic Ca (Ca^{2+}) but this is rarely done.
      4. 1.0 g albumin carries 0.8 mg bound Ca^{2+}
   D. Promote urinary excretion of Ca
      1. Isotonic NaCl fluid of choice
      2. Furosemide 5 mg/kg initially, then 5 mg/kg/hr thereafter
   E. Glucocorticoids
      1. Limit bone resorption
      2. Decrease intestinal absorption of calcium
      3. Increase renal excretion of calcium
      4. Direct cytolytic effect on some tumor cells, i.e., lymphosarcoma. Primary hyperparathyroidism not responsive to steroid therapy.
   F. Surgical exploration of neck—when all other causes of hypercalcemia have been eliminated

HYPOPARATHYROIDISM

I. Etiology
   A. Iatrogenic—due to removal of thyroid and inadvertent removal of parathyroid or damage to blood supply of the parathyroid glands

    B. Idiopathic

    C. Congenital

    D. Autoimmune disease

 II. In canine population, hypoparathyroidism is rare.

III. Clinical signs

    A. Tetany

    B. Unsteady gait

    C. Sluggish

    D. Pain when mobile

 IV. Laboratory

    A. Low Ca—any value <8.5 mg/dl. Always evaluate serum magnesium levels in hypocalcemic patients

    B. High phosphorus

    C. Complete laboratory evaluation including complete blood count (CBC), urinalysis (UA), chemistry panel

 V. Treatment

    A. Primary aim of treatment is to return serum Ca to low normal range (9.0 mg/dl)

    B. Severe hypocalcemia—may see muscle tremors, tetany, managed with IV administration of 10% calcium gluconate (0.5–1.5 ml/kg up to 10 ml total)

      1. Slow administration (15–30 minutes)

      2. Monitor with electrocardiogram.

      3. Stop calcium administration if

        a) Bradycardia

        b) Elevation of ST segment

        c) Shortening of QT interval

      4. Can repeat dose at 6- to 8-hour intervals, if needed.

    C. Vitamin D administration

      1. Several forms available

      2. Long-term management

      3. Dihydroxytachysterol in oil (Hytakerol)

        a) Relatively inexpensive and widely available

        b) Daily maintenance dose of 0.007–0.010 mg/kg administered orally

        c) May require 1–2 weeks to restore normocalcemia

    D. Monitor serum calcium levels every 2 weeks.

ADRENAL CORTEX

HYPERFUNCTION—CANINE CUSHING'S SYNDROME

Endocrine Interrelations

 I. Steroids secreted by adrenal cortex are classified into five groups

    A. Aldosterone—almost all from the subcapsular zona glomerulosa

B. Corticosteroids—cortisol and corticosterone
C. Progesterone
D. Androgens
E. Estrogens
II. In several species (dogs, cows, guinea pigs, human beings) more cortisol is produced than corticosterone (Table 19-3).
III. Summary of adrenocortical control mechanisms for cortisol production (Fig. 19-1).

Clinical features

I. Polyuria and polydipsia are usually the first changes noted by the owner, who may see an increased appetite, anestrous of long duration in female, symmetrical alopecia, muscle weakness, and lethargy or pot belly.
II. Incidence of clinical signs (Table 19-4).

Clinical Pathologic Findings

I. Hematologic
   A. Elevated packed cell volume in 33% of patients (7 of 21 patients studied by Rijnberk et al., 1968)
   B. Total leucocyte count usually elevated with an elevation of neutrophils
      Capen et al., 1967 reported in 16 dogs an average total leucocyte count of 18,100/mm^3 with over 92% neutrophils.
   C. Absolute lymphopenia and eosinopenia
      1. Rijnberg et al., 1968 reported eosinopenia in 16 of 21 and lymphopenia in 12 of 21 dogs
      2. Capen et al., 1967 reported eosinophils below 82/mm^3 in 16 of 16 patients and lymphocytes averaged 1,200/mm^3
   D. Summary of hematologic changes
      1. Steroids cause rapid destruction of lymphocytes in blood, lymphoid

TABLE 19-3.   RATIO OF CORTISOL TO
CORTICOSTERONE PRODUCTION IN
DIFFERENT SPECIES

Species	Cortisol:Corticosterone
Dog	2:1–5:1
Cat	5:1
Guinea pig	2:1
Sheep	3:1–10:1
Man	4:1–10:1
Rat	0:10
Rabbit	1:10

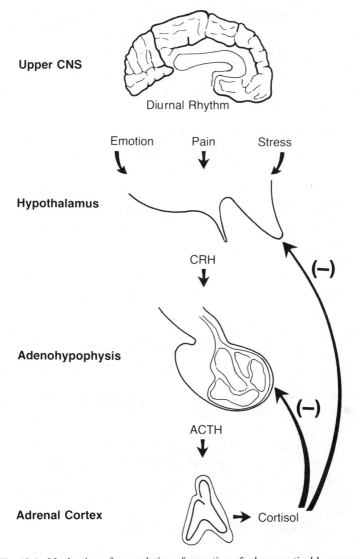

Upper CNS

Diurnal Rhythm

Emotion   Pain   Stress

Hypothalamus

CRH

(–)

Adenohypophysis

ACTH

(–)

Adrenal Cortex → Cortisol

Fig. 19-1. Mechanisms for regulation of secretion of adrenocortical hormones.

tissue, and thymus. Also reduce the blood eosinophils without affecting the marrow eosinophil count.
2. Polymorphonuclear leucocyte and platelet counts are increased by steroids, also steroids decrease migration into area of infection.
3. Red cell mass increased by steroids
II. Blood chemistry
  A. Serum Na^+, K^+, and Cl^- usually within normal limits
  B. Hypokalemia reported but rare. Hypokalemia is also infrequent in

TABLE 19-4.　INCIDENCE OF CLINICAL SIGNS

Clinical Sign	Lubberink (71)*	Rijnberk (21)	Capen (26)	Schechter (18)
Polydipsia	61	21	24	18
Polyphagia	62	21	3	12
Abdominal enlargement	68	21	8	18
Enlarged liver (roentgenogram)	65	19	—	11
Lethargy	45	16	7	14
Obesity	40	12	10	—
Alopecia	39	11	9	18
Absence of estrus (14 bitches)	30 (35)	10	—	—
Intolerance to heat	29	9	—	—
Muscle weakness	50	9	10	12
Exophthalmos	34	6	—	—
Pigmentation	—	5	5	12
Calcinosis cutis	3	3	4	10
Acne	4	3	—	9
Skin atrophy	63	—	—	—

*Number of dogs in study.

human patients but is reported to occur with very high cortisol production rates as might occur with an adrenal tumor.

    C. Plasma cholesterol elevated

            i) 216–509 mg/dl (Siegel et al., 1970)

            ii) Elevated serum alkaline phosphatase levels

III. Urinalysis

    A. Most consistent alteration is a low osmolality or specific gravity of the urine.

    B. Mechanism of polyuria in Cushing's disease unknown

       1. Possibly associated with

          a) Depression of renal tubular permeability to water

          b) Partial inhibition of ADH release

          c) Elevation of responsive threshold of osmoreceptors

       2. Probably not associated with:

          a) Osmotic diuresis

          b) Absolute lack of ADH due to destruction of neurohypophysis

IV. Summary of laboratory findings (Table 19-5)

 V. Endocrinologic parameters

    A. Steroids in the urine—has been shown that at least 60% of the metabolites of cortisol present in the glucuronide fraction of canine urine are

TABLE 19-5. SUMMARY OF LABORATORY FINDINGS

Abnormality	Approximate cases (%)
Eosinopenia	90
Elevated alkaline phosphatase	80
Subnormal T3	80
Lymphopenia	75
Neutrophilia	60
Subnormal T4	50
Elevated GPT	50
Elevated Na	35
Elevated GOT	30
Elevated K	15
Hyperglycemia/glucosuria	10

Data from Lubberink AAME: Diagnosis and Treatment of Canine Cushing's Syndrome. Drukherij Elinwijk BV, Utrecht, 1977.
Abbreviations: GOT, glutamic oxaloacetic transaminase; GPT, glutamic pyruvic transaminase.

reduced at C-20. Thus Porter-Sibler reaction less suitable in canine than in human patients.

B. Hormone levels in the plasma
 1. Competitive protein binding
  Measures cortisol, thus values reported will be lower than values obtained by fluorometric method.
 2. Fluorometric method
  Measure cortisol and corticosterone (11β-hydroxycorticosteroids) (11β-OHCS) and may be subject to more substances causing false elevations of values. Also lacks sensitivity in the lower ranges.
 3. Radioimmunoassay method
  Very sensitive method, specifically measures cortisol. Use laboratory that has standardized the assay for dogs. Use range of normal and abnormal values established by the laboratory you are using when interpreting results.
 4. Important to note that there is considerable overlap between normal and Cushing's syndrome when only resting values are considered.
 5. Stimulation tests
  A good method at the present for separating normal from Cushing's syndrome dog is to use the ACTH stimulation test. There are multiple doses for ACTH use in literature and variable times of testing after ACTH. In addition, the final results vary with the method [(CPB); (Fl); radioimmunoassay (RIA)] used.

    a) IM stimulation test:
      (1) Use ACTH gel (10–40 IU).
      2) Take pre-ACTH sample.
      (3) Plasma sample 2 hours later.
    b) IV ACTH stimulation test (superior to the IM test)
      (1) Use 0.25 mg (10–20 U) aqueous ACTH solution IV.
      (2) Take control value immediately before ACTH administration
      (3) Post-ACTH injection sample 2 hours after ACTH

6. Suppression tests

    Use of dexamethasone (oral or IV) has been used primarily for the differentiation of bilateral adrenocortical hyperplasia from an autonomously hyperfunctioning adrenal tumor and to establish the diagnosis of canine hyperadrenocorticism.

    a) Dexamethasone screening test is indicated to establish the diagnosis of hyperadrenocorticism. Administer dexamethasone IV (0.01 mg/kg) after collection of a blood sample for a baseline cortisol value. Eight hours postinjection, collect a second sample. The baseline cortisol value may or may not be within the normal range. In normal dogs, the plasma cortisol value will be reduced to below 10 ng/ml in the 8-hour postinjection sample, often near zero values. In dogs with hyperadrenocorticism, minimal suppression will be noted, if at all.

    b) High-dose dexamethasone suppression is used to differentiate adrenocortical tumors from pituitary-dependent hyperadrenocorticism. For the suppression test, inject dexamethasone IV at a dose of 0.1 mg/kg and collect blood immediately before and 3 hour postinjection.

    c) In dogs with pituitary-dependent hyperadrenocorticism, plasma cortisol is suppressed to near zero within 8 hours. In dogs with an adrenal tumor, there is little or no change in plasma cortisol levels.

Treatment

  I. Bilateral adrenalectomy
    A. Is a good procedure, but it requires surgical skill and knowledge of the surgical field involved. Adrenal glands are quite closely attached to postcava in some cases.
    B. Paracostal approach preferred to a ventral midline approach
    C. Requires more precise medical management of the patient both pre and post-operatively
  II. Pituitary gland ablation
    A. Is preferred method of treatment when a pituitary tumor is suspected cause of disease
    B. Difficult procedure in brachiocephalic breeds

C. Use pharyngeal route

D. Replacement therapy post-operative is oral glucocorticoids and thyroid hormone.

E. Most patients will develop postoperative transient DI which must be controlled with exogenous antidiuretic hormone (ADH) therapy.

III. Chemotherapy

Mitotane (Lysodren)

A. An adrenocorticolytic drug which acts mainly on the zona fasciculata and reticularis. Zona glomerulosa is relatively resistant.

B. Several methods available for using the drug

1. Method 1

a) Patient carefully monitored as to water consumption and lymphocyte count prior to start of therapy

b) Dosage—50 mg Lysodren/kg once daily and continue until water consumption starts to fall and absolute lymphocyte counts are in normal range.

c) Therapy should continue for minimum of 5 days and may take 18–21 days before a response is noted.

d) After response is obtained, maintain patient on dose of 50 mg/kg once every 2 weeks.

2. Method 2

a) Daily dose of 50 mg/kg is divided and given $\frac{1}{2}$ in the morning and $\frac{1}{2}$ in the evening for 10 continuous days.

b) Three days after initiation of Lysodren therapy, patient started on 5 mg oral prednisolone once daily for 10 consecutive days.

c) Put patient on maintenance dose of 50 mg/kg once every 2 weeks or as needed

3. In some dogs occasional toxic signs may be observed. If seen, stop drug and wait at least 1 week before restarting therapy (anorexia, depression, ataxia, vomiting)

4. Monitor patient with occasional CBC, chemistry screen.

5. An occasional patient may have total destruction of its adrenal cortex in which case it will be necessary to replace mineralocorticoids as in Addison's disease.

HYPOFUNCTION—HYPOADRENOCORTICISM, ADDISON'S DISEASE

Summary of Aldosterone Control
Mechanisms (Fig. 19-2)

Clinical Features (Mineralocorticoid
Deficiency)

I. Depression, weakness

II. Anorexia

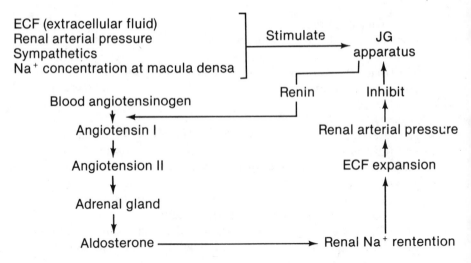

Fig. 19-2. Summary of aldosterone control mechanisms.

III. Hypotension (weak femoral pulse)
IV. Dehydration
 V. Vomition and/or diarrhea
VI. Bradycardia (only when serum K^+ levels severely elevated)

Primary versus Secondary Hypoadrenocorticism

  I. Primary adrenocortical insufficiency—results from a disease process which destroys most of the adrenal cortex resulting in a deficiency of aldosterone and glucocorticoids. The clinical picture is primarily due to aldosterone loss.
 II. Secondary adrenocortical insufficiency—occurs due to a lack of ACTH and may be associated with prolonged glucocorticoid therapy or occasionally with panhypopituitarism. Clinical signs are a combination of Cushing's syndrome appearance with acute or subacute shock syndrome due mainly to cortisol deficiency; aldosterone production remains normal.

Clinical Pathologic Findings

  I. Hematologic
    A. Erythrocyte parameters may show a normochromic normocytic anemia
    B. Usually within normal limits
    C. Total leucocyte count usually normal although may range from 9,850 to 66,000/mm³
    D. Eosinophilia not a consistent change
    E. Lymphocytosis also not a consistent finding
    F. Elevation of serum proteins usually a reflection of the degree of dehydration.

II. Blood chemistry
  A. Electrolytes (see chapter 2)
    1. Serum K^+ levels elevated (renal retention)
      a) Normal values in the dog 3.5–5.0 mEq/L.
      b) Elevations above 5.5 mEq/L are suggestive.
      c) Elevations above 6.0 mEq/L are moderate.
      d) Elevations above 7.0 mEq/L are severe.
    2. Serum Na^+ values are low (Cl^- parallels Na^+).
      a) Normal values in dog 137–149 mEq/L.
      b) Values may range as low as 115 mEq/L.
  B. Blood urea nitrogen
    1. Mild to severe elevation in almost all patients, especially in those showing definite clinical signs.
    2. Associated with the lowered renal arterial pressure, and reduced glomerular filtration rate (GFR)
  C. Hypoglycemia does not appear to be a consistent finding in hypoadrenocorticism in dogs as it may be in human patients.
III. Urinalysis
  Usually no specific or significant changes on a routine urinalysis
IV. Plasma cortisol levels
  A. Due to the acute nature of the disease, it is often not possible to carry out extensive stimulation tests (ACTH) to evaluate a patient in an acute shock-like state.
  B. In acute primary hypoadrenocorticism, plasma cortisol values will be very low and there will be no response to exogenous ACTH.

Treatment

  I. Aims of treatment
    A. Replace deficient mineralocorticoids.
    B. Correct dehydration.
    C. Return renal function to normal.
    D. Supplement glucocorticoids.
 II. Acute adrenal crisis is an emergency.
    A. Immediately infuse isotonic saline solution through IV jugular catheter (also insert urethral catheter to monitor urine flow).
    B. Supplement IV fluids with a soluble IV glucocorticoid.
    C. Administer 1–5 mg desoxycorticosterone acetate (DOCA) by IM route.
    D. Parenteral hydrocortisone succinate will supply both gluco- and mineralocorticoid activity.
III. Maintenance therapy
    A. Some form of mineralocorticoid replacement is needed. Patient needs both gluco- and mineralocorticoids.
      1. Fludrocortisone tablets, 0.1 mg tablets (Florinef); dosage—$\frac{1}{2}$ to three tablets daily. Begin with once-daily administration. Occasional pa-

tient requires greater amount or twice daily administration for proper maintenance.
   2. Desoxycorticosterone pivalate (DOCP), 25 mg/ml. Twenty-five milligrams DOCP will release equivalent of approximately 1 mg of desoxycorticosterone per day. Each dose will last 3–4 weeks. Adjust dosage, based on serum electrolyte levels.
B. Glucocorticoids are needed for daily maintenance.
   Oral prednisolone tablets, 5 mg, or oral prednisone tablets, 20 mg once daily. Dose is approximately 0.25–0.5 mg/kg once daily.

PHARMACOLOGY OF ADRENOCORTICOSTEROIDS

Metabolic Actions

I. Glucocorticoids have significant effects on metabolism of glucose, proteins, and lipids
II. Effects on glucose
   Increase blood glucose level—due in part to gluconeogenesis, antiinsulin effects of glucocorticoids, and altered lipid metabolism
III. Effects on proteins
   A. Reduction in peripheral protein synthesis
   B. Relative increase in protein catabolism
IV. Effects on lipid metabolism
   A. Inhibition of long-chain fatty acid synthesis
   B. Mobilization of free fatty acids from fat stores

Structure

I. Cortisol (hydrocortisone) naturally secreted glucocorticoid of the adrenal cortex
II. Basic steroid nucleus. Carbon skeleton common to all steroid hormones (Fig. 19-3).
III. Structure of cortisol (hydrocortisone)
   Structural features essential for glucocorticoid activity are circled with dotted line (Fig. 19-4).
IV. Modifications of the molecular structure can be made as long as the basic C-skeleton and the above four features are not altered, to produce glucocorticoids of different potency, duration of action, protein binding affinity and relative glucocorticoid/mineralocorticoid ratios.

Transport of Glucocorticoids

I. May be transported in blood stream as free steroid or bound to plasma proteins

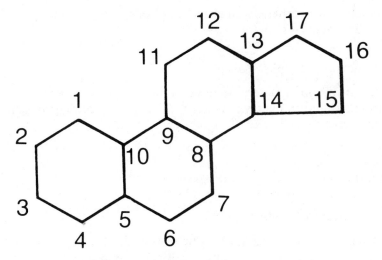

Fig. 19-3. Nucleus common to all steroidal hormones.

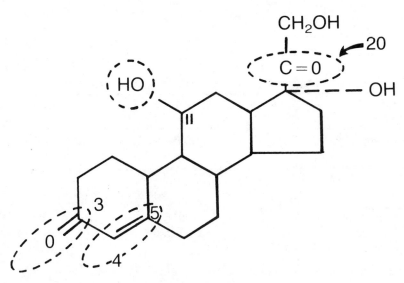

Fig. 19-4. Structure of cortisol. Structural features essential for glucocorticoid activity are circled by dotted lines.

A. May bind nonspecifically to albumin
    B. May bind to corticosteroid-binding globulin
 II. Synthetic glucocorticoids, in general, are less avidly bound.
III. Only free glucocorticoid is active.

Esters of Glucocorticoids (Bases)

Glucocorticoids in parenteral solution available as esters that vary in water
solubility. Esters affect mainly the rate at which the glucocorticoid is absorbed
from injection site (Table 19-6).

Comparison of glucocorticoid anti-inflammatory Potency and Durations of Action. See table 19-7 and chapter 5.

Rational use of corticosteroids

I. Fundamental reasons for use of glucocorticoids
    A. Specific replacement therapy to correct a deficiency
        1. Primary adrenocortical insufficiency
        2. Hypopituitarism resulting in low ACTH output
    B. Exert a pharmacologic effect in the treatment of a specific disease
        1. Collagen disorders
        2. Inflammatory conditions
        3. Allergic states
        4. Neoplastic diseases
        5. Immune complex disorders
        6. Other

TABLE 19-6.   ESTERS OF GLUCOCORTICOIDS

Ester	Water Solubility	Route of Administration	Complete Absorption
Hemisuccinate	Very high	IV, IM, SQ	30–60 min
Phosphate	Very high	IV, IM, SQ	30–60 min
Acetate	Poor	Intraarticular,	Slow—2–14 days
Diacetate	Poor	intralesional,	Slow—2–14 days
Tebutate	Poor	or IM	Slow—2–14 days
Acetonide	Poor	Topical, IM	Very slow
Hexacetonide	Poor	IM, intralesional, intraarticular	Slow
Valerate	Poor	Topical	Slow

TABLE 19-7. COMPARISON OF GLUCOCORTICOID AND ANTIINFLAMMATORY
POTENCY AND DURATIONS OF ACTION

Glucocorticoid Base	Antiinflammatory Potency	20-kg Dog Dose[a] (mg)	Duration of HPA Suppression (hr)	Mineralopotency
Short-acting				
Hydrocortisone	1	20	<12	+ +
Cortisone	0.8	25	<12	+ +
Intermediate-acting				
Prednisolone	4.0	5	12–36	+
Prednisone	3.5	5	12–36	+
Methyl prednisolone	5.0	4	12–36	0
Triamcinolone	5.0	4	12–36	0
Long-acting				
Dexamethasone	30	0.75	>48	0
Betamethasone	25	0.6	>48	0
Paramethasone	10	2	>48	0

[a] Physiologic replacement.

II. Replacement steroid therapy

Corticosteroid daily secretion rate in dog (Table 19-8) *Doses:* two to three times normal daily output may be used safely as intermittent therapy provided that the steroid compound being used is a short-acting glucocorticoid.

III. Alternate-day steroid therapy

A. The general principle of alternate-day steroid therapy is that of administering a single dose of a short- or intermediate-acting steroid on alternate mornings in quantities equivalent to the total dose being employed over a 48-hour period.

B. Forms of glucocorticoids that can be used for alternate-day steroid therapy in dogs include:

1. Hydrocortisone—short-acting
2. Cortisone—short-acting

TABLE 19-8. CORTICOSTEROID DAILY
SECRETION RATE IN DOG

Cortisol	758	μg/kg
Corticosterone	321	μg/kg
Desoxycortisol	88	μg/kg
Desocylcorticosterone	6	μg/kg
Aldosterone	8	μg/kg
Total	1.2	mg/kg

TABLE 19-9.   TAPERING THE DOSE

Day	Prednisolone (mg)
1	17.5
2	12.5
3	20
4	10
5	22.5
6	7.5
7	25
8	5
9	25
10	5
11	30
12	0
13	30
14	0
15	30
16	0
17	25
18	0
19	25
20	0
21	20
22	0

    3. Prednisone—intermediate-acting
    4. Prednisolone—intermediate-acting
C. Definition: The action of the drug is based on the length of pituitary-adrenal suppression (biological half-life)
    1. Short—Less than 12 hr
    2. Intermediate—12–36 hr
    3. Long—Greater than 48 hr
D. It should be kept in mind that even though methylprednisolone and triamcinolone are classified as intermediate-acting steroids in people, there is no conclusive proof that the same is also true for the dog. Triamcinolone has the longest half-life of the intermediate-acting preparations. Until further proof is obtained, do not use methylprednisolone or triamcinolone for alternate-day steroid therapy.
E. The alternate-day concept involves administering an exogenous glu-

cocorticoid in a manner that mimics the normal diurnal cycle of cortisol and thereby minimizes both hypothalamic-pituitary suppression and certain undesired tissue side effects.

1. Administer steroid around 7–8 A.M. on alternate days.
2. In patients that have been on long-term steroids, taper to an alternate-day program over 2-week period rather than change suddenly.
3. Find daily dose that will control clinical signs first.

F. Example of "tapering the dose" (Table 19-9): 15-kg dog with atopic dermatitis that requires continuous year-round glucocorticoids. Pruritus is presently being controlled with 15 mg prednisolone per day. To switch to alternate-day program, follow the protocol shown in the table.

SUGGESTED READINGS

Belshaw BG, Rijnberk A: Radioimmunoassay of plasma T4 and T3 in the diagnosis of primary hypothyroidism in dogs, J Am Anim Hosp Assoc 15:17, 1979

Burke TJ: Hormone and corticosteroid therapy. Vet Clin N Am 12(1):1–150, 1982

Capen CC, Martin SL, and Koestner A: Neoplasms in the adenohypophysis in dogs, Path Vet 4:301, 1967

Chew DJ, Meuteu DJ: Disorders of calcium and phosphorus metabolism. Vet Clin Am 12:411, 1982

Lees GE: Hypoparathyroidism. p. 876. In Kirk RW (ed): Current Veterinary Therapy, VIII. WB Saunders, Philadelphia, 1983

Lubberink AAME: Diagnosis and Treatment of Canine Cushing's Syndrome. Drukkerij Elinwijk BV, Utrecht, 1977

Meijer JC: An investigation of the pathogenesis of pituitary-dependent hyperadrenocorticism in the dog. Ph.D Thesis, University of Utrecht, the Netherlands, 1980

Mulnix JA: Diabetes insipidus. p. 850. In Kirk RW (ed): Current Veterinary Therapy, VIII. WB Saunders, Philadelphia, 1983

Parker WM, Scott DW: Growth hormone responsive alopecia in the mature dog: a discussion of 13 cases. J Am Anim Hosp Assoc 16:824, 1980

Rijnberk A: Iodine Metabolism and Thyroid Disease in the Dog. Drukkerij Elinkwijk-Utrecht, 1971

Rijnberk A, Derkinderen PJ, and Thijssen JHH: Spontaneous Hyperadrenocorticism in the Dog: J Endocrinol 41:397, 1968

Scott DW: Dermatologic use of glucocorticoids. Vet Clin N Am 12(1):19, 1982

Schechter RD, Stabenfeldt GH, Gribble DM, and Ling GU: Treatment of Cushing's Syndrome in the Dog with an Adrenocorticolytic Agent (o,p' DDD), J Am Vet Med Assoc 162:629, 1973

Siegel ET, Kelly DF, and Berg P; Cushing's Syndrome in the Dog: J Am Vet Med Assoc 157:2081, 1970

20

Reproductive Disorders
Thomas J. Burke, D.V.M.

THERAPEUTIC INTERVENTIONS IN THE HEALTHY BITCH AND QUEEN

Estrus Control

General Considerations

The best means of estrus control is overiohysterectomy. Pharmacologic methods have been developed for owners who, for a variety of reasons (some justifiable) will not subject their animals to surgery.

Treatment

I. Progestogens
   A. Long-term progestional therapy in both the bitch and queen may lead to cystic endometrial hyperplasia, mammary neoplasia, and development of diabetes mellitus.
   B. Megestrol acetate is the only approved progestogen for this indication in the United States.
      1. Bitch
         a) To stop a cycle in proestrus the dose is 2.2 mg/kg SID for 8 days beginning during the first 3 days of proestrus. The timing of the next cycle is quite variable but may be prolonged by giving 2.2 mg/kg/day for 4 days followed by 0.55 mg/kg/day for 16–20 days.
         b) To postpone an anticipated cycle megestrol is given at 0.55 mg/kg/day for 32 days beginning at least 7 days prior to the onset of proestrus. British veterinarians prescribe a dose of 0.1–0.2 mg/kg twice weekly for up to 4 months following a postponement course of therapy for prolonged suppression. The patient should then be allowed to have an unmedicated cycle before being re-treated.

605

2. Queen
   Megestrol is not approved for use in cats in the United States at this time. British recommendations are:
   a) Anestrus—2.5 mg/cat/week for up to 18 months
   b) Diestrus—2.5 mg/cat/day for up to 60 days
   c) Estrus—5.0 mg/cat/day for 3–5 days then place on diestrus regimen

   Cats treated with either long-term regimen should have an unmedicated cycle before being retreated.

II. Androgens
   A. Mibolerone, a synthetic, androgenic, anabolic, 19-norsteroid is the only compound currently approved for estrus suppression in the bitch in the United States. The dosage ranges from 30 μg per dog per day for dogs up to 12 kg to 180 μg per dog per day for those weighing over 45 kg. German shepherds and German shepherd-crosses require twice as much drug as other breeds of similar size. This is the only known breed variation and its reason is unknown. Treatment must be begun at least 30 days prior to proestrus. Mibolerone will not arrest proestrus. Currently the drug is approved for a 2-year treatment period but current work shows promise that lifelong therapy may be possible.
   B. Side effects include clitoral hypertrophy with concomitant vaginitis (worse in prepuberal bitches), deepening of the voice, and exacerbation of preexisting seborrheic dermatitis. If given to pregnant bitches severe masculinization of female fetuses will result. Abnormal liver function tests are seen in some patients. Clinical signs of liver disease have not been reported. All side effects disappear after cessation of therapy except that mild residual clitoral hypertrophy may be noted. Bitches that experience estrus while on therapy for more than 30 days may need to have their dose increased by 20–50% *after* firmly establishing that they are not pregnant.
   C. Precaution—*mibolerone should not be used in cats.*

THERAPEUTIC ABORTION

General Considerations

There are no approved drugs for this purpose at this time. An established pregnancy is difficult to interrupt.

Treatment

I. Surgery
   Bilateral ovariectomy will result in abortion within 8 days.

II. Glucocorticoids

Dexamethasone caused either resorption or abortion in bitches given 0.14–0.17 mg/kg SID IM for 10 days starting at day 30 and 45, respectively. This has not been tried in the cat.

III. Prostaglandins

A. Prostaglandin $F_{2\alpha}$ given at 20 μg/kg IM TID for 2 days produced abortion in four of seven bitches that were at least 25 days pregnant.

B. Other prostaglandins are being tested and some look promising.

C. Prostaglandin $F_{2\alpha}$ given to cats past day 42 of pregnancy at doses of 0.5–1.0 mg/kg for 1 day or 2 days will result in abortion if the patient has been stressed prior to treatment or is pretreated with adrenocorticotropic hormone (ACTH).

MISMATING

General Considerations

Therapy should be begun as soon after the misalliance as is practical, certainly within 72 hours for maximum efficacy.

Treatment

I. Estrogens

A. Diethylstilbestrol (DES)

1. Repositol injection of 0.5 mg/kg IM. Administer only once. Total dose not to exceed 24 mg.

2. Tablets daily for 5 days; total daily dose of 0.1–1.0 mg/dog.

B. Estradiol-17-cyclopentyl propionate (ECP). *One* IM dose of 0.02 mg/kg. For cats use 0.25 mg total dose/cat.

C. Estradiol benzoate or valerate. One IM dose of 0.1 mg/kg (not to exceed 3 mg total).

All estrogens may produce bone marrow suppression. Young dogs are more resistant to this effect. In addition, an increased risk of cystic endometrial hyperplasia and subsequent pyometritis is produced, perhaps as high as 30%. Cats are relatively resistant to the effects on bone marrow. Diethylstilbestrol may be hepatotoxic in cats.

II. Megestrol acetate

When administered at 2.2 mg/kg for at least 3 days prior to mating, megestrol has a contraceptive effect in bitches if the treatment is continued for another 5 days at 3.0–4.0 mg/kg. In cats a single dose of 2.5 mg/kg given within 12 hours of mating has prevented pregnancy.

III. Prostaglandins

Prostaglandins have proven ineffective in preventing pregnancy when administered in the early postcoital period.

ESTRUS INDUCTION

General Considerations

Patient selection is critical for induction of estrus by injection of exogenous gonadotrophic hormones. Be certain that the owner is knowledgeable about heat detection. The patient must be at least 24 months old, have normal ovaries, normal thyroid function, and baseline serum progesterone levels. Pregnant mare serum gonadotrophin has been widely used but the author has experienced some difficulty with its use probably as a result of batch-to-batch and/or shelf-life potency variation.

Treatment—bitch

Porcine pituitary follicle-stimulating hormone FSH (FSH-P) 0.75 mg/kg IM once daily for 10 days. Follow with human chorionic gonadotrophin (HCG) 100–200 IU/kg/day IM for 3 days, beginning on day 10. Breed whenever the patient will stand. If this occurs before day 10 continue therapy as above. Some animals may not breed until several days after the cessation of therapy. Some bitches will establish a normal cycle after one treatment. Conception rates have been about 80%. Ovulation may also be produced with gonadotrophin-releasing hormone (GnRH) 50–200 µg per dog (each dose) IM. Two doses are given 6 hours apart on day 11.

Treatment—queen

I. Porcine pituitary follicle-stimulating hormone given IM at total dose of 2.0 mg per cat daily for up to 5 days. Stop if behavioral estrus occurs before day 5. If no estrus is observed by day 5 repeat treatment in 6–8 weeks. To help insure ovulation administer one dose of GnRH 25 µg per cat IM on the day of breeding.
II. The reader is referred to the list of Suggested Readings at the end of this chapter for other regimens that have been successful for other authors.

FEMALE REPRODUCTIVE DISORDERS

PROLONGED ESTRUS (NYMPHOMANIA)

General Considerations

Expression of estrus for more than 2 weeks is generally caused by ovarian cysts that produce estrogens. Ovariohysterectomy is immediately curative.

Treatment

Therapeutic attempts at causing ovulation of the cysts are indicated in breeding animals.

I. Gonadotrophin-releasing hormone
   A. Fifty to 200 μg IM daily for up to 5 days in the bitch. Twice daily injections may improve the efficacy.
   B. Twenty-five micrograms IM daily for 2 days in queens.
   C. Repeat in 1 week if unsuccessful.
II. Human chorionic gonadotrophin
   A. Fifty to 200 IU/kg IM daily for up to 9 days in the bitch.
   B. Two hundred and fifty IU per cat IM daily for 2 days in queens.
   C. Repeat in 1 week if unsuccessful.
III. Surgery
   Aspiration of the cysts at surgery is often successful when medical therapy has failed.

FALSE PREGNANCY

General Considerations

The cause of this common syndrome remains an enigma. Serum progesterone levels are normal. Also it is not uncommon to see signs in bitches spayed during the luteal phase of the cycle. Spontaneous regression of signs is the rule and therapeutic intervention is warranted only when the owners demand it.

Treatment

I. Progestogens
   Megestrol acetate 2.2 mg/kg/day for 8–10 days. Some cases rebound after treatment. Re-treat as above and then treat at 0.55 mg/kg/day for 21 days.
II. Androgens
   A. Testosterone propionate at 2.5 mg/kg IM. Repeat in 2–4 weeks if necessary.
   B. Mibolerone at 35 μg/kg/day for 7–10 days. If patient rebounds re-treat as above and put on estrus prevention dose for 1 to 2 months.
III. Estrogens
   Not recommended

ABORTION RESULTING FROM EARLY LUTEOLYSIS

I. General Considerations
   This syndrome results from lack of endogenous progesterone during pregnancy. Affected females are usually habitual aborters with no other demonstrable cause for the abortions. The diagnosis is based upon finding baseline levels of serum progesterone (by radioimmunoassay) at the time of abortion *and* finding no other possible cause.

II. Progesterone in oil is given IM beginning about a week prior to the anticipated abortion based upon the patient's history. The dose is 1.0 mg/kg. It is repeated weekly up to the 53rd–55th day of gestation. Prolonged pregnancies are not uncommon even when the injections are stopped by day 55 and Caesarean delivery may be necessary.

Progestogens have been shown to masculinize female fetuses. The owner should be forewarned of this possibility but the author has not seen this occur using progesterone in oil.

ENDOMETRITIS

General Considerations

Low-grade bacterial infection of the uterus is a common cause of infertility. The patient is usually asymptomatic. In some animals the proestrual discharge contains excessive numbers of neutrophils. The diagnosis is based on recovery of a significant growth of bacteria from the area of the cervix during proestrus or from the uterus at surgery. A long-guarded culture instrument should be used with a speculum to minimize contamination with normal vaginal flora.

Treatment

I. Antibiotics

The choice of therapy depends upon culture and sensitivity results. Treatment should be continued for a minimum of 3 weeks. If breeding is anticipated during the treatment period one should choose the safest possible drug. In the author's experience semisynthetic penicillins and cephalosporins have neither affected conception nor been teratogenic. The tetracyclines, chloramphenicol, and long-acting sulfonamides are to be avoided if at all possible.

II. Infusions

Infusions of antibacterial compounds or antibiotics are of questionable value as they probably do not reach the site of infection.

PYOMETRA-PYOMETRITIS

General Considerations

Generally a disease of the luteal phase of the cycle, this is a polysystemic disease resulting from the bacteremia and/or toxemia with the uterus as the focus of infection. Gram-negative rods are the usual culprit with *Escherichia coli* being the most commonly isolated organism. Culture and sensitivity testing are prerequisites for rational therapy in all animals. Culture methods should be adequate to recover both anaerobes and aerobes.

Treatment

I. Surgery

Ovariohysterectomy is the treatment of choice in those patients that have little or no value as breeding animals. An alternative to salvage the uterus is to perform a hysterotomy, flush the uterus with an antiseptic, place catheters through the cervix to facilitate postoperative uterine lavage, and remove the corpora lutea from the ovaries.

II. Antibiotics

Therapy should be based on culture and sensitivity results and should continue for at least 3 weeks. Based on retrospective studies, the following antibiotics are listed in descending order of percent of sensitivity to guide the clinician in choice of an antibiotic while the initial culture results are pending: gentamicin, cephalosporins, ampicillin. Renal function should be monitored if an aminoglycoside is chosen. In cases of severe sepsis combined therapy with gentamicin and carbenicillin should be considered.

III. Prostaglandins

Prostaglandin $F_{2\alpha}$ has been shown to have uterotropic effects. It causes myometrial contraction thus emptying the uterus, increases uterine blood flow thus enhancing antibiotic levels at the site of infection, and either directly or indirectly opens the cervix. The dose is 250 µg/kg once daily. Treatment is continued until there is little or no discharge seen in the first hour postinjection. About 5 days after the last dose another injection is given to insure that the uterus is not filling with pus. Side effects seen have included vomiting, loose (cow pie) stool, weakness, hyperpnea, collapse, salivation, and pupillary constriction, or dilation. All are temporary and will vary in occurrence and severity within a treatment period. The dose given above is for prostaglandin $F_{2\alpha}$ THAM salt [Dinoprost Tromethamine (Upjohn)] only. Other formulations may require other doses.

IV. Ancillary therapy

A. Fluids

Appropriate rehydration should be undertaken immediately regardless of the choice of therapy.

B. Hormones

The use of either estrogens or progestogens is contraindicated. If the patient is anemic the use of androgens to stimulate erythropoeisis may be considered.

Prognosis

Medical therapy with prostaglandins results in avoiding surgery in nearly 97% of patients. Slightly over 75% have had normal litters.

ECLAMPSIA

General Considerations

Hypocalcemic tetany occurs in small- to medium-size bitches. It generally occurs during the first few weeks of lactation but may occur in late pregnancy. Signs vary from nervousness and anxiety early to muscle tetany or spastic lateral recumbency late in the course. High fever is a routine finding. Death results from hyperthermic cerebral edema or respiratory failure. Epileptiform seizures, hypoglycemia, and strychnine toxicosis should be ruled out.

Treatment

I. Calcium
   A. Calcium borogluconate or lactate (10%) should be administered IV to effect. One to 5 ml is usually adequate. It should be given *slowly* and stopped if cardiac arrhythmias occur.
   B. A SQ bolus equal to the amount needed to control the tetany is given. Calcium lactate is less irritating than gluconate or borogluconate.
   C. Oral calcium is dispensed; 1–3 g calcium gluconate SID. *Do not* supplement with vitamin D as hypercalcemia may result.
II. Hyperthermia
   Cool patient with baths or alcohol rubs and/or cold water enemas until the rectal temperature has decreased to 103°F.
III. Glucocorticoids
   Glucocorticoids should not be used in the treatment of this disease. They tend to lower serum calcium and antagonize vitamin D thus inhibiting intestinal absorption of calcium.
IV. Puppies
   The puppies should be raised as orphans since recurrence is high if they are allowed to continue nursing.
V. Lactation
   Lactation may be decreased by not allowing the puppies to nurse, reduction in daily caloric intake, administration of diuretics, especially furosemide, and androgenic steroids if necessary.
VI. Seizures
   If the patient has tetany to the point that the clinician cannot "hit a vein," parenteral injection of diazepam, phenobarbital, or pentobarbital (in descending order of preference) may be given to allow a clysis to be established.

Precaution

Be sure you are not dealing with hypoglycemia.

VAGINAL HYPERPLASIA

General Considerations

Considered by some to represent prolapse of the vagina, this condition is an exaggerated response of the vaginal mucosal and submucosal tissue to normal levels of estrogen. It occurs during proestrus, especially in brachiocephalic breeds. There is a protrusion of pink, turgid tissue through the vulva. Normally it is the floor of the vagina but the lateral and dorsal surfaces may be involved. It naturally disappears with the onset of the luteal phase of the cycle. It tends to recur with each cycle. If breeding is desired artificial insemination must be performed.

Treatment

I. The exposed tissue needs to be protected from drying and trauma. Methylcellulose drops are often all that is necessary. If the tissue does not look healthy an antibiotic may be applied topically. Some patients require suturing the vulvar labia together over the tissue to protect it.
II. Progestogens will hasten the involution if breeding is not planned. Oral megestrol acetate at 2.2 mg/kg SID until resolution has occurred is preferred.

VAGINITIS

General Considerations

I. Bacterial infection is but one cause of vaginitis. Others include viral (herpes) infection, androgen-induced clitoral hyperplasia, neoplasia, and foreign bodies. Clinical signs include abnormal discharge, excessive licking of the vulva, tenderness on palpation, and discomfort when sitting. Vaginal discharge may originate from the vagina, but may also come from the cervix or uterus. Uninformed owners may consider normal proestral bleeding to be a sign of infection. Other diseases of the perineum and anal sacs may cause signs similar to vaginitis.
II. Diagnosis is based upon history, physical examination, cytology, and vaginoscopy. Cultures must be interpreted with caution as the vagina normally harbors a wide variety of bacteria. As a rule the lower vagina harbors more organisms than the anterior portion and mixed cultures with low numbers of bacteria are most frequent. A speculum should be employed to guide the swab past the lower vagina into the mid or anterior vagina. Both aerobes and anaerobes should be cultured. Recovery of one or perhaps two organisms with moderate to heavy growth should be considered significant.

III. Prepuberal vaginitis usually disappears with the onset of puberty. Bacterial vaginitis in postpuberal bitches is frequently a recurrent disease requiring periodic therapy. When present during proestrus and bleeding is anticipated it should be treated vigorously as the organisms and/or their "toxins" are spermicidal.

Treatment

I. Antibiotics

Antibiotic therapy should be based on culture and sensitivity results. The minimum treatment period is 2 weeks. (See section on Endometritis, above if breeding is anticipated during the treatment period.) Currently there is no treatment approved for use in dogs for herpesvirus.

II. Infusions

Infusions of antimicrobial agents, including antibiotics, are beneficial. Povidone iodide, chlorhexidine, half-strength Lugol's solution, gentamicin, neomycin, and furacin have all been used with success. If antibiotics are chosen they should be diluted so that the infusate contains the parenteral dose for the patient based upon its body weight. Infusions should continue on a BID basis until there is clinical or cytologic improvement. They should be stopped 72 hours prior to breeding.

MALE REPRODUCTIVE DISORDERS

LACK OF LIBIDO

General Considerations

This condition may be caused by low testosterone production. If serum testosterone levels are normal then a behavioral problem must be suspected. If the testes are abnormal other causes should be investigated.

Treatment

Patients must have normal testes and normal thyroid function. Supraphysiologic doses of testosterone may cause spermatogenic arrest and potentiate prostatic disease. Use oral testosterone at 0.1–0.25 mg/kg/day. Expect a response in 10–30 days.

BRUCELLOSIS

General Considerations

Caused by a small gram-negative coccobacillus, this highly contagious disease may reach epidemic proportions in some kennels. It is transmissible to people. Clinical signs include last-trimester abortion and epididymitis leading to orchitis and scrotal dermatitis from excessive licking. Some animals are asymptomatic and only have a history of reproductive failure. The diagnosis is based on serologic tests and culture. Note that CO_2 *inhibits* the growth of this *Brucella*.

Treatment

Euthanasia is recommended for all proven-positive cases. Antibiotic therapy readily suppresses the bacteremia, however, recrudescence is common. Spaying or castration will eliminate the major source of organism shedding. Some long-term cures have been effected using:

I. Tetracycline HCl 30 mg/kg (each dose) TID for 21 days. No treatment for 21 days. Repeat tetracycline for 21 days adding streptomycin 20 mg/kg BID IM.
II. Minocycline HCl 12.5 mg/kg BID for 14 days with streptomycin 10 mg/kg BID IM for the first 7 days.

Prophylaxis

Currently there is no vaccine available.

BALANOPOSTHITIS

General Considerations

Virtually all male dogs will have a low-grade bacterial infection of the glans penis and adjacent preputial mucosa. A small amount of purulent discharge is considered normal. In severe cases the patient licks excessively (do not confuse with masturbation) and/or the amount of discharge is of concern to the owner. Diagnosis is based upon physical examination to rule out preputial pyoderma, foreign bodies, neoplasia (especially transmissible venereal tumor), masturbation, urethritis, prostatic disease, lower urinary tract disease including uroliths, and herpesvirus infection. Biopsy, urinalysis, radiography, cytology, and culture may be necessary.

Treatment

I. Since this disease tends to recur treatment is rarely curative on a long-term basis. Local therapy is usually sufficient. Infusions of an antibiotic-corticosteroid lotion or solution BID work well. If lymphoid follicles are present they may be rubbed with copper sulfate crystals followed by infusions as described above. Successful topical chemotherapy has included infusions of 1:10,000 potassium permanganate, 1.0% silver nitrate, or Lugol's solution followed by antibiotic-corticosteroid lotion.

II. Treatment is continued until the patient is clinically improved and repeated as necessary.

SUGGESTED READINGS

Burke TJ (ed): Hormone and corticosteroid therapy. Vet Clin N Am 12:79, 1982

Jones DE, Joshua JO: Reproductive Clinical Problems in the Dog. Wright PSG, Bristol, England, 1982

Kirk RW (ed): Current Veterinary Therapy. VIII. WB Saunders, Philadelphia, 1983

Morrow DA (ed): Current Therapy in Theriogenology. WB Saunders, Philadelphia, 1980

21

Dermatologic Diseases
Danny W. Scott, D.V.M.

BACTERIAL DERMATOSES

ACUTE MOIST DERMATITIS

I. General comments

   Acute moist dermatitis (pyotraumatic dermatitis, "hot spot") is an acute, localized, rapidly progressive, painful and pruritic, self-induced, erosive to ulcerative dermatosis with secondary superficial bacterial infection. Underlying disorders known to initiate the itch-scratch/lick cycle include allergies (flea, inhalant, food), ectoparasitisms, infections, foreign bodies, trauma, anal sacculitis, and otitis externa.

II. Treatment

   Acute moist dermatitis is a benign but uncomfortable and disfiguring dermatosis. The aims of therapy are to clean and dry the lesion, prevent further self-mutilation, and to alleviate the underlying cause.

   A. Clean and dry.

   The lesion should be gently clipped and cleaned with antiseptic solutions such as povidone-iodine (Betadine) or chlorhexidine (Nolvasan). As these lesions are often very painful, cleansing the animal may require sedation. Drying is accomplished with astringents such as 5% tannic acid with 5% salicylic acid in 70% isopropyl alcohol (Tan Sal: *single* application) or aluminum acetate (Domeboro solution: 10- to 15-minute soaks TID until dry).

   B. Prevent further self-mutilation.

   This is usually accomplished with systemic glucocorticoids: oral prednisone or prednisolone at 1 mg/kg SID for 5–7 days, or a single IM injection of 1 mg/kg methylprednisolone acetate (Depo-Medrol).

SKIN FOLD DERMATITIS

I. General comments

   Skin fold dermatitis (skin fold pyoderma, intertrigo) is due to localized anatomic skin defects which result in frictional dermatitis, maceration, and secondary superficial bacterial infection.

II. Treatment

    A. Skin fold dermatitis is benign, but unsightly and malodorous. The aims of therapy are to control superficial infection and to surgically extirpate the folds.

    B. Clean and dry

        The area should be gently clipped and cleaned with antiseptics (povidone-iodine, chlorhexidine). Drying is accomplished with astringents (aluminum acetate, tannic acid or salicylic acid). Once the dermatitis is clean and dry, surgical extirpation is curative.

IMPETIGO

  I. General comments

     Impetigo (superficial pustular dermatitis) is a superficial, nonfollicular pustular skin infection of dogs and cats less than 6 months of age. In dogs, the usual cause is a coagulase-positive staphylococcus, while in cats the usual organisms involved are β-hemolytic streptococci and *Pasteurella multocida*. Poor nutrition, filthy environment, and infectious diseases are occasional predisposing factors.

  II. Treatment

     Impetigo is a totally benign dermatosis. Many patients with mild cases undergo spontaneous remission. Patients with more severe cases are usually easily cured by daily washing with antiseptic solutions such as povidone-iodine, chlorhexidine, or benzoyl peroxide (OxyDex shampoo). Povidone-iodine and benzoyl peroxide can be irritating to many cats.

FOLLICULITIS, FURUNCULOSIS, AND CELLULITIS

  I. General comments

     Folliculitis, furunculosis, and cellulitis represent increasingly deep and severe stages of bacterial hair follicle infection which may be localized (face, pressure points, feet) or generalized. In dogs, the most commonly isolated organism from initial infections is a coagulase-positive Staphylococcus. In cats, the most commonly isolated organisms are β-hemolytic streptococci and *Pasteurella multocida*. Chronic and recurrent cases may be associated with underlying diseases, such as demodicosis, dermatophytosis, allergy, seborrhea, hypothyroidism, and feline leukemia virus infection.

  II. Treatment

     Whereas folliculitis is usually a benign dermatosis, furunculosis and cellulitis may be life-threatening (septicemia). The aims of therapy are to treat the infection with specific systemic antibiotics, clean and dry the skin, establish surgical drainage where necessary, and alleviate any underlying disease.

A. Systemic antibiotics

Specific antibiotic therapy is best determined by culture and sensitivity. In the dog, commonly used effective oral antibiotics include erythromycin (6–10 mg/kg TID: administered with a little food—may cause vomiting); lincomycin (20 mg/kg BID: may cause vomition or diarrhea); oxacillin (10 mg/kg TID: may cause vomition); chloramphenicol (40 mg/kg TID); and cephalexin (30 mg/kg BID). In cats, commonly used antibiotics include ampicillin (20 mg/kg TID), amoxicillin (10 mg/kg BID), and cephalexin (30 mg/kg BID). Superficial infections (folliculitis) should be treated for 3 weeks, whereas deep (furunculosis, cellulitis) or recurrent infections should be treated for a minimum of 6–8 weeks.

B. Clean and dry.

Gentle cleansing, drying, and relief of pruritus and pain are accomplished with topical antiseptics such as daily chlorhexidine or benzoyl peroxide shampoos, or daily wet soaks (15–30 minutes BID) or whirlpool baths with chlorhexidine (1 oz per bathtub of body-temperature water).

FUNGAL DERMATOSES

DERMATOPHYTOSIS

I. General comments

Dermatophytosis ("ringworm") is a localized or generalized superficial fungal skin infection which usually follows a benign, self-limited course with spontaneous remission often occurring within 1–3 months. The aims of treatment are to reduce contagion to the environment and other animals and/or people, and to eradicate the infection.

A. Reduce contagion

Hair should be clipped from affected areas (localized) or from the entire body (generalized) and carefully disposed of. The entire body should be treated with an antifungal solution such as povidone-iodine shampoo (Betadine), chlorhexidine (Nolvasan), 2% lime sulfur dip (Orthorix: may dry skin and coat; smells like "rotten eggs"; stains jewelry), or 3% captan (Orthocide: contact-sensitizer in people). Isolated skin lesions can be treated daily with antifungal ointments or creams such as povidone-iodine, chlorhexidine, or miconazole (Conofite). The environment should be carefully cleaned, where possible, by thorough vacuuming and application of fungicidal agents (povidone-iodine, chlorhexidine, 0.5% sodium hyposulfite, 2% lime sulfur) on a weekly basis until 2 weeks after clinical cure.

B. Eradicate the infection.

Due to self-limiting nature of most infections, the therapeutic steps taken in (a), above usually suffice. Severe or chronic cases are treated with oral griseofulvin (Fulvicin) at 50–100 mg/kg SID or divided BID. Griseofulvin should be given with a fatty meal, and continued for 2 weeks beyond clinical cure. Griseofulvin is teratogenic and may occasionally produce anorexia, depression, vomiting, diarrhea, dermatitis, or anemia.

PARASITIC DERMATOSES

CHEYLETIELLOSIS

I. General comments

Cheyletiellosis is a pruritic or nonpruritic, dorsally distributed papulo-crustous and/or scaling dermatitis of dogs and cats caused by the large surface mites, *Cheyletiella blakei, C. parasitivorax*, and *C. yasguri*. The disease is potentially transmissible to people.

II. Treatment

Cheyletiellosis is usually easy to cure. The aims of therapy are to kill the mites on the patient, all in-contact dogs and cats, and in the animal's environment.

A. Kill mites on animals.

Cheyletiella mites are usually susceptible to most topical parasiticidal agents. Animals may be bathed with pyrethrin (Mycodex) or carbamate (Mycodex with carbaryl) shampoos once weekly, or dipped with 2% lime sulfur- (Orthorix), carbamate- (Sendran) or organophosphate- (Dermaton II) containing products once weekly. Treatments should be administered for 4 weeks. Most carbamates, organophosphates, and organochlorines are potentially toxic to cats.

B. Kill mites in environment.

The use of parasiticidal sprays or foggers is highly recommended, especially in kennel or cattery situations, or in patients with recurrent infection.

CANINE SCABIES

I. General comments

Canine scabies (sarcoptic mange) is an intensely pruritic, papulocrustous dermatitis, especially involving the ears, limbs, and ventrum, caused by the burrowing mite, *Sarcoptes scabei var canis*. The disease is potentially transmissible to people.

II. Treatment

Canine scabies is usually easy to cure. The aims of therapy are to kill the mites on the patient and all in-contact dogs. Canine scabies mites appear to have developed regional differences in susceptibility to certain classes of topical parasiticides. Dogs should be a) Clipped (if thick- or long-haired) b) Bathed with a gentle soap (Allergroom, HyLyt*EFA) to remove crusts and debris c) Dipped weekly until 2 weeks after clinical cure with 2% lime sulfur (Orthorix) or lindane (Gamma R-X)

FELINE SCABIES

I. General comments

Feline scabies (notoedric mange) is an intensely pruritic, papulocrustous dermatitis, especially involving the head, neck, and ears, caused by the burrowing mite, *Notoedres cati*. The disease is potentially transmissible to people.

II. Treatment

Feline scabies is usually easy to cure. The aims of therapy are to kill the mites on the patient and all in-contact cats. Cats should be:

A. Clipped (if long-haired)

B. Bathed with a gentle shampoo (Allergroom; HyLyt*EFA) to remove crusts and debris

C. Dipped weekly until 2 weeks after clinical cure with 2% lime sulfur (Orthorix)

CANINE DEMODICOSIS

I. General comments

Canine demodicosis (demodectic mange) is a pruritic or nonpruritic papulocrustous dermatitis, especially involving the face and feet, caused by the hair follicle mite, *Demodex canis*.

II. Treatment

Localized canine demodicosis in the dog less than one year of age usually spontaneously regresses within three months. Therapy is not recommended for such cases. Localized demodicosis in older dogs or generalized demodicosis in any age dog may require aggressive miticidal and systemic antibiotic therapy (Where pyoderma is a complicating factor: see Folliculitis, Furunculosis, and Cellulitis, above.) Miticidal therapy is accomplished with amitraz (Mitaban) according to manufacturer's instructions. Amitraz may cause transient lethargy and depression as well as severe cellulitis in affected areas. Some cases of generalized demodicosis are never cured. Because of the genetic predilection associated with most cases of canine generalized demodicosis, it is strongly recommended that affected dogs be neutered as soon as their health permits.

PEDICULOSIS

I. General comments

Pediculosis (lice) is a pruritic or nonpruritic, papulocrustous and/or scaling dermatitis, especially involving the dorsum of dogs and cats caused by biting or sucking lice. Pediculosis is often associated with filth, crowding, and debilitation.

II. Treatment

Pediculosis is usually easy to cure. The aims of therapy are to kill the lice on the patient and all in-contact animals of the same species, and correct any underlying causes. Lice are usually susceptible to most topical parasiticidal agents. Animals may be bathed with pyrethrin- (Mycodex) or carbamate- (Mycodex with carbaryl) containing shampoos once a week, or dipped with 2% lime sulfur (Orthorix) or carbamate- (Sendran) containing solutions once a week. Treatments are continued for 4 weeks. Most carbamates, organophosphates, and organochlorines are potentially toxic in cats.

FLEAS

I. General comments

Fleas may produce a mildly pruritic and papulocrustous dermatitis through simple trauma and irritation (flea bite dermatitis) or an intensely pruritic, papulocrustous dermatitis, especially involving the tailhead, caudomedial thighs, and neck through a process of sensitization (flea bite hypersensitivity). Dogs, cats, and people may be affected.

II. Treatment

Fleas and their related dermatoses may be extremely difficult to control in warmer areas of the country. The aims of therapy are to kill fleas on the patient, on all in-contact dogs and cats, and in the animal's environment. In the animal with flea bite hypersensitivity, systemic glucocorticoids and/or hyposensitization to fleas may also be required.

A. Kill fleas on animals

Fleas have developed regional differences in susceptibility to certain classes of topical parasiticides. In some cases, flea control may be easily accomplished with persistent topical applications of carbamate (Ortho Sevin Garden Dust), or pyrethrin-carbamate (Diryl) powders two to three times per week or the weekly administration of carbamate (Sendran) or organophosphate (Dermaton II) dips. In other cases, the use of systemic organophosphates, such as cythioate (Proban; administered orally according to manufacturer's directions) may be preferable. Flea collars, flea shampoos, and natural products such as brewer's yeast, thiamine, and garlic are virtually worthless for flea control.

B. Kill fleas in environment

This is best accomplished with sprays (malathion, dioxathion, chlorpyrifos) or foggers (Vet-Fog, Siphotrol 10, or Siphotrol Plus) *indoors* every 1–2 months or as needed, and with sprays (malathion, chlorpyrifos, propetamphos) outdoors every 1–2 months or as needed. In many instances, professional exterminators offer a superior and less expensive eradication program.

C. Treat the allergy

Animals with flea bite hypersensitivity often require concurrent systemic glucocorticoid therapy to control severe pruritus and self-mutilation. This may be accomplished on a short-term basis (1–3 weeks) with the daily administration of oral prednisone or prednisolone at 1 mg/kg or a single IM injection of 1 mg/kg methylprednisolone (Depo-Medrol). If chronic administration of systemic glucocorticoids is required, *only* prednisone or prednisolone should be used, and *only* on an alternate-day steroid regimen (see Chapters 5 and 19 and Suggested Readings following this chapter). Although flea hyposensitization is still in the clinical evaluation stage, it is worth trying in otherwise hopeless cases. One milliliter of flea antigen (Flea Antigen 1:100, Greer) is administered intradermally once weekly until a response is seen, or until no response is seen after 3 months of treatment. "Booster" injections are administered as needed (every 3–8 weeks).

Pelodera Dermatitis

I. General comments

Pelodera (rhabditic) dermatitis is a pruritic papular dermatitis affecting the contact areas of dogs, and is caused by the free-living nematode, *Pelodera strongyloides*.

II. Treatment

Pelodera dermatitis is easily cured. The aims of therapy are to kill the nematodes in the skin, eradicate the nematodes in the animal's environment, and prevent self-mutilation.

A. Kill nematodes in the skin.

Dogs should be dipped weekly for 3 weeks with a carbamate (Sendran), organophosphate (Dermaton II), or organochlorine (Gamma R-X) solution.

B. Kill nematodes in the environment

Decaying organic debris should be avoided or removed. Contaminated areas can be sprayed with numerous parasiticidal preparations such as chlorpyrifos, malathion, dixathion, or propetamphos.

C. Control self-mutilation

Severely pruritic dogs may be treated with systemic glucocorticoids such as oral prednisone or prednisolone at 1 mg/kg/day for 7–10 days, or with a single IM injection of 1 mg/kg methylprenisolone acetate (Depo-Medrol).

IMMUNOLOGIC DERMATOSES

ATOPY

I. General comments

Atopy is a genetically-predilected, seasonal or nonseasonal pruritic dermatosis of dogs and, probably, cats. Offending allergens are usually inhaled, and the face, ears, feet, and ventrum are usually affected.

II. Treatment

Atopy is a chronic but benign disorder. The aims of therapy are to avoid the allergens, relieve pruritus and self-mutilation with systemic glucocorticoids or hyposensitization, and to control complicating factors.

A. Avoidance of allergens

This can only be accomplished if intradermal skin testing has been done (see Suggested Readings).

B. Relief of pruritus

This is usually best achieved with systemic glucocorticoids. Induction doses of oral prednisone or prednisolone should approximate 1 mg/kg/day for 5–7 days. If chronic administration of systemic glucocorticoids is required, the above oral steroids should be administered on an alternate-day basis *only* (see Chapters 5 and 19 and Suggested Readings, this chapter). Antihistamines are usually of minimal benefit. If steroid therapy is unsuccessful or accompanied by unacceptable side effects (polyuria, polydipsia, polyphagia, obesity, behavioral abnormalities, panting, urinary incontinence, hepatopathy, myopathy, pancreatitis, and so forth), *hyposensitization* is indicated. This is only possible if intradermal skin testing has been performed (see Suggested Readings for details).

C. Control complicating factors.

Because pruritus is an additive phenomenon, it becomes very important to alleviate concurrent dermatologic problems in the allergic patient. Thus, dry skin should be managed, as needed, with emollient shampoos (Allergroom; HyLyt EFA) and rinses (Humilac); secondary pyodermas should be treated quickly (see section on Folliculitis, Furunculosis, and Cellulitis, above); and flea infestations should be vigorously controlled (see section on Fleas, above).

FOOD HYPERSENSITIVITY

I. General comments

Food hypersensitivity is a nonseasonal, pruritic, pleomorphic cutaneous eruption of dogs and cats. Gastrointestinal signs may or may not be present.

II. Treatment

The aims of therapy are to avoid offending dietary allergens, and to prevent self-mutilation. Hypoallergenic diets will differ from patient to patient, and may take several months to define. Self-mutilation is best prevented with systemic glucocorticoids (see section on Atopy, above).

Contact Dermatitis

I. General comments

Contact dermatitis may be due to primary skin irritants (most common) or allergic sensitization (rare). Both are usually characterized by a variably pruritic dermatitis affecting thinly-haired, contact areas.

II. Treatment

The aims of therapy are to avoid the offending contactant(s), and to prevent self-mutilation. Pruritus, depending on its severity, may be controlled with systemic glucocorticoids (see section on Atopy, above) or with topical glucocorticoids, such as betamethasone-17-valerate (Valisone ointment, cream, or lotion: apply two or three times daily until controlled, then as needed).

Urticaria

I. General comments

Urticaria may be caused by immunologic (bugs, drugs, diet) or nonimmunologic (infections, heat, cold, psychogenic) factors. It is characterized by multifocal to generalized wheals which may or may not be pruritic.

II. Treatment

The aims of therapy are to eliminate the cause and to suppress the cutaneous reaction. Elimination of the cause is often all that is necessary with the urticaria regressing within hours to a few days. If severe, the cutaneous reaction is best treated with epinephrine (0.1–0.5 ml of a 1:1,000 solution SQ) with or without systemic glucocorticoids (2 mg/kg prednisone or prednisolone orally or IM).

Pemphigus and Pemphigoid

I. General comments

Pemphigus and pemphigoid are autoimmune skin disorders in dogs and cats. These disorders are often severe, and may be life-threatening. They are usually chronic, requiring life-long therapy with potentially hazardous drugs.

II. Treatment

The aim of therapy is to suppress the autoimmune tissue reaction with systemic "immunosuppressive" or "immunomodulating" drugs. This may be accomplished with large doses of glucocorticoids, with or without other concurrent immunomodulating drugs, such as azathioprine (Imuran), chlorambucil (Leukeran), or aurothioglucose (Solganal). Side effects with these drugs are common, varying from mild to severe, and close physical and hematologic monitoring of the patient is critical. The reader is referred to Chapter 6 and the Suggested Readings for details.

DISCOID LUPUS ERYTHEMATOSUS

I. General comments

Discoid lupus erythematosus (nasal solar dermatitis, "collie nose") is a photoaggravated immune-mediated disorder which primarily affects the nose and occasionally the face, ears, and oral cavity of dogs. It is a chronic disease which usually requires lifelong therapy.

II. Treatment

The aims of therapy are to suppress the inflammatory reaction and to avoid ultraviolet light exposure.

A. Suppress inflammation

This is usually best accomplished with systemic glucocorticoids (oral prednisone or prednisolone at 2 mg/kg/day until controlled, then on an alternate-day basis for maintenance). If systemic steroids are unacceptable for some reason, large doses of vitamin E may be used (dl-α-tocopheryl acetate is given orally at 400 IU twice daily). The vitamin E should be given on an empty stomach and has a 30- to 60-day "lag period" before clinical effect is appreciated. Systemic glucocorticoids may be used as needed during this lag phase. In mild cases, topical glucocorticoids (Valisone ointment or cream, applied two to three times daily) may suffice.

B. Avoidance of ultraviolet light

This is accomplished by avoiding sun exposure between 8 A.M. and 5 P.M. during the day, and using topical sunscreens when sun exposure is unavoidable. Topical paraminobenzoic acid derivatives (Sundown) are applied 2 hours before sun exposure and again at the time of exposure.

PSYCHOGENIC DERMATOSES

CANINE ACRAL LICK DERMATITIS

I. General comments

Acral lick dermatitis ("lick granuloma," "neurodermatitis") is a chronic "bad habit" of dogs, wherein solitary or multiple excoriated plaques or nodules, especially on the distal limbs, are maintained by the dog's licking and chewing. Precipitating causes include trauma, foreign bodies, allergies, infections, and numerous "displacement phenomena."

II. Treatment

The aims of therapy are to identify and eliminate the initiating factor(s) wherein possible, and to break the "bad habit" (see Chapter 17). Depending on the severity of the lesions and the dog's dedication to self-mutilation, treatments for the lesions may include various combinations of protective bandaging, topical "antichew" preparations (Bitter Apple; Obtundia), topical glucocorticoids (Valisone cream or ointment; Synotic), or sublesional glucocorticoids (10–40 mg Depo-Medrol). Severe cases may require the concurrent administration of behavior-modifying drugs such as phenobarbital (2–6 mg/kg orally twice daily), diazepam (Valium; 1.25–20 mg total dose orally, once or twice daily), or megestrol acetate (Ovaban or Megace: 1 mg/kg orally once daily until controlled, then 0.25–1 mg/kg every two or three days). These drugs may cause side effects, such as depression, anxiety, polydipsia, polyuria, and polyphagia in any given dog. Although effective in certain cases, surgical excision, cryosurgery, radiation therapy, cobra venom injections, orgotein (Palosein) injections, and acupuncture are not highly recommended.

FELINE PSYCHOGENIC ALOPECIA AND DERMATITIS

I. General comments

Psychogenic alopecia and dermatitis ("neurodermatitis") are chronic "bad habits" of cats wherein solitary or multiple excoriated plaques or areas of alopecia only are maintained by the cat's licking and chewing. Precipitating factors are as described in the section on Canine Acral Lick Dermatitis, above.

II. Treatment

The aims of therapy are as described in the section Canine Acral Lick Dermatitis, above. Where drug therapy is required to break the habit, only systemic behavior-modifying agents are routinely successful in cats. Such drugs may include phenobarbital (2–6 mg/kg orally twice daily), diazepam (1.25–5 mg total dose, once or twice daily), megestrol acetate (Ovaban or Megace at 2.5–5 mg total dose orally every other day until controlled, then every 1–2 weeks), or medroxyprogesterone acetate (Depo-Provera, 100 mg total dose, SQ every 2–6 months). Progestagens are not approved for this use in cats or dogs, and may produce a plethora of side effects including polyuria, polydipsia, polyphagia, obesity, pyometra, diabetes mellitus, mammary gland hyperpalsia/neoplasia, Cushing's syndrome, and adrenocortical suppression (see Suggested Readings and Chapter 17).

SEBORRHEIC DERMATOSES

SEBORRHEIC SKIN DISEASE

I. General comments

Seborrhea is characterized by localized or generalized areas of altered keratinization (scaling) with or without excessive glandular secretion, dermatitis, and pruritus. Seborrhea is almost always a secondary disorder associated with hormonal disturbances, allergies, nutritional abnormalities, environmental conditions, ecto- or endo-parasitism, systemic diseases, and so forth (see Suggested Readings). Seborrheic skin is predisposed to bacterial infection.

II. Treatment

A. The aims of therapy are to alleviate the underlying cause(s) wherein possible, to control the altered state of keratinization and/or glandular secretion, and to control secondary pyoderma (see section on Folliculitis, Furunculosis, and Cellulitis, above).

B. Antiseborrheic therapy

Selection of the appropriate antiseborrheic agent is based on the gross morphology of the skin lesions present, patient idiosyncracies, and species considerations (see Suggested Readings). Antiseborrheic shampoos are usually administered every 2 or 3 days until the dermatitis is controlled. They should be thoroughly lathered, left on the patient for 5–15 minutes, and thoroughly rinsed off. For maintenance therapy, shampoos are given as needed (every 1–4 weeks). "Dry" seborrheas are best treated with emollient shampoos (Allergroom; HyLyt*EFA) and rinses (Humilac). "Oily" seborrheas usually respond well to benzoyl peroxide (OxyDex) or selenium sulfide (Selsun Blue). When follicular plugging and/or pyoderma are prominent, benzoyl peroxide (OxyDex) or sulfur (Sebbafon) are indicated. *Coal tar* products may be irritating to dogs and are contraindicated in cats. Benzoyl peroxide may be irritating to some dogs and cats.

ACNE

I. General comments

Acne is a common benign disorder of keratinization manifested by comedones, papules, and pustules predominently on the chin and lips of dogs and cats.

II. Treatment

The aims of therapy are to remove the comedones and to treat any secondary bacterial infection. In dogs, many animals will achieve spontaneous remission with maturity. Other dogs, pending the severity of the acne, may require topical "follicular flushing" agents, such as benzoyl peroxide (OxyDex gel or shampoo) or vitamin A acid (Retin-A) once or twice daily, as needed. Secondary bacterial infections may necessitate systemic antibiotics (see section Folliculitis, Furunculosis, and Cellulitis, above). In cats, acne is usually chronic and persistent. Mild cases may require no therapy. More severe cases benefit from topical benzoyl peroxide (OxyDex gel or shampoo) or chlorhexidine (Nolvasan shampoo) applied once or twice daily, as needed. Benzoyl peroxide may be irritating to some cats. Secondary bacterial infections may require appropriate systemic antibiotic therapy.

MISCELLANEOUS DERMATOSES

FELINE EOSINOPHILIC GRANULOMA COMPLEX

I. General comments

The eosinophilic granuloma complex is a common, often idiopathic group of dermatoses in cats. Some cases are associated with flea bite hypersensitivity, food hypersensitivity, or atopy.

II. Treatment

The aims of therapy are to alleviate any underlying cause(s) and to suppress inflammation. Solitary lesions may respond to topical (Valisone lotion, cream, or ointment applied two to three times daily) or sublesional (10–20 mg of Depo-Medrol) glucocorticoids. Other patients will require systemic glucocorticoids (20 mg DepoMedrol SQ, repeat in 2 weeks, then repeat as needed) or progestagens (Ovaban or Megace, 2.5–5 mg orally every other day until controlled, then every 1–2 weeks if needed: or 100 mg Depo-Provera SQ every 2–6 months, as needed). Progestagens are not approved for use in cats, and may be associated with numerous side effects (see section Feline Psychogenic Alopecia and Dermatitis, above). Procedures such as surgical excision, cryosurgery, and radiation therapy are effective in selected patients, but are not generally recommended.

FELINE MILIARY DERMATITIS

I. General comments

Miliary dermatitis is a cutaneous reaction pattern in the skin of the cat. Most cases of miliary dermatitis are associated with an underlying cause, such as flea bite hypersensitivity, ecto-or endoparasitism, food hypersensitivity, atopy, dermatophytosis, and bacterial folliculitis (see Suggested Readings). Some cases are idiopathic.

II. Treatment

The aims of therapy are to alleviate any underlying cause(s) and to suppress inflammation. In idiopathic cases, the drugs of choice are progestagens, as described in the section Feline Eosinophilic Granuloma Complex, above.

PANNICULITIS

I. General comments

Panniculitis, in dogs and cats, may be due to infections, foreign bodies, vitamin E deficiency, concurrent immunologic disorders (lupus erythematosus), pancreatic disease, or may be sterile and idiopathic.

II. Treatment

The aims of therapy are to alleviate any underlying cause(s), and, for the sterile idiopathic variety to suppress inflammation. Sterile idiopathic ("nodular'') panniculitis usually responds well to large doses of systemic glucocorticoids (oral prednisone or prednisolone, 2–4 mg/kg/day). Animals less than 1 year of age will often undergo long-term, drug-free remissions. Older animals often require prolonged alternate-day steroid therapy.

ZINC-RESPONSIVE DERMATOSIS

I. General comments

Zinc-responsive dermatoses are usually nonpruritic skin disorders characterized by severe crusting and hyperkeratosis especially affecting the face, pinnae, mucocutaneous junctions, pressure points, and feet. The etiology may be dietary or idiopathic.

II. Treatment

The aims of therapy are to correct any dietary imbalances (zinc deficiency and/or calcium/phytate excess), or, in idiopathic cases, to supply a daily source of zinc. Daily zinc therapy may be accomplished with oral zinc sulfate (220–440 mg/day: administer with food; if using tablets, crush first; may cause vomition) or zinc methionine (Zinpro: one tablet/10 kg/day). Idiopathic cases often require prolonged therapy.

JUVENILE CELLULITIS

I. General comments

Juvenile cellulitis (''puppy strangles'') is an idiopathic disorder of dogs less than 6 months of age. Although mortality is very low, residual scarring can be significant.

II. Treatment

The aims of therapy are to suppress inflammation and to treat secondary bacterial infection, if present.

A. Suppress inflammation.

This is usually accomplished with systemic glucocorticoids [oral or SQ dexamethasone (Azium) at 0.2 mg/kg once daily for 7–10 days] and topical astringent wet soaks [aluminum acetate (Domeboro solution)] in body-temperature water; apply for 10–15 minutes three or four times daily).

B. Treat secondary infection

This is accomplished with systemic antibiotics (see Folliculitis, Furunculosis, and Cellulitis, above) for 3 weeks.

SUBCORNEAL PUSTULAR DERMATOSIS

I. General comments

Subcorneal pustular dermatosis is an idiopathic, pruritic, or nonpruritic sterile pustular skin disease of dogs. Although benign, the disorder tends to be chronic.

I. Treatment

The aim of therapy is to suppress the sterile pustule formation, and, when present, the pruritus. The drug of choice is dapsone (Avlosulfon) given orally, with a little food, at 1 mg/kg three times daily. After the dermatosis is controlled (1–4 weeks), a maintenance regimen is determined (1 mg/kg once daily, twice weekly). Dapsone is a potentially toxic drug (anemia, leukopenia, thrombocytopenia, vomition, dermatitis, and hepatopathy) and treatment must be closely monitored (see Suggested Readings).

SUGGESTED READINGS

Muller GH, Kirk RW, Scott DW: Small Animal Dermatology. 3rd Ed. WB Saunders, Philadelphia, 1983

Scott DW: Dermatologic use of glucocorticoids: topical and systemic. Vet Clin N Am 12:19, 1982

Scott DW: Chrysotherapy. p. 448. In Kirk RW (ed): Current Veterinary Therapy VIII. WB Saunders, Philadelphia, 1983

22

Clinical Monitoring of Drug Concentrations
Carol A. Neff-Davis, M.S.

INTRODUCTION

I. The rational use of drugs requires that the proper drug be administered (based on correct diagnosis) in proper amounts. The latter requirement necessitates that dosage regimens be individualized for each patient.

II. Recommended dosage regimens are based on an "average" and are intended as guidelines or starting points. By selecting therapeutic objectives (observable end-points), therapy can be initiated in a directed manner.

III. Some drugs do not elicit a well-defined, or quantifiable response, making it difficult to know when therapeutic end-points are achieved. Too often dosage corrections are based on having observed toxicity and realizing that the dose was too high. By monitoring the concentration of a drug in the plasma during therapy, the dosage regimen can be modified before toxicity appears.

IV. Many of the adverse effects due to drug overdose have drastic effects on the disposition, elimination, and bioavailability of the drug being given, which may make the therapy more difficult to control and contribute to therapeutic failure.

RATIONALE FOR MONITORING DRUG PLASMA CONCENTRATIONS

GENERAL COMMENTS

I. It has been well established that the pharmacologic effect of a drug is directly related to the concentration in the plasma and by measuring the concentration required to produce a given effect, therapeutic ranges (minimum and maximum serum concentrations needed to produce a given effect) have been established for a number of drugs.

633

II. Since the establishment of drug monitoring services in the clinic, it has become apparent that most therapeutic failures are not due to lack of pharmacologic effect at the site of action, but due to failure to maintain the appropriate drug concentrations.

III. By measuring the plasma concentration achieved following a prescribed dosage regimen, the dosage can be individualized for the needs of the patient.

FACTORS IINFLUENCING PLASMA CONCENTRATIONS

Individual variation and species differences in pharmacokinetic processes
  I. Route of administration (rate and extent of absorption from pharmaceutical preparation)
  II. Food composition and consumption
  III. Gastrointestinal pH
  IV. Gastric emptying
  V. Splanchnic blood flow
  VI. Volume of distribution
  VII. Protein binding
  VIII. Renal function
  IX. Rate and extent of drug metabolism (hepatic and nonhepatic)

EFFECT OF PATHOPHYSIOLOGY ON DRUG DISTRIBUTION AND ELIMINATION

Cardiac Disease

I. Reduction in cardiac output results in reduced blood flow to various organs (less drug at site of action).
II. Heart failure will result in reduced drug protein binding.

Pulmonary Disease

  I. Hemodynamic effect
  II. Gas deficiency produces pH changes (which affect tissue distribution and renal clearance).
  III. Hypoxia will affect organ blood flow.

Hepatic Disease

  I. Reduction in intrinsic clearance of a drug ($\downarrow$ blood flow)
  II. Reduction in drug metabolism ($\downarrow$ liver enzyme activity)
  III. Reduction in drug protein binding (chronic hepatic insufficiency)

Renal Disease

Uremia may have a profound effect on extent of protein binding, volume of distribution, and rate of drug metabolism

Thyroid Disease

I. Many drugs will have a reduced rate of elimination due to hypothyroidism.
II. Reduction in gastrointestinal motility
III. Reduction in organ blood flow and volume of distribution

Hypoalbuminemia

I. Albumin is the major serum protein that binds drugs.
II. Although hypoalbuminemia is not a disease per se, many different disease processes can lead to a reduction in serum albumin (heart failure, chronic hepatic insufficiency, or any disease that results in reduced production).

SITUATIONS WHERE DRUG MONITORING CAN BE USEFUL

I. Suspected owner noncompliance
II. Drug has narrow therapeutic range
III. Change in regimen or dosage form
IV. Lack of therapeutic effect
    Some individuals may attain adequate concentrations, but are unresponsive and would require different therapy.
V. Concomitant drug therapy
    A. Drug-drug interaction
    B. Drug liver enzyme induction
    C. Reduction in drug protein binding (displacement)
VI. Patient has impaired renal function.
VII. Patient has acute or chronic liver dysfunction.
VIII. Obese animals
IX. Older animals
X. To confirm toxicity
XI. To avoid drug accumulation by individualization of drug therapy
XII. To confirm inadequate dosage regimen

PROCEDURES FOR THERAPEUTIC DRUG MONITORING

POSSIBLE LOCATIONS FOR THERAPEUTIC DRUG MONITORING SERVICE

I. Local human hospital clinical laboratory
II. Local clinical reference laboratory

III. College or school of veterinary medicine teaching hospital
IV. State diagnostic laboratory

ANALYTICAL METHODS USED IN THERAPEUTIC
DRUG MONITORING

Microbiologic Assay (Bioassay)

  I. Good method for determination of total antimicrobial activity.
  II. Requires moderately large serum sample (4–5 ml)
  III. Sample must be taken and clot removed aseptically.
  IV. Long turnaround time limits its use in therapeutic monitoring situations
     (1–2 days).

Chromatographic Analysis

  I. Include both high performance liquid chromatography (HPLC) and gas-
     liquid chromatography (GLC)
  II. Good method for determination of therapeutic concentrations of drugs.
  III. Sample volume required is modest (1–2 ml serum)
  IV. Methods provide high degree of specificity, but some drugs (if being ad-
     ministered at same time) may interfere with assay
  V. Short turnaround time (same day or within 24 hours of receipt of sample)

Immunologic Assay

  I. One of the fastest growing analytical techniques available
  II. There are several modes available and many commercial kits on the market
     today.
    A. Radioimmunoassay (RIA)
    B. Enzyme-linked immunoassays
  III. Methods provide high sensitivity (nanogram/milliter)
  IV. Methods are highly specific (no interference with other drugs being ad-
     ministered)
  V. Short turnaround time (within 12 hours, depending on laboratory proce-
     dures)

Caveat

  All analytical procedures used in therapeutic drug monitoring require strict
controls and validation. Many laboratories have set up methods to evaluate
drug concentrations in human serum only, and have not validated their methods
in other animal species. Methods that have not been validated in species of
interest should be interpreted with caution.

HOW TO SUBMIT SAMPLE FOR ANALYSIS

I. Contact the laboratory that will perform the analysis and indicate you would like to send samples.
II. Inquire whether the method they are using has been validated in dogs and cats. For results to have any interpretative meaning (other than a spot check for toxicity), normal ranges will have to be established for species of interest.
III. Request information about what volume of samples will be needed and how samples should be sent to laboratory.
IV. To check whether plasma concentrations are within therapeutic range, make sure a constant dosing protocol has been followed and that adequate time has elapsed since initiation of therapy for establishment of steady-state concentrations. (See length of time required for steady-state conditions under specific drugs)
V. Record when animal received last dose and when sample was taken. (See section Time of Collection, Drug Information Tables, below.)
VI. Record and submit following clinical information
A. Species
B. Age, sex
C. Weight
D. Dosage rate, formulation, route
E. Time of last dose
F. Time blood sample was taken
G. General clinical status (hepatic or renal function, state of hydration, nutrition, and so forth)
H. Other drugs being administered
I. Whether toxicity is suspected

SAMPLING REQUIREMENTS AND PRECAUTIONS
FOR DRUG ANALYSIS

I. If giving IV infusions, do not take sample for analysis from vein being used for infusion.
II. For sample to have any interpretative value, sample should be taken at specified collection time following drug administration.
III. Collect adequate blood samples so that enough serum or plasma is obtained. Many methods have a minimum volume requirement.
IV. Collect blood sample and remove serum or plasma as soon as possible.
A. Cells should not be allowed to sit in serum for any extended period of time because drugs which normally partition into red blood cells will diffuse out and result in higher than normal serum concentrations.
B. The use of heparin as an anticoagulant should be avoided, as it may interfere with some methods of analysis.

V. Put sample in appropriate container, glass or plastic. Some drugs will adsorb onto certain material. (Check Drug Information Tables, below.)

VI. Samples should be refrigerated or frozen until they can be analyzed. Some drugs will be destroyed if not stored properly.

VII. Care should be taken to prevent hemolysis. Drug concentrations can be higher (or lower) than normal depending on drug red blood cell distribution.

VIII. Vacutainer tubes should be avoided. The plastizers (found in the stoppers) can leak out and displace drug bound to serum protein and cause a redistribution into the red blood cells.

INTERPRETATION OF RESULTS (FIG. 22-1)

Initial Dosing Period

I. After each dose, drug concentration will increase during absorption phase and begin to fall during elimination phase.

II. If additional doses are given, peak and trough levels will continue to rise after each dose until "steady-state" concentrations are achieved (amount of drug taken in equals amount of drug eliminated).

III. The amount of time required for achievement of steady-state concentration

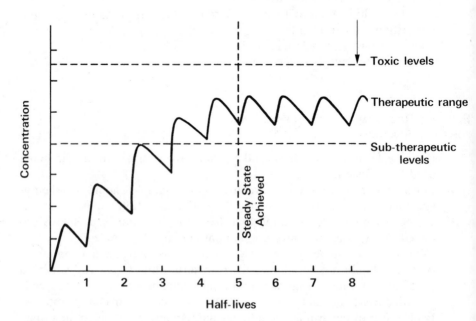

Fig. 22-1. Theoretical representation of accumulation of drug in serum following multiple, fixed doses of drug.

depends on biological half-life (T½) of drug and will occur only after therapy has been followed for five to six half-lives.

STEADY-STATE DRUG CONCENTRATIONS

  I. Can be subtherapeutic
 II. Can be within therapeutic range
III. Can be above the therapeutic range and might have accumulated in the animal to toxic levels

SAMPLING DURING STEADY STATE

  I. Peak or trough levels can be taken for evaluation.
 II. Peak levels are harder to evaluate due to wide individual variation in absorption and amount of time required for peak concentrations.
III. Determination of trough levels reduces variation and the results can be interpreted easier.
 IV. Once the drug plasma concentration is known, it can be compared to values that represent normal therapeutic ranges.
  V. The amount of drug given can be adjusted up or down to provide optimum therapeutic serum concentration for that particular animal.

INDIVIDUALIZATION TECHNIQUES

  I. Select initial dosage regimen based on normal population data and modified for clinical status of animal.
 II. Monitor plasma concentration after steady state is established.
III. Modify dose based on observed plasma concentration.
   A. If plasma concentration at steady state is subtherapeutic, increase dose based on following equation

$$\text{New dose} = \frac{C_{ss}}{C_{OBS}} \times \text{old dose}$$

  where C_{ss} is desired plasma concentration and C_{OBS} is the concentration observed.
   B. If plasma concentration is too high, reduce dose using same equation.
   C. If levels are very high, a withdrawal time may have to be used to allow levels to fall more quickly before additional drug is administered.
 IV. After new regimens are instituted, additional plasma concentrations should be analyzed to confirm new steady-state levels.
  V. Do not collect sample until new dosing regimen has been followed for 5 half-lives and new "steady-state" conditions are established.

GENERAL COMMENTS ON HOW TO
USE DRUG INFORMATION TABLES

    I. The following tables have been compiled to provide pharmacokinetic, therapeutic, toxicologic, and sample collection information. The list is limited to drugs that are commonly monitored in clinical situations.

   II. Pharmacokinetic Information

       These are values that have been reported in the literature and have been determined in adult, healthy animals. Unfortunately, there is little information about the elimination of these drugs in cats. The values should be used as guidelines, and allowances must be made for the influence of disease processes on the drug elimination in dogs and cats.

  III. Therapeutic ranges and toxic levels

       For the most part, the values reported have been taken from human data. Although not correlated to plasma concentrations, many of the toxic signs reported in humans have been observed in animals.

  IV. Dosage

       This information is provided for comparative purposes and are based on recommended dosages reported in formularies published by Purdue University and Colorado State University veterinary medical teaching hospitals. The dosage regimens are to be used as guidelines only.

    V. Sample collection

       Different methods require different sample volumes and these are indicated in this section. Specific laboratory requirements should be followed when samples are collected for drug evaluation.

  VI. Time to steady state

       Samples should be taken only after steady state is established. This requires dosing an animal for *at least five half-lives* before taking any samples for analysis.

$$\text{Time to steady state (hours)} = T\tfrac{1}{2} \times 5$$

 VII. Time of collection

       This will depend on the route of administration, but usually the most optimum time to collect sample is just before next dose is given.

DRUG INFORMATION TABLES

CHLORAMPHENICOL (pKa = 5.5)

Dosage Guidelines

  I. Dog
    A. IM, oral: 50 mg/kg, q8h
    B. IV: 35 mg/kg, q6h

II. Cat
   A. IM, oral: 50 mg/kg, q12h
   B. IV: 50 mg/kg, q10h

Pharmacokinetic Constants (see Davis et al., 1972, Suggested Readings)

   I. Dog
      A. $T\frac{1}{2}$ = 4.2 hr
      B. V'd = 1.8 L/kg
  II. Cat
      A. $T\frac{1}{2}$ = 5.1 hr
      B. V'd = 2.4 L/kg

Procedure for Monitoring Chloramphenicol Concentrations

   I. Select desired dosage regimen and administer drug until steady-state concentrations are established.
  II. Length of time required for steady-state conditions
      A. Dog—21.0 hours
      B. Cat—26.0 hours
 III. Collect 5–6 ml of blood just before next dose (6–12 hours after last dose, depending on dosage regimen).
  IV. Remove and store serum (or plasma) in container (glass or plastic). Several methods require a minimum of 2 ml serum or plasma.
   V. Record appropriate clinical data and exact time of last dose and time of sample collection.
  VI. Submit sample to laboratory for drug analysis.
 VII. Common methods used for chloramphenicol analysis include HPLC and EIA.

Interpretation of Results

   I. Therapeutic range
      5–15 μg/ml (*Note*: optimum serum concentrations should be based on MIC data.)
  II. Toxicity usually occurs at concentrations >20 μg/ml.
 III. Toxic signs include aplastic anemia, thrombocytopenia, leukopenia, and cardiovascular collapse (usually in neonate and due to immature liver enzyme system).

Dosage Modification

   Can be made if inappropriate concentrations are reported. Confirm new steady-state concentrations after change in dosage (see IIIA., Individualization Techniques).

DIGITOXIN [pKa = not applicable (glycoside)]

Dosage Guidelines

I. Dog
   A. Oral: 0.033 mg/kg
   B. q8h
II. Cat
   Not recommended

Pharmacokinetic Constants (See Flasch and Heinz, 1979, Peters et al., 1981 Suggested Readings)

I. Dog
   A. $T\frac{1}{2}$ = 8.2 hr
   B. V'd = 1.5 L/kg
II. Cat
   A. $T\frac{1}{2}$ = 31.8 hr
   B. V'd = 1.2 L/kg
      Although this is a recent study of cats using RIA methods, cross-reactivity of antibody to digoxin (metabolite of digitoxin) was not evaluated. Reported $T\frac{1}{2}$ may be the result of digitoxin and digoxin serum concentrations.

Procedure for Monitoring Digitoxin Concentrations

I. Select desired dosage regimen and administer drug until steady state is established.
II. Length of time required for steady-state conditions
   A. Dog—41.0 hours
   B. Cat—6.7 days
III. Collect 1–2 ml blood before next dose.
IV. Remove and store serum (or plasma) in glass container only (cardiac glycosides are known to adsorb to plastic).
V. Record appropriate clinical data and exact time of last dose and time of sample collection.
VI. Submit sample to laboratory for analysis.
VII. Common methods used for determination of digitoxin include RIA and EIA.

Interpretation of Results

I. Therapeutic range
   15–35 ng/ml

II. Toxicity usually occurs at levels >40 ng/ml.
III. Toxic signs include anorexia, nausea, vomition, cardiac arrhythmias, muscle weakness, and depression.

Modification in Dosage

Should be made if inappropriate concentrations are reported. Confirm new steady-state concentrations after changing dosage regimen. (see IIIA., Individualization Techniques).

Digoxin [pKa = not applicable (glycoside)]

Dosage Guidelines

I. Dog
    A. Oral: 0.011 mg/kg
    B. q12h
II. Cat
    A. Oral: 0.008 mg/kg
    B. q12h

Pharmacokinetic Constants (see Breznock, 1973; Bolton and Powell, 1982 in Suggested Readings)

I. Dog
    A. $T\frac{1}{2}$ = 31.3 hr
    B. V'd = 19.0 L/kg
II. Cat
    A. $T\frac{1}{2}$ = 33.5 hr
    B. V'd = 14.5 L/kg
        Some work seems to indicate that the elimination process for digoxin in the cat involves saturation kinetics and $T\frac{1}{2}$ in the cat may be dose-dependent.

Procedure for Monitoring Digoxin Concentrations

  I. Select desired dosage regimen and administer drug until steady state is established.
 II. Length of time required for steady-state conditions
    A. Dog—6.5–7.0 days
    B. Cat—7.0–7.5 days
III. Collect 1- to 2 ml blood sample before next dose (or at least 8 hours after dosing). It is recommended that additional serum samples be taken at time

of drug determination for evaluation of electrolytes. These data will aid in the interpretation of serum concentrations

IV. Remove and store serum (or plasma) in *glass container only* (cardiac glycosides are known to adsorb to plastic).

V. Record appropriate clinical data and exact time of last dose and time of sample collection.

VI. Submit sample to laboratory for analysis.

VII. Common methods used for determination of digoxin include RIA and EIA.

Interpretation of Results

I. Therapeutic range
  A. Dog—0.9–3.0 ng/ml
  B. Cat—0.9–2.0 ng/ml

II. Toxicity usually occurs at levels >3.0 ng/ml (dog) and >2.4 ng/ml (cat).

III. Toxic signs include anorexia, nausea, vomition, cardiac arrhythmias, muscle weakness, and depression.

Factors Affecting Myocardial Sensitivity

Result in greater response at given serum concentration
  I. Hypothyroidism
  II. Hypokalemia
  III. Hypercalcemia
  IV. Hypomagnesia
  V. Hypoalbuminemia
  VI. Hypoxia
  VII. Alkalosis
  VIII. Renal disease
  IX. Hepatic disease

Drugs Affecting Serum Concentration

Can expect elevated (↑) or reduced (↓) levels
  I. Chloramphenicol ↑
  II. Furosemide ↓
  III. Phenobarbital ↓
  IV. Phenylbutazone ↓
  V. Primidone ↓
  VI. Quinidine ↑
  VII. Tetracyclines ↑

Modification of Dosage

May be made if inappropriate concentrations are reported. Confirm new steady-state concentration after changing dosage regimen (see IIIA., Individualization Techniques).

GENTAMICIN (pKa = 8.2)

Dosage Regimen

I. Dog
   A. IM: 2–3 mg/kg
   B. q8h
II. Cat
   A. IM: 2–3 mg/kg
   B. q12h

Pharmacokinetic Constants (see Riviere, Suggested Readings)

I. Dog
   A. $T\frac{1}{2}$ = 0.9–1.3 hr
   B. V'd = 0.3 L/kg
II. Cat (not available)
   A. $T\frac{1}{2}$ = not available
   B. V'd = not available

Procedure for Monitoring Gentamicin Concentrations

I. Select desired dosage regimen and administer drug until steady state is established.
II. Length of time required for steady-state conditions
      Dog—6.5 hours
III. Collect 1–2 ml blood at 1–2 hours after dosing (for peak concentration determinations) or just before next dose (for trough determinations). Heparinized tubes should not be used due to interference in assay.
IV. Remove and store serum (or plasma) in *plastic container only* (aminoglycosides are known to adsorb to glass).
V. Record appropriate clinical data and exact time of last dose and time of sample collection.
VI. Submit sample to laboratory for analysis and indicate if peak or trough determination.
VII. Common methods used for gentamicin determinations include RIA and EIA.

Interpretation of Results

I. Therapeutic range
   A. Peak: 5–8 μg/ml
   B. Trough: 0.5–1.5 μg/ml

II. Optimum serum concentrations should be based on MIC data of infecting organism.

III. Toxicity usually occurs at
   A. Peak levels >12–15 μg/ml
   B. Trough levels >2 μg/ml

IV. Toxic signs include nystagmus, vertigo (ototoxicity), elevated blood urea nitrogen (BUN), and elevated serum creatinine (nephrotoxicity).

V. Incidence of both ototoxicity and nephrotoxicity is associated with trough levels greater than 2 μg/ml for prolonged periods of time. Risk is reduced by monitoring trough levels and maintaining below 2 μg/ml.

Modification of Dosage

May be made if inappropriate concentrations are reported. Confirm new steady-state concentrations after changing dosage regimen (see IIIA, Individualization Techniques).

LIDOCAINE (pKa = 7.85)

Dosage Guidelines

I. Dog
   A. IV: loading dose 4 mg/kg
   B. Infusion 50 μg/kg/min

II. Cat
   A. IV: 1–3 mg/kg
   B. Infusion rate not available

Pharmacokinetic Constants (see Wilcke et al. 1983 in Suggested Readings)

I. Dog
   A. $T\frac{1}{2}$ = 0.9 hr
   B. V'd = 1.4 L/kg

II. Cat
   A. $T\frac{1}{2}$ = not available
   B. V'd = not available

Procedure for Monitoring Lidocaine Concentrations

I. Select desired dosage regimen and administer drug until steady state is established.

II. Length of time required for steady-state conditions: Dog—5 hours

III. Collect 5 ml blood sample and store serum (or plasma) in container (glass or plastic).
IV. If infusing lidocaine, obtain blood sample from opposite limb from infusion catheter.
V. Record appropriate clinical data and exact time of last dose and time of sample collection.
VI. Submit sample to laboratory for analysis and indicate if you would like analysis of lidocaine only or whether analysis should be done for lidocaine and active metabolites.
VII. Common methods used for lidocaine determination include HPLC, GLC, and EIA.

Interpretation of Results

I. Therapeutic range
   Dog: 2–6 µg/ml
II. Lidocaine is rapidly metabolized by liver to two active metabolites [monoethylglycinexylidide (MEGX) and glycinexylidide (GX)].
III. Total pharmacologic effect results from the concentration of lidocaine and active metabolites in the serum.
IV. Toxicity usually occurs (in the dog) at >8 µg/ml.
V. Toxic signs include apprehension, vocalization, intermittent running activity, tonic muscular extension, coma, and respiratory arrest.

Modification of Dose (or Infusion)

May be made if inappropriate concentrations are reported. Confirm new steady-state concentration after changing dosage regimen.

PHENOBARBITAL (pKa = 7.3)

Dosage Guidelines

I. Dog
   A. Oral: 2 mg/kg, q12h
   B. IV: 6 mg/kg, p.r.n. (status epilepticus)
II. Cat
   Oral: 4 mg/kg, q12h
III. See chapter 16.

Pharmacokinetic Constants (see Pedersoli, Suggested Readings)

I. Dog
   A. $T_{\frac{1}{2}}$ = 53.0 hr
   B. V'd = 7.4 L/kg

II. Cat
   A. $T\frac{1}{2}$ = not available
   B. V'd = not available
III. There is a wide range in individual $T\frac{1}{2}$ reported in literature (32–75 hours).
IV. Individuals should be monitored to establish appropriate dose.
 V. Animals on long-term phenobarbital medication have shortened $T\frac{1}{2}$ values for other drugs that are metabolized and eliminated by liver enzyme oxidative pathways.

Procedure for Monitoring
Phenobarbital Concentrations

 I. Select desired dosage regimen and administer drug until steady-state is established.
II. Length of time required for steady-state conditions
   A. Dog—16 days
   B. Cat—NA
III. Collect 5 ml blood sample and store serum (or plasma) in container (glass or plastic).
IV. Record appropriate clinical data and exact time of last dose and time of sample collection.
 V. Submit sample to laboratory for analysis.
VI. Common methods used for phenobarbital concentrations include HPLC, GLC, and EIA.

Interpretation of Results

 I. Therapeutic range 15–40 µg/ml
II. Toxicity usually occurs at >40 µg/ml

Modification of Dose

  May be made if inappropriate concentrations are reported. Confirm new steady-state concentration after changing dosage regimen (See IIIA, Individualization Techniques).

PHENYTOIN (pKa = 8.3)

Dosage Guidelines

 I. Dog
   A. Oral: 6–30 mg/kg, q8h
   B. IV: 5 mg/kg, *slowly*
II. Cat—Oral 10 mg/kg

Pharmacokinetic Constants (see Frey and Loscher, and Kowaleyck, Suggested Readings)

I. Dog
    A. $T_{\frac{1}{2}}$ = 3.3 hr
    B. V'd = 1.5 L/kg
II. Cat
    A. $T_{\frac{1}{2}}$ > 24.0 hr
    B. V'd = not available

Procedure for Monitoring Phenytoin Concentrations

    I. Select desired dosage regimen and administer drug until steady-state concentrations are established.
  II. Length of time required for steady-state conditions
    A. Dog—22.0 hours
    B. Cat—5–6 days
 III. Collect 5–6 ml blood sample just before next dose.
 IV. Remove and store serum (or plasma) in container (glass or plastic).
  V. Record appropriate clinical data and exact time of last dose and time of sample collection.
 VI. Submit sample to laboratory for analysis.
VII. Common methods used for determination of phenytoin include HPLC and EIA.

Interpretation of Results

  I. Therapeutic range 10–20 µg/ml
 II. Toxicity usually occurs at levels >20 µg/ml.
III. Toxic signs include agitation, emesis, and incoordination.

Modification of Dose

May be made if inappropriate concentrations are reported. There is considerable variation in bioavailability for phenytoin. Confirm new steady-state concentrations after changing dosage regimen (see IIIA, Individualization Techniques).

PRIMIDONE (pKa = NA)

Dosage Guidelines

I. Dog
        Oral: 25 mg/kg, q12h

II. Cat

     Oral: 20 mg/kg, q12h

       Some work has been done with primidone in cats which indicates that primidone may not be contraindicated in cats, as previously thought (see Sawchuk, Suggested Readings).

Pharmacokinetic Constants (see Frey, Cunningham, Suggested Readings)

  I. Dog

    A. $T\frac{1}{2}$ = 6.1 hr

    B. V'd = not available

 II. Cat

    A. $T\frac{1}{2}$ = not available

    B. V'd = not available

Procedures for Monitoring Primidone Concentrations

    I. Select desired dosage regimen and administer drug until steady-state concentrations are established.

   II. Length of time required for steady-state conditions (based on phenobarbital)

       Dog—16 days

  III. Collect 5–6 ml blood sample just before next dose.

  IV. Remove and store serum (or plasma) in container (glass or plastic).

   V. Record appropriate clinical data and exact time of last dose and time of sample collection.

  VI. Submit sample to laboratory for analysis.

 VII. Common methods used for determination of primidone include HPLC and EIA.

VIII. Some laboratories can quantitate primidone and its active metabolites.

  IX. Phenobarbital is the major metabolite of primidone in the dog and should be monitored rather than primidone.

Interpretation of Results

  I. Therapeutic range

     0.6–1.1 μg/ml (dog)

 II. Toxicity usually occurs due to high phenobarbital levels.

III. Toxic signs are similar to phenobarbital toxic signs.

Modification

Can be made if inappropriate concentrations are reported. Confirm new steady-state concentrations after changing dosage regimen (see IIIA, Individualization Techniques).

PROCAINAMIDE (pKa = 9.2)

Dosage Guidelines

I. Dog
   A. Oral: 125–500 mg/dog, q6–8h
   B. IM: 125–250 mg, total dose
II. Cat
   Dose not available

Pharmacokinetic Constants (see Kaufman et al., Suggested Readings)

$T\frac{1}{2}$ for procainamide has not been determined. Some studies using oral administration indicate a fairly short $T\frac{1}{2}$ (less than 4 hours).

Procedure for Monitoring Procainamide Concentrations

   I. Select desired dosage regimen and administer until steady-state concentrations are established.
   II. Length of time required for steady state-conditions: Dog—20.0 hours (approximately)
   III. Collect 5–6 ml blood sample just before next dose.
   IV. Remove and store serum (or plasma) in container (glass or plastic).
   V. Record appropriate clinical data and exact time of last dose and time of sample collection.
   VI. Submit sample to laboratory for analysis.
   VII. Common methods used for determination of procainamide include HPLC, GLC, EIA, and FIA.
   VIII. Most laboratory methods can determine procainamide and its major metabolite, n-acetylprocainamide.

Interpretation of Results

   I. Therapeutic range
      4–10 μg/ml
   II. Toxicity usually occurs at levels >10 μg/ml

III. Toxic signs include cardiac depression, nausea, vomition, anorexia, and hypotension.

IV. Some multiple dosing studies indicate that dogs do not metabolize procainamide to n-acetylprocainamide and most pharmacologic effects are due to procainamide concentrations.

Modification of Dose

Can be made if inappropriate concentrations are reported. Confirm new steady-state concentrations after changing dosage regimen (see IIIA, Individualization Techniques).

QUINIDINE (pKa = 8.4)

Dosage Guidelines

I. Dog
Oral: 10–20 mg/kg, q8h
II. Cat
Oral: 10–20 mg/kg, q6h

Pharmacokinetic Constants (see Neff et al., Suggested Readings)

I. Dog
A. $T\frac{1}{2}$ = 5.6 hr
B. V'd = 2.9 L/kg
II. Cat
A. $T\frac{1}{2}$ = 1.9 hr
B. V'd = 2.2 L/kg

Procedure for Monitoring Quinidine Concentrations

I. Select desired dosage regimen and administer drug until steady-state concentrations are established.
II. Length of time required for steady-state conditions
A. Dog—28.0 hours (approximately)
B. Cat—10.0 hours
III. Collect 5–6 ml blood sample just before next dose.
IV. Remove and store serum (or plasma) in container (glass or plastic).
V. Record appropriate clinical data and exact time of last dose and time of sample collection.

VI. Submit sample to laboratory for analysis.
VII. Common methods used for determination of quinidine include HPLC, GLC, EIA, and FIA.

Interpretation of Results

 I. Therapeutic range
      2.5–5.0 µg/ml
 II. Toxicity usually occurs at levels >10 µg/ml
III. Toxic signs include nausea, vomition, and diarrhea.
IV. Modification can be made if inappropriate concentrations are reported.
 V. Confirm new steady-state concentrations after changing dosage regimen.

THEOPHYLLINE (pKa = 8.8)

Dosage Guidelines

 I. Dog
        Oral: 11.0 mg/kg, q8h
II. Cat
        Oral: 5 mg/kg, q12h

Pharmacokinetic Constants (see Neff et al., McKiernan et al., Suggested Readings)

 I. Dog
    A. $T\frac{1}{2}$ = 5.7 hr
    B. V'd = 0.82 L/kg
II. Cat
    A. $T\frac{1}{2}$ = 7.9 hr
    B. V'd = 0.46 L/kg

Procedure for Monitoring Theophylline Concentrations

  I. Select desired dosage regimen and administer drug until steady-state concentrations are established.
 II. Length of time required for steady-state conditions
     A. Dog—30.0 hours (approximately)
     B. Cat—40.0 hours
III. Collect 5–6 ml blood sample just before next dose.
IV. Remove and store serum (or plasma) in container (glass or plastic).

   V. Record appropriate clinical data and exact time of last dose and time of
      sample collection.
  VI. Submit sample to laboratory for analysis.
 VII. Common methods used for determination of procainamide include HPLC,
      GLC, EIA, and FIA.

Interpretation of Results

   I. Therapeutic range
         10–20 μg/ml
  II. Toxicity usually occurs at levels >25 μg/ml.
 III. Toxic signs include nausea, insomnia, gastric acid secretion and diarrhea.
      Seizures usually associated with serum concentrations greater than 35
      μg/ml.

Modification of Dose

   Can be made if inappropriate concentrations are reported. Confirm new-
steady state concentrations after changing dosage regimen (see IIIA, Individualization Techniques).

SUGGESTED READINGS

   Amlie JP, Storslim L, Helclaas O: Correlation between pharmacokinetics and iso-
tropic and electrophysiologic responses to digitoxin in the intact dog. J Cardiovasc
Pharmacol 1:529, 1979
   Baggot JD: Principles of drug distribution in domestic animals. WB Saunders, Philadelphia, 1977
   Bolton GR, Powell AA: Plasma kinetics of digoxin in the cat. Am J Vet Res 43:1994,
1982
   Breznock EM: Application of canine kinetics of digoxin and digitoxin in the ther-
apeutic digitalization in the dog. Am J Vet Res 34:993, 1973
   Cunningham JG, Hardukewych D, Jensen HA: Therapeutic serum concentrations
of primidone and its metabolites, phenobarbital and phenylethylmalonamide in epileptic
dogs. J Am Vet Med Assoc, 182:1091, 1983
   Davis LE, Neff CA, Baggot JD, Powers TE: Pharmacokinetics of chloramphenicol
in domesticated animals. Am J Vet Res 33:2259, 1972
   El-Sayed MA, Loscha W, Frey HH: Pharmacokinetics of ethosuximide in the dog.
Arch Intern Pharmacodyn 234:180, 1978
   Flasch H, Heinz H: Pharmacokinetics of dihydrodigitoxin in the cat. A comparison
with digitoxin. Naunyn Schmiedebergs Arch Pharmacol 310(2):147, 1979
   Frey HH, Gobel W, Loscher W: Pharmacokinetics of primidone and its active me-
tabolites in the dog. Arch Intern Pharmacodyn Ther 242:14, 1979
   Frey HH, Loscher W: Clinical pharmacokinetics of phenytoin in the dog: a re-
evaluation. Am J Vet Res 41:1635, 1980
   Gibaldi M, Prescott LF (eds): Handbook of clinical pharmacokinetics. ADIS Health
Science Press, New York, 1983

Hamlin RL: Basis for selection of a cardiac glycoside for dogs. Proceedings 1st Symp Vet Pharmacol Ther, Baton Rouge, LA, 1978

Kaufman GM, Weirich WE, Mayer PR: The pharmacokinetics of regular and sustained release procainamide in the dog. Proc Am Coll Vet Intern Med (abstr) July 1983

Kowalczyk DF: Correlation of serum phenytoin concentrations (diphenylhydantoin) with the administration of oral and intravenous phenytoin in dogs. J Vet Pharmacol Ther 3:237, 1980

Lai CM, Reynolds RD, Kanaath BL et al: Effect of coronary artery ligation on the pharmacokinetics of n-acetylprocainamide in dogs. Res Commun Clin Pathol Pharmacol 29:369, 1980

McKiernan BC, Neff-Davis CA, Koritz GD, Davis LE, Pheris DR: Pharmacokinetic studies of theophylline in dogs. J Vet Pharmacol Ther 4:103, 1981

McKiernan BC, Neff-Davis CA, Koritz GD, Davis LE: Pharmacokinetics of theophylline in cats. J Vet Pharmacol Ther 6:99, 1983

Neff CA, Davis LE, Baggot JD: A comparative study of pharmacokinetics of quinidine. Am J Vet Res 33:1521, 1972

Pedersoli W, Ravis, Nachreiner R: Pharmacokinetics of phenobarbital in dogs following multiple oral administration. Am J Vet Res (submitted for publication)

Peters DN, Hamlin RL, Powers JD: Absence of pharmacokinetic interaction between digitoxin and quinidine in the dog. J Vet Pharmacol Ther 4:271, 1981

Riviere JE, Coppoc GL, Hinsman EJ, Carlton WW: Gentamicin pharmacokinetics changes in induced acute canine nephrotoxic glomerulonephritis. Antimicrob Agents Chemother 20:387, 1981

Sadée W, Beelen GC: Drug Level Monitoring. Analytical Techniques, Metabolism and Pharmacokinetics, John Wiley & Sons, New York, 1980

Sawchuk SA: Evaluation of primidone in the cat. M.S. thesis, University of Illinois, Urbana, 1980

Wilcke JR, Davis LE, Neff-Davis CA, Koritz GD: Pharmacokinetics of lidocaine and its active metabolites in the dog. J Vet Pharmacol Ther 6:49, 1983

23

Clinical Management of Toxicoses and Adverse Drug Reactions

J. Edmond Riviere, D.V.M.

GENERAL COMMENTS

I. Diseases induced by reactions to foreign chemicals and drugs are becoming more common in veterinary practice.

II. Primary therapeutic objective in acute poisonings are
   A. Preservation of life
   B. Stabilization of vital signs
   C. Elimination of the toxin

III. Toxin-induced damage of specific organ systems may result in their failure. Refer to appropriate chapters elsewhere in this book for discussion of management.

IV. Additional information may be found in the Suggested Readings or the practitioner may call the University of Illinois Veterinary Toxicology Hotline (217) 333-3611 for specific information concerning a patient. This chapter is not a comprehensive review of clinical toxicology but rather is designed to be a brief clinical summary of the material oriented to the practitioner.

GENERAL PRINCIPLES OF TREATMENT

EMERGENCY TREATMENT

I. Establish and maintain a patent airway.

II. Provide ventilation.

III. Restore cardiac function.

IV. Insert IV catheter for administration of
   A. Fluids and electrolytes
   B. Emergency drugs
      1. Specific antidotes if available
      2. Use of additional drugs should be kept at a minimum to avoid adverse interactions.
 V. Respiratory and cardiac support
   A. Intubation with a cuffed endotracheal tube is necessary in comatose animals for anesthesia or if enterogastric lavage is to be performed.
   B. Artificial respiration administered by means of a mechanical ventilator or AMBU bag.
   C. The routine use of pharmacologic respiratory stimulants is discouraged since positive respiratory assistance is usually sufficient.
   D. In the event of cardiac arrest, appropriate measures should be instituted:
      1. Inotropic or chronotropic drugs
      2. External or internal cardiac massage
      3. Electrical defibrillation
   E. Fluid therapy should be administered if volume contraction is present.
   F. Correct acid-base or electrolyte disturbances (see chapter 2).
   G. The use of external heat or cooling sources is preferred to pharmacologic intervention in correcting hypothermia or hyperthermia.
   H. Maintenance of normal homeostasis by the above supportive procedures will usually protect against further toxin-induced injury and will support renal and hepatic function so that elimination of systemically absorbed toxin can occur.
 VI. Anticonvulsant therapy
   A. Convulsions can be controlled by inducing light anesthesia with an ultra-short-acting barbiturate. However, these agents are respiratory depressants and may worsen a toxicant-induced respiratory depression.
   B. If the animal is to be anesthetized with an inhalational agent, further anticonvulsant therapy is not required.
   C. Diazepam, methocarbamol, or glyceryl guaiacolate dosed to effect may be effective in controlling convulsions.
   D. Placing the animal in a quiet, darkened environment is often an effective anticonvulsant measure.
   E. See chapter 16.
VII. Alleviation of pain
   A. Administration of the above procedures can be difficult if the animal is suffering from pain as a result of the intoxication. Pain is also a major source of stress which can seriously hamper recovery.
   B. Analgesics such as morphine or meperidine have been suggested. However, narcotic-induced respiratory depression may be an adverse reaction (see chapter 1).

General comments

Once the animal is stable, it is imperative to prevent further absorption of the agent into the body. The methods employed to achieve this goal are dependent upon the source and route of exposure as well as on the physiochemical and pharmacologic characteristics of the compound. In all cases, the animal should immediately be physically separated from the source of the poison. This could be as simple as removing food or restraining the individual.

Percutaneous Exposure

I. Washing the animal's skin is an effective remedy to prevent further absorption. Care should be taken to protect persons performing this procedure from being exposed to the poison. Baths with large volumes of water are the preferred method.

II. Intensive scrubbing leading to abrasion or the use of lipid-solubilizing solutions (oil or hydrocarbon solvents) are discouraged since both of these procedures may increase percutaneous absorption. However, mild scrubbing with soapy solutions may be necessary to remove lipid-soluble compounds.

Oral Exposure

I. Induction of emesis
 A. Contraindicated if
  1. Poison is a corrosive agent, a volatile hydrocarbon, or a petroleum distillate.
  2. The patient is in a semicomatose or unconscious state.
  3. Convulsions are present.
  4. Aspiration pneumonia is a serious complication in animals not possessing a cough reflex.
 B. If the time interval between exposure to toxin and presentation to the veterinarian is greater than a few hours, emesis will not be effective.
 C. As a general rule, vomitus should be saved for subsequent chemical analysis.
 D. Emetic agents. See table 23-1.
  1. Emesis should be induced within 15–25 minutes with these agents.
  2. Respiratory depression or protracted emesis caused by apomorphine can be reversed with narcotic antagonists.
  3. Syrup of ipecac should never be used if activated charcoal is administered since the effectiveness of the charcoal will be greatly reduced.
  4. If emesis does not occur after two doses of ipecac, gastric lavage

TABLE 23-1. EMETIC DRUGS

Drug	Route	Dose
Apomorphine (dogs only)	IV	0.04 mg/kg
	IM, SQ	0.08 mg/kg
Syrup of ipecac	PO	1–2 ml/kg
Table salt	PO	1–3 tsp in warm water
Hydrogen peroxide	PO	5–25 ml
Xylazine (cats)	IM	0.44 mg/kg

should be instituted since absorption of ipecac may result in cardiac toxicity.

II. Gastric and enterogastric lavage
   A. Animals must be unconscious or under light anesthesia, and have a cuffed endotracheal tube in place before these procedures are instituted. This technique is most effective when
   1. A large-size stomach tube is employed.
   2. Large volumes of lavage fluid are used (5–10 ml/kg).
   3. The procedure is performed less than 2 hours after ingestion of the poison.
   B. Contraindications include a weakened stomach wall.
   C. Suitable lavage fluids are warm saline or tap water. The addition of activated charcoal increases the effectiveness of the procedure.
   D. After infusion, contents should be aspirated and another cycle of infusion started in 5–10 minutes. This procedure may be repeated 10–15 times.
   E. An alternate procedure which may be more effective is enterogastric lavage in conjunction with a high-gravity warm water enema. A retrograde filling of the intestines occurs by applying digital pressure on the anus. This procedure is continued until clear fluid is flowing from the gastric tube. Note that care must be taken to avoid serious electrolyte disturbances.
   F. These procedures should only be instituted if emesis cannot be induced or is contraindicated.

III. Adsorbent therapy
   A. Absorption can also be prevented by physically binding the toxicant to a nonabsorbable carrier.
   B. Two to 8 g/kg of activated vegetable charcoal given at a concentration of 1 g/5–10 ml water administered by stomach tube should be followed in 30 minutes by a cathartic unless a lavage is being performed.
   C. This regimen is ineffective against cyanide intoxication.
   D. Syrup of ipecac decreases its effectiveness as does MgO and tannic acid, components of the "universal antidote."

IV. Catharsis. Administration of sodium sulfate orally at a dose of 1 g/kg effectively hastens the gastrointestinal transit of toxicants. This drug is more effective and safer than magnesium sulfate. If lipid-soluble toxicants are involved, mineral oil or vegetable oil followed by a saline cathartic may be effective.

ENHANCE ELIMINATION

General Comments

Once an animal's condition has been stabilized and attempts to decrease further absorption of compound have been instituted, the final step short of specific antidotal therapy is to enhance the rate of elimination of absorbed compound from the body by augmenting the normal physiologic mechanisms.

Renal Excretion

I. Diuresis
   A. For compounds that normally undergo tubular reabsorption, an increased rate of urine flow may increase clearance of the compound from the body.
   B. Mannitol at a dose of 2 g/kg/hr or furosemide at a dose of 5 mg/kg every 6–8 hours.
   C. If urine output does not increase after giving these agents, further doses should not be given since systemic toxicity may result.
   D. The supportive fluid therapy by itself may increase urine output sufficiently to enhance elimination of drug.

II. Urinary pH
   A. For toxicants that undergo nonionic renal tubular reabsorption, changing urinary pH may significantly change the rate of renal clearance.
   B. For weak acids such as aspirin and some barbiturates, alkalinizing the urine will "trap" the compounds in the renal tubule in their ionized form thereby preventing reabsorption and increasing clearance.
   C. Acidifying the urine will increase the clearance of weak bases such as amphetamines, procainamide, or quinidine.
   D. A brisk rate of urine flow is required for these maneuvers to be optimal.
   E. Ammonium chloride appears to be an effective acidifying agent while sodium bicarbonate is an efficient alkalinizing agent for this purpose.

III. Dialysis
   A. Compounds that are capable of being dialyzed include alcohols, glycols, barbiturates, many antibiotics, metals, halides, alkaloids, glycosides, and some endogenous toxins.
   B. The efficiency of dialysis in removing these toxicants is a function of
      1. The size of the molecule
      2. The degree of serum protein binding
      3. The efficiency of the dialyzer

    4. The pharmacokinetics of the drug in the animal. For instance, compounds that have a large volume of distribution, i.e., digoxin, are not efficiently dialyzed since only a small fraction of free drug is available for elimination.

  C. Hemodialysis and hemoperfusion are still not practical procedures for most veterinary clinics, however with the advent of the new column-disk peritoneal catheter and with better control of peritonitis, this mode of therapy is becoming an alternative.

Hepatic Elimination

Reliable methods are not presently available to enhance clearance of compounds from the body eliminated primarily by the liver. If toxicity is a result of metabolites which are eliminated by the kidney, then the above procedures may be beneficial. Phenobarbital given in low doses is a potent inducer of hepatic microsomal enzymes and may find a use in treating chronic intoxication of compounds biotransformed by these enzymes, i.e., chlorinated hydrocarbons.

COMMONLY ENCOUNTERED TOXICANTS

GENERAL COMMENTS

   I. Small animal poisonings can be broadly divided into two classes, those arising from accidental exposure and those occurring as an adverse reaction to the therapeutic use of a veterinary drug. In the first case, the diagnosis may not be evident while in the latter case, the identity of the toxicant is often known.

  II. Compounds causing accidental poisonings include owner's prescription drugs, rodenticides, insecticides, herbicides, household and industrial chemicals, environmental contaminants, and various biotoxins.

 III. The general treatment regimens outlined above are often utilized in poisonings resulting from these sources.

 IV. Many of these toxicants have specific target organs in man and animals including

    A. The kidney (see table 23-2)

    B. The liver (see table 23-3)

    C. The hematopoietic system (see table 23-4)

    D. These may suggest general treatment protocols.

  V. The aim of the present section is to present specific therapeutic protocols which may be beneficial in treating these poisonings.

TABLE 23-2. DRUGS PRODUCING NEPHROTOXICITY

Antimicrobial drugs
    Ampicillin, I
    Amphotericin B, T
    Bacitracin, T
    Cephaloridine, T
    Colistin, T
    Gentamicin, T
    Kanamycin, T
    Methicillin, I
    Neomycin, T
    Oxacillin, I
    Penicillin, I, V
    Polymyxin B, T
    Sulfonamides, O, I
    Tetracyclines, T, V
    Tobramycin, T

Heavy metals
    Arsenicals, T, N
    Bismuth, T
    Cadmium, T
    Copper, T
    Gold salts, T, N
    Mercurials, T, N
    Uranium, T

Analgesics
    Ibuprofen, I
    Naproxen, I
    Phenacetin, T
    Phenylbutazone, T, V
    Salicylates, T

Antineoplastic drugs
    Adriamycin, N
    Cis-platin, T
    Cyclophosphamide, T, V
    Daunorubicin, N
    Methotrexate, O
    Mithramycin, T

Diuretics
    Furosemide, I
    Mannitol, T
    Thiazides, I, V

Miscellaneous
    Captopril, N
    Dextrans, V
    EDTA, T
    Lithium, N
    Penicillamine, N
    Phenazopyridine, T
    Phenindione, I
    Probenecid, N

Mechanisms are indicated by I, interstitial; N, nephrotic; O, obstructive; T, tubular; V, vasculitis.
From Davis LE: Veterinary Clinical Pharmacology. WB Saunders, Philadelphia (in press).

RODENTICIDES

Warfarin and Other Anticoagulants (see table 23-5)

I. Mechanisms of action

A. These agents competitively inhibit the regeneration of active vitamin K which results when vitamin K epoxide is generated as a byproduct of its participation in the carboxylation of clotting factors II, VII, IX, and X.

B. As a result of this inhibition, the production of these active clotting factors is inhibited resulting in their gradual depletion over a period of several days.

C. The result is hemorrhage in multiple areas of the body.

D. Massive doses of warfarin may cause acute death secondary to vascular collapse.

E. Also see chapter 8.

TABLE 23-3.   DRUGS CAUSING HEPATOTOXICITY

Anesthetics	Cardiovascular
Chloroform	Procainamide
Halothane	Quinidine
Methoxyflurane	Warfarin
Anticonvulsants	Antineoplastics
Carbamazepine	Busulfan
Phenobarbital	Cyclophosphamide
Primidone	L-Asparginase
Valproic acid	6-Mercaptopurine
	Methotrexate
Antimicrobial drugs	Mithramycin
Ampicillin	Urethane
Carbenicillin	
Erythromycin estolate	Endocrine agents
5-Fluorocytosine	Anabolic steroids
Griseofulvin	(C-17 alkylated)
Isoniazid	Corticosteroids
Nitrofurantoin	Methimazole
Quinacrine	Propylthiouracil
Tetracyclines	
	Tranquilizers
Analgesics	Diazepam
Acetaminophen	Haloperidol
Ibuprofen	Phenothiazines
Indomethacin	
Naproxen	Other drugs
Phenylbutazone	Cimetidine
Salicylates	Danthron
	Dapsone
	Iodochlorhydroxyquin
	Nicotinamide
	Stibofen
	Thiabendazole
	Vitamin A

From Davis LE: Veterinary Clinical Pharmacology. WB Saunders, Philadelphia, (in press).

II. Clinical signs
  A. Hemorrhage, including petechiae and ecchymoses
  B. Pale and cyanotic mucous membranes
  C. Weak and rapid pulse
  D. Additional signs include weakness, dyspnea, prostration, and occasional bloody vomitus, feces, or urine.
III. Treatment
  A. The primary aim of therapy is to replace vitamin K so that clotting factors can gradually be replenished.
  B. If massive hemorrhage is present, citrated whole blood should be given.
  C. Vitamin K_1 and vitamin K_2 are the compounds of choice since they are more active than vitamin K_3 and vitamin K_4 preparations.
    1. Synonyms for vitamin K_1 include phytonadione, phylloquinone, and phytomenadione.

   2. Vitamin K_1 can be given IV, IM, or SQ at a dose of 5 mg/kg for dogs and a total dose of 2.5–5 mg/kg for cats.

   3. When given IV, a small-gauge needle should be used and a pressure wrap applied after injection.

   4. Rate of IV infusion should not exceed 0.02 mg/min/kg.

  D. Supportive therapy should be given as indicated.

Strychnine

This alkaloidal rodenticide is a common agent used to maliciously poison small animals due to its widespread availability. The compound is readily absorbed orally and can produce clinical signs within 1–5 hours with food delaying onset of signs.

  I. Mechanism of action

    A. Selective and reversible inhibition of glycine-mediated postsynaptic neurotransmission in the inhibitory spinal cord neurons.

    B. This results in loss of spinal cord reflex inhibition causing extensor reflex hyperexcitability in dogs and cats when external sensory stimuli are present.

TABLE 23-4. DRUGS THAT HAVE CAUSED APLASTIC ANEMIA

Antineoplastic	Endocrine agents
Busulfan	Estrogens
Cyclophosphamide	Thiouracil
Cytosine arabinoside	Thiocyanate
Methotrexate	Methimazole
Mustargen	Tolbutamide
Vinblastine	
Vincristine	Tranquilizers
	Meprobamate
Antimicrobials	Phenothiazines
Amphotericin B	
Chloramphenicol	Antihistamines
Methicillin	Chlorpheniramine
Pyrimethamine	Tripelennamine
Quinacrine	
Sulfonamides	Miscellaneous
Tetracyclines	Benzene
	Carbamazepine
Analgesics	Carbon tetrachloride
Phenylbutazone	Chlordane
Phenacetin	DDT
Indomethacin	Disophenol
	γ-Benzene hexachloride
Heavy metals	
Organic arsenicals	
Gold salts	
Colloidal silver	

From Davis LE: Veterinary Clinical Pharmacology. WB Saunders, Philadelphia (in press).

TABLE 23-5.   VITAMIN K ANTAGONIST
DRUGS AND RODENTICIDES

Acenocoumarol
Anisindione
Brodifacoum
Bromadialone
Chlorophacinone
Coumachlor
Coumafuryl (Fumarin)
Coumatetralyl
Cyclocloumarol
Dicumarol
Difenacoum
Diphenadione (Diphacinone)
Ethyl biscoumacetate
Naphthylindanedione
Phenindione
Phenprocoumon
Pindone
Sulfaquinoxaline
Valone
Warfarin

II. Clinical signs
   A. Initially, poisoned animals demonstrate anxiety and an increased sensitivity to external stimuli.
   B. This is followed by an increased extensor muscle tone and then by tonic convulsions induced by auditory, tactile, or visual stimuli. Opisthotonus, orthotonus, and *risus sardonicus* are observed.
   C. Breathing may stop and the eyes are generally fixed and pupils dilated.
   D. Convulsions last from 30 seconds to a few minutes followed by a period of relaxation until the next convulsion is induced.
III. Treatment
   A. Standard regimens for convulsion control should be instituted. Agents commonly used include pentobarbital, diazepam, methocarbamol, or inhalational anesthesia.
   B. Gastric lavage and tannic acid administered orally may be helpful. Body temperature should be maintained during anesthesia.
   C. Since strychnine is a weakly basic compound, acidifying the urine will increase clearance.

IV. Prognosis is excellent so long as vital functions are maintained during the period of convulsion control. An important step to take in treating the strychnine-poisoned animal is to keep it in a quiet, dark environment to minimize convulsions until appropriate therapy is given.

ANTU

α-Naphthyl thiourea (ANTU) poisoning has decreased in incidence due to the use of other rodenticides.
  I. Mechanism of action
       α-Naphthyl thiourea rapidly produces pulmonary edema in susceptible animals by increasing pulmonary capillary permeability. In animals that can vomit, ANTU often induces emesis which may decrease the amount of drug absorbed.
 II. Clinical signs
      A. Initially, vomition and salivation a few minutes to hours after ingestion.
      B. This is followed by diarrhea, coughing, dyspnea, depression, and weakness.
      C. The respiratory difficulty can worsen from the accumulation of fluid to produce extreme cyanosis, and ultimately a comatose state can occur by 10–12 hours after ingestion.
      D. Death may occur as early as 2–4 hours after ingestion.
III. Treatment
       No specific antidote for ANTU poisoning is available. If the animal survives for longer than 12 hours, the prognosis is favorable. Initial efforts should be directed at removing any nonabsorbed toxin from the gastrointestinal tract. Once pulmonary edema is present, therapy is supportive. Furosemide and high-oxygen tension may be beneficial. (See Chapter 11 for treatment of pulmonary edema.)

Sodium Fluoroacetate

  I. General comments
       This extremely toxic rodenticide (compound 1080) is an odorless, tasteless, water-soluble compound. It and a derivative, fluoroacetamide, can kill dogs and cats that consume rodents poisoned by the drug. Because of this relay toxicity, use of these compounds has decreased in recent years.
 II. Mechanism of action
       These compounds act by blocking the tricarboxylic acid cycle through the formation of fluorocitric acid which inhibits aconitase activity. This effectively prohibits the cell from producing metabolic energy which causes cell death.
III. Clinical signs
      A. After a latent period of a few hours, the animal appears restless and vomition usually occurs.

    B. Hyperactivity of the gastrointestinal tract occurs followed by aimless running and barking in dogs or crying in cats.

    C. This leads to violent tonic-clonic convulsions lasting for approximately a minute. The interval between these convulsive episodes decreases as the syndrome progresses.

    D. Cats may develop cardiac arrhythmias.

    E. Eventually, the animal cannot recover from the convulsions and exhaustion, prolonged coma, and continuous muscular spasms lead to death in about 12 hours after ingestion.

IV. Treatment

    A. There is no effective antidote for compound 1080 poisoning.

    B. Treatment is supportive, being directed at controlling the convulsive episodes and maintaining vital functions.

    C. IV calcium gluconate and glucose therapy may be beneficial.

    D. Some workers have suggested combating the citrate accumulation by administering acetate as glyceryl monoacetate IM at a dose of 0.55 g/kg.

V. Prognosis is grave.

Thallium

I. General comments

    This heavy metal rodenticide is not frequently encountered. Because of its physicochemical stability, the compound is persistent in the environment and the host after absorption from the skin or gastrointestinal tract.

II. Mechanism of action

    A. Thallium interacts with sulfhydryl enzymes in various tissues of the body, inhibiting oxidative phosphorylation.

    B. May exchange with potassium in excitable tissues

    C. The compound is extensively distributed in the body and persists for periods measured in months.

III. Clinical signs

    A. Signs usually appear within 2–3 days after ingestion.

    B. Emesis followed by diarrhea, thirst, anorexia, lethargy, progressive weakness, and cachexia follow.

    C. Mucous membranes are congested, conjunctival vessels may be injected, and the body temperature is usually elevated.

    D. The animal may die acutely with signs of hyperexcitability, paresis, and convulsions.

    E. Animals that survive for several days demonstrate periodic episodes of gastrointestinal distress, incoordination, and depression.

    F. Dry, crusty erythematous skin with hair loss and exudation is usually present in this chronic phase.

    G. During the terminal stages, hyperexcitability, apprehension, ataxia, and vocalization occur culminating in death within 10–14 days of ingestion.

IV. Treatment
   A. If the animal is examined during the acute phases, removal of unab-
      sorbed toxin should be attempted.
   B. An antidote that increases the clearance of thallium from the body,
      diethyldithiocarbamate (dithizone) may be efficacious in dogs, although
      the compound may be toxic to cats.
   C. In chronic cases, oral prussian blue (potassium ferric hexacyanoferrate
      II) has been suggested as a specific antidote.
   D. Oral potassium chloride is also a useful adjuvant therapy.
   E. Of utmost importance is aggressive fluid and electrolyte therapy and
      nutritional and nursing care.
   F. IV parenteral alimentation and vitamin therapy are suggested.
   G. Specific antibiotic therapy may also be indicated if secondary infections
      develop.

Vacor

   I. General comments
         This recently introduced rodenticide (N-3-pyridylmethyl-N-p-nitro-
      phenyl urea) may cause toxicity in small animals, especially cats since they
      appear to be more sensitive.
  II. Mechanism of action. Nicotinamide antagonism.
 III. Clinical signs
   A. Glycosuria and shock may occur.
   B. Rats generally die in 4–6 hours after a period of inactivity.
  IV. Treatment
   A. Steps to prevent toxin absorption should be instituted.
   B. IM nicotinamide should be given and supportive therapy instituted.

Zinc Phosphide

   I. Mechanism of action.
         This compound mixes with water and hydrochloric acid in the stomach
      to liberate phosphine gas which causes severe gastrointestinal irritation a
      few days after exposure.
  II. Clinical signs
   A. In acute cases, colic, anorexia, lethargy, emesis, an increased rate and
      depth of respiration, asphyxiation, and coma
   B. Chronic poisoning is due to a combination of phosphine gas and zinc
      toxicity with renal and hepatic dysfunction.
 III. Treatment
         Vital functions should be supported and further toxin absorption pre-
      vented if the animal is examined during the acute phase.

PESTICIDES

Metaldehyde

    I. General comments.

        This compound is a widely used snail and slug bait which has been reported to cause poisonings in dogs and cats.

   II. Mechanism of action

        Hydrolysis in the stomach yields acetaldehyde which is responsible for clinical signs.

  III. Clinical signs

      A. Exposure results in signs of anxiety, sialosis, incoordination, polypnea, and tachycardia.

      B. Muscle fasciculations or continuous muscle spasms and collapse can occur.

      C. Nystagmus is common in cats.

      D. Death usually results from respiratory failure.

      E. Acidosis is often present.

  IV. Treatment. Therapy is largely symptomatic and supportive.

Chlorinated Hydrocarbons

    I. General comments

      A. This is a very large class of insecticides which include aldrin, benzene hexachloride, chlordane, dieldrin, dichloro-diphenyl trichloroethane (DDT), endrin, heptachlor, kelthane, lindane, mirex, and toxaphene.

      B. These agents are slowly metabolized and eliminated from the body resulting in persistence in tissue for extremely long periods of time.

      C. They are also very resistant to environmental degradation.

      D. Use has been severely curtailed due to this persistence and toxicity.

   II. Mechanism of action

      A. These very lipid-soluble compounds primarily cause central nervous system stimulation or depression.

      B. Hepatotoxicity, renal toxicity, and myocardial toxicity may also occur.

  III. Clinical signs

      A. These insecticides generally cause extreme excitement but may also cause profound depression.

      B. Muscle tremors and fasciculations occur initially in the head and neck and progress posteriorly.

      C. Periods of violent convulsions followed by depression can occur.

      D. Sialosis, anorexia, and diarrhea are common.

      E. Cats may be more sensitive to cutaneous exposure because of their grooming habits.

  IV. Treatment

      A. Phenobarbital given at an oral dose of 15–60 mg has been reported to be an effective regimen for controlling hyperactivity due to these compounds.

B. This barbiturate's ability to induce hepatic microsomal enzymes should also increase the rate of degradation of these insecticides.

C. If the animal is presented in convulsions, barbiturates or diazepam should be administered.

D. The animal should be bathed to remove residual insecticide from skin and coat.

E. Additional therapy is supportive.

Organophosphates and carbamates

I. General comments

   A. These classes of insecticides have largely replaced the chlorinated hydrocarbons because they are not biologically or environmentally persistent.

   B. The number of these compounds is staggering and animals are often simultaneously exposed to multiple agents. Table 23-6 is a partial listing.

II. Mechanism of action

   A. Inhibition of acetylcholinesterase activity at neurotransmitter junctions results in synaptic accumulation of acetylcholine and persistent neuronal activity.

   B. The inhibition of organophosphates is irreversible while that of the carbamates is reversible.

   C. A syndrome of delayed neurotoxicity may also occur with some compounds.

TABLE 23-6. ORGANOPHOSPHATE AND
CARBAMATE INSECTICIDES

Organophosphates	Carbamates
Azinphosmethyl	Aldicarb
Carbophenothion	Carbaryl
Chlorfenvinphos	Carbofuran
Chlorthion	Metalkamate
Coumaphos	Methomyl
Diazinon	Propoxur
Dichlorvos	
Dimethoate	
Dioxathion	
Disulfoton	
Ethion	
Famophos	
Fenthion	
Malathion	
Parathion	
Ronnel	
Ruelene	
Trichlorfon	

III. Clinical signs
  A. The primary clinical signs of intoxication are those of muscarinic cholinergic stimulation.
    1. Salivation
    2. Lacrimation
    3. Urination
    4. Defecation
    5. Dyspnea
    6. Skeletal muscle fasciculations followed by weakness and paralysis may occur.
    7. Tonic-clonic convulsive seizures may be present.
    8. Severe depression may also be observed in some animals.
    9. Onset of signs can be from a few minutes to a few hours after exposure.
    10. Death is usually attributed to respiratory failure.
IV. Treatment
  A. Atropine should be dosed to effect.
  B. The acetylcholinesterase regenerator pralidoxime (2-PAM) (2-pyridine-aldoxime methiodide) should be given concurrently.
    1. This therapy is contraindicated with carbamate intoxication.
    2. It is most effective if administered shortly after exposure before the organophosphate-enzyme complex has "aged."
    3. Pralidoxime therapy is only required for 24–36 hours if aging has not occurred.
  C. Supportive therapy, especially respiratory, is crucial for recovery.

METALS

Arsenic

  I. General comments
     This classic toxin has been used as a rodenticide, insecticide, herbicide, and as a malicious poison. It can also be found in some mineral and emerald green paints, in therapeutic agents such as Fowler's solution or organic arsenical heartworm medication (i.e. thiacetarsamide), or in the environment secondary to contamination from smelters. It is commonly found in ant and roach poisons.
  II. Mechanism of action
    A. Arsenic inhibits essential sulfhydryl group-containing enzymes and uncouples oxidative phosphorylation by substituting for phosphorous in normally stable phosphorylated intermediates to produce labile arsenylated oxidation byproducts.
    B. These actions can be lethal to cellular metabolism.
    C. Primary target organs include the gastrointestinal tract, kidney, liver, spleen, lung, and skin.

   D. Arsenic is generally rapidly eliminated from the body in the urine and feces.
III. Clinical signs
   A. The primary presenting signs in an acute case of arsenic poisoning in small animals is a sudden onset of hemorrhagic gastroenteritis.
   B. Restlessness, vomition, and abdominal pain accompany the bloody diarrhea and death may occur in 12–20 hours.
   C. In the terminal stages, the animal will appear weak, dehydrated, and anemic.
   D. If a sublethal dose is absorbed, the syndrome is protracted and a toxic nephrosis may be the primary clinical problem.
IV. Treatment
   A. If gastrointestinal signs are not present but an animal is known to have eaten an arsenic-containing compound, gastric lavage is indicated.
   B. If gastroenteritis is the presenting sign, then the chelator dimercaprol [British antilewisite (BAL)] should be given IM three times daily at a dose of 6–7 mk/kg or four times daily at 3–4 mg/kg. Intervals between doses can be increased on the third day and twice daily administration of the lower dose can be given on the 4th through 10th days.
   C. Aggressive supportive therapy including fluids and electrolytes should be administered.
   D. If the animal is uremic, the animal should be handled as an acute renal failure patient (see chapter 12).
   E. Analgesics and antibacterials should be administered as needed.

Lead

  I. General comments
   A. Lead poisoning is one of the most common toxicoses diagnosed in small animals, especially puppies less than 1 year of age.
   B. It does not appear to be common in cats.
   C. Sources in the environment are numerous, however, the most common is lead-containing paint.
   D. The route of exposure is usually oral.
 II. Mechanism of action. Target organs include the bone marrow, central nervous system, liver, and kidney.
III. Clinical signs
   A. Gastrointestinal distress marked by vomiting, abdominal pain, and anorexia usually precede neurologic signs such as convulsions, hysteria, behavioral abnormalities, ataxia, blindness, and biting actions.
   B. Hematologic changes include anemia, erythrocyte basophilic stippling, and a left-shift neutrophilia.
   C. In chronic cases, anorexia and progressive weight loss may be present accompanied by depression and generalized weakness.

IV. Treatment
   A. Therapy is first aimed at removing nonabsorbed lead from the gastrointestinal tract by emetics, enemas, or lavage techniques.
   B. Attempts should then be made to increase the rate of elimination of stored lead from the body by administering chelating drugs which effectively mobilize lead body stores so that lead-chelate complexes can be eliminated rapidly in the urine or bile.
      1. Calcium EDTA (ethylenediaminetetraacetate) is given SQ at a dosage of 25 mg/kg every 6 hours for 2–5 days.
      2. Treatment can be repeated in 2 weeks.
      3. An alternative chelation agent available is penicillamine given orally at a dose of 100 mg/kg daily for 1–2 weeks. Use of this drug may be accompanied by anorexia, vomition, or listlessness, signs which are minimal if the drug is administered on an empty stomach in divided doses or if antiemetics such as a phenothiazine are given.
      4. Penicillamine should be given only if the toxicosis is mild or as follow-up therapy to EDTA treatment.
      5. Neurologic signs should be treated symptomatically by the general measures previously outlined (see chapter 16) and supportive therapy instituted as required.
      6. The environmental source of lead should be removed.
      7. Children in the household may also be at risk to lead poisoning.

Mercury

I. General comments
   Intoxication by this heavy metal is not often encountered in veterinary practice today although exposure to mercurial ointments (mercuric chloride) or use of mercury-containing diuretics may produce toxicoses.
II. Clinical signs
   Toxicity is primarily attributed to gastroenteritis or renal failure.
III. Treatment is supportive, however, the prognosis is poor since the disease is often advanced before a diagnosis is made.
IV. Cats are susceptible to environmental methylmercury poisoning (Minamata disease) and have served as environmental sentinels for it. Signs are of severe neurologic dysfunction and treatment is futile.

Thallium

See above discussion.

MISCELLANEOUS TOXINS

Cyanide

I. General comments
   This lethal poison, also referred to as prussic or hydrocyanic acid, is

utilized in industry and is employed as a vermicide and as a fumigant. Low doses of the chemical can be tolerated.

II. Mechanism of action
   A. Cyanide interacts with cytochrome oxidase to form a stable complex which blocks electron transport, and thus cellular respiration.
   B. Endogenous thiosulfate combines with cyanide to form thiocyanate which can be eliminated by the kidney.

III. Clinical signs
   A. Usually lethal doses of cyanide will produce sudden death in a few minutes without preceding clinical signs.
   B. If the animal is alive, excitement, muscle tremors, dyspnea, and possibly salivation and fecal and urine voiding will be seen.
   C. Characteristically, mucous membranes will be bright red.

IV. Treatment. If the animal is presented alive, 20% sodium nitrite and 20% sodium thiosulfate at dose of 10 mg/kg nitrite and 30 mg/kg thiosulfate should be administered IV without delay.

Ethylene Glycol

I. General comments
   A. This compound is the toxic ingredient of antifreeze and is a common cause of poisoning in small animals.
   B. Its sweet taste is attractive to pets.
   C. Cats appear to be more sensitive than dogs.

II. Mechanism of action
   A. Acute acidosis. If massive amounts are absorbed or if the animal is presented within approximately 24 hours after ingestion, metabolic conversion to a series of acids has occurred. Clinical signs are due to a combination of these acids (i.e., glycolic and glyoxylic acid) and ethylene glycol itself.
   B. Subacute uremic syndrome. If the animal has survived the acute phase, clinical signs are due to an acute renal failure induced by metabolism of ethylene glycol to nephrotoxic metabolites (i.e., oxalic acid). Clinical deterioration in the acute phase would exacerbate this uremic state.

III. Clinical signs
   A. Acute phase
      1. The animal is generally presented in a moderately depressed, incoordinated, and ataxic state.
      2. Vomition frequently occurs.
      3. This is followed by paresis and coma.
      4. Examination of urine sediment 6 hours or longer after ingestion will demonstrate oxalate crystals.
      5. Convulsions are not common.
      6. A state of hyperosmolemia is often present.

B. Subacute phase
1. Dogs surviving 24 hours may have serum urea nitrogen values greater than 200 mg/dl.
2. Signs seen during the acute phase may be present to a less severe degree.
3. Progressive depression and ataxia may develop over a period of a few weeks.
4. Oliguria or anuria may be present.
5. Muscle fasciculations, paddling, and episodes of generalized muscle contractions accompanying the uremia may be present.
6. If urine is being voided, oxalate crystals will be present.

IV. Treatment
A. Acute phase
1. Specific therapy should be instituted as rapidly as feasible.
2. Administer a 20% ethanol solution IV at a dose of 5.5 ml/kg accompanied by 8 ml/kg of a 5% sodium bicarbonate solution intraperitoneally.
3. This protocol should be repeated every 4 hours for one day and then every 6 hours for an additional 1–2 days.
4. Alternatively, 50% ethanol may be administered until the animal is insensitive to a toe-pinch reflex. Pure ethanol, and not denatured alcohol must be used. As much ethanol as the animal will tolerate must be given to effectively block the hepatic oxidation of the ethylene glycol by alcohol dehydrogenase.
5. Fluid balance must be carefully monitored to prevent overhydration in the oliguric or anuric patient.
6. Success of this regimen is dependent upon its prompt initiation.
7. Prognosis is good if the animal responds within 12–16 hours.
B. Subacute phase. The above treatment is not effective in the uremic state. The only feasible therapy is peritoneal dialysis, or if available, hemodialysis.

Herbicides

I. General comments. As a class of chemicals, these compounds have a fairly low order of toxicity to companion animals. Signs of poisoning are nonspecific and include mild gastrointestinal distress, weakness, or contact dermatitis. Treatment is symptomatic and supportive.
II. 2,4-Dichlorophenoxyacetic acid (2,4-D). Dogs may be particularly sensitive to poisoning by this compound according to the University of Illinois Animal Poison Control Center.

THERAPEUTIC AGENTS

Acetaminophen

I. General comments
A. This analgesic has been reported to cause numerous poisonings in cats.

    B. Cats appear to be sensitive because of deficiencies in detoxifying mechanisms (glucuronide and glutathione conjugation) coupled with an inherent sensitivity of feline erythrocytes to oxidative damage.

    C. Neonatal erythrocytes also appear to be sensitive to oxidant effects.

II. Mechanism of action

    A. Acetaminophen inhibits prostaglandin synthesis in susceptible tissues.

    B. Oxidation of hemoglobin to methemoglobin results in Heinz body formation and hemolysis.

    C. Toxic intermediates form which covalently bind to hepatic lysosomal membranes due to the limited availability of glutathione. This results in hepatic necrosis.

III. Clinical signs

    A. Many of the clinical signs are attributed to methemoglobin formation and other hematologic signs. Cyanosis, facial edema, Heinz body anemia, hemoglobinuria, and jaundice may be seen.

    B. Signs attribute to hepatic necrosis are also seen.

IV. Treatment. In addition to supportive therapy, i.e., fluid and oxygen, the most effective treatment of toxicosis is the oral administration of acetylcysteine at a dose of 1.4 ml/kg of a 10% solution. This serves as an exogenous sulfhydryl donor to enhance detoxification. Charcoal inactivates acetylcysteine.

Aspirin

I. General comments.

    A. This commonly employed salicylate has been reported to cause toxicity in both dogs and cats.

    B. Cats appear particularly sensitive because of a deficiency in dotoxification enzymes.

    C. A dose of 5–25 mg/kg for 15 days does not induce adverse reactions. However, a five-grain aspirin tablet contains 324 mg, therefore a single tablet given to a 3-kg cat will result in a dose of 108 mg/kg and probably toxicosis.

    D. Children's aspirin tablets contain 1.25 grain which is equivalent to 81 mg of drug.

II. Mechanism of action

    A. Toxicologic action is primarily an extension of aspirin's pharmacologic activity of inhibiting prostaglandin synthesis.

    B. Can induce acidosis in large doses

    C. Is capable of uncoupling oxidative phosphorylation

III. Clinical signs

    A. Initially a respiratory alkalosis occurs secondary to a direct stimulation of the respiratory center with hyperventilation.

    B. This is followed by a profound metabolic acidosis.

    C. Hyperpyrexia occurs due to the uncoupling of oxidative phosphorylation.

    D. The animal may vomit from stimulation of the chemoreceptor trigger zone.

    E. Gastrointestinal ulceration and bleeding may be seen.

    F. Anorexia and coma may be seen.

IV. Treatment

    A. Unabsorbed drug should be removed from the stomach by gastric lavage.

    B. Elimination of absorbed drug can be hastened by alkalinizing the urine with parenteral sodium bicarbonate administration. Inducing osmotic diuresis with mannitol will enhance this action.

    C. Acidosis must be controlled.

    D. Supportive therapy should be instituted.

Aminoglycosides

I. General comments

    A. This class of therapeutically essential antibiotics include amikacin, dihydrostreptomycin, gentamicin, kanamycin, neomycin, and tobramycin.

    B. Toxicity is minimal when given orally for local effect since oral absorption generally does not occur.

II. Mechanism of action

    A. Ototoxicity is difficult to diagnose in veterinary practice.

        1. Vestibular toxicity is generally reversible.

        2. Cochlear toxicity is generally permanent.

        3. Ototoxicity may occur when treating otititis externa with gentamicin in a patient with a perforated tympanic membrane.

    B. Oral neomycin therapy may induce a malabsorption syndrome.

    C. Aminoglycosides may induce a neuromuscular blockade

        1. Curariform-like

        2. Inhibition of release of acetylcholine from presynaptic motor neurons due to impairment of calcium influx is contributory.

        3. Primarily occurs as an adverse interaction with other curariform neuromuscular blocking agents.

    D. The most common toxicosis is nephrotoxicity.

        1. Dependent on both dose and length of drug administration

        2. Nephrotoxicosis is predisposed by prior renal insufficiency, volume depletion, acidosis, and the concurrent use of other nephrotoxic drugs or the high-ceiling diuretics such as furosemide.

        3. The primary site of damage is the proximal renal tubule.

    E. Depression of cardiac contractility may also occur.

III. Clinical signs. Signs of early renal toxicity include polyuria and decreased urine osmolarity, cylindruria, and enzymuria followed by azotemia and uremia.

IV. Treatment
  A. Nephrotoxicity is reversible if drug therapy is stopped and aggressive fluid therapy instituted.
  B. Serial monitoring of urine osmolarity or enzyme activity (N- acetyl-β-D-glucosaminidase) or serum urea nitrogen concentrations will allow early detection of toxicosis.
  C. Protection against toxicity may be afforded by maintaining hydration and alkalinizing urine; the latter also will increase antibacterial activity of aminoglycosides.
  D. In the presence of prior renal insufficiency, drug should be administered using a fixed-dose, increased-interval dosage adjustment regimen based on creatinine clearance.
  E. Full doses of drug should be administered in the presence of life-threatening infections as the threat of toxicosis should not deter from the therapeutic goal of eradicating the infectious agent.
  F. If serum drug concentrations can be determined (see chapter 22), gentamicin and tobramycin trough concentrations should be maintained less than 2 μg/ml (10 μg/ml for amikacin and kanamycin). Peak concentrations do not appear to be directly correlated to nephrotoxicity.
  G. Streptomycin is minimally toxic while neomycin should not be administered parenterally.
  H. Neuromuscular blockade should be treated with neostigmine and calcium administration.
  I. Ototoxicity can only be handled by removal of drug.

Chloramphenicol

  I. General comments
    A great deal has been written on the propensity of this drug to produce a dose-independent irreversible depression of bone marrow activity. The drug has a low order of toxicity in adult companion animals.
 II. Mechanism of action
  A. A dose-related bone marrow depression occurs with prolonged use of the drug in dogs and cats.
  B. Cats appear relatively sensitive to this effect because of the feline deficiency in glucuronide conjugation which results in a decreased ability to eliminate the drug. Likewise, the young of any species have a deficiency in clearance of this compound.
  C. Therapeutic doses of chloramphenicol decreases the rate of hepatic biotransformation of many drugs normally metabolized by the liver.
  D. This drug's ability to inhibit protein synthesis may interfere with immunoglobin production and wound healing.
III. Clinical signs
  A. Bone marrow depression will be manifested by vacuolation of many of

the early cells of the myeloid and erythroid series, neutropenia, and lymphocytopenia.

B. Common signs include inappetence, depression, vomition, and sometimes diarrhea.

C. The effects of decreased drug biotransformation will be reflected in prolonged barbiturate anesthesia. Other drugs affected include digoxin, codeine, phenytoin, and tolbutamide.

IV. Treatment

Therapy is symptomatic and supportive after stopping drug administration (see chapter 8).

Amphotericin

This widely employed antifungal agent regularly induces azotemia when employed clinically. This effect is secondary to a direct tubular toxicity coupled with renal vasoconstriction. Therapy should be discontinued if the serum urea nitrogen (SUN) exceeds 40–50 mg/dl. Concurrent mannitol administration may be protective. Emesis is a common side effect which can be used to titrate the dose.

Griseofulvin

The administration of 35 mg/kg of this antifungal drug to cats in the first trimester of pregnancy was teratogenic as evidenced by kittens with cleft palate and multiple congenital malformations of the skeleton and brain.

Urinary Antiseptics

I. Methylene blue

Cats appear sensitive to this oxidizing drug since methemoglobinemia and Heinz body formation may occur.

II. Nalidixic acid

When human doses of drug are administered to small animals, signs of neurotoxicity, gastrointestinal disturbances, and dermatotoxicity may be observed.

III. Nitrofurantoin

The following may result from systemic use of this drug: polyneuritis, gastrointestinal disturbances, pulmonary infiltrates, and hemolytic anemia.

IV. Methenamine mandelate

Gastrointestinal distress, crystalluria, and systemic acidosis may be associated with the use of this agent.

Anthelminthics

I. Organophosphates and carbamates

See section above. Since many of these agents are available, toxicity may occur when multiple drugs are employed in the same animal.

II. Disophenol (DNP)

This hookworm drug has been associated with emesis, a transient lens opacity, and at high doses, hyperthermia, polypnea, dyspnea, polydipsia, polyuria, tachycardia, and tetany. These latter effects are caused by a drug-induced uncoupling of oxidative phosphorylation. Hyperthermia should be treated with ice baths rather than pharmacologic agents.

III. Dithiazanine iodide

Vomition, diarrhea, and weakness are commonly associated with use of this drug. Hepatotoxicity and nephrotoxicity have also been reported.

IV. Levamisole

Acute intoxication resembles acute nicotine poisoning which is manifested by signs of organophosphate poisoning and central nervous system excitability, arrhythmias, and respiratory distress. Atropine and ganglionic blocking agents may be effective therapy.

Cancer Chemotherapeutic Agents

I. General comments

A. Toxicity is directed against tissues with rapid rates of cellular turnover (i.e., bone marrow, gastrointestinal tract mucosa, hair follicle, basal dermal epithelium).

B. Signs of toxicosis include immunosuppression, hematologic disturbances, diarrhea, vomition, alopecia, and local dermatitis.

C. Drugs used to treat tumors of the endocrine system may produce related endocrine dysfunction.

D. Some additional target organs have been identified for specific drugs. See tables 23-2 through 23-4.

II. Doxorubicin—heart (congestive cardiomyopathy, dysrhythmias)

III. Bleomycin—Lung (interstitial pneumonitis)

This drug does not cause significant bone marrow or gastrointestinal toxicity.

IV. Cis-platin—kidney (dose-related nephrotoxicity)

V. Cyclophosphamide—urinary bladder (sterile cystitis)

VI. 5-Fluorouracil—cerebellum

VII. Glucocorticoids

Numerous adverse reactions have been associated with this class of compounds. With chronic dosing, immunosuppression, gastric ulcers, osteoporosis, iatrogenic Cushing's syndrome, and hepatopathy may be seen. Alternate-day administration of these drugs may decrease the incidence of adverse reactions.

VIII. Methotrexate—kidney, liver, lung
 IX. Streptozocin—pancreas, kidney
  X. Vincristine—peripheral nervous system

Anticonvulsants

Evidence in support of adverse drug reactions to these drugs in the veterinary literature is scant. The drugs listed below, and phenobarbital, are capable of inducing hepatic microsomal drug-metabolizing enzymes.
 I. Phenytoin
    Megaloblastic anemia secondary to folate deficiency.
II. Primidone
    Cirrhosis with chronic therapy.

HYPERSENSITIVITY REACTIONS

 I. In addition to the specific chemical and drug toxicities described above, immunologic mechanisms can be responsible for chemical-induced illness. This is particularly important for some adverse drug reactions.
 II. So-called drug allergy usually requires a previous exposure and sensitization to the drug. Subsequent exposure to the agent results in a antigen-antibody reaction with release of various inflammatory mediators such as histamine, serotonin, kinins, and so forth. These reactions may be immediate or delayed. The highest incidence of immediate untoward effects (i.e., anaphylaxis) after a first exposure to a drug is via the IV route. Penicillins have been associated with many forms of drug allergic reactions.
III. Chapters 5 and 6 should be consulted for more specific details on diagnosis and treatment.
IV. Typical drug-induced immunologic reactions include
    A. Anaphylaxis, acute gastrointestinal distress, fever
    B. Urticaria, hives
    C. Rhinitis, asthma, dyspnea
    D. Angioneurotic edema
    E. Interstitial nephritis
    F. Hemolytic anemia
 V. Treatment
    A. For life-threatening anaphylaxis, IV or IM epinephrine and aggressive supportive therapy is indicated.
    B. Specific antihistamine therapy may help prevent relapse.
    C. Nonspecific corticosteroid therapy is not optimal.

SUGGESTED READINGS

Aronson AL, Riviere JE: Toxicology and pharmacology. p. 61. In Pratt PW (ed): Feline Medicine. American Veterinary Publications, Santa Barbara, CA, 1982

Booth NH, McDonald LE (eds): Veterinary Pharmacology and Therapeutics. 5th Ed. Iowa State University Press, Ames, 1982

Buck WB, Hoskins JD: Diseases caused by chemical and physical agents. p. 141. In Catcott EJ (ed): Canine Medicine. 4th Ed. American Veterinary Publications, Santa Barbara, CA, 1979

Colloquium on clinical pharmacology. J Am Vet Med Assoc 176:1041, 1980

Davis LE: Hypersensitivity reactions induced by antimicrobial drugs. J Am Vet Med Assoc 185:1131, 1984.

Davis LE (ed): Topics in drug therapy. Monthly feature of J Am Vet Med Assoc 175: 1979 and monthly to date.

Doull J, Klaassen CD, Amdur MO: Toxicology, the Basic Science of Poisons. 2nd Ed. Macmillan, New York, 1980

English PB: Antimicrobial chemotherapy in the dog. III. Possible adverse reactions. J Sm Anim Pract 24:423, 1983

Gilman AG, Goodman LS, Gilman A (eds): The Pharmacological Basis of Therapeutics. Macmillan, New York, 1980

Ndiritu CG, Enos LR: Adverse reactions to drugs in a veterinary hospital. J Am Vet Med Assoc 171:335, 1977

Oehme, FW (ed): Chemical and physical disorders p. 75–167 In Kirk RW (Ed.): Current Veterinary Therapy. VIII. WB Saunders, Philadelphia, 1983

Oehme FW: Toxicologic disorders. p. 80. In Ettinger SJ (ed): Textbook of Veterinary Internal Medicine. WB Saunders, Philadelphia, 1982

Riviere JE: Toxicity and interactions. p. 204. In Johnston D (ed): Bristol Veterinary Handbook of Antimicrobial Therapy. Veterinary Learning Systems, Princeton Junction, NJ, 1982

Riviere JE, Davis LE: Renal handling of drugs in renal failure. p. 643. In Bovee KC (ed): Canine Nephrology. Harwal Publishing, Media, PA 1984

Thornhill JA: Peritoneal dialysis in the dog and cat: an update. Comp Contin Ed Pract Vet 3:20, 1981

APPENDIX Usual Dose of Drugs Mentioned in Text

Drug	DOGS Dose	DOGS Interval	DOGS Route	CATS Dose	CATS Interval	CATS Route
Acepromazine	0.1 mg/kg	q 8h	IV, IM	0.1 mg/kg	sid	IM, IV
Acetaminophen	10 mg/kg	q 12h	PO	NOT RECOMMENDED		
Acetazolamide	7 mg/kg	q 8h	PO	7 mg/kg	q 8h	PO
Acetohydroxamic acid	10–15 mg/kg	q 12h	PO	NOT ESTABLISHED		
ACTH	2 U/kg	sid	IM	2 U/kg	sid	IM
Albendazole	25 mg/kg	q 12h	PO	NOT ESTABLISHED		
Allopurinol	10 mg/kg	q 8h	PO	NOT ESTABLISHED		
Aluminum hydroxide	15–45 mg/kg	bid	PO	15–45 mg/kg	bid	PO
Amikacin	5 mg/kg	q 6–8h	IV, IM, SQ	5 mg/kg	q 6–8h	IV, IM, SQ
Aminophylline	10 mg/kg	q 12h	PO	5 mg/kg	q 12h	PO
Amitriptyline	1–2 mg/kg	sid	PO	5–10 mg total	sid	PO
Ammonium chloride	200 mg/kg	q 8h	PO	40 mg/kg	q 8h	PO
Amoxicillin	11 mg/kg	q 12h	PO, IM	11 mg/kg	q 12h	PO, IM
Amphotericin B	0.15–0.5 mg/kg	sid	IV on alternate days	0.15–0.25 mg/kg	sid	IV on alternate days
Ampicillin,	10–20 mg/kg	q 6h	PO	10–20 mg/kg	q 6h	PO
	5–10 mg/kg	q 6h	IV, IM	5–10 mg/kg	q 6h	IV, IM
Amprolium	110–220 mg/kg	sid	in feed	NOT ESTABLISHED		
Antineoplastic drugs	SEE TABLE 7-1					
Apomorphine	0.08 mg/kg	once	IM, SQ	DO NOT USE		

(Continued)

APPENDIX Usual Dose of Drugs Mentioned in Text (*Continued*)

Drug	DOGS			CATS		
	Dose	Interval	Route	Dose	Interval	Route
Aprindine	1–2 mg/kg	q 8h	PO	NOT ESTABLISHED		
	100 µg/kg/min	continuous infusion	IV			
Arecoline acetarsol	5 mg/kg	once	PO	5 mg/kg	once	PO
Aspirin	10 mg/kg	q 12h	PO	10 mg/kg	q 48h	PO
Atropine	0.04 mg/kg	q 6h	IV, SQ	0.04 mg/kg	q 6h	IV, SQ
Aurothioglucose	1 mg/kg	weekly	IM	NOT ESTABLISHED		
Azathioprine	2.2 mg/kg	sid	PO	2.2 mg/kg	sid	PO
Bendroflumethiazide	0.2–0.4 mg/kg	sid	PO	0.2–0.4 mg/kg	sid	PO
Betamethasone	0.15 mg/kg	once	IM	NOT ESTABLISHED		
Bethanechol	50 µg/kg	once	SQ	2.5–5 mg total dose	q 8–12h	PO
	0.5–1 mg/kg	q 6h	PO			
Bismuth subsalicylate	10–30 ml	q 6h	PO	NOT ESTABLISHED		
Bunamidine	25–50 mg/kg	once	PO	25–50 mg/kg	once	PO
Butamisole	2.4 mg/kg	once	SQ	NOT RECOMMENDED		
Butorphanol	0.05–0.1 mg/kg	q 8h	SQ	NOT ESTABLISHED		
Calcitonin	4–8 IU/kg	q 12h	IM	NOT ESTABLISHED		
Calcium carbonate	100 mg/kg	sid	PO	100 mg/kg	sid	PO
Calcium EDTA	25 mg/kg	q 6h	IV	25 mg/kg	q 6h	IV
Calcium gluconate	50–150 mg/kg	prn	IV slowly	50–150 mg/kg	prn	IV slowly

Drug	Dose	Interval	Route	Dose	Interval	Route
Calcium lactate	0.5–2.0 g	sid	in feed	0.2–0.5 g	sid	in feed
Captopril	1–2 mg/kg	q 8h	PO	NOT ESTABLISHED		
Carbenicillin	15–50 mg/kg	q 6h	IV	15–50 mg/kg	q 6h	IV
Cascara sagrada extract	1–4 ml	prn	PO	0.5–1.5 ml	prn	PO
Castor oil	5–25 ml	prn	PO	3–10 ml	prn	PO
Cefamandole	25 mg/kg	q 6h	IM, IV	25 mg/kg	q 6h	IM, IV
Cefazolin	20–25 mg/kg	q 6–8h	IM, IV	20–25 mg/kg	q 6–8h	IM, IV
Cefoxitin	25 mg/kg	q 4–6h	IM, IV	25 mg/kg	q 4–6h	IM, IV
Cephradine	20 mg/kg	q 6h	PO	20 mg/kg	q 6h	PO
	10 mg/kg	q 6h	IM, IV	10 mg/kg	q 6h	IM, IV
Cephadroxil	10 mg/kg	q 12h	PO	10 mg/kg	q 12h	PO
Cephalexin	8–30 mg/kg	q 8h	PO	8–30 mg/kg	q 8h	PO
Cephalothin	20–35 mg/kg	q 6–8h	IV, IM, SQ	20–35 mg/kg	q 6–8h	IV, IM, SQ
Chlorambucil	0.2 mg/kg	sid	PO for 10 d	0.2 mg/kg	sid	PO for 10 d
THEN	0.1 mg/kg	sid	PO	0.1 mg/kg	sid	PO
Chloramphenicol	25–50 mg/kg	q 8h	PO, IM, IV	25–50 mg/kg	q 12h	PO, IM, IV
Chlorothiazide	20–40 mg/kg	q 12h	PO	20–40 mg/kg	q 12h	PO
Chlorpheniramine	1 mg/kg	q 12h	PO	1 mg/kg	q 12h	PO
Chlorpromazine	3 mg/kg	q 12h	PO	3 mg/kg	q 12h	PO
	0.5 mg/kg	q 12h	IV or IM	0.5 mg/kg	q 12h	IV or IM
Chlorpropamide	10–40 mg/kg	sid	PO	NOT ESTABLISHED		
Cimetidine	10 mg/kg	q 8h	PO	2.5 mg/kg	q 12h	PO
	5 mg/kg	q 12h	IV			
Clindamycin palmitate	3 mg/kg	q 6h	PO	3 mg/kg	q 6h	PO

(Continued)

APPENDIX Usual Dose of Drugs Mentioned in Text (*Continued*)

Drug	DOGS			CATS		
	Dose	Interval	Route	Dose	Interval	Route
Clindamycin phosphate	5 mg/kg	q 8h	IV, IM	5 mg/kg	q 8h	IV, IM
Cloxacillin	10 mg/kg	q 6h	PO, IM	10 mg/kg	q 6h	PO, IM
Codeine	2 mg/kg	q 6h	PO	NOT ESTABLISHED		
Colistin	10 mg/kg	q 6h	PO (not absorbed)	10 mg/kg	q 6h	PO (not absorbed)
Colistimethate	1–2 mg/kg	q 12h	IM, IV	1–2 mg/kg	q 12h	IM, IV
Cyclophosphamide	< 5 kg–2.5 mg/kg	sid	PO	2.5 mg/kg	sid	PO
	5–25 kg–2.2 mg/kg	sid	PO			
	>25 kg–1.5 mg/kg	sid	PO			
Danthron	35 mg/kg	prn	PO	20 mg/kg	prn	PO
Dantrolene	1–5 mg/kg	q 8h	PO	0.5–2 mg/kg	q 12h	PO
Dapsone	1 mg/kg	q 12h	PO	NOT ESTABLISHED		
Desmopressin acetate	1 drop	q 8h	intranasally or conjuct. sac	NOT ESTABLISHED		
Dexamethasone	0.25 mg/kg	once	IV, IM	0.25 mg/kg	once	IV, IM
Dextroamphetamine	0.2–1.3 mg/kg	sid	PO	NOT ESTABLISHED		
Dextromethorphan	1–2 mg/kg	q 6h	PO	1–2 mg/kg	q 6h	PO
Diazepam (anticonvulsant)	1 mg/kg	prn	IV to effect	1 mg/kg	prn	IV to effect
Diazepam (anxiolytic)	0.25 mg/kg	q 8h	PO	0.25 mg/kg	q 8h	PO

Drug	Dose	Frequency	Route	Dose	Frequency	Route
Diazoxide	10 mg/kg	q 12h	PO	NOT ESTABLISHED		
Dichlorophen	300 mg/kg	once	PO	150 mg/kg	once	PO
Dichlorphenamide	2–5 mg/kg	q 8h	PO	10–25 mg total	q 8h	PO
Dichlorvos	11 mg/kg	once	PO	11 mg/kg	once	PO
Dicloxacillin	10–25 mg/kg	q 8h	PO, IM	10–25 mg/kg	q 8h	PO, IM
Diethylcarbamazine (prevent ascarids)	6.6 mg/kg	sid	PO	6.6 mg/kg	sid	PO
Diethylcarbamazine (treat ascarids)	55–110 mg/kg	once	PO	55–110 mg/kg	once	PO
Diethylstilbestrol	0.5 mg/kg	once	IM	NOT RECOMMENDED		
	0.1–1.0 mg total dose	sid	PO			
Digitoxin	0.03–0.04 mg/kg	q 12h	PO	NOT RECOMMENDED		
Digoxin	0.22 mg/m^2	q 12h	PO tabs	0.01 mg/kg	sid	PO
	0.18 mg/m^2	q 12h	PO elixir			
Dihydrotachysterol	0.007–0.01 mg/kg	sid	PO	NOT ESTABLISHED		
Dimenhydrinate	8 mg/kg	q 8h	PO	12.5 mg total dose	q 8h	PO
Dimercaprol	6 mg/kg	q 8h	IM	6 mg/kg	q 8h	IM
Diphenhydramine	4 mg/kg	q 8h	PO	4 mg/kg	q 8h	PO
Diphenidol	1 mg/kg	q 8h	IM, IV	NOT ESTABLISHED		
Diphenoxylate	0.063 mg/kg	q 8h	PO	0.063 mg/kg	q 12h	PO
Diphenylthiocarbazone	70 mg/kg	q 8h	PO	NOT RECOMMENDED		
Dipyrone	25 mg/kg	q 8h	IM	NOT RECOMMENDED		
Disophenol	0.22 ml/kg	once	SQ	NOT RECOMMENDED		

(*Continued*)

APPENDIX Usual Dose of Drugs Mentioned in Text (*Continued*)

Drug	DOGS			CATS		
	Dose	Interval	Route	Dose	Interval	Route
Disopyramide	7–30 mg/kg	q 2h	PO	NOT ESTABLISHED		
Dithiazanine iodide	22 mg/kg	sid	PO for 7 d	NOT RECOMMENDED		
Dobutamine	5–40 μg/kg/min	Continuous infusion	IV	NOT ESTABLISHED		
Docusate	2 mg/kg	sid	PO	2 mg/kg	sid	PO
Dopamine	10 μg/kg/min	Continuous infusion	IV	10 μg/kg/min	Continuous infusion	IV
Doxapram	1–5 mg/kg	once	IV	1–5 mg/kg	once	IV
Doxycycline	5 mg/kg	q 12h	PO	5 mg/kg	q 12h	PO
Ephedrine	2–4 mg/kg	q 8h	PO	5 mg total	q 8h	PO
Epinephrine	10 μg/kg	prn	IV, IM	10 μg/kg	prn	IV, IM
Erythromycin	5–20 mg/kg	q 8h	PO	5–20 mg/kg	q 8h	PO
Estradiol benzoate	0.1 mg/kg	once	IM	0.25–0.5 mg total	once	IM
Fenbendazole	50 mg/kg	sid	PO for 3 d	NOT ESTABLISHED		
Flucytosine	25–38 mg/kg	q 6h	PO	25–38 mg/kg	q 6h	PO
Fludrocortisone	0.2–1.0 mg total	sid	PO	0.1–0.2 mg total	sid	PO
Flumethasone	0.05–0.25 mg total	sid	PO, IV, IM	0.03–0.1 mg total	sid	PO, IV, SQ
Flunixin meglumine	1 mg/kg	sid no more than 3 d		NOT ESTABLISHED		

	Dose	Frequency	Route	Dose	Frequency	Route
FSH	0.75 mg/kg	sid	IM	2 mg total	sid	IM
Framycetin	20 mg/kg	q 6h	PO (not absorbed)	20 mg/kg	q 6h	PO (not absorbed)
Furosemide	2–4 mg/kg	q 8h	PO	2–4 mg/kg	q 8h	PO
	2–8 mg/kg	q 6h	IV	2–8 mg/kg	q 6h	IV
Gentamicin	4 mg/kg	q 12h	IV, IM	4 mg/kg	q 12h	IV, IM
Glibenclamide	0.2 mg/kg	sid	PO	NOT ESTABLISHED		
Glipizide	0.25–0.5 mg/kg	q 12h	PO	NOT ESTABLISHED		
Glucagon	0.03 mg/kg	prn	IV	NOT ESTABLISHED		
Glycerin	1–1.5 g/kg	q 6h	PO	NOT ESTABLISHED		
Glycobiarsol	220 mg/kg	sid	PO	NOT ESTABLISHED		
Glycopyrrolate	0.01 mg/kg	q 8h	IM, SQ	NOT ESTABLISHED		
Gonadotrophin-releasing hormone	50–200 µg total dose	once	IM	25 µg	once	IM
Griseofulvin	50–100 mg/kg	sid	PO	50–100 mg/kg	sid	PO
Growth hormone	5–10 U	every other day, 5–15 treatments	IM	NOT ESTABLISHED		
Haloperidol	0.02 mg/kg	q 12h	IM	NOT ESTABLISHED		
Heparin	500 U/kg	q 8h	SQ, IV	250 U/kg	q 8h	SQ
Human chorionic gonadotropin	100–200 IU/kg	sid	IM	NOT ESTABLISHED		
Hydralazine	1 mg/kg	q 12h	PO	2.5–10 mg total dose	q 12h	PO

(Continued)

APPENDIX Usual Dose of Drugs Mentioned in Text (*Continued*)

Drug	DOGS			CATS		
	Dose	Interval	Route	Dose	Interval	Route
Hydrochlorothiazide	2–4 mg/kg	q 12h	PO	2–4 mg/kg	q 12h	PO
Hydrocortisone	5 mg/kg	q 12h	PO, IV, IM	5 mg/kg	q 12h	PO, IV, IM
Imidocarb dipropionate	5 mg/kg	once	SQ	NOT ESTABLISHED		
Insulin (protamine zinc)	1 U/kg	sid	SQ	0.5 U/kg	sid	SQ
Insulin (regular)	0.25 U/kg	adjust prn	IM			
Isoproterenol	0.01 mg/kg	prn	IV	0.01 mg/kg	prn	IV
Isosorbide dinitrate	1 mg/kg	q 6h	PO	NOT ESTABLISHED		
Kanamycin	5–15 mg/kg	q 6–8h	IM, IV, SQ	5–15 mg/kg	q 6–8h	IM, IV, SQ
Kaolin-pectin	1–2 ml/kg	q 6h	PO	1–2 ml/kg	q 6h	PO
Ketamine	NOT RECOMMENDED			11–33 mg/kg	once	IM
				2–4 mg/kg	once	IV
Ketoconazole	10–30 mg/kg	q 8h	PO	10–30 mg/kg	q 8h	PO
Levamisole	11 mg/kg	sid	PO for 6–12 days	20–40 mg/kg	every other day	PO
Levarterenol	1–2 ml/250 ml D5W	infuse to effect	IV	1–2 ml/250 ml D5W	infuse to effect	IV
Lidocaine	4 mg/kg	initial bolus	IV	NOT ESTABLISHED		
	50 µg/kg/min	continuous infusion	IV			

Drug	Dose	Freq	Route	Dose	Freq	Route
Lidocaine (continued)	6 mg/kg	q 1h	IM	10–25 mg/kg	q 12h	PO
Lincomycin	10–25 mg/kg	q 12h	PO	10 mg/kg	q 12h	IV, IM
Lithium citrate	7 mg/kg	q 8h	PO	NOT ESTABLISHED		
Magnesium hydroxide	5–30 ml	prn	PO	2–5 ml	prn	PO
Magnesium sulfate	5–25 g	prn	PO	2–5 g	prn	PO
Mebendazole	22 mg/kg	sid for 3 d	PO	NOT ESTABLISHED		
Medroxyprogesterone	10 mg/kg	once	IM, SQ	NOT ESTABLISHED		
Megestrol acetate	1–2 mg/kg	sid	PO	5–10 mg	sid	PO 7–10 days
				THEN 5 mg	weekly for 1 month	PO
				THEN 2.5 mg	weekly for 1 month	PO
Melphalan	0.1 mg/kg	sid 10 d	PO	0.1 mg/kg	sid for 10 d	PO
THEN	0.05 mg/kg	sid	PO	THEN 0.5 mg/kg	sid	PO
Meperidine	10 mg/kg	prn	IM	5 mg/kg	prn	IM
Metaproterenol	0.5 mg/kg	q 6h	PO	0.5 mg/kg	q 6h	PO
Metaraminol	100 µg/kg	prn	IV, IM	100 µg/kg	prn	IV, IM
Methenamine mandelate	10 mg/kg	q 6h	PO	NOT ESTABLISHED		
Methicillin	20 mg/kg	q 6h	IM, IV	20 mg/kg	q 6h	IM, IV
Methionine	0.2–1.0 g/kg	q 8h	PO	0.2–1.0 g/kg	q 8h	PO
Methoxamine	100 µg/kg	prn	IV	100 µg/kg	prn	IV
Methylphenidate	2–4 mg/kg	sid	PO	NOT RECOMMENDED		
Methylprednisolone	1 mg/kg	sid	PO, IM	1 mg/kg	sid	PO, IM

(Continued)

693

APPENDIX Usual Dose of Drugs Mentioned in Text (*Continued*)

Drug	DOGS			CATS		
	Dose	Interval	Route	Dose	Interval	Route
Metoclopramide	0.5 mg/kg	q 8h	PO	0.5 mg/kg	q 8h	PO
Metronidazole	60 mg/kg	sid	PO	NOT ESTABLISHED		
Mibolerone	3 μg/kg	sid	PO	NOT RECOMMENDED		
Miconazole	10 mg/kg	q 8h	IV	NOT ESTABLISHED		
Milrinone	1 mg/kg	q 8h	PO	NOT ESTABLISHED		
Minocycline	5 mg/kg	q 12h	PO	5 mg/kg	q 12h	PO
Mitotane (Lysodren)	50 mg/kg	sid	PO	NOT ESTABLISHED		
Morphine	0.25 mg/kg	q 5h or prn	IM	0.1 mg/kg	q 6h or prn	IM
Nafcillin	25 mg/kg	q 6h	PO, IV, IM	25 mg/kg	q 6h	PO, IV, IM
Nalidixic acid	3 mg/kg	q 6h	PO	3 mg/kg	q 6h	PO
Nalorphine	1 mg/kg	prn	IV	1 mg/kg	prn	IV
Naloxone	40 μg/kg	prn	IV	40 μg/kg	prn	IV
Nandrolone decanoate	1–1.5 mg/kg	weekly	IM	1–1.5 mg/kg	weekly	IM
Neomycin	20 mg/kg	q 6h	PO (not absorbed)	20 mg/kg	q 6h	PO (not absorbed)
Neostigmine	0.02 mg/kg	q 6h	IM	NOT ESTABLISHED		
Niclosamide	71.4 mg/kg	once	PO	71.4 mg/kg	once	PO
Nitrofurantoin	4 mg/kg	q 8h	PO	4 mg/kg	q 8h	PO
Nitrofurantoin	3 mg/kg	q 8h	IM	3 mg/kg	q 8h	IM
Nitroprusside sodium	1–5 μg/kg/min	continuous infusion	IV	NOT ESTABLISHED		

Drug	Dose	Interval	Route	Dose	Interval	Route
Noscapine	0.5–1.0 mg/kg	q 6–8 h	PO			
Nystatin	100,000 U	q 6h	PO (not absorbed)	100,000 U	q 6h	PO (not absorbed)
Oxacillin	10–15 mg/kg	q 6h	PO, IV, IM	10–15 mg/kg	q 6h	PO, IV, IM
Oxymorphone	0.03–0.05 mg/kg	q 6h	IM	NOT RECOMMENDED	q 6h	IM
Oxytocin	5–10 U	15–30 min	IV, IM	0.5–3 U	once	IV, IM
Paregoric	2–15 ml	q 6h	PO	NOT RECOMMENDED	q 6h	PO
Penicillamine	10–15 mg/kg	q 12h	PO	NOT ESTABLISHED	q 12h	PO
Penicillin G (Na or K)	20,000–40,000 U/kg	q 4h	IV, IM, SQ	20,000–40,000 U/kg	q 4h	IV, IM, SQ
Penicillin G (procaine)	20,000 U/kg	q 12–24h	IM	20,000 U/kg	q 12–24h	IM
Pentobarbital (sedation)	2–4 mg/kg	q 6h	PO	2–4 mg/kg	q 6h	PO
Petrolatum, liquid	5–30 ml	prn	PO	2–5 ml	prn	PO
Phenobarbital (anticonvulsant)	2–6 mg/kg	q 8–12h	IM, IV	2–6 mg/kg	q 8–12h	IM, IV
Phenobarbital (sedation)	2 mg/kg	q 12h	PO	2 mg/kg	q 12h	PO
Phenoxybenzamine	0.25–0.5 mg/kg	q 6–12h	PO	0.25 mg/kg	q 8h	PO
Phenylbutazone	22 mg/kg	q 8h	PO	NOT RECOMMENDED		PO
Phenylephrine	0.15 mg/kg	prn	IV	0.15 mg/kg	prn	IV

(*Continued*)

APPENDIX Usual Dose of Drugs Mentioned in Text (*Continued*)

Drug	DOGS			CATS		
	Dose	Interval	Route	Dose	Interval	Route
Phenylpropanolamine	3 mg/kg	q 12h	PO	NOT ESTABLISHED		
Phenytoin	30 mg/kg	q 8h	PO	2–3 mg/kg	q 24h	PO
	10 mg/kg	q 8h	IV			
Phthalofyne	180 mg/kg	once	PO	NOT RECOMMENDED		
Piperazine	20–30 mg/kg	once	PO	20–30 mg/kg	once	PO
Pitressin	1–2 U	q 4–6h	SQ	1–2 U	q 4–6h	SQ
Pitressin tannate	1–2 U	q 36–72h	SQ or IM	NOT ESTABLISHED		
Polymixin B	2 mg (20,000 U)/kg	q 12h	IM	NOT RECOMMENDED		
Potassium chloride	5–15 mEq	sid	PO	2.5–7 mEq	sid	PO
Pralidoxine	10–50 mg/kg	prn	IM, IV	10–50 mg/kg	prn	IM, IV
Prazosin < 15 kg BW	1 mg	q 8h	PO	NOT ESTABLISHED		
> 15 kg BW	2 mg	q 8h	PO			
Prednisolone	1 mg/kg	sid	PO, IM	1 mg/kg	sid	PO, IM
Prednisone	0.5 mg/kg	sid	PO	0.5 mg/kg	sid	PO
Primidone	11–22 mg/kg	q 8h	PO	11–22 mg/kg	q 8h	PO
Procainamide	6 mg/kg	q 4h	PO	NOT RECOMMENDED		
	6 mg/kg	bolus	IV			
FOLLOWED BY	10–40 µg/kg/min	continuous infusion	IV			

Drug	Dose	Route	Frequency	Dose	Frequency	Route
Procainamide (*Continued*)	8–10 mg/kg	IM	q 4h	0.13 mg/kg	q 12h	IM
Prochlorperazine	0.13 mg/kg	IM	q 6h	0.13 mg/kg	sid	IM or IV
Promazine	2–4 mg/kg	IM or IV	sid	2–4 mg/kg		
Promethazine	2 mg/kg	PO	sid	NOT ESTABLISHED		
Propantheline	0.5–1 mg/kg	PO	q 8h	7.5 mg total dose	q 72h	PO
Propranolol	5–40 mg/kg	PO	q 6h	< 6 kg BW 2.5–5.0 mg	q 8h	PO
	0.5–1.5 mg/kg	IV	prn	> 6 kg BW 5.0–7.5 mg	q 8h	PO
Prostaglandin F$_{2\alpha}$ tromethamine	250 µg/kg	IV slowly	sid	NOT ESTABLISHED		
Psyllium	3–10 g	in feed	sid	3 g	sid	in feed
Pyrantel	5 mg/kg	PO	once	10 mg/kg	once	PO
Pyridostigmine < 5 kg BW,	45 mg	PQ	q 6h	NOT ESTABLISHED		
5–25 kg,	45–90 mg	PQ	q 6h			
> 25 kg,	90–135 mg	PQ	q 6h			
Pyrimethamine	0.5–1.0 mg/kg	PO	sid	0.5–1.0 mg/kg	sid	PO
Quinacrine	50–100 mg total	PO	q 12h	10 mg/kg	sid	PO
Quinidine	6–20 mg/kg	PO	q 8h	NOT RECOMMENDED		
Sodium EDTA	25–75 mg/hr	IV	continuous infusion	NOT ESTABLISHED		
Spectinomycin	5–10 mg/kg	IM	q 12h	NOT ESTABLISHED		
Spironolactone	2–4 mg/kg	PO	sid	2–4 mg/kg	sid	PO
Streptomycin	10 mg/kg	IM, SQ	q 6h	10 mg/kg	q 6h	IM, SQ

(*Continued*)

APPENDIX Usual Dose of Drugs Mentioned in Text (Continued)

Drug	DOGS Dose	DOGS Interval	DOGS Route	CATS Dose	CATS Interval	CATS Route
Streptozotocin	14.5 mg/kg	sid infusion	IV (see Ch. 15)	NOT ESTABLISHED		
Sulfadiazine	110 mg/kg	q 12h	PO	110 mg/kg	q 12h	PO
Sulfadiazine-Trimethoprim	30 mg/kg	q 12h	PO	30 mg/kg	sid	PO
Sulfadimethoxine	25 mg/kg	sid	PO, IV, IM	25 mg/kg	sid	PO, IV, IM
Sulfamethizole	50 mg/kg	q 8h	PO	50 mg/kg	q 8h	PO
Sulfasalazine	15 mg/kg	q 6h	PO	NOT ESTABLISHED		
Sulfisoxazole	50 mg/kg	q 8h	PO	50 mg/kg	q 8h	PO
Styrylpyridium-diethyl-carbamazine	5.5 mg/kg	once	PO	NOT ESTABLISHED		
Terbutaline	10 µg/kg	q 4h	SQ	10 µg/kg	q 4h	SQ
	30 µg/kg	q 8h	PO	30 µg/kg	q 8h	PO
Testosterone propionate	2.5 mg/kg	once	IM	2.5 mg/kg	once	IM
Tetrachlorethylene	0.22 ml/kg	once	PO	0.22 ml/kg	once	PO
Tetracycline	25 mg/kg	q 8h	PO	25 mg/kg	q 8h	PO
Thenium closylate	5–10 mg/kg	q 12h	IV	5–10 mg/kg	q 12h	IV
	2.3–4.5 kg, 250 mg	q 12h	PO	NOT RECOMMENDED		
	OVER 4.5 kg, 500 mg	sid	PO			
Theophylline	5–7 mg/kg	q 8h	PO	3 mg/kg	q 12h	PO
Thiabendazole	15–35 mg/kg	q 12h	in feed	NOT ESTABLISHED		

698

Drug	Dose	Interval	Route	Dose	Interval	Route
Thiacetarsamide	2.2 mg/kg	q 12h, 2 days	IV	NOT RECOMMENDED		
Thiamine	2 mg/kg	sid	PO	4 mg/kg	sid	PO
Thyroid, dessicated	15–20 mg/kg	sid	PO	15–20 mg/kg	sid	PO
Thyroxin	20–32 µg/kg	sid	PO	50–100 µg total dose	sid	PO
Ticarcillin	15–25 mg/kg	q 8h	IM, IV	15–25 mg/kg	q 8h	IM, IV
Tobramycin	1 mg/kg	q 8h	IV, IM	1 mg/kg	q 8h	IV, IM
Tocainide	50–100 mg/kg	q 8h	PO	NOT ESTABLISHED		
Toluene	0.22 ml/kg	once	PO	0.22 ml/kg	once	PO
Triamcinolone	0.25 mg/kg	sid	IM, PO	0.25 mg/kg	sid	IM, PO
Triamterene	1–2 mg/kg	q 12h	PO	NOT ESTABLISHED		
Triflupromazine	0.2 mg/kg	q 8h	PO	NOT ESTABLISHED		
Trifluoperazine	0.03 mg/kg	q 12h	IM	NOT ESTABLISHED		
Triidothyronine	4.4 µg/kg	q 8h	PO	4.4 µg/kg	q 8h	PO
Trimethobenzamide	4 mg/kg	q 6h	IM	NOT ESTABLISHED		
Tylosin	5–10 mg/kg	q 12h	IV, IM	5–10 mg/kg	q 12h	IV, IM
	10 mg/kg	q 8h	PO	10 mg/kg	q 8h	PO
Valproic acid	60 mg/kg	q 8h	PO	NOT ESTABLISHED		
Vancomycin	10 mg/kg	q 6–8h	PO, IV	10 mg/kg	q 6–8h	IV
Verapamil	0.1 mg/kg	q 8h	IV	NOT ESTABLISHED		
Vinblastine	0.05 mg/kg	weekly	IV	0.05 mg/kg	weekly	IV
Vincristine	0.01–0.025 mg/kg, max. dose 1.5 mg	every 4–7 d	IV	0.01–0.025 mg/kg max. dose 1.5 mg	every 4–7 d	IV
Vitamin D	70–175 IU	sid	PO 7 days	70 IU	sid	PO 7 days

(Continued)

APPENDIX Usual Dose fo Drugs Mentioned in Text (*Continued*)

Drug		Dose	DOGS Interval	Route	Dose	CATS Interval	Route
Vitamin K₁		1 mg/kg	q 8h	PO, SQ	1 mg/kg	q 8h	PO, SQ
Warfarin sodium		0.2 mg/kg initially	sid	PO	NOT RECOMMENDED		
	THEN	0.05–1.0 mg/kg	sid	PO			
Xylazine		0.5–1.0 mg/kg	once	IV	0.5–1.0 mg/kg	once	IV
		1–2 mg/kg	once	IM	1–2 mg/kg	once	IM

INDEX

Page numbers followed by f represent figures; Those followed by t represent tables.